Women's Health Review

Women's Health Review

A Clinical Update in Obstetrics-Gynecology

Philip J. Di Saia, MD

The Dorothy J. Marsh Chair in Reproductive Biology, Professor, Department of Obstetrics and Gynecology, Division of Gynecologic Oncology, University of California Irvine Medical Center, Orange, California

Gautam Chaudhuri, MD, PhD

Distinguished Professor and Executive Chair, Department of Obstetrics and Gynecology, Distinguished Professor, Department of Molecular and Medical Pharmacology, David Geffen School of Medicine at UCLA, Los Angeles, California

Linda C. Giudice, MD, PhD, MSc

Distinguished Professor and Chair, Department of Obstetrics, Gynecology, and Reproductive Sciences, The Robert B. Jaffe, MD Endowed Professor in the Reproductive Sciences, University of California, San Francisco, San Francisco, California

Thomas R. Moore, MD

Professor and Chairman, Department of Reproductive Medicine, University of California, San Diego, School of Medicine, San Diego, California

Manuel Porto, MD

Professor and Chairman, The E.J. Quilligan Endowed Chair, Department of Obstetrics and Gynecology, University of California, Irvine, School of Medicine, Orange, California

Lloyd H. Smith, MD, PhD

Professor, Department of Obstetrics and Gynecology, University of California, Davis, School of Medicine, Sacramento, California

ELSEVIER
SAUNDERS

ELSEVIER
SAUNDERS

1600 John F. Kennedy Blvd.
Ste 1800
Philadelphia, PA 19103-2899

WOMEN'S HEALTH REVIEW: A CLINICAL UPDATE IN OBSTETRICS-GYNECOLOGY   ISBN: 978-1-4377-1498-2

Copyright © 2012 by Saunders, an imprint of Elsevier Inc. All rights reserved.

Notices

Knowledge and best practice in this field are constantly changing. As new research and experience broaden our understanding, changes in research methods, professional practices, or medical treatment may become necessary.

Practitioners and researchers must always rely on their own experience and knowledge in evaluating and using any information, methods, compounds, or experiments described herein. In using such information or methods they should be mindful of their own safety and the safety of others, including parties for whom they have a professional responsibility.

With respect to any drug or pharmaceutical products identified, readers are advised to check the most current information provided (i) on procedures featured or (ii) by the manufacturer of each product to be administered, to verify the recommended dose or formula, the method and duration of administration, and contraindications. It is the responsibility of practitioners, relying on their own experience and knowledge of their patients, to make diagnoses, to determine dosages and the best treatment for each individual patient, and to take all appropriate safety precautions.

To the fullest extent of the law, neither the Publisher nor the authors, contributors, or editors, assume any liability for any injury and/or damage to persons or property as a matter of products liability, negligence or otherwise, or from any use or operation of any methods, products, instructions, or ideas contained in the material herein.

Library of Congress Cataloging-in-Publication Data

Women's health review : a clinical update in obstetrics-gynecology / Philip J. Di Saia ... [et al.].
    p. ; cm.
  Includes bibliographical references and index.
  ISBN 978-1-4377-1498-2 (pbk. : alk. paper)
I. Di Saia, Philip J., 1937-
  [DNLM: 1. Genital Diseases, Female. 2. Pregnancy Complications. 3. Women's Health. WP 100]
  618.1--dc23   2011043934

Senior Content Strategist: Stefanie Jewell-Thomas
Content Development Specialist: Sabina Borza
Publishing Services Manager: Patricia Tannian
Senior Project Manager: Sharon Corell
Senior Book Designer: Ellen Zanolle

Printed in the United States of America
Last digit is the print number: 9 8 7 6 5 4 3 2 1

We the authors would like to express our gratitude to our students and patients who have trusted us with their education and care as we nurtured the tree of knowledge contained in this text.

Contributors

Carolyn J. Alexander, MD
Associate Director of the Residency Program
Assistant Clinical Professor, Obstetrics and Gynecology
Department of Obstetrics and Gynecology
Division of Reproductive Endocrinology and Infertility
David Geffen School of Medicine at UCLA
Cedars-Sinai Medical Center
Los Angeles, California

Sara Arian, MD
Research Associate
Department of Obstetrics and Gynecology
Division of Maternal Fetal Medicine
University of California Irvine Medical Center
Orange, California;
Obstetrics and Gynecology Resident
University of Texas Health Science Center at Houston
Houston, Texas

Shannon R. Bales, MD
Clinical Fellow
Department of Internal Medicine
Division of Endocrinology
UCLA Center for Health Sciences
Los Angeles, California

Kathleen Brennan, MD
Assistant Clinical Professor
Division of Reproductive Endocrinology and
    Infertility
Department of Obstetrics and Gynecology
University of California, Los Angeles
Los Angeles, California

Marcelle I. Cedars, MD
Professor and Director
Division of Reproductive Endocrinology and Infertility
Department of Obstetrics, Gynecology and Reproductive
    Sciences
University of California, San Francisco
San Francisco, California

John K. Chan, MD
Associate Professor and Director
Division of Gynecologic Oncology
Department of Obstetrics, Gynecology, and Reproductive
    Sciences
University of California, San Francisco
San Francisco, California

Gautam Chaudhuri, MD, PhD
Distinguished Professor and Executive Chair
Department of Obstetrics and Gynecology
Distinguished Professor
Department of Molecular and Medical Pharmacology
David Geffen School of Medicine at UCLA
Los Angeles, California

Angela Y. Chen, MD, MPH
Assistant Professor
Family Planning, Chief of Service & Fellowship Director
Department of Obstetrics and Gynecology
David Geffen School of Medicine at UCLA
Los Angeles, California

Inder J. Chopra, MD
Professor
Department of Internal Medicine
Division of Endocrinology
University of California, Los Angeles
UCLA Center for Health Sciences
Los Angeles, California

Tatiana Stanisic Chou, MD
Junior Specialist
Department of Obstetrics and Gynecology
University of California, Irvine
Orange, California;
Resident
Department of Obstetrics and Gynecology
Kaiser Permanente
Oakland, California

Judith H. Chung, MD, PhD
Assistant Professor
Department of Obstetrics and Gynecology
University of California Irvine Medical Center
Orange, California

Deborah Cohan, MD, MPH
Associate Professor
Department of Obstetrics, Gynecology and Reproductive
    Sciences
University of California, San Francisco;
Medical Director
Bay Area Perinatal AIDS Center;
Associate Director
National Perinatal HIV Hotline and Clinicians Network
San Francisco, California

Craig R. Cohen, MD, MPH
Professor
Department of Obstetrics, Gynecology and Reproductive
    Sciences
University of California, San Francisco
San Francisco, California

Deirdre A. Conway, MD
Clinical Fellow
Department of Obstetrics and Gynecology
Division of Reproductive Endocrinology and Infertility
University of California, Los Angeles
Los Angeles, California;
Clinical Instructor
Department of Obstetrics and Gynecology
Division of Reproductive Endocrinology and Infertility
University of California, San Diego
San Diego, California

John L. Dalrymple, MD
Associate Professor
Division Director, Gynecologic Oncology
Department of Obstetrics, Gynecology and Reproductive
    Sciences
The University of Texas Medical School Houston
Houston, Texas

Philip D. Darney, MD, MSc
Distinguished Professor
Department of Obstetrics, Gynecology and Reproductive
    Sciences
Director
Bixby Center for Global Reproductive Health
University of California, San Francisco
San Francisco, California

Khady Diouf, MD
Reproductive Infectious Disease Fellow
Department of Obstetrics and Gynecology
University of California San Francisco
San Francisco, California;
Instructor
Harvard Medical School;
Associate OB/GYN Physician
Division of Global Obstetrics and Gynecology
Department of Obstetrics and Gynecology
Brigham and Women's Hospital
Boston, Massachusetts

Robert M. Ehsanipoor, MD
Assistant Professor
Department of Gynecology and Obstetrics
Division of Maternal Fetal Medicine
Johns Hopkins University School of Medicine
Baltimore, Maryland

Tania F. Esakoff, MD
Assistant Clinical Professor
Department of Obstetrics and Gynecology
Division of Maternal Fetal Medicine
David Geffen School of Medicine at UCLA
Cedars Sinai Medical Center
Los Angeles, California

Robin Farias-Eisner, MD, PhD
Professor
Vice Chair, Administration;
Director, Gynecologic Oncology
Department of Obstetrics and Gynecology
David Geffen School of Medicine at UCLA
Los Angeles, California

Christine K. Farinelli, MD
Clinical Instructor
Department of Obstetrics and Gynecology
Division of Maternal Fetal Medicine
University of California, Irvine
Orange, California

Nicole D. Fleming, MD
Assistant Professor
Gynecologic Oncology
MD Anderson Cancer Center
Houston, Texas

Esther Friedrich, MD
Assistant Clinical Professor
Department of Obstetrics and Gynecology
Division of Maternal Fetal Medicine
University of California, Irvine, School of Medicine
Orange, California;
Staff Perinatologist
Maternal-Fetal Medicine and Genetics
Southern California Permanente Medical Group
Los Angeles, California

Katherine Cynthia Fuh, MD
Gynecologic Oncology Fellow
Department of Obstetrics and Gynecology
University of California, San Francisco
San Francisco, California;
Stanford University
Stanford, California

Afshan B. Hameed, MD, FACOG, FACC
Associate Professor of Clinical Obstetrics and Gynecology
Associate Professor of Clinical Cardiology
Medical Director of Obstetrics
University of California, Irvine
Orange, California

Tamera J. Hatfield, MD, PhD
Assistant Professor
Department of Obstetrics and Gynecology
Division of Maternal Fetal Medicine
University of California Irvine Medical Center
Orange, California

J. Seth Hawkins, MD, MBA
Assistant Professor
Department of Obstetrics and Gynecology
University of California, Irvine, School of Medicine
Irvine, California

Stephen Hebert, MD
Associate Clinical Professor
Department of Reproductive Medicine
Division of Perinatal Medicine
University of California, San Diego
San Diego, California;
Honorary Staff
Department of Obstetrics and Gynecology
Scripps Memorial Hospital, La Jolla
La Jolla, California

Kathryn P. Hirst, MD
H.S. Assistant Clinical Professor
Department of Family and Preventive Medicine
Department of Psychiatry
Department of Pediatrics
Director of UC San Diego Maternal Mental Health
    Clinic
University of California, San Diego
San Diego, California

Heather Huddleston, MD
Assistant Professor
Department of Obstetrics, Gynecology and Reproductive
    Sciences
University of California, San Francisco
San Francisco, California

Andrew D. Hull, BMedSci, BMBS, FRCOG, FACOG
Professor of Clinical Reproductive Medicine
Director, Maternal Fetal Medicine Fellowship
Department of Reproductive Medicine
University of California, San Diego
San Diego, California

Erica Boiman Johnstone, MD, MHS
Assistant Professor
Department of Obstetrics and Gynecology
University of Utah
Salt Lake City, Utah

Jennifer A. Jolley, MD
Assistant Professor
Department of Obstetrics and Gynecology
Division of Maternal Fetal Medicine
University of Washington Medical Center
Seattle, Washington

Daniel Kahn, MD, PhD
Assistant Professor
Division of Maternal Fetal Medicine
Department of Obstetrics and Gynecology
David Geffen School of Medicine at UCLA
Los Angeles, California

Thomas F. Kelly, MD
Clinical Professor and Chief
Department of Reproductive Medicine
Division of Perinatal Medicine
University of California, San Diego, School of Medicine;
Director of Maternity Services
University of California San Diego Medical Center
La Jolla, California

Caron Kim, MD, MSc
Physician
Department of Obstetrics and Gynecology
David Geffen School of Medicine at UCLA
Los Angeles, California

Jae H. Kim, MD, PhD
Associate Professor of Pediatrics
Attending Neonatologist
Division of Neonatology
Department of Pediatrics
University of California San Diego Medical Center
San Diego, California

D. Yvette LaCoursiere, MD, MPH
Assistant Professor
Department of Reproductive Medicine
Division of Perinatal Medicine
University of California, San Diego
San Diego, California

Felicia L. Lane, MS, MD
Associate Health Sciences Professor
Associate Residency Program Director
Department of Obstetrics and Gynecology
Division of Female Pelvic Medicine and Reconstructive
    Surgery
University of California, Irvine, School of Medicine
Irvine, California

Jennifer K. Lee, MD
Clinical Instructor
Department of Obstetrics and Gynecology
Division of Urogynecology
University of California, Irvine, School of Medicine
Irvine, California

Carol A. Major, MD
Professor and Residency Program Director
Department of Obstetrics and Gynecology
Division of Maternal Fetal Medicine
University of California, Irvine
Orange, California;
Director of Perinatal Services
Department of Obstetrics and Gynecology
Fountain Valley Regional Hospital
Fountain Valley, California

Ruchi Mathur, MD, FRCPC
Director, Diabetes Outpatient Treatment and Education
    Center
Division of Endocrinology, Diabetes and Metabolism
Department of Medicine
Cedars Sinai Medical Center;
Assistant Professor of Medicine
David Geffen School of Medicine at UCLA
Los Angeles, California

Bradley J. Monk, MD, FACS, FACOG
Professor
Division of Gynecologic Oncology
Department of Obstetrics and Gynecology
Creighton University School of Medicine at
St. Joseph's Hospital and Medical Center
Phoenix, Arizona

Thomas R. Moore, MD
Professor and Chairman
Department of Reproductive Medicine
University of California, San Diego, School of Medicine
San Diego, California

Susannah May Mourton, MBChB, MS
Gynecologic Oncologist
Sutter Medical Group
Sacramento, California

Lauren Nathan, MD
Professor
Department of Obstetrics and Gynecology
David Geffen School of Medicine at UCLA
Los Angeles, California

Erica Oberman, MD
Physician
Department of Obstetrics and Gynecology
David Geffen School of Medicine at UCLA
Los Angeles, California

Joanne L. Perron, MD, FACOG
Fellow, Occupational and Environmental Medicine
Program on Reproductive Health and the Environment
University of California, San Francisco
San Francisco, California

Nicole M. Petrossi, BS
Executive Assistant
Department of Obstetrics and Gynecology
Division of Maternal Fetal Medicine
University of California Irvine Medical Center
Orange, California

Manuel Porto, MD
Professor and Chairman
The E.J. Quilligan Endowed Chair
Department of Obstetrics and Gynecology
University of California, Irvine, School of Medicine
Orange, California

Kristen H. Quinn, MD, MS, FACOG
Assistant Professor
Department of Obstetrics and Gynecology
Division of Maternal Fetal Medicine
Medical College of Wisconsin
Milwaukee, Wisconsin

Gladys A. Ramos, MD
Associate Physician
Department of Reproductive Medicine
Division of Perinatology
University of California, San Diego;
Faculty Attending
Department of Reproductive Medicine
University of California San Diego Health System
San Diego, California

Andrea J. Rapkin, MD
Professor of Obstetrics and Gynecology
Executive Vice Chair
Department of Obstetrics and Gynecology
David Geffen School of Medicine at UCLA;
Director, UCLA Pelvic Pain Clinic
UCLA Medical Center
Los Angeles, California

Katherine A. Rauen, MD, PhD
Associate Professor
Department of Pediatrics
Department of Obstetrics, Gynecology and Reproductive
    Sciences
University of California, San Francisco
UCSF Helen Diller Family Comprehensive Cancer Center
San Francisco, California

Anne O. Rodriguez, MD
Gynecologic Oncology Specialists
Coastal Communities Cancer Center
Ventura, California

Wendy Satmary, MD
Assistant Clinical Professor
Department of Obstetrics and Gynecology
David Geffen School of Medicine at UCLA
Los Angeles, California;
Medical Doctor
Department of Obstetrics and Gynecology
Kaiser Permanente
Panorama City, California

David B. Schrimmer, MD
Clinical Professor
Department of Reproductive Medicine
Division of Perinatal Medicine
University of California, San Diego
San Diego, California

Brian L. Shaffer, MD
Assistant Professor
Department of Obstetrics and Gynecology
Division of Maternal Fetal Medicine
Oregon Health and Science University
Portland, Oregon

Mousa I. Shamonki, MD
Director, In Vitro Fertilization and Assisted
  Reproduction
Department of Obstetrics and Gynecology
Division of Reproductive Endocrinology and
  Infertility
UCLA Fertility and Health Care Center
Los Angeles, California

Amanda Skillern, MD
Clinical Fellow
Division of Reproductive Endocrinology and Infertility
Department of Obstetrics, Gynecology and Reproductive
  Sciences
University of California, San Francisco
San Francisco, California

Lloyd H. Smith, MD, PhD
Professor
Department of Obstetrics and Gynecology
University of California, Davis, School of Medicine
Sacramento, California

Karen Smith-McCune, MD
Professor
Department of Obstetrics, Gynecology and Reproductive
  Sciences
University of California, San Francisco
San Francisco, California

Andrew H. Spencer, MD
Maternal Fetal Medicine Fellow
Department of Reproductive Medicine
University of California, San Diego
San Diego, California

Carolyn B. Sufrin, MD, MA
Assistant Professor
Department of Obstetrics, Gynecology and Reproductive
  Sciences
University of California, San Francisco
San Francisco General Hospital
UCSF Bixby Center for Global Reproductive Health
San Francisco Department of Public Health, Jail Health
  Services
San Francisco, California

Patrice M. Sutton, MPH
Research Scientist
Program on Reproductive Health and the Environment
Department of Obstetrics, Gynecology and Reproductive
  Sciences
University of California, San Francisco
San Francisco, California

Christopher Tarnay, MD
Associate Professor
Director
Division of Female Pelvic Medicine and Reconstructive
  Surgery
Department of Obstetrics and Gynecology
David Geffen School of Medicine at UCLA
Los Angeles, California

Maryam Tarsa, MD, MAS
Associate Clinical Professor
Department of Reproductive Medicine
University of California, San Diego;
Faculty Attending
Department of Reproductive Medicine
University of California San Diego Medical Center
San Diego, California

Krishnansu S. Tewari, MD, FACOG, FACS
Associate Professor
Director of Research
Principal Investigator, Gynecologic Oncology Group
University of California, Irvine;
Co-Chair, Clinical Trials Protocol Review & Monitoring
  Committee;
The Chao Family NCI-Designated Comprehensive Cancer
  Center
Division of Gynecologic Oncology
Department of Obstetrics and Gynecology
University of California Irvine Medical Center
Orange, California

Mari-Paule Thiet, MD
Professor and Director
Division of Maternal Fetal Medicine
Vice Chair of Patient Safety and Quality Assurance
Department of Obstetrics, Gynecology and Reproductive
  Sciences
University of California, San Francisco
San Francisco, California

Julianne S. Toohey, MD
Clinical Professor
Department of Obstetrics and Gynecology
Division of Maternal Fetal Medicine
University of California Irvine Medical Center
Orange, California

Steven A. Vasilev, MD, MBA, FACOG, FACS
Clinical Professor
Department of Obstetrics and Gynecology
University of California, Los Angeles
Los Angeles, California;
Chief of Service
Director, Surgical and Radiation Oncology Clinical Trials
Department of Obstetrics and Gynecology/Gynecologic
  Oncology
Kaiser Permanente Los Angeles Medical Center
Los Angeles, California

Carrie M. Wambach, MD
Fellow Physician
Department of Reproductive Endocrinology and Infertility
University of California, Los Angeles
Los Angeles, California

Deborah A. Wing, MD
Professor
Director
Department of Obstetrics and Gynecology
Division of Maternal Fetal Medicine
Director, Maternal-Fetal Medicine Fellowship
University of California Irvine Medical Center
Orange, California

Douglas A. Woelkers, MD
Associate Clinical Professor
Department of Reproductive Medicine
Division of Perinatal Medicine
University of California, San Diego, School of Medicine
San Diego, California

Richard B. Wolf, DO, MPH, FACOG
Associate Clinical Professor
Department of Reproductive Medicine
University of California, San Diego, School of Medicine;
Attending Perinatologist
Department of Reproductive Medicine
University of California San Diego Medical Center
La Jolla, California

Lynlee M. Wolfe, MD
Fellow
Department of Reproductive Medicine
Division of Maternal Fetal Medicine
University of California, San Diego
La Jolla, California

Tracey J. Woodruff, PhD, MPH
Professor and Director
Program on Reproductive Health and the Environment
Department of Obstetrics, Gynecology and Reproductive
    Sciences
University of California, San Francisco
San Francisco, California

Shagufta Yasmeen, MD
Associate Professor
Department of Obstetrics and Gynecology
University of California Davis Health System
Sacramento, California

Peter Yuan, MD
Fellow
Division of Endocrinology
Department of Medicine
Cedars-Sinai / VA Greater Los Angeles Program;
Clinical Instructor
Department of Internal Medicine
David Geffen School of Medicine at UCLA
Los Angeles, California

Preface

The clinical practice of obstetrics and gynecology requires constant vigilance in updating our knowledge base. A few years ago, the five chairs—Gautam Chaudhuri, Linda Giudice, Thomas Moore, Manuel Porto, and Lloyd Smith—of the five Departments of Obstetrics and Gynecology in the five University of California (UC) medical schools agreed to produce a text designed to update the clinical science with emphasis on the last 10 years of our science. I was "volunteered" to serve as senior editor, and we have restricted authorship to only UC faculty as of 2010, realizing some members have moved on since the project began. The authors have strived to keep the information current and very readable to accommodate the schedules of busy clinicians. All of the proceeds from this work will be used to create a fund for seed research grants to University of California faculty in women's health on a peer review basis.

I would like to personally thank the authors and editors who also volunteered their time and efforts: Carolyn Alexander, Sara Arian, Shannon R. Bales, Kathleen Brennan, Marcelle Cedars, John Chan, Gautam Chaudhuri, Angela Chen, Inder Chopra, Tatiana Stanisic Chou, Judith Chung, Deborah Cohan, Craig Cohen, Deirdre Conway, John Dalrymple, Philip Darney, Khady Diouf, Robert M. Ehsanipoor, Tania Esakoff, Robin Farias-Eisner, Christine Farinelli, Nicole D. Fleming, Esther Friedrich, Katherine Fuh, Linda C. Giudice, Afshan Hameed, Tamera J. Hatfield, J. Seth Hawkins, Stephen Hebert, Kathryn Hirst, Heather Huddleston, Andrew D. Hull, Erica Boiman Johnstone, Jennifer Jolley, Daniel Kahn, Thomas Kelly, Caron Kim, Jae H. Kim, D. Yvette LaCoursiere, Felicia Lane, Jennifer Lee, Carol A. Major, Ruchi Mathur, Bradley Monk, Thomas R. Moore, Susannah Mourton, Lauren Nathan, Erica Oberman, Joanne Perron, Nicole M. Petrossi, Manuel Porto, Kristen H. Quinn, Gladys A. Ramos, Andrea Rapkin, Katherine Rauen, Anne Rodriguez, Wendy Satmary, David Schrimmer, Brian Shaffer, Mousa Shamonki, Amanda Skillern, Lloyd Smith, Karen Smith-McCune, Andrew H. Spencer, Carolyn Sufrin, Patrice Sutton, Christopher Tarnay, Maryam Tarsa, Krishnansu Tewari, Mari-Paule Thiet, Julianne Toohey, Steven Vasilev, Carrie M. Wambach, Deborah Wing, Douglas Woelkers, Richard Wolf, Lynlee Wolfe, Tracey Woodruff, Shagufta Yasmeen, and Peter Yuan.

"Education never ends, Watson. It is a series of lessons with the greatest effort for the last."

SIR ARTHUR CONAN DOYLE **(1859-1930)**
His Last Bow, "The Adventure of the Red Circle"

Philip J. Di Saia

Gautam Chaudhuri

Linda C. Giudice

Thomas R. Moore

Manuel Porto

Lloyd H. Smith

Acknowledgments

All authors acknowledge our many patients and teachers who have enriched our enthusiasm for learning the state of our science. We also express a special note of appreciation to the many clerical assistants who have helped produce the many chapters. We are especially grateful to Sabina Borza, Stefanie Jewell-Thomas, and Lisa Kozik for their tireless efforts in getting this text ready for print.

Contents

Women's Health Review

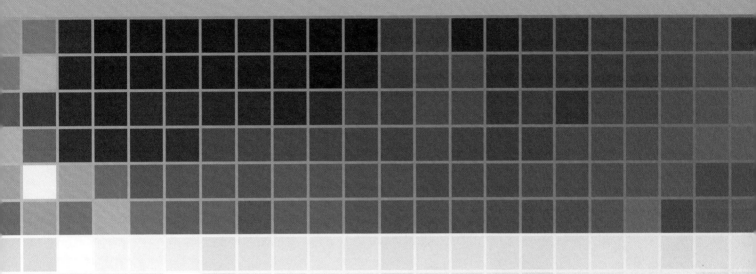

SECTION 1

Female Development

Reproductive Genetics

BRIAN L. SHAFFER • KATHERINE A. RAUEN

KEY UPDATES

1 Screening for carriers of single gene disorders—is it time for expansion?

2 Women of Eastern European/Ashkenazi Jewish descent should be offered carrier screening for Tay-Sachs, Canavan, familial dysautonomia, and cystic fibrosis.

3 Women at risk for having a fetus affected with a hemoglobinopathy should be offered screening with a complete blood count, and hemoglobin electrophoresis or high-performance liquid chromatography.

4 The performance of screening for cystic fibrosis depends on the geographic ancestry and number of mutations assessed in molecular testing.

5 Women with a family history of undiagnosed cognitive disability, autism, or premature ovarian failure should be offered carrier screening for Fragile X.

6 Universal carrier screening for spinal muscular atrophy (SMA) is controversial and currently should be offered to those with a family history.

7 All pregnant women should be offered invasive prenatal diagnosis.

8 Risks of invasive prenatal diagnosis may be lower than previously reported.

9 Chromosomal analysis with array comparative genomic hybridization (CGH) offers unique advantages and disadvantages and may be warranted in certain clinical circumstances.

10 Private umbilical cord blood banking may be used to treat a number of genetic, hematologic, and malignant disorders but should be considered investigational.

11 Noninvasive prenatal diagnosis may be possible in determining the fetal sex and blood type.

Screening for Carriers of Single Gene Disorders

UPDATE #1

The role of the obstetrician-gynecologist providing prenatal care continues to expand, and the discussion of carrier screening in the preconception or early prenatal period is necessary. The goal of a carrier-screening program is to provide risk assessment and to offer timely and cost-effective testing with the choice of prevention or preparation for the birth of an affected child. Such screening has traditionally been based on geographic ancestry, although others advocate offering screening to all patients (ACOG Committee on Genetics, Committee Opinion No. 442, 2009; Norton, 2008; Musci, 2005).

ROLE OF THE OBSTETRICIAN-GYNECOLOGIST

1. The obstetrician-gynecologist provides care for women at nearly every stage of their lives; thus we have a unique opportunity to assess the potential risk for genetic disease prior to or during early pregnancy.
2. Women who are determined to have a family history of genetic disease should be referred for formal genetic counseling. Those who are determined to be at risk based on geographic ancestry are offered appropriate screening testing either by the obstetrician-gynecologist or in the setting of formal genetic counseling. Recently, advocacy groups and some authorities have recommended expansion of carrier screening (ACOG Committee on Genetics, Committee Opinion No. 442, 2009; Musci, 2005; Norton, 2008).

CHARACTERISTICS FOR A SUCCESSFUL SCREENING PROGRAM

1. To warrant screening for carrier status of single gene disorder, the disorder must be of considerable clinical severity and frequency to warrant screening.
2. A timely, cost-effective, or relatively inexpensive test must be available that affords reliable carrier diagnosis and prenatal diagnosis.
3. Further, as carriers are asymptomatic and typically have a negative family history (and thus often have no personal experience with the disorder), appropriate nondirective genetic counseling and education must be provided such that appropriate decision-making occurs.

4. The main goal of a genetic carrier screening program includes prevention, which may be accomplished in a number of ways once carriers are identified: forgoing pregnancy, adoption, in-vitro fertilization (IVF) with preimplantation diagnosis (PGD), gamete donation, or prenatal diagnosis with termination of an affected pregnancy.

5. In addition to prevention, other benefits of prenatal diagnosis include adequate time for education and preparation for the birth of an affected child, and a planned delivery in a center where the neonate may receive immediate and appropriate care (Musci, 2005).

ETHNICITY-BASED SCREENING: GEOGRAPHIC ANCESTRY VERSUS UNIVERSAL SCREENING

1. Screening for different disorders may be universal or based on different "ethnic" groups because a mutation associated with the disorder occurred originally in a small population (founder effect) that was isolated for religious, geographic, or political reasons or in some instances offered an advantage. Therefore, these "gene changes" or genetic mutations are present in a higher frequency in that population (e.g., those of Ashkenazi and Eastern European Jewish descent). It is important to be mindful that it is not the "ethnicity" per se that is causative but one's "geographic ancestry" that determines the risk for carrying different mutations/variants, and the provider's language should reflect these details (ACOG Committee on Genetics, Committee Opinion No. 442, 2009; Musci, 2005; Norton, 2008).

2. A number of professional organizations, advocacy groups, and carrier screening companies recommend an expansion of heterozygote screening for interested couples because of lower costs, indistinction of ethnicity, and geographic ancestry, among other reasons. We will discuss these details in the key updates that follow.

Carrier Screening Based on Ashkenazi Jewish Ancestry

UPDATE #2

Carrier screening for Tay-Sachs, Canavan, familial dysautonomia, and cystic fibrosis should be offered to all women of Ashkenazi Jewish ancestry (ACOG Committee on Genetics, Committee Opinion No. 442, 2009). Some professional organizations recommend screening for additional disorders, which vary in incidence, clinical severity, and availability of treatment (Gross et al, 2008; Monaghan et al, 2008). After considering patient population characteristics, local resources (e.g., formal genetic counseling), and a discussion with the local/regional prenatal diagnosis provider, providers may determine if they will offer additional testing.

A. The current American College of Obstetricians and Gynecologists (ACOG) screening recommendations suggest offering testing for Tay-Sachs, Canavan, familial dysautonomia, and cystic fibrosis to individuals of Ashkenazi Jewish descent (ACOG Committee on Genetics, Committee Opinion No. 442, 2009).

B. Individuals may inquire about other disorders with an increased incidence in those of Ashkenazi Jewish descent (Table 1-1) and may be referred for formal genetic counseling and testing.

C. ACOG does not currently recommend screening for all the disorders listed in Table 1-1. The authors cite decreasing carrier frequency and in some cases diminished severity (e.g., Gaucher disease) of the disorder with limited or no limitations on cognitive performance and increased availability of treatment (e.g., enzyme replacement therapy for Gaucher) in support of the policy. Advocacy groups and those with a family history of Gaucher have supported offering screening to all individuals at an increased risk (ACOG Committee on Genetics, Committee Opinion No. 442, 2009).

TABLE 1-1   Ashkenazi Jewish/East European—Geographic Ancestry-Based Carrier Screening

Disorder	Disease Incidence	Carrier Frequency	Detection Rate
Tay-Sachs*	1/3000	1/30-31	98% by HEX A enzyme 92%-99% by DNA
Canavan*	1/6400-9100	1/40-48	98%
Familial dysautonomia*	1/3600	1/31-32	99%
Cystic fibrosis*	1/2500-3000	1/24-29	94%-97%
Fanconi anemia- group C	1/32,000	1/89	98%-99%
Niemann-Pick, type A	1/32,000	1/90	94%-97%
Mucolipidosis, type IV	1/62,500	1/127	90%-95%
Bloom	1/40,000	1/107	99%
Gaucher	1/900	1/15-18	89%-95%
French Canadian/Cajun*			
Tay-Sachs	1/675-360,000	1/13-300	Varies

*ACOG recommendation: Clinicians should offer carrier screening for each disorder. Patients may inquire about the other disorders.
ACMG recommends offering screening for all disorders listed in Table I to all individuals of Ashkenazi Jewish descent.
Carrier frequency, detection rates and prevalence from Monaghan KG, Feldman GL, Palomaki GE, et al: Technical standards and guidelines for reproductive screening in the Ashkenazi Jewish population, *Genet Med* 10:57-72, 2008.
Modified from March of Dimes: *Genetic screening pocket facts,* White Plains, NY, 2001, March of Dimes.

D. In contrast, because of the high detection rates and reliable DNA-based and enzyme testing, the American College of Medical Genetics (ACMG) recommends offering testing for each of the disorders listed in Table 1-1 to those at an increased risk. Furthermore, the organization concludes that each disorder meets the criteria for inclusion in a screening program (see Characteristics for a successful screening program, in the preceding list) (Gross, Pletcher, Monaghan, 2008).

E. At times, clinicians may be placed in a difficult position and may have to choose between conflicting sets of recommendations to determine how to best serve their patients. We suggest discussing this with your local prenatal diagnosis provider(s) or referral center to determine what is routinely offered in that setting.
   1. More specifically, the ob-gyn can offer a concise statement to each patient of Ashkenazi descent about these disorders and refer any patients who express any interest or concern for additional education and potential testing.

F. In the future, screening for genetic disorders may become more widespread because of the indistinction of traditional ethnic groups. Specifically, admixing of populations in which individuals often have grandparents of different ethnicities/geographic ancestries make specific risk calculations less accurate and more complex to determine.

G. If one individual in a couple is of a high-risk group, that individual should be screened first. If that person is a determined to be a carrier, then the partner (regardless of ethnicity) should be offered screening (ACOG Committee on Genetics, Committee Opinion No. 442, 2009).

H. The relatively low cost of performing such screening may afford properly counseled individuals (and their partners) the ability to undergo carrier testing for a number of conditions in the near future. For instance, one commercial company offers carrier screening for more than 100 autosomal recessive disorders, at a cost that is slightly more than screening for cystic fibrosis at a traditional commercial laboratory. This and other companies offer such testing and directly advertise to consumers, including women (and their families) who are pregnant or are planning a pregnancy or in-vitro fertilization (IVF). Such screening may eventually become commonplace as the cost of carrier screening and additional testing continues to decrease in cost. It is critical that women and their families undergo appropriate genetic counseling to understand the risks and benefits of such testing and that each disorder meet the criteria for a carrier screening program.
   1. For instance, inclusion of hereditary hemochromatosis (HH) in a universal carrier screening program is somewhat problematic. HH is an autosomal recessive disorder with a carrier frequency of approximately one in nine in those of European descent. The disorder leads to inappropriate absorption of iron and typically manifests late in adulthood. Most individuals who are homozygous for the common disease-causing alleles do not have end-organ disease, so it is difficult for most authorities to advocate for universal screening.

Carrier Screening for Disorders of Hemoglobin

UPDATE #3

Hemoglobinopathies continue to affect a significant proportion of neonates born in the United States, resulting in considerable morbidity and mortality. Effective carrier screening utilizing traditional geographic-based ancestry screening with mean corpuscular volume (MCV) and hemoglobin electrophoresis in those without iron deficiency anemia can efficiently identify those at risk for having an affected child (ACOG Committee on Genetics, Practice Bulletin No. 78, 2007).

A. Screening for hemoglobinopathies based on specific ethnic groups, race, or geographic ancestry may be of limited value, as the geographic and ethnic distribution of hemoglobinopathies has broadened.

B. Hemoglobin S or sickle cell is well known and quite common in those of certain geographic ancestry. Additional hemoglobin variants (e.g., hemoglobin C, E, B, or D) may also result in serious sequelae.

C. ACOG recommends that individuals at increased risk of carrying a hemoglobinopathy should be offered screening.

D. Individuals from a Northern European, Japanese, Native American, Inuit, and Korean background are considered at low risk for a hemoglobinopathy, likely because of a common limited ancestral exposure to malaria, as hemoglobin S offers a survival advantage to those infected with malaria (ACOG Committee on Genetics, Practice Bulletin No. 78, 2007) (Table 1-2).

E. Screening for variant forms of hemoglobin (e.g., Hb S) is best accomplished by hemoglobin electrophoresis or high-performance liquid chromatography (HPLC). Additional forms of testing employed, such as solubility testing (Sickledex), cannot detect additional clinically important hemoglobin variants (e.g., Hb C, E, B, D, or β thalassemia) and are thus less useful in screening for hemoglobinopathies and prenatal diagnosis.

F. Mean corpuscular volume (MCV) is employed as a screen for those at risk for thalassemia. Most authorities have proposed a cutoff of 80 fL, which is overall considered to be sensitive; however, others suggest that in high prevalence areas (e.g., those of Southern Chinese or Thai descent) a cutoff of 85 fL be considered (Chan et al, 2001).

G. Those with a low MCV and a normal hemoglobin electrophoresis or HPLC without iron deficiency anemia are at risk of α thalassemia, and partner testing and molecular diagnosis should be offered.

H. Iron deficiency anemia can mislead clinicians and can be diagnosed via serum ferritin, zinc protoporphyrin or a number of other diagnostic tests.

I. Use of MCV in combination with hemoglobin electrophoresis can be diagnostic for β thalassemia. A detailed algorithm for carrier screening is proposed later (Musci, 2005). (Figure 1-1)

TABLE 1-2   **Ethnic/Geographic Ancestry at Significant Risk for Hemoglobinopathies**

Disorder	Important Disease Causing Genotypes	Diagnostic Tests
Sickle Cell Anemia		
African American, African, Mediterranean (Greek, Italian), Turkish, Arabic, Southern Iranian, Asian Indian, Brazilian, Central American	HbSS HbSC HbS/β^0-thalassemia	Hgb electrophoresis (both cellulose acetate and citrate agar electrophoresis) High-performance liquid chromatography (HPLC) Thin layer isoelectric focusing with solubility test
Alpha Thalassemia		
Southeast Asian, Pacific Islander, Middle Eastern, Indian, Chinese Mediterranean, African (not African American)	(--/--) Barts (α-/--) Hb H disease α -thalassemia trait hypochromic/microcytic anemia (α-/α-) African (trans) (--/$\alpha\alpha$) SE Asian (cis)	MCV <80 fL MCV <85 fL (in highest risk) Normal Hb electrophoresis Molecular diagnostic testing: gap-PCR (common deletions), multiplex ligation-dependent amplification (MLPA)
Beta Thalassemia		
Mediterranean (Italy, Greece), East Asian (China, Thailand), Middle Eastern (Turkey, Pakistan), Central Asia (West India), African American	β^0-thalassemia β^+-thalassemia HbE/β-thalassemia	MCV<80 fL Elevated HbA$_2$ ($\geq$3.5%) Molecular diagnostic testing: PCR, allele-specific oligonucleotides (ASO), others

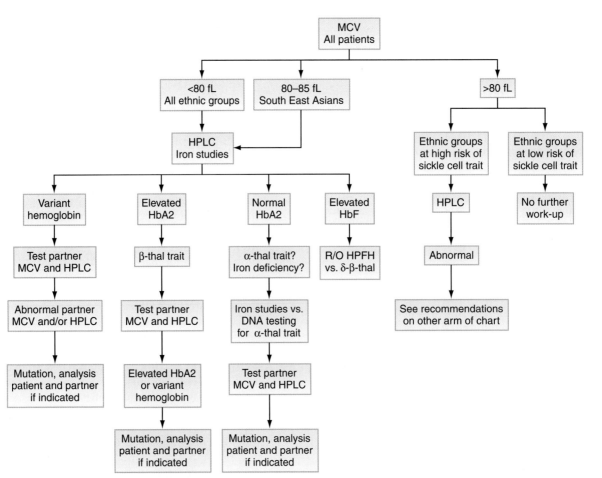

Figure 1-1. Carrier evaluation for prenatal patients at risk of hemoglobinopathy. Hemoglobin electrophoresis can be substituted for high-performance liquid chromatography (HPLC). MCV = Mean corpuscular volume; HPFH = Hereditary persistence of fetal hemoglobin. (From Musci TJ: Screening for single gene genetic disease, *Gynecol Obstet Invest* 60:19-26, 2005.)

Carrier Screening for Cystic Fibrosis

UPDATE #4

Carrier screening for cystic fibrosis (CF) is common, and many individuals regardless of geographic ancestry undergo screening during the preconception or prenatal period. Providers should counsel patients that depending on their specific ancestry and the number of mutations assessed in the panel, the performance of the test varies for each couple. Specifically, the highest sensitivity is obtained in those of Ashkenazi or Northern European descent, whereas information is limited in those of Asian descent. Specific risks may be calculated for an individual patient and her partner (Committee on Genetics, American College of Obstetricians and Gynecologists, Committee Opinion No. 325, 2005).

A. Obstetricians have been routinely offering cystic fibrosis screening to patients for nearly 10 years. Initially, testing was limited to those of Caucasian ancestry. In a more recent survey, two thirds of obstetricians routinely offered carrier screening to all patients, regardless of the patient's ethnicity (Morgan et al, 2005).
B. Obstetricians report finding increasing difficulty in assigning a single ethnicity.
C. Providers felt that offering carrier screening with decreased sensitivity was acceptable as long as the patient understood the limitations of testing (Table 1-3).
D. Specifically, negative carrier screening reduces but does not eliminate the risk of being a carrier.
E. Residual risks can be calculated and provided to women and their partners.
F. For those at risk of having an affected child, a definitive phenotype is very difficult to predict.
G. ACOG supports the practice of offering screening to all women as long as women are aware of their risk and the limitations of testing are reviewed.
H. Offering testing to all individuals will not afford a greater understanding of the patient's true ethnic or geographic ancestry; however, if no mutations are detected, the patient's risk of having an affected child decreases.

Further, if a mutation is detected, appropriate workup may continue; thus, ACOG has supported this approach.
I. Although there are more than 1300 known mutations in the cystic fibrosis gene, ACMG currently recommends a 23 mutation panel for carrier screening, which includes the most common mutations (i.e., those accounting for more than 0.1% of all cases of cystic fibrosis) found in those with cystic fibrosis.
J. A number of commercial laboratories offer expanded panels of up to 97 different mutations. These panels have increased sensitivity, but there is an additional cost (Watson et al, 2004).
K. Expanded screening or gene sequencing should be considered when one partner is a carrier and the other is not of Caucasian ancestry or when there are features suggestive but not diagnostic on prenatal ultrasound (e.g., echogenic bowel). Residual risks can be calculated and discussed with the couple (Norton, 2008).
L. Specific variants of note:
   1. If and only if an R117H gene variant mutation is detected, proceed with 5T/7T/9T variant testing. Both 7T and 9T are considered polymorphisms, whereas 5T is a variably penetrant mutation.
   2. Classic CF occurs when 5T is found on the same chromosome as R117H and there is a classic mutation (e.g., ΔF508) on the other chromosome.
   3. In a female with 5T on one chromosome and a classic mutation on the other, no clinical significance is predicted; however, males with this same mutation configuration will likely have congenital absence of the vas deferens and resultant infertility.
   4. Carriers of R117H will likely benefit from genetic counseling.
   5. The I148T variant was on the initial ACMG panel and does not appear to be a disease-causing mutation. The most recent ACMG guidelines recommend removing this variant from screening panels; however, commercial laboratories may still report this genetic variant.
   6. The mutation 3199del6 is a disease-causing mutation but occurs in less than 0.1% of those with CF and is not included on the ACMG panel. Clinicians often proceed with 3199del6 testing in the setting of I148T variant because of its association with I148T (Watson et al, 2004).

Screening for Fragile X Syndrome

UPDATE #5

Because of the frequency, severity, and lack of effective treatment, advocates recommend expanding carrier screening to all women (Musci, 2005), rather than only to women with the traditional indications such as a family history of Fragile X, tremor/ataxia syndrome, unexplained autism or cognitive disability, or a personal history of an unexplained learning disability or premature ovarian failure. However, because of the relative genetic complexity of the disorder, formal genetic counseling should be offered prior to universal carrier testing (American College of Obstetricians and Gynecologists Committee on Genetics, Committee Opinion No. 469, 2010; Norton 2008).

TABLE 1-3   **Cystic Fibrosis: Incidence, Carrier Risks and Detection Rates***

Group	Incidence	Carrier Risk	Detection	After One Negative Parental Risk of Affected Fetus
Ashkenazi	1/2270	1/24	94%	1/83,000
Caucasian	1/2500	1/25	88%	1/21,000
Hispanic	1/13,500	1/58	72%	1/18,000
African American	1/15,100	1/61	64%	1/54,000
Asian American	1/35,100	1/94	49%	1/75,000

*Detection rates derived from using ACMG 23 mutation panel.

A. Fragile X is the most common form of inherited mental retardation, and those affected often have cognitive disability, craniofacial dysmorphisms, speech and language difficulties, and behavior abnormalities such as autism or autistic-like features.

B. Fragile X affects individuals from a variety of ethnic backgrounds and is inherited in an X-linked manner; however, the molecular genetics are complex. Fragile X occurs secondary to hypermethylation and results in an altered transcription of the Fragile X mental retardation 1 (*FMR1*) gene.

C. Hypermethylation occurs with expansion of a trinucleotide repeat (cytosine-guanine-guanine, or CGG). Though each commercial laboratory may have slightly different numbers, a general classification for CGG repeats is listed here (Table 1-4):
   1. *Unaffected* individuals have fewer than 40 CGG repeats.
   2. *Intermediate* or "gray zone" alleles range from 41 to 60.
   3. Individuals with 61 to 200 CGG repeats have a *premutation* and are *phenotypically* normal.
      a. Women with premutations are at increased risk for premature ovarian failure (POF) and having an affected child.
      b. Males are at risk of a late-onset neurodegenerative disorder characterized best by tremor and ataxia. This condition is known as Fragile X–Ataxia (FXTAS). Women are also at risk of FXTAS, but have a lower risk of exhibiting signs and symptoms.
         (1) Approximately 17% of men exhibit signs and symptoms of FXTAS prior to age 60.
         (2) The risk for women is less, but precise estimates are not currently available.
      c. The risk of expansion to a full mutation is greater with an increased number of CGG repeats.
      d. The lowest number of CGG repeats to expand to a full mutation in a single generation (i.e., mother to child) is 56 repeats.
      e. Consideration of prenatal diagnosis and genetic counseling is warranted in those with gray zone alleles with 56 or more CGG repeats (Sherman, et al, 2005; Murray, et al, 2001; American College of Obstetricians and Gynecologists Committee on Genetics, Committee Opinion No. 469, 2010; Saul et al, 2010).

D. Those with >200 CGG repeats have a *full mutation*, and all males and approximately 50% of females are affected with Fragile X syndrome. Women with full mutations are at risk of having an affected child.

E. Who should be offered carrier screening for Fragile X?
   1. Women with a family history of Fragile X, autism, unexplained learning disability or unexplained mental retardation should be offered screening.
   2. Prenatal diagnosis should be offered to known premutation and full mutation carriers and to those with known affected relatives to assess their own reproductive risks.
   3. Offer screening to all women with a personal history of a learning disability, premature ovarian failure, or elevated follicle-stimulating hormone (FSH) at age <40.
   4. At the present time, the ACMG and ACOG do not currently endorse population screening because of the complexities of inheritance and variation in phenotype in females in addition to the requirements for formal genetic counseling and the potential limited geographic availability of such testing. Further, in one study about the feasibility of universal testing, not all women could understand the complex genetic risks despite being in favor of such testing (American College of Obstetricians and Gynecologists Committee on Genetics, Committee Opinion No. 469, 2010; Sherman et al, 2005).
   5. Because of reliable diagnostic testing, the severity of the phenotype, the presumed cost-effectiveness, and prior study participants' desire to undergo screening in a number of research settings, some centers routinely offer Fragile X screening to all women of reproductive age. In addition, routine screening occurs in Israel, and several reports of universal screening success and acceptability have been published (Toledano-Alhadef et al, 2001). Additional reports from prenatal diagnosis centers where Fragile X screening is routine with available genetic counseling including concise education is eagerly awaited prior to the adoption of universal screening for Fragile X syndrome for all women of reproductive age.

TABLE 1-4   **Fragile X CGG Repeat Expansion, Risks, and Clinical Phenotype**

Mutation Type	CGG Trinucleotide Repeats	Risk of Transmission to Full Mutation	Methylation Status (*FMRI*)	Phenotype	
				Men	Women
Normal	<40	None	Unmethylated	Normal	Normal
Intermediate "Gray Zone"	41-60	Risk of transmission at 56 repeats	Unmethylated	Normal	Normal
Premutation	60-200	Yes Increases with repeat number	Unmethylated	At risk for Fragile X-Ataxia (17% by age 60)	At risk for Fragile X Ataxia and premature ovarian failure (POF risk 21%)
Full Mutation	>200	Approximately 100%	Methylated	Fragile X syndrome 100% with mental retardation	50% with normal intellect; 50% with mental retardation

Carrier Screening for Spinal Muscular Atrophy (SMA)

UPDATE #6

SMA is the second most common fatal autosomal recessive disorder, and screening should be offered to all those with a family history of SMA. Some organizations have proposed universal screening because of the clinical severity, incidence, and limited treatment options, but others have opposed this idea because of the lack of appropriate educational and cost-effectiveness analysis studies, widespread availability of genetic counseling, and testing limitations such as the inability to predict phenotype in the absence of a family history and testing challenges such as a considerable false negative rate (ACOG Committee on Genetics, Committee Opinion No. 432, 2009; Prior et al, 2008).

A. SMA is an autosomal recessive disorder that leads to progressive muscle weakness and paralysis. The α motor neurons in the anterior horn of the spinal cord are affected.

B. SMA is the second most common fatal autosomal recessive disorder and is characterized by three clinical courses.
   1. SMA I (Werdnig-Hoffman) is the most severe and typically results in death secondary to respiratory failure at 2 years of life.
   2. Survival improves in those affected with SMA II, but children are unable to sit, stand, or walk unaided. This is the most common form of SMA, and these individuals often die of respiratory failure in adolescence.
   3. Those with SMA III (Kugelberg-Welander) are able to learn to walk unaided, and the onset usually occurs after 18 months. The signs and symptoms of SMA III can be quite variable, and these individuals may have a normal life expectancy (ACOG Committee on Genetics, Committee Opinion No. 432, 2009; Prior et al, 2008).

C. SMA is usually caused by deletion on both copies of survival motor neuron 1 (*SMN1*). A second gene, survival motor neuron 2 (*SMN2*), is nearly identical to *SMN1* but does not produce protein. There may be zero to two copies of *SMN2*, which influences the severity of SMA. In addition, 15% of normal individuals may have no copies of *SMN2*.

D. Carrier detection is problematic in 3% to 4% of the population, as these individuals have no phenotypic features of SMA and have two *SMN1* copies on one chromosome and none on the other. Because of testing limitations, these individuals are not identified as carriers but are still at risk of having an affected child.

E. Carrier detection is also a challenge in that SMA arises from a *de novo* mutation event in 2% of cases (Table 1-5).

F. Because of the severity of the disease, limited treatment, reliable DNA-based testing, and relatively high panethnic carrier frequency, universal carrier screening has been proposed.

G. The ACMG recommends offering routine carrier screening to all couples; however, at present, ACOG does not recommend universal screening for SMA.
   1. The rationale proposed by ACOG supporting the limitation of universal screening prior to launching universal screening is as follows:
      a. Limitations in predicting the type (i.e., I, II or III) of SMA in the absence of a family history.
      b. A lack of study data relating to education and counseling, patient preferences, and utility measurements enabling an appropriate cost effectiveness analysis.
      c. Availability and logistics for patients to obtain appropriate genetic counseling services.

H. Consideration of universal screening may be warranted if couples understand the genetics of SMA and the limitations of testing (i.e., false negative rate) in the setting of formal genetic counseling.
   a. With such a severe illness, studies on patient preferences, cost utility, and feasibility will hopefully be forthcoming (Prior et al, 2008).

Invasive Prenatal Diagnosis

UPDATE #7

All women should be offered screening or invasive prenatal testing for aneuploidy via amniocentesis or chorionic villus sampling (CVS). Each woman should be provided risks of aneuploidy or other genetic disorder based on her age-related risk or those derived from serum or ultrasound screening. Women should be offered counseling to individually weigh the risks of a procedure related loss with the risk of having an affected fetus (American College of Obstetricians and Gynecologists, Practice Bulletin No. 88, 2007).

A. The ACOG recently recommended that invasive prenatal diagnosis be made available to all women regardless of maternal age.
   1. Pretest counseling should consist of a detailed discussion of screening compared with invasive testing including the following:
      a. Screening counseling should include which disorders have reliable screening, including the anticipated sensitivity and specificity of carrier screening.
      b. Invasive testing counseling should review the disorders that may be detected (i.e., aneuploidy other than Down syndrome), the prognosis, and the risks and specific options (CVS and amniocentesis) of invasive testing.

TABLE 1-5   Carrier Screening for Spinal Muscular Atrophy

Disorder	Disease incidence	Carrier frequency	Detection Rate
Spinal muscular atrophy	1/10,000	1/40-60	90%-98% Dual *SMN1* copy deletion 2%-5% Compound heterozygotes

2. Several studies have illustrated that women weigh the risk of having an affected fetus, the risk of a procedure-related loss, and the consequences of having an affected child differently, and each should be offered clear and accurate information in an unbiased manner (American College of Obstetricians and Gynecologists, Practice Bulletin No. 88, 2007).

Risks of Invasive Prenatal Diagnosis

UPDATE #8

Procedure-related loss caused by invasive testing has traditionally been quoted as 1 in 200, but recent studies indicate that this is an overestimation. The procedure-related loss rate for invasive testing does not appear to be different by procedure type (CVS versus amniocentesis) or route (CVS by transabdominal or trans-cervical) and is approximately 1 in 300 to 500 in experienced centers. Early CVS (<9 weeks) or amniocentesis (<14 weeks) can be associated with increased rates of malformations or pregnancy loss (American College of Obstetricians and Gynecologists, Practice Bulletin No. 88, 2007; Caughey et al, 2006; Eddleman et al, 2006, Odibo et al, 2008).

A. Update on Chorionic Villus Sampling (CVS)
　1. Procedure-related pregnancy loss rate
　　a. The attributable loss rate after CVS will always be higher than amniocentesis secondary to the increased background loss rate at earlier gestational ages. Recent studies have suggested that the gap of procedure-related loss may be closing, and in an experienced center, may actually be closer to expectant management than previously understood.
　　　(1) In one recent retrospective cohort study spanning two decades, the procedure-related loss rate was highest in the earliest years and lowest more recently—the loss rate associated with CVS was 1 in 360, which was not different than amniocentesis but higher than expectant management (Caughey et al, 2006).
　　　(2) A meta-analysis suggested that pooled total pregnancy loss rates were similar for amniocentesis and CVS
　　　　(a) Improved provider skill and ultrasound technology are proposed as potential ameliorating factors in improved loss rates.
　　　(3) The route of CVS, transcervical or transabdominal, does not appear to affect the miscarriage rate after CVS.
　2. Fetal injury/malformation associated with CVS
　　a. CVS should not be performed prior to 9 completed weeks.
　　　(1) Limb reduction defects and oromandibular hypoplasia have been associated with early CVS performed at 7 weeks or at earlier gestational ages.
　　　(2) Transverse limb defects and oromandibular hypoplasia are not expected to occur at greater than background in women who choose to undergo CVS at 9 to 14 weeks' gestation.

　　b. Maternal complications
　　　(1) Vaginal spotting or bleeding occurs in approximately 30% to 35% of women after CVS, and those undergoing the procedure should be counseled appropriately.
　　　(2) Infection or amniotic fluid leakage is estimated to be approximately 0.5% after CVS.
B. Update on invasive prenatal diagnosis with amniocentesis
　1. Attributable pregnancy loss rate associated with amniocentesis
　　a. Traditionally, the miscarriage rate after amniocentesis has been quoted as 1 in 200 and several publications have recently suggested that the true risk may actually be lower.
　　b. The risk of pregnancy loss related to amniocentesis in one prospective unmatched trial was 1 in 1600 (Eddleman et al, 2006).
　　　(1) Criticisms of this assessment included that the termination rate in those with amniocentesis was nearly 3% versus 0.2% in those who had no such procedure. In addition, the loss rate was defined as pregnancy loss at less than 24 weeks, whereas other studies have used 28 weeks or even until delivery at term to define pregnancy loss. These limitations may underestimate the true risk associated with amniocentesis.
　　c. Is the loss rate different in those with and without invasive prenatal diagnosis?
　　　(1) In several studies, the loss rate after amniocentesis was not different than it was for those who did not have an amniocentesis.
　　　(2) In one retrospective cohort study in which women had amniocentesis for abnormal serum screening, the loss rate was actually lower in the amniocentesis group compared with the control group (Odibo et al, 2008).
　　d. What is the true pregnancy loss rate associated with amniocentesis?
　　　(1) As noted earlier, a prospective trial of unselected patients to detect the sensitivity of aneuploidy screening reported a procedure-related loss rate of 1 in 1600.
　　　(2) Several centers recently reported on their experience in retrospective cohort studies, and the risk for a loss attributable to the amniocentesis ranged from 1 in 370 to 1 in 769 (Caughey et al, 2006; Odibo et al, 2008).
　　　(3) In the ACOG bulletin on invasive prenatal testing, the estimated pregnancy loss rate attributable to amniocentesis is estimated to be 1 in 300 to 500.
　　　(4) Performed by an individual skilled at performing amniocentesis, with direct visualization using ultrasound and a 22-gauge needle, an estimate of a risk of miscarriage of 1 in 300 to 500 is likely correct.
　　e. Early amniocentesis (performed at less than 14 weeks) results in higher rates of miscarriage and other complications such as talipes equinovarus and amniotic fluid culture failure. As a result, ACOG suggests that early amniocentesis should not be offered to women.

2. What are the other risks of amniocentesis?
   a. Leakage of fluid occurs in less than 2% of women undergoing amniocentesis.
   b. The risks of direct fetal injury are quite low with proper technique. There may be a low risk of indirect fetal injury as a result of removing amniotic fluid, such as respiratory insufficiency, or orthopedic issues (e.g., talipes equinovarus or congenital hip dislocation is low with the risk likely <1%). These risks may be increased with removal of excessive amounts of amniotic fluid.
   c. Major congenital malformations do not appear to be increased in the long-term follow-up of children after prenatal amniocentesis compared with those whose mothers had no amniocentesis.
   d. Culture failure occurs in less than 1% of all specimens (American College of Obstetricians and Gynecologists, Practice Bulletin No. 88, 2007).

Chromosomal Analysis with Array CGH

UPDATE #9

Array CGH offers unique advantages and disadvantages for detection of chromosomal abnormalities and may be warranted in certain clinical circumstances. The conventional karyotype remains the gold standard for chromosome number and structural abnormalities. Chromosomal microarray is a promising technique that can detect clinically significant deletions and duplications on cultured or uncultured material at a higher resolution more rapidly compared with the conventional karyotype. Specific limitations including the possibility of copy number variants of uncertain significance, the inability to detect balanced rearrangements, and low level mosaicism, and increased costs compared with karyotype will need to be addressed prior to the widespread application of array CGH to prenatal diagnosis (American College of Obstetricians and Gynecologists, Committee Opinion No. 446, 2009).

A. The conventional karyotype analysis still remains the gold standard, at present, for the evaluation of chromosome number and structural anomalies in prenatal diagnosis. The benefits of this standard technique include the detection of the following:
   1. Whole chromosome aneuploidy, which is defined as an abnormal number of chromosomes, such as trisomy 21 (Down syndrome)
   2. Very large deletions or duplications (> 10 to 15 Mb of chromosome material), which may be interstitial or terminal
   3. Balanced translocations (apparently) in which no chromosome material appears to be missing or duplicated
   4. Mosaicism, which is defined as the presence of two populations of cells with different genotypes in one individual who has developed from a single fertilized egg (e.g., mosaic Klinefelter's syndrome wherein some of the patient's cells contain XY chromosomes and some contain XXY chromosome)
   5. Marker chromosomes, which are small, structurally abnormal chromosomes in which no part can be identified by standard G-banding (American College of Obstetricians and Gynecologists, Committee Opinion No. 446, 2009)

B. The conventional karyotype does have some limitations in the prenatal setting
   1. Banding resolution from a CVS or amniocentesis sample is approximately 400 to 450 bands. Therefore, smaller deletions or duplications can be missed.
      a. Submicroscopic balanced rearrangements, which are not uncommon, can be missed.
   2. Although standard karyotyping may identify the presence of a marker chromosome, it may not aid in the identification of the marker's origin without the use of additional molecular-cytogenetic techniques, such as FISH.
   3. Turnaround time for the standard karyotype analysis can take up to 2 weeks because of special preparation and culturing of the specimen (American College of Obstetricians and Gynecologists, Committee Opinion No. 446, 2009).

C. A new technology called the "microarray," which utilizes comparative genomic hybridization (array CGH), is a chip-based technology that has much higher resolution and, therefore, is able to scan the genome for submicroscopic copy number variation that is missed by conventional karyotyping. This technology has become more widespread with its application in the postnatal analysis of individuals with neurocognitive delay and multiple congenital anomalies. Although array CGH is not currently used as the first line of chromosomal analysis in the prenatal setting, its acceptance is becoming more widespread as it becomes more commercially available. Its use does have advantages:
   1. The "targeted" microarray is a chip whereby the genomic probes encompass areas of known chromosomal abnormalities (e.g., subtelomeres or 22q11.2) and also include probes scanning the genome at a higher resolution than conventional karyotyping but at a lower resolution than an oligonucleotide array (discussed later). This targeted array, at the present time, is preferred for prenatal analysis in the setting of multiple congenital anomalies on ultrasound or a family history that is suspicious for a known submicroscopic deletion syndrome (e.g., 22q11.2). The advantage of a targeted approach is that it decreases the likelihood of identifying a copy number variant of unknown significance.
   2. A high-resolution oligonucleotide array is the array of choice in the postnatal setting, but it is not the first line of chromosome analysis in the prenatal setting unless there is a specific, identified chromosome abnormality in the family (e.g., an apparent balanced translocation) or a prenatal karyotypic anomaly (e.g., marker chromosome, unbalanced rearrangement) that has been identified and one wishes to gain more information.
   3. The microarray will be able to identify submicroscopic deletions and duplications that conventional prenatal chromosome analysis cannot pick up.
   4. Although it is common practice to utilize cultured material for the microarray, it is not necessary; thus, uncultured tissues such as products of conception can be run on the microarray.

5. Compared with traditional karyotype, the turnaround time is faster. The microarray takes days as opposed to weeks.
6. The microarray may be able to identify a marker chromosome if there is genomic material present on the marker, which is covered by the microarray probes (Manning, et al, 2007).

D. Array CGH, despite its higher resolution, does have limitations:
1. There may be copy number variants identified in the fetus that are of unclear significance. It is highly recommended to obtain parental blood samples in case an unknown variant is identified.
2. There is limited availability of the microarray in that not all institutions offer this technology and insurance may not pay for the use of this new technology.
3. The microarray does not detect balanced rearrangements such as balanced translocations or inversions because there is no gain or loss of genomic material.
4. The microarray does not detect triploidy or tetraploidy.
   a. Low-level mosaicism down to approximately 20% to 25% can be missed.
   b. At present, the microarray costs more than a standard karyotype (American College of Obstetricians and Gynecologists, Committee Opinion No. 446, 2009; Manning et al, 2007).

Umbilical Cord Blood Banking

UPDATE #10

Umbilical cord blood banking may potentially treat a number of devastating illnesses; however, prospective parents must carefully consider a number of potential issues before choosing to use a private umbilical cord blood bank. Advantages of high rates of engraftments and limited graft versus host disease rates with umbilical cord blood transplant are balanced by a smaller number of hematopoietic cells, and longer time to engraftment as well as the cost and ethical challenges of private banking must be addressed to maximize this useful resource (Committee on Obstetric Practice, Committee on Genetics, Committee Opinion No. 399, 2008; Moise, 2005).

A. Umbilical cord blood contains hematopoietic stem cells, which could potentially be used for future transplantation.
B. There are several advantages of umbilical cord blood over bone marrow or peripheral blood.
C. Many disorders could potentially benefit from hematopoietic stem cell transplantation including inborn errors of metabolism, hematopoietic malignancies, and genetic disorders of the blood and immune system (Table 1-6).
D. The first successful transplant from an umbilical cord blood transfusion was performed in 1988, and it is estimated that more than 7000 transplants have been performed since.
E. Advantages of umbilical cord blood

TABLE 1-6 Indications, Past and Potential, for Umbilical Cord Blood Transplant

Thalassemias	Immune Deficiencies
α-thalassemia	Ataxia telangiectasia
β-thalassemia	Chronic granulomatous disease
E-β°-thalassemia	DiGeorge syndrome
E-β⁺-thalassemia	Hypogammaglobulinemia
Sickle Cell	Mucolipidosis, type II
HbSS, HbSC	X linked immunodeficiency
HbS/β°-thalassemia	Severe combine immunodeficiency
HbS/β⁺-thalassemia	
Oncologic Disorders	**Metabolic Disorders**
Acute lymphoblastic leukemia	Adrenoleukodystrophy
Acute myeloid leukemia	Gaucher
Chronic myeloid leukemia	Metachromatic leukodystrophy
Burkitt lymphoma	Krabbe disease
Familial histiocytosis	Gunther disease
Hemophagocytic lymphohistiocytosis	Hurler syndrome
Hodgkin's disease	Hurler-Scheie
Non-Hodgkin's lymphoma	Hunter syndrome
Hematologic Disorders	Sanfilippo syndrome
Autoimmune neutropenia	Maroteaux-Lamy syndrome
Diamond Blackfan anemia	Mucolipidosis, types II and III
Pancytopenia	Alpha mannosidosis
Kostmann's syndrome	Niemann-Pick, type A and B
Fanconi's anemia	Sandhoff disease
Glanzmann's disease	Tay-Sachs disease
Thrombocytopenia with absent radius (TAR syndrome)	

Adapted from Moise KJ: Umbilical cord stem cells, *Obstet Gynecol* 106:1393-1407, 2005.

1. High rates of success of engraftment and less graft-versus-host disease (GvHD), even in the setting of human leukocyte antigen (HLA) mismatch.
   a. HLA matching of four to six out of six antigens may be sufficient for treatment, resulting in a higher number of available donors and a simpler more rapid matching process.
   b. Lower rates of CMV infection may lead to lower rates of GvHD.
2. High concentration of highly proliferative hematopoietic stem cells, which can reconstitute hematopoiesis in the recipient.
3. Collection is safe, easy, and pain free without morbidity for the donor.
4. Is almost immediately available when needed and there is a nearly limitless supply. Further, ethnic diversity should match the birth rate and supply (Committee on Obstetric Practice, Committee on Genetics, Committee Opinion No. 399, 2008; Moise, 2005).

F. Disadvantages of umbilical cord blood
1. The number of hematopoietic stem cells must be great enough to allow for engraftment and in most units is only adequate for children or small adults.
2. Engraftment occurs over a longer period of time in umbilical cord cells compared with bone marrow. This disadvantage leads to higher rates of morbidity because of infection or bleeding.

3. There may be a weakened response to leukemia cells in those derived from cord blood compared to marrow transplant.

4. There are additional donor cells for leukocyte infusion or second transplant (Committee on Obstetric Practice, Committee on Genetics, Committee Opinion No. 399, 2008; Moise, 2005).

G. Umbilical cord blood banks: public versus Private
   1. Public umbilical cord blood banks generally promote allogenic donation.
   2. Units are available to anyone with an appropriate indication and HLA matching.
   3. Cord blood may be donated when a neonate is delivered at a hospital associated with a public bank.
      a. The cell count, HLA profile, and other relevant information is kept in a public database.
      b. Rigorous screening and testing for infectious disease is governed by the U.S. Food and Drug Administration.

H. Private cord blood banks
   1. Family members pay a fee for the collection and yearly storage of cord blood, and the unit may be accessed if the child or an additional family member requires such therapy.
   2. In general, these units are often saved as an "insurance policy" to potentially treat disease later in life.
      a. However, if a child later develops leukemia or an inborn error of metabolism, the unit could not be used to treat that child, as these abnormalities would be present in stem cells.
      b. The likelihood of using an autologous unit of blood is estimated to be 1 in 2700 or potentially even lower.
      c. A recent cost-effectiveness analysis found that private cord blood banking was not cost effective and only would become cost effective if the entire cost of blood banking was $262 or less or the risk of the child requiring a hematopoietic stem cell transplantation (HSC) was more than 1 in 110 (Kaimal et al, 2009).

I. Directed banking
   1. This most often occurs when a child is affected by a specific disorder and has a younger sibling. The unit is processed and kept for treatment of the sibling.

J. Private versus public: ethical challenges
   1. Several concerns have been raised regarding the private use of cord blood including quality control, long-term availability, costs, and the ethics of limiting use for those who have saved a unit privately versus using it for anyone with an indication for transplant.
   2. Some private banks have quoted the chance of utilization of a unit at 1 in 27 and in the future a much higher rate of use is expected, estimated at 50%.
      a. ACOG recently released a committee opinion on umbilical cord banking, in which the authors wrote, "Parents should not be sold this service without a realistic assessment of their likelihood of return on their investment."
      b. Public banks afford greater access for the general population and have stringent procedures for collecting, testing, and processing specimens, and

advocacy groups and professional organizations are proponents of expanding public umbilical cords banking.

   c. When patients request information on cord blood donation, a detailed discussion with the following elements should be considered:
      (1) Review the advantages and disadvantages of private versus public donation including the costs, quality-control concerns, and the likelihood of utilizing the cord blood (~1 in 2700).
      (2) Review of information and testing (genetic and infectious), the potential outcome of the utilization of poor units, and that demographic data will be maintained on the patient.
      (3) Some states have passed legislation regarding informing patients about private blood banking and clinicians should obtain this information from their state medical board about specific requirements.
      (4) There is strong consideration of directed donation when a family member has a condition potentially treatable with HSC (Committee on Obstetric Practice, Committee on Genetics, Committee Opinion No. 399, 2008; Kaimal, et al 2009; Moise, 2005).

Noninvasive Diagnosis of Fetal Material

UPDATE #11

Noninvasive prenatal diagnosis may be helpful in determination of fetal RhD status or sex to determine if a fetus is at risk for iso-immunization or an X-linked disorder. In addition, reliable results for paternally derived genetic disorders are possible. However, cost and reliability of these has limited widespread application of these techniques. The detection of fetal aneuploidy via maternal serum remains a challenge, and several trials are ongoing to determine the feasibility of this important technology (Norbury et al, 2008).

A. Invasive prenatal diagnosis has associated risks; the foremost is procedure-related miscarriage.

B. The quest for an accurate, rapid, cost-effective test for the prenatal diagnosis of fetal sex, fetal RhD status, genetic disorders, and aneuploidy has many advantages, the most important being safety for the pregnancy.

C. Fetal cells and fragments of genetic material (e.g., DNA and RNA) exist in the maternal circulation.
   1. Fetal cells are unlikely to lead to genetic diagnosis because they are rare, technically difficult to work with, and persist from prior pregnancies and as such cannot afford accurate prenatal diagnosis.
   2. Fragments of fetal DNA and RNA have a short half-life (e.g., ~16 minutes) and thus are specific to the current pregnancy. In fact, cell-free fetal DNA is undetectable approximately 2 hours after delivery.
   3. Fetal DNA exists in maternal circulation because of apoptosis of placental cells and potentially fetal blood

cells and is available at the 9th to 10th postmenstrual week, allowing for early prenatal diagnosis.

4. Fetal DNA and RNA represent a small proportion of the material in the maternal blood, thus complicating the ability to reliably detect certain genetic abnormalities (Norbury et al, 2008).

   a. Successful approaches have utilized detection of sequences on the Y chromosome or specific mutations or sequences inherited from the father.

     (1) Fetal sex determination is technically possible and important in X-linked disease (e.g., ornithine transcarbamylase deficiency, among many others) by about 10 weeks of gestation.

     (2) Fetal sex determination allows for appropriate medication administration when a female fetus is at risk for congenital adrenal hyperplasia (CAH) and requires maternal administration of dexamethasone beginning at 8 to 9 weeks of gestation.

   b. Detection of maternally inherited sequences is problematic and has limited success with differing methylation patterns.

   c. DNA fragments can be detected and amplified using polymerase chain reaction (PCR).

     (1) Can be successful and accurate if the target of interest is paternally inherited (Y chromosome).

       (a) RhD testing is available, is sensitive, and can limit the need for RhoGAM and increased surveillance if the fetus is not RhD positive (Gautier et al, 2005; Moise et al, 2005).

       (b) Paternally derived autosomal dominant and recessive mutations are detectable using PCR techniques.

         (i) Achondroplasia, β-thalassemia, CAH, cystic fibrosis, myotonic dystrophy, and Huntington's disease have all been detected using cell-free fetal DNA from the maternal plasma.

     (2) Limitations of this technique are time and cost, as many reactions must occur for accurate diagnosis and this has hampered the development of a reliable test for fetal aneuploidy (Norbury et al, 2008).

   d. Detection of fetal aneuploidy

     (1) Fetal DNA levels in the maternal circulation are higher when the fetus is affected with trisomy 21 and 13.

     (2) Most aneuploidy is derived from maternal meiotic nondisjunction, making the detection challenging.

     (3) Researchers who employ intensive PCR techniques are able to compare the ratio of fetal copies of chromosome 21 to maternal copies, but this investigation is hampered by high cost and is time consuming (Chiu et al, 2009).

     (4) Promising results have been obtained from other researchers who have attempted to detect aneuploidy by using differently imprinted ratios of mRNA (Ghanta et al, 2010).

     (5) It may be a number of years before accurate cost-effective detection of fetal genetic disorders including trisomy 21 is available in singleton pregnancies, but the potential to eliminate many procedure-related miscarriages requires continual research and innovation until prenatal diagnosis is made safer for all women who desire such information.

SUGGESTED READINGS

Screening for Carriers of Single Gene Disorders

American College of Obstetricians and Gynecologists Committee on Genetics: ACOG committee opinion no. 442: preconception and prenatal carrier screening for genetic diseases in individuals of Eastern European Jewish descent, *Obstet Gynecol* 114(4):950–953, 2009.

Musci TJ: Screening for single gene genetic disease, *Gynecol Obstet Invest* 60(1):19–26, 2005.

Norton ME: Genetic screening and counseling, *Curr Opin Obstet Gynecol* 20(2):157–163, Apr 2008.

Carrier Screening Based on Ashkenazi Jewish Ancestry

American College of Obstetricians and Gynecologists Committee on Genetics: ACOG committee opinion no. 442: preconception and prenatal carrier screening for genetic diseases in individuals of Eastern European Jewish descent, *Obstet Gynecol* 114(4):950–953, 2009.

Gross SJ, Pletcher BA, Monaghan KG: Carrier screening in individuals of Ashkenazi Jewish descent, *Genet Med* 10(1):54–56, 2008.

Monaghan KG, Feldman GL, Palomaki GE, et al: Technical standards and guidelines for reproductive screening in the Ashkenazi Jewish population, *Genet Med* 10(1):57–72, 2008.

Carrier Screening for Hemoglobinopathies

American College of Obstetricians and Gynecologists Committee on Obstetrics: ACOG practice bulletin no. 78: hemoglobinopathies in pregnancy, *Obstet Gynecol* 109(1):229–237, 2007.

Chan LC, Ma SK, Chan AY, et al: Should we screen for globin gene mutations in blood samples with mean corpuscular volume (MCV) greater than 80fL in areas with high prevalence of thalassemia? *J Clin Pathol* 54(4):317–320, 2001.

Musci TJ: Screening for single gene genetic disease, *Gynecol Obstet Invest* 60(1):19–26, 2005.

Carrier Screening for Cystic Fibrosis

Committee on Genetics: American College of Obstetricians and Gynecologists: ACOG committee opinion no. 325, December 2005: update on carrier screening for cystic fibrosis, *Obstet Gynecol* 106(6):1465–1468, 2005.

Morgan MA, Driscoll DA, Zinberg S, et al: Impact of self-reported familiarity with guidelines for cystic fibrosis carrier screening, *Obstet Gynecol* 105(6):1355–1361, 2005.

Norton ME: Genetic screening and counseling, *Curr Opin Obstet Gynecol* 20(2):157–163, 2008.

Watson MS, Cutting GR, Desnick RJ, et al: Cystic fibrosis population carrier screening: 2004 revision of the American College of Medical Genetics mutation panel, *Genet Med* 6(5):387–391, 2004.

Carrier Screening for Fragile X

American College of Obstetricians and Gynecologists Committee on Genetics: ACOG committee opinion no. 469: carrier screening for fragile X syndrome, *Obstet Gynecol* 116(4):1008–1010, 2010.

Murray J, Cuckle H: Cystic fibrosis and fragile X syndrome: the arguments for antenatal screening, *Comb Chem High Throughput Screen* 4(3):265–272, 2001.

Musci TJ: Screening for single gene genetic disease, *Gynecol Obstet Invest* 60(1):19–26, 2005.

Norton ME: Genetic screening and counseling, *Curr Opin Obstet Gynecol* 20(2):157–163, 2008.

Saul RA, Tarleton JC: FMRI-related disorders. In Pagon RA, Bird TD, Dolan CR, Stephens K, editors: *Gene Reviews* [Internet], Seattle, University of Washington (website), www.genetests.org. Accessed March 8, 2010.

Sherman S, Pletcher BA, Driscoll DA: Fragile X syndrome: diagnostic and carrier testing, *Genet Med* 7(8):584–587, 2005.

Toledano-Alhadef H, Basel-Vanagaite L, Magal N, et al: Fragile-X carrier screening and the prevalence of premutation and full mutation carriers in Israel, *Am J Hum Genet* 69(2):351–360, 2001.

Carrier Screening for Spinal Muscular Atrophy

American College of Obstetricians and Gynecologists Committee on Genetics: ACOG committee opinion no. 432: spinal muscular atrophy, *Obstet Gynecol* 113(5):1194–1196, May 2009.

Prior TW: Carrier screening for spinal muscular atrophy, *Genet Med* 10(11):1–3, Nov 2008.

Prior TW, Russman BS: Spinal muscular atrophy. In Pagon RA, Bird TD, Dolan CR, Stephens K, editors: *Gene Reviews* [Internet], Seattle, University of Washington (website), www.genetests.org. Accessed March 8, 2010.

Invasive Prenatal Testing

American College of Obstetricians and Gynecologists: ACOG committee opinion no. 446: array comparative genomic hybridization in prenatal diagnosis, *Obstet Gynecol* 114(5):1161–1163, 2009.

American College of Obstetricians and Gynecologists: ACOG practice bulletin no. 88, December 2007: invasive prenatal testing for aneuploidy, *Obstet Gynecol* 110(6):1459–1467, 2007.

Caughey AB, Hopkins LM, Norton ME: Chorionic villus sampling compared with amniocentesis and the difference in the rate of pregnancy loss, *Obstet Gynecol* 108(3 Part 1):612–616, 2006.

Eddleman KA, Malone FD, Sullivan L, et al: Pregnancy loss rates after midtrimester amniocentesis, *Obstet Gynecol* 108(5):1067–1072, 2006.

Manning M, Hudgins L: Use of array based technology in the practice of medical genetics, *Genet Med* 9(11):650–653, 2007.

Odibo AO, Gray DL, Dicke JM, et al: Revisiting the fetal loss rate after second-trimester genetic amniocentesis: a single center's 16-year experience, *Obstet Gynecol* 111(3):589–595, 2008.

Chromosomal Analysis with Array CGH

Array Comparative Genomic Hybridization in Prenatal Diagnosis: ACOG Committee Opinion, No. 446. American College of Obstetricians and Gynecologists, *Obstet Gynecol* 114:1161–1163, 2009.

Manning M, Hudgins L: Use of array based technology in the practice of medical genetics, *Genet Med* 9:650–653, 2007.

Umbilical Cord Blood Banking

Committee on Obstetric Practice: Committee on Genetics: ACOG committee opinion no. 399, February 2008: umbilical cord blood banking, *Obstet Gynecol* 111(2 Part 1):475–477, 2008.

Kaimal AJ, Smith CC, Laros RK, Caughey AB, Cheng YC: Cost-effectiveness of private umbilical cord blood banking, *Obstet Gyencol* 114(4):848–855, 2009.

Moise KJ Jr: Umbilical cord stem cells, *Obstet Gynecol* 106(6):1393–1407, 2005.

Noninvasive Testing Genetic

Chiu RW, Cantor CR, Lo YM: Non-invasive prenatal diagnosis by single molecule counting technologies, *Trends Genet* 25(7):324–331, 2009.

Gautier E, Benachi A, Giovangrandi Y, et al: Fetal RhD genotyping by maternal serum analysis: a two-year experience, *Am J Obstet Gynecol* 192(3):666–669, 2005.

Ghanta S, Mitchell ME, Ames M, et al: Non-invasive prenatal detection of trisomy 21 using tandem single nucleotide polymorphisms, *PLoS One* 5(10):e13184, 2010.

Moise KJ: Fetal RhD typing with free DNA in maternal plasma, *Am J Obstet Gynecol* 192(3):663–665, 2005.

Norbury G, Norbury CJ: Non-invasive prenatal diagnosis of single gene disorders: how close are we? *Semin Fet Neonat Med* 13(2):76–83, 2008.

References

Please go to expertconsult.com to view references.

Chapter 2

Reproductive Environmental Health

JOANNE L. PERRON • PATRICE M. SUTTON • TRACEY J. WOODRUFF

KEY UPDATES

1 Trends in reproductive health outcomes document that many indicators of reproductive health are under strain.

2 Women of childbearing age incur ubiquitous contact to toxic environmental contaminants that can expose the fetus through placental transfer, and maternal exposure can continue in the newborn through breast-feeding.

3 The fetus and developing human are highly vulnerable to exposure from environmental contaminants, and adverse health impacts can manifest across the life span of individuals and generations.

4 Hormone receptor types and functions, including those involved in metabolism, obesity, and brain signaling, can be targets of endocrine disrupting chemicals (EDCs), which are encountered in the daily lives of all women of childbearing age.

5 A wide range of adverse reproductive and developmental health outcomes are linked to environmental contaminants encountered in the daily lives of ob-gyn patients.

6 The majority of chemicals in commerce have entered the marketplace without comprehensive and standardized information on their reproductive, developmental, or other chronic toxicities. In 2009, the U.S. Environmental Protection Agency established "Essential Principles for Reform of Chemicals Management Legislation" to help inform legislative efforts now under way to reauthorize and significantly strengthen the effectiveness of chemical regulation.

7 Current recommendations for identifying, managing, and preventing preconception and prenatal exposure to environmental toxicants include (1) routinely taking a patient's environmental exposure history and (2) providing patient education on how to take steps to reduce exposure.

Reproductive Environmental Health

SCOPE

Reproductive environmental health addresses exposures to environmental contaminants (synthetic chemicals and metals), particularly during critical periods of development (such as prior to conception and during pregnancy), and their potential effects on all aspects of future reproductive health throughout the life course, including conception, fertility, pregnancy, child and adolescent development, and adult health (Woodruff, Carlson, et al 2008).

The Environment Is a Key Determinant of Health

- *Infectious disease.* Interventions to improve water and waste sanitation in the beginning of 21st century contributed to great advancements in health.
- *Acute illness.* Environmental pollution in the mid- to latter part of the 20th century caused a wide range of morbidity and mortality (i.e., "killer smogs" in Donora, Pennsylvania,

and London, UK; industrial chemical releases in Bhopal, India; the burning of the Cuyahoga River in Ohio).

- *Cancer.* A substantial body of human evidence has accumulated since the 1950s linking cancer to environmental and occupational exposures (President's Cancer Panel, 2010; Brody, 2007).

UPDATE #1

Trends in reproductive health outcomes document that many indicators of reproductive health are under strain. The full spectrum of female and male reproductive disorders as well as poor birth outcomes and childhood disorders are increasing: 12% of women with diminished fecundity (7.3 million) in the United States (Chandra et al, 2005); persistent decline in age of thelarche and menarche onset from 1940 to 1994 in the United States (Euling et al, 2008); testicular cancer increase in Europe (1% to 6%) since the 1950s with an increase of approximately 60% in the United States since the 1970s (Bray et al, 2006; Shah et al, 2007); declining sperm counts in Scandinavian countries (Jorgensen et al, 2006); declining testosterone levels in multiple countries (Andersson et al, 2005;

Jørgensen et al, 2011; Travison et al, 2007); cryptorchidism and hypospadias becoming more common birth defects (Baskin et al, 2001; Foresta et al, 2008), an increase in premature birth (Davidoff et al, 2006) and gestational diabetes mellitus in the United States (Getahun, 2008); an increase in preeclampsia in Norway (Dahlstrøm et al, 2006); gastroschisis increase in California (Vu et al, 2008); congenital hypothyroidism increase in New York (Harris et al, 2007); an increase in the rate of certain childhood cancers (acute lymphoblastic leukemia, central nervous system tumors, non-Hodgkin's lymphomas) (USEPA, 2006); and an increase in childhood behavioral disorders (Pastor et al, 2008) and autism prevalence (Rice, 2009). These trends in reproductive health have occurred in roughly the same time frame in which human exposure to both natural and synthetic chemicals has dramatically increased. More than 80,000 chemical substances are listed by the Environmental Protection Agency (EPA) as manufactured or processed in the United States, or imported into the country, (USEPA, 2011; USEPA 2007) but this is probably an overestimate of the number of chemicals currently in commercial use. The EPA believes that not all of these chemicals are being produced or imported at any given time, and it is currently reassessing the total (USEPA 2011).

Approximately 700 new industrial chemicals are introduced each year (USEPA 2007). About 3,000–4,000 chemicals are identified as high volume chemicals, meaning that more than a million pounds of each of them are manufactured or imported annually (USEPA 2011). These may pose special risks by virtue of their volume.

Exposure to Environmental Contaminants Is Ubiquitous

- Environmental chemicals with reproductive, fertility or developmental health effects are distributed throughout homes, workplaces, and communities and contaminate food, water, air, and consumer products (Woodruff et al, 2010) (Table 2-1).
- Everyone in the United States has measurable levels of multiple environmental contaminants in their body (see Update #2) (Centers for Disease Control and Prevention, 2009).

UPDATE #2

Women of childbearing age incur ubiquitous contact to toxic environmental contaminants that can result in exposure of the fetus through placental transfer, and maternal exposure can continue in the newborn through breast-feeding (Diamanti-Kandarakis et al, 2009). Consider the following examples. A 2011 study using population-based data from the National Health and Nutrition Examination Survey documented ubiquitous exposure among pregnant women in the U.S. to multiple chemicals. The study found that virtually all pregnant women have measured levels of all of the following chemicals that can be harmful to human reproduction and/or development in their bodies: lead, mercury, toluene, perchlorate, bisphenol A (BPA), and some phthalates, pesticides, perfluorochemicals (PFCs), polychlorinated biphenyls (PCBs) and polybrominated diphenol ethers (PBDEs) (Woodruff, 2011). An analysis of second trimester amniotic fluid samples from 51 women found the presence of at least one environmental contaminant (Foster et al, 2000). Pesticides have been detected in human urine (Riederer et al, 2008), semen (Kumar et al, 2000), breast milk (Jaga et al, 2003; Solomon et al, 2002), ovarian follicular fluid

(Baukloh et al, 1985; Younglai, 2002), cord blood (Tan, 2003, 2009), and amniotic fluid (Bradman, 2003; Foster et al, 2000). Population-based studies conducted by the U.S. Centers for Disease Control and Prevention between 2003 and 2006 document that about 3% of U.S. women of childbearing age have a blood level of mercury that places their child at some increased risk of adverse health effects (U.S. Environmental Protection Agency, 2010).

The Fetus and Developing Human Are Highly Vulnerable to Exposure to Exogenous Chemicals

- Fetal and child vulnerability is due to their high metabolic rate, underdeveloped liver detoxifying mechanisms, immune system, and blood brain barrier (Newbold, 2010); childrens' vulnerability is also due to the fact that they eat and drink more per unit of body weight than adults and their normal behaviors put them into closer contact with the environment (Miller et al, 2002).

KEY EXAMPLES

- Maternal alcohol abuse associated with fetal alcohol syndrome (Calhoun, 2007).
- Tobacco exposure is a risk factor for adverse birth and neurodevelopmental outcomes (Corneilus 2009; Raatikainen 2007).
- In the 1950s, methylmercury exposure in utero resulted in severe neonatal neurologic impairment in children after pregnant mothers consumed high levels of methylmercury-contaminated fish and shellfish from toxic industrial releases in Minamata, Japan; (Rusyniak, 2005) developmental and cognitive effects can occur in children exposed prenatally to mercury at low doses that do not result in effects in the mother; (Grandjean 1997, 1998, 1999) the adverse neurologic effects of methylmercury exposure may be delayed (Commission on Life Sciences, 2010; U.S. Environmental Protection Agency, 2010).
- In the 1960s, thalidomide, a drug given to pregnant women for morning sickness, with no adverse maternal consequences, when taken day 28 to day 42 postconception, resulted in a high rate of congenital limb and gastrointestinal malformations (Taussig, 1962; McBride, 1961, 1977).
- In the 1970s, diethylstilbestrol (DES) prescribed in up to 10 million pregnancies from 1938 to 1971 to prevent miscarriage was found to be a "transplacental carcinogen" causally linked to postpubertal benign and malignant reproductive tract abnormalities in the daughters and sons of DES-exposed mothers; harm was manifested decades after exposure (NIH, 1999; Newbold, 2004). Established health impacts include vaginal clear cell adenocarcinoma, vaginal epithelial changes, reproductive tract abnormalities (e.g., gross anatomic changes of the cervix, T-shaped and hypoplastic uteri), ectopic pregnancies, miscarriages, premature births, and infertility in females exposed in utero, reproductive tract abnormalities (e.g., epididymal cysts, hypoplastic testis, cryptorchidism) in males exposed in utero, and an increased risk for breast cancer in women who took the drug while pregnant (NIH, 1999). Recent cohort studies

TABLE 2-1   **Selected Examples of Contaminants Linked to Reproductive, Fertility, or Developmental Problems**

Types of Contaminants and Examples	Sources and Exposure Circumstances
Metals	
Mercury*	Occurs from energy production emissions and naturally enters the aquatic food chain through a complex system. Primary exposure by consumption of contaminated seafood
Lead*	Occupational exposure occurs in battery manufacturing/recycling, smelting, car repair, welding, soldering, firearm cleaning/shooting, stained glass ornament/jewelry making; nonoccupational exposure occurs in older homes where lead-based paints were used, in or on some toys/children's jewelry, water pipes, imported ceramics/pottery, herbal remedies, traditional cosmetics, hair dyes, contaminated soil, toys, costume jewelry
Organic Compounds	
Solvents	Used for cleaning, degreasing, embalming, refinishing and paint systems in a wide range of industries; found in automotive products, degreasers, thinners, preservers, varnish and spot removers, pesticides (inert component), and nail polish
Ethylene oxide	Occupational exposure to workers sterilizing medical supplies or engaged in manufacturing
Pentachlorophenol	Wood preservative for utility poles, railroad ties, wharf pilings; formerly a multiuse pesticide. Found in soil, water, food, breast milk
Bisphenol-A (BPA)	Chemical intermediate for polycarbonate plastic and resins. Found in consumer products and packaging. Exposure through inhalation, ingestion, and dermal absorption
Polychlorinated biphenyl (PCB)	Used as industrial insulators and lubricants; banned in the 1970s, but persistent in the aquatic and terrestrial food chains resulting in exposure by ingestion
Dioxins*	Dioxins and furans are multiple toxic chemicals formed by trash and waste incineration involving chlorine and categorized as a persistent organic pollutants (POPs), pervasive chemicals that bioconcentrate as they move up the food chain; found in dairy products, meat, fish, and shellfish
Perfluorooctane sulfonate (PFOS)*	Perfluorinated compound used in consumer products as stain and water repellents; persists in the environment; occupational exposure to workers and general population exposure by inhalation, ingestion, and dermal contact
Polybrominated diphenyl ethers (PBDEs)	Flame retardants that persist and bioaccumulate in the environment; found in furniture, textiles, carpeting, electronics, and plastics that are mixed into, but not bound to, foam or plastic
Di-(2 ethyl hexyl) phthalate (DEHP) diethylphthalate (DEP), di-n-butyl phthalate (DBP)	Synthetically derived, phthalates are used in a variety of consumer goods such medical devices, cleaning and building materials, personal care products, cosmetics, pharmaceuticals, food processing, and toys
	Exposure occurs through ingestion, inhalation, and dermal absorption
Pesticides	Applied in large quantities in agricultural community and household settings; in 2001, more than 1.2 billion pounds of pesticide active ingredients were used in the United States; pesticide can be ingested, inhaled, and absorbed by the skin the pathways of pesticide exposure include food, water, air, dust, and soil
Chlorpyrifos	Organophosphate pesticide used in agricultural production and for home pest control (home uses are now restricted)
Dichlorodiphenyltrichloroethane (DDT)*	Organochlorine insecticide, banned in the United States in the 1970s, is still used for malaria control overseas
	Present in the food chain
Air Contaminants	
Environmental tobacco smoke (ETS)	Burning of tobacco products, exposure by inhalation from active or passive smoking
Particulate matter (PM), ozone, lead	Sources include combustion of wood and fossil fuels, and industrial production
	Exposure by inhalation
Glycol ethers	Used in enamels, paints, varnishes, stains, electronics, cosmetics; occupational and general population exposure by inhalation, ingestion, and dermal contact

Adapted from Fox MA, Aoki Y: Environmental contaminants and exposure. In Woodruff TJ, Janssen SJ, Guillette LJ Jr, Giudice LC: *Environmental impacts on reproductive health and fertility.* Cambridge, UK, 2010, Cambridge University Press, pp 8-22.
From ATSDR, 2002; ATSDR, 2004; Committee on the Health Risks of Phthalates, 2010; Hanke, 2004; Hauser, Sokol, 2008; Kiely, 2009; Meeker, 2010; National Library of Medicine, 2010; USEPA, 2006; World Health Organization, 2010; Woodruff, 2008.
*Chemical is persistent and/or bioaccumulative.

CHILD DEVELOPMENT AND
WINDOWS OF SUSCEPTIBILITY

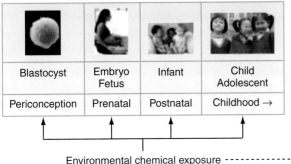

Blastocyst	Embryo Fetus	Infant	Child Adolescent
Periconception	Prenatal	Postnatal	Childhood →

Environmental chemical exposure - - - - - - - - - →
Immediate and long term
consequences

Figure 2-1. Critical and sensitive windows of susceptibility. A *critical window of susceptibility* is a unique time period during development when exposures to environmental contaminants can disrupt or interfere with the physiology of a cell, tissue, or organ (Grandjean, Bellinger, Bergman et al, 2008). Exposures during this window may result in adverse, permanent effects that can have lifelong and even intergenerational impacts on health. In contrast, during a *sensitive window of susceptibility* exposures may still affect development or result in eventual adult disease, but with reduced magnitude compared with the effect of exposure during other time periods (Morford, Henck, Breslin et al, 2004). The periconception window is defined as the inclusive span preceding, including, and immediately after conception (Louis, Cooney, Lynch et al, 2008). Given that development continues after birth, critical and sensitive windows are seen during periconception, pregnancy, infancy, childhood, puberty, pregnancy, and lactation. (Modified from Louis, Cooney, Lynch et al: Periconception window: advising the pregnancy-planning couple, *Fertil Steril* 89[2, Suppl 1]:e119-e121, 2008).

indicate that women who were exposed to DES prenatally have an increased risk of breast cancer after age 40 (Palmer, 2006). Animal data predict intergenerational impacts (i.e., among granddaughters of DES-exposed women) to date supported by limited human data (Newbold, 2010).

UPDATE #3

The fetus and developing human are highly vulnerable to exposure to environmental contaminants, and adverse health impacts can manifest across the life span of individuals and generations (Figure 2-1). It has been traditionally assumed that environmental exposures experienced by an average person living in the United States would be below levels of reproductive harm. However, a rapidly expanding body of scientific evidence has upended this assumption about the benign nature of "low-level" environmental exposures (Committee on the Health Risks of Phthalates, 2009). In general, the human reproductive system is vulnerable to biologic perturbations, particularly when these changes occur during critical windows of development. Even subtle perturbations caused by chemical exposures may lead to important functional deficits and increased risks of disease and disability in infants, children, and across the span of human life (Crain, Janssen, Edwards et al, 2008; Grandjean, Bellinger, Bergman et al, 2008; Woodruff, Carlson, Schwartz et al, 2008); the strength of the evidence is sufficiently high that leading scientists, reproductive health providers, and other health care practitioners have called for timely action to prevent harm (Grandjean et al, 2008; Woodruff, Carlson, Swartz et al, 2008; Diamanti-Kandarakis et al, 2009; President's Cancer Panel, 2010).

Mechanisms of Action

- *The Developmental Basis of Adult Disease/Dysfunction* describes links between the in utero environment, the external environment, an individual's genes, and the propensity to develop disease or dysfunction later in life (Diamanti-Kandarakis et al, 2009).
  - Perinatal influences on chronic adult disease were first described in the field of nutrition (Barker, 1995) with the evidence base independently evolving in the field of developmental toxicology (Table 2-2) (Newbold, 2010).
  - It is now apparent from animal studies that the in utero and neonatal developmental periods constitute "a critical window" for both nutrition and for exposure to environmental chemicals (Heindel et al, 2009).
  - This convergence underlies the hypothesis that in addition to nutritional impacts on fetal growth, environmental endocrine disrupting chemicals can act as "obesogens" that can permanently derange developing regulatory systems required for body weight homeostasis (Heindel et al, 2009).
  - DES is the well-documented example of the developmental origins of the disease/dysfunction paradigm (Newbold et al, 2010).
- *The "epigenetic" mechanism* is one type of mechanism that influences developmental programming (i.e., mechanisms that alter gene activity without mutating the DNA sequence and lead to modifications that can be transmitted to daughter cells) (see Table 2-2) (Weinhold, 2006). The most common epigenomic alterations are methylation of the DNA at cytosine with subsequent gene silencing or modification of the DNA histone support, which affects chromatin folding and attachment (Weinhold, 2006).
- *"Endocrine disruption"* is a related mechanism of action of environmental contaminants. Endocrine disrupting compounds (EDCs) act by perturbing the synthesis, secretion, transport, binding, action, or elimination of natural hormones in the body that are responsible for the maintenance of homeostasis, reproduction, development, and behavior (Woodruff and Giudice, 2010).
  - EDCs are associated with wide-ranging effects on male and female reproduction, breast development and cancer, prostate cancer, neuroendocrinology, thyroid, metabolism and obesity, and cardiovascular endocrinology (Diamanti-Kandarakis et al, 2009).
  - EDCs act through traditional nuclear hormone receptor pathways (estrogen, progesterone, androgen, thyroid, and retinoid) and more diverse avenues such as non-nuclear, neurotransmitter, or orphan receptors and enzymatic pathway interference (Diamanti-Kandarakis et al, 2009).
  - EDCs can have multiple hormonal effects; for example, dichlorodiphenyltrichloroethane (DDT) is an estrogen disruptor, whereas its metabolite, dichloro diphenyldichloroethylene (DDE) is an androgen antagonist (Diamanti-Kandarakis et al, 2009). BPA perturbs both estrogen and thyroid hormones (Vandenberg et al, 2009).
  - The molecular structures of EDCs can generally contain a central ring that mimics steroid hormones and often has added halogen groups (chlorine, bromine, fluorine) (Diamanti-Kandarakis et al, 2009), which confer various material properties such as molecular stability.

TABLE 2-2   Features of "Developmental Origins of Disease and Dysfunction" Paradigm Common to Both Nutritional and Environmental Exposure Studies

- Time-specific (vulnerable window) and tissue-specific effects may occur with both nutritional and environmental chemical exposures.
- The initiating in utero environmental insult (nutritional or environmental chemical) may act alone or in concert with other environmental stressors. That is, there could be an in utero exposure that would lead by itself to pathophysiology later in life, or there could be in utero exposure combined with a neonatal exposure (same or different environmental stressor[s] or adult exposure that would trigger or exacerbate the pathophysiology).
- The pathophysiology may manifest as the occurrence of a disease that otherwise would not have happened, an increase in risk for a disease that would normally be of lower prevalence, or either an earlier onset of a disease that would normally have occurred or an exacerbation of the disease.
- The pathophysiology may have a variable latent period from onset in the neonatal period, to early childhood, to puberty, to early adulthood, to late adulthood depending on the environmental stressor, time of exposure, and tissue/organ affected.
- Either altered nutrition or exposure to environmental chemicals can lead to aberrant developmental programming that permanently alters gland, organ, or system potential. These states of altered potential or compromised function (regardless of the stressor—nutritional or chemical exposure) are likely to result from epigenetic changes (e.g., altered gene expression resulting from the effects on imprinting) and the underlying methylation-related protein-DNA relationships associated with chromatin remodeling. The result is an individual that is sensitized such that it will be more susceptible to certain diseases later in life.
- The effect of either developmental nutrition or environmental chemical exposures can be transgenerational, affecting future generations.
- Although the focus of nutritional changes during development has been on low birth weight, effects of in utero exposure to toxic environmental chemicals or nutritional changes may both occur in the absence of reduced birth weight. The lack of a specific easily measurable biomarker for these effects that is similar to birth weight makes it more difficult to assess developmental effects. Thus, for both exposures, newer and more sensitive biomarkers of exposure are needed.
- Extrapolation of risk from both nutritional studies and environmental exposures may be difficult because effects may not follow a monotonic dose-response relationship. Nutritional effects that result in low birth weight are different from those that result in high birth weight. Similarly, low dose effects of environmental chemicals may not be the same as the effects that occur at higher doses. Also, the environmental chemical or nutritional effects may have an entirely different effect on the embryo, fetus, or perinatal organism, compared to the adult.
- Exposure of one individual to an environmental stressor (environmental chemical or nutritional or combinations) may have little effect, whereas another individual will develop overt disease or dysfunctions because of differences in genetic background including genetic polymorphisms.
- The toxicant (or nutritional)-induced pathogenic responses are most likely the result of altered gene expression or altered protein regulation associated with altered cell production and differentiation that are involved in the interactions between cell types and the establishment of cell lineages. These changes may lead to abnormal morphologic or functional characteristics of the tissues, organs, and systems. These alterations may be due, at least in part, to altered epigenetics. One example of epigenetic chromatin remodeling is changes in the underlining methylation-related protein-DNA relationships. Effects may occur in a time-specific (i.e., vulnerable window) or tissue-specific manner, and the changes may not be reversible. The result is an organism that is sensitized such that it will be more susceptible to specific diseases later in life.

Adapted from Newbold RR, Heindal JJ: Developmental exposures and implications for disease. In Woodruff TJ, Janssen SJ, Guillette LJ Jr, Giudice LC: *Environmental impacts on reproductive health and fertility.* Cambridge, UK, 2010, Cambridge University Press, pp 92-102.

- EDCs may exert dose-response curves that are not linear (Diamanti-Kandarakis et al, 2009), where low-dose exposure during critical and sensitive periods of development may be more potent than higher-dose exposures.
- *Mutagenic mechanisms.* DNA damage can adversely affect reproduction and development. A well-documented example is radiation-induced cancer resulting from exposure to ionizing radiation.
  - It is generally believed that complex forms of DNA double-strand breaks are the most biologically important type of lesions induced by ionizing radiation, and these complex forms are likely responsible for subsequent molecular and cellular effects (Committee to Assess Health Risks from Exposure to Low Levels of Ionizing Radiation, 2006).
  - There is growing concern about the sharp rise in the use of computed tomography scans in medicine as a result of the non-negligible radiation exposures involved, particularly for pediatric patients (Chodick, 2009).

UPDATE #4

Hormone receptor types and functions, including those involved in metabolism, obesity, and brain signaling, can be targets of endocrine disrupting chemicals that all women of childbearing age encounter in their daily lives (Diamanti-Kandarakis et al, 2009).

Reproductive and Developmental Health Impacts of Environmental Exposures

- There are three authoritative U.S. lists/sources of information about chemicals with reproductive and developmental toxicity: the U.S. National Toxicology Program, Center for Evaluation of Risks to Human Reproduction (NTP/CERHR) (CERHR, 2010), the U.S. Environmental Protection Agency (U.S. EPA) (EPA, 2011), and the California Environmental Protection Agency (Cal-EPA) (CalEPA, 2010), Chemicals

Known By the State of California to Cause Cancer or Reproductive Toxicity.

KEY EXAMPLES

- *Pesticides.* Some pesticide exposures can interfere with all developmental stages of reproductive function in adult females (Mendola et al, 2008) and are associated with adverse outcomes that occur throughout the life course of males and females, including sterility in males, spontaneous abortion, diminished fetal growth and survival, and childhood and adult cancer (Infante-Rivard et al, 2007; Whorton et al, 1977, 1988; Wigle et al, 2008, 2009).

- *Solvents.* Occupational solvent exposure has been associated with a low sperm count (Cherry et al, 2001) and reduced overall semen quality (Tielemans et al, 1999), impaired fertility in women (Sallmén et al, 1995; Wennborg et al, 2001), and increased risk of spontaneous abortion with maternal occupational exposure to ethylene glycol (Wigle et al, 2008). Prenatal solvent exposure is associated with birth defects (Stillerman et al, 2008).

- *Lead.* Lead exposure has been associated with adverse effects on male reproductive function (Hauser et al, 2008), pubertal delay in females (Mendola et al, 2008), increased risk of spontaneous abortion, hypertension during pregnancy, impaired offspring neurodevelopment, and reduced fetal growth (Bellinger, 2005).

- *Bis-phenol A (BPA).* There is significant animal evidence that exposure during critical windows of development can result in permanent alterations to the reproductive system in a number of ways, thus increasing the risk of future health problems, including rodent hematopoietic and testicular cancers as well as preneoplastic lesions of the breast and prostate (Keri, et al, 2007). BPA alters the "epigenetic programming" of genes in experimental animals and wildlife. Specifically, prenatal or neonatal exposure to low doses of BPA results in organizational changes in the prostate, breast, testis, mammary glands, body size, brain structure and chemistry, and behavior of laboratory animals; there is also experimental animal evidence that adult exposure to BPA results in substantial neurobehavioral effects and reproductive effects in both males and females. A central concern is that these adverse effects are occurring in animals within the range of exposure to BPA typical of the U.S. population (vom Saal, et al 2007).

- *Dioxin.* The developing individual is extensively sensitive to exposure to dioxin, with effects ranging from altered thyroid and immune status; altered neurobehavior at the level of hearing, psychomotor function, and gender-related behaviors; altered cognition, dentition, and development of reproductive organs; and delays in breast development, in addition to altered sex ratios among the exposed offspring (White et al, 2009; WHO, 2010). Developmental exposures to dioxin are of great concern, in part because effects documented in human studies occur at the high end of the exposures experienced by the general population (White et al, 2009). Dioxin exposures have been linked to intergenerational health impacts (Mocarelli, 2008; White et al, 2009).

- *Phthalates.* By inhibition of 5α-reductase (Greathouse, 2010), phthalates perturb androgen mechanisms in rodents creating a "phthalate syndrome" of numerous male reproductive abnormalities, including infertility, decreased sperm count, shortened anogenital distance (AGD), hypospadias, cryptorchidism, and other malformations (Swan, 2008; Committee on the Health Risks of Phthalates, 2010). According to the National Academy of Sciences, phthalate syndrome has many similarities to the hypothesized testicular dysgenesis syndrome (poor semen quality, testicular cancer, cryptorchidism, and hypospadias [Skakkebak et al, 2001]) in humans (Committee on the Health Risks of Phthalates, 2010). Additionally, preconception phthalate exposure is associated with cognitive and behavioral disorders in children (Engel et al, 2008), altered play behavior in boys (Swan, 2010), and diminished female neonatal motor skills (Engel et al, 2009).

- *Polychlorinated biphenyls (PCBs).* Mechanisms of perturbed thyroid functioning and signaling occur through transport disruption, enhanced hepatic catabolism, inhibition of thyroid hormone, and direct or indirect agonist or antagonist action on the thyroid receptor (Woodruff, Zeise, Axelrad et al, 2008). A statistically significant inverse relationship between levels of thyroid hormones and PCBs and organochlorine pesticides in pregnant women was found (Chevrier, et al 2008), suggesting that current exposure levels to PCBs and chlorinated pesticides can affect thyroid function during pregnancy. These findings have important implications in that maternal T4 is the only source of thyroid hormone during the first trimester to the developing brain, and thus thyroid hormones of maternal origin play an essential role in fetal neurodevelopment (Morreale de Escobar, 2000). A relative state of hypothyroidism in the developing fetus may contribute to the neurotoxic effects of PCBs (Diamanti-Kandarakis et al, 2009). PCB androgen disruption is a risk factor for changes in sperm morphology, count, penetration efficacy, and motility (Guo, et al 2000; Hauser, 2006; Hsu et al, 2003).

- *Polybrominated diphenyl ethers (PBDEs).* There is an association between levels of PBDEs and thyroid, reproductive, and behavioral effects in animals (Agency for Toxic Substances and Disease Registry [ATSDR], 2004). Several recent studies document body burden and adverse health outcomes; several PBDE congeners were associated with lower scores on tests of mental and physical development at 12 to 48 and 72 months (Herbstman, 2010) and delay in time to pregnancy (Harley, 2010).

UPDATE #5

A wide range of adverse reproductive and developmental health outcomes are linked to environmental contaminants encountered in the daily lives of ob-gyn patients. A recent assessment of the evidence by Slama et al. (2010) based on human epidemiologic evidence for fetal loss, fetal growth, gestational length, complications of pregnancy, secondary sex ration, and congenital malformations found sufficient evidence for one or more of these adverse outcomes for atmospheric pollution, passive smoking, lead, mercury, perfluorooctane sulfonate (PFOS) and perfluorooctanoate (PFOA), glycol ethers, aromatic solvents, and low-dose ionizing radiation (Table 2-3).

TABLE 2-3 Overview of Considered Reproductive Outcomes and Level of Evidence for a Possible Sensitivity to Specific Environmental Pollutants in Humans

Pollutant	Fetal Loss Early (<20 weeks)	Late	Fetal Growth	Gestational Length	Complications of Pregnancy	Secondary Sex Ratio	Congenital Malformations
Atmospheric pollutants		Limited	Limited/ sufficient	Limited/ sufficient	Limited (preeclampsia)	Inadequate	Limited (cardiac malformations)
Passive smoking (ETS)	Limited	Limited	Sufficient	Sufficient	Inadequate	Inadequate	Limited/ sufficient
Water pollutants							
Chlorination by-products	Inadequate	Inadequate	Limited/ sufficient	Inadequate	Inadequate	Inadequate	Limited
Nitrates	Inadequate		Inadequate	Inadequate			Inadequate
Other Chemical Compounds							
Metals							
Lead	Sufficient Limited (pat.)		Limited/ sufficient Limited (pat.)	Limited/ sufficient Limited (pat.)	Sufficient/ limited (gestational hypertension)	Limited/ Sufficient (pat.)	Inadequate
Mercury	Limited (pat.)		Inadequate	Limited			Sufficient
Cadmium	Limited		Inadequate	Inadequate			
Arsenic							Limited
PCB, PCDD, PCDF			Limited (PCB)	Inadequate (PCB)		Limited (pat. TCDD)	Limited (PCBs)
Flame Retardants PBDE							
Perflourinated chemicals (PFOS, PFOA)			Limited/ sufficient	Inadequate			
Organochlorine pesticides							
DDT, DDE	Limited	Inadequate (pat.)	Limited	Limited		Inadequate (pat.)	Limited
Other organochlorines		Inadequate	Inadequate	Limited			Limited
Organophosphate pesticides		Inadequate	Limited	Limited			
Phthalates				Inadequate			Inadequate
Solvents							
Glycolethers	Sufficient						Limited
Chlorinated	Limited/ sufficient						Limited
Aromatic	Limited (pat.)		Inadequate	Limited/ sufficient			
Radiations (low doses)							
Ionizing		Limited (pat.)	Limited/ sufficient		Inadequate	Limited	Limited/ sufficient
Non-ionizing	Inadequate						

The level of evidence has been classified as *sufficient* (several good-quality studies by different groups, or an expert panel already considered the level of proof as sufficient), *limited* (evidence is suggestive of an association, e.g. based on at least one good quality study, but remains limited), or *inadequate* (available studies are of sufficient quality, consistency or statistical power to permit a conclusion regarding the presence or absence of an association), as a modification of what has been suggested elsewhere. *pat* indicates that the level of evidence relates to a possible effect of paternal exposures.

Adapted from Slama, R., Cordier, S: Environmental contaminants and impacts on healthy and successful pregnancies. In Woodruff TJ, Janssen SJ, Guillette LJ Jr, Giudice LC: *Environmental impacts on reproductive health and fertility,* Cambridge, UK, 2010, Cambridge University Press, pp 125-144.

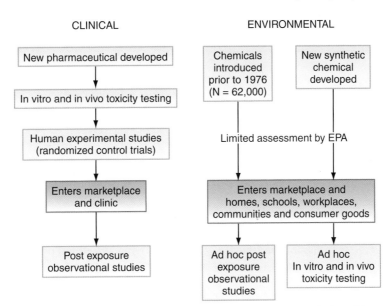

Figure 2-2. **Comparison of streams of evidence in clinical and environmental health sciences.** (Adapted from Woodruff TJ, Sutton P; Navigation Guide Work Group. An evidence-based medicine methodology to bridge the gap between clinical and environmental health sciences. *Health Aff (Millwood)*. 2011 May;30(5):931-7.

Identification of Chemicals with Reproductive and Developmental Toxicity

- There are critical differences between clinical and environmental health sciences in the types of evidence generally available and how decisions to expose populations and patients are made.
- Clinicians cannot assume as they do with pharmaceuticals that adequate in vitro and in vivo testing of environmental contaminants has been undertaken and considered by regulatory agencies before widespread human exposure occurs (Figure 2-2). Patient exposure to most environmental contaminants occurs in the absence of information about reproductive and developmental toxicity.
- Human exposure to pharmaceuticals does not occur in the absence of some potential benefit greater than the known risks. The gold standard for informing clinical risk-benefit decisions about medical interventions is a well-conducted randomized controlled trial. There is no comprehensive comparable weighing of health benefits and risks in the environmental arena.
- The benefits of environmental chemicals are largely unrelated to patient health, and exposures are generally unintentional and highly variable. Randomized controlled trials on environmental contaminants are virtually precluded from the evidence stream in environmental health science because of ethical considerations.
- The reliability of experimental animal data for reproductive and developmental health has been well established. One of the earliest and most thorough sources of evidence is a technical report from 1984 for the National Center for Toxicological Research (Kimmel et al, 1984). This study, along with others, concluded there is concordance of developmental and reproductive effects and that humans are as sensitive as or more sensitive than the most sensitive animal species (National Research Council, 2000).

- Human epidemiologic studies of environmental chemicals provide the most direct evidence of the relationship between exposure and increase risk of adverse health outcomes, and are often the basis of regulatory and policy decision making. However, human epidemiologic studies require that we wait for people to develop clearly identified diseases from exposure, and thus represent a failure of prevention.

UPDATE #6

The majority of chemicals in commerce have entered the marketplace without comprehensive and standardized information on their reproductive, developmental or other chronic toxicities (Wilson et al, 2006). The U.S. Environmental Protection Agency established "Essential Principles for Reform of Chemicals Management Legislation" to help inform legislative efforts now underway to reauthorize and significantly strengthen the effectiveness of chemical regulation (U.S. Environmental Protection Agency, 2010).

Clinical Management

- Identifying patients with hazardous exposures, advising all patients on prevention measures, and referring patients when necessary are all essential parts of clinical management.
- Patient risk is a function of the toxicity of the compound and exposure. Routes of exposure are dermal, ingestion, and/or inhalation. Key determinants of exposure are: concentration, frequency and duration, and patient vulnerability, including any underlying health conditions (Fox et al, 2010).
- Women of reproductive age with occupational exposures to substances with reproductive and developmental toxicity are at high risk and susceptible to adverse reproductive outcomes (Figa-Talamanca, 2006).

TABLE 2-4   Occupational and Environmental Exposure History

Work/Hobbies

What is your occupation? What are your hobbies?

What are the occupations and hobbies of other members of your household?

Are you exposed to any of the following substances at work, home, or school: fumes, vapors, dusts, pesticides, painting materials, lead, mercury or other metals?

Have you ever felt sick after contact with a chemical?

Do you wear personal protective equipment at work or while doing hobbies?

Do your symptoms get better away from work/hobbies?

Residence

Was your home built before 1978? If so, has it been tested for lead paint?

If your home has lead paint, is it flaking? Have you done any recent remodeling?

Where does your drinking water come from?

Have you had your water tested for lead?

If you have a private well, has the water been tested?

Do you know of any industrial emissions near your house (hazardous waste sites, dry cleaners, auto repair shops)?

Do you live in an agricultural area?

Do you use pesticides? In your home? Garden? On pets?

Do you use any traditional medications or remedies?*

Do you ever smell chemical odors while you are at home?

Do your symptoms get better away from home?

Diet

What kind of fish do you eat? How often do you eat fish?

Do you or anyone in your home fish in local waters?

Do you eat a lot of foods high in animal fats (fast food, ice cream, cheese, whole milk, fatty meats)?

Do you grow your own vegetables? Has the soil been tested?

Do you take any dietary supplements?*

---

*May involve exposure to heavy metals such as mercury or lead.
Adapted from Solomon GM, Janssen SJ: (2010). Communicating with patients and the public about environmental exposures and reproductive risk. In Woodruff TJ, Janssen SJ, Guillette LJ Jr, Giudice LC: *Environmental impacts on reproductive health and fertility*, Cambridge, UK, 2010, Cambridge University Press, pp 214-226.

• Socioeconomic and racial disparities exist with regard to environmental contaminant exposures; understanding the environment of patient population can help target high risk exposures (Morello-Froschm et al 2006).

UPDATE #7

Current recommendations for identifying, managing, and preventing preconception and prenatal exposure to environmental toxicants: (1) routinely take a patient's environmental exposure history (Table 2-4) (Solomon, 2010) and (2) provide patient education on how to take steps to reduce exposure (Program on Reproductive Health and the Environment from Advancing Science to Ensure Prevention [FASTEP], 2011). A detailed list of recommendations can be found at http://www.prhe.ucsf.edu/prhe/tmlinks.html.

SUGGESTED READINGS

Barker DJP: Fetal origins of coronary heart disease, *BMJ* 311(6998):171–174, 1995.

Centers for Disease Control and Prevention: *Fourth national report on human exposure to environmental chemicals 2009*, Atlanta, GA, 2009, Centers for Disease Control and Prevention.

Committee on the Health Risks of Phthalates: *Phthalates and cumulative risk assessment* (website). www.nap.edu/catalog.php?record_id=12528. Accessed April 20, 2010.

Committee to Assess Health Risks from Exposure to Low Levels of Ionizing Radiation: National Research Council: *Health risks from exposure to low levels of ionizing radiation: BEIR VII Phase 2*, Washington, DC, 2006, National Academies Press.

Crain DA, Janssen SJ, Edwards TM, et al: Female reproductive disorders: the roles of endocrine-disrupting compounds and developmental timing, *Fertil Steril* 90(4):911–940, 2008.

Davidoff MJ, Dias T, Damus K, et al: Changes in the gestational age distribution among U.S. singleton births: impact on rates of late preterm birth, 1992 to 2002, *Semin Perinatol* 30(1):8–15, 2006.

Diamanti-Kandarakis E, Bourguignon J-P, Giudice LC, et al: Endocrine-disrupting chemicals: an Endocrine Society scientific statement, *Endocr Rev* 30(4):293–342, 2009.

European Environment Agency: *Late lessons from early warnings: the precautionary principle 1896–2000* (website). www.eea.europa.eu/publications/environmental_issue_report_2001_22/issue-22-part-00.pdf. Accessed May 26, 2011.

Figa-Talamanca I: Occupational risk factors and reproductive health of women, *Occup Med (Lond)* 56(8):521–531, 2006.

Fox MA, Aoki Y: Environmental contaminants and exposure. In Woodruff TJ, Janssen SJ, Guillette LJ Jr, Giudice LC, editors: *Environmental impacts on reproductive health and fertility*, Cambridge, 2010, Cambridge University Press, pp 8–22.

Gibb S: Toxicity testing in the 21st century: a vision and strategy, *Reprod Toxicol* 25(1):136–138, Jan 2008.

Grandjean P, Bellinger D, Bergman A, et al: The faroes statement: human health effects of developmental exposure to chemicals in our environment, *Basic Clin Pharmacol Toxicol* 102(2):73–75, 2008.

Greathouse KL, Walker CL: Mechanisms of endocrine disruption. In Woodruff TJ, Janssen SJ, Guillette LJ Jr, Giudice LC, editors: *Environmental impacts on reproductive health and fertility*, Cambridge, 2010, Cambridge University Press, pp 72–91.

Heindel JJ, vom Saal FS: Role of nutrition and environmental endocrine disrupting chemicals during the perinatal period on the aetiology of obesity, *Mol Cell Endocrinol* 304(1-2):90–96, 2009.

Infante-Rivard C, Weichenthal S: Pesticides and childhood cancer: an update of Zahm and Ward's 1998 review, *J Toxicol Environ Health B Crit Rev* 10(1-2):81–99, 2007.

Kimmel CA, Holson JF, Hogue CJ, Carlo G: *Reliability of experimental studies for predicting hazards to human development*, Jefferson, AR, 1984, National Center for Toxicological Research, NCTR Technical Report for Experiment No. 6015.

Louis GMB, Cooney MA, Lynch CD, Handal A: Periconception window: advising the pregnancy-planning couple, *Fertil Steril* 89(2 Suppl 1):e119–e121, 2008.

Meeker JD, Hauser R: Environmental contaminants and reproductive and fertility effects in the male: adult exposure. In Woodruff TJ, Janssen SJ, Guillette LJ Jr, Giudice LC, editors: *Environmental impacts on reproductive health and fertility*, Cambridge, 2010, Cambridge University Press, pp 154–160.

Mendola P, Messer LC, Rappazzo K: Science linking environmental contaminant exposures with fertility and reproductive health impacts in the adult female, *Fertil Steril* 89(2 Suppl):e81–e94, Feb 2008.

Miller MD, Marty MA, Arcus A, et al: Differences between children and adults: implications for risk assessment at California EPA, *Int Journal Toxicol* 21(5):403–418, 2002.

Morello-Frosch R, Lopez R: The riskscape and the color line: examining the role of segregation in environmental health disparities, *Environ Res* 102(2):181–196, 2006.

National Research Council: *Scientific frontiers in developmental toxicology and risk assessment*, Washington, DC, 2000, National Academies Press.

Newbold RR, Heindal JJ: Developmental exposures and implications for disease. In Woodruff TJ, Janssen SJ, Guillette LJ Jr, Giudice LC, editors: *Environmental impacts on reproductive health and fertility*, Cambridge, 2010, Cambridge University Press, pp 92–102.

President's Cancer Panel: *Reducing environmental cancer risk: what we can do now*, Bethesda, MD, 2010, Department of Health and Human Services, National Institutes of Health, National Cancer Institute.

Program on Reproductive Health and the Environment from Advancing Science to Ensure Prevention (FASTEP): *Toxic Matters* (website). prhe.ucsf.edu/prhe/pdfs/ToxicMatters.pdf. Accessed May 26, 2011.

Slama R, Cordier S: Environmental contaminants and impacts on healthy and successful pregnancies. In Woodruff TJ, Janssen JS, Guillette LJ Jr, Giudice LC, editors: *Environmental impacts on reproductive health and fertility*, Cambridge, 2010, Cambridge University Press, pp 125–144.

Solomon GM, Janssen SJ: Communicating with patients and the public about environmental exposures and reproductive risk. In Woodruff TJ, Janssen SJ, Guillette LJ Jr, Giudice LC, editors: *Environmental impacts on reproductive health and fertility*, Cambridge, 2010, Cambridge University Press, pp 214–226.

Stillerman KP, Mattison DR, Giudice LC, Woodruff TJ: Environmental exposures and adverse pregnancy outcomes: a review of the science, *Reprod Sci* 15(7):631–650, 2008.

Sutton P, Giudice LC, Woodruff TJ: Reproductive environmental health, *Curr Opin Obstet Gynecol* 22(6):517–524, Dec 2010.

Sutton P, Wallinga D, Perron J, Gottlieb M, Sayre L, Woodruff T: Reproductive health and the industrialized food system: a point of intervention for health policy, *Health Aff (Millwood)* 30(5):888–897, 2011 May.

U.S. Environmental Protection Agency: *America's Children and the Environment (ACE): Measure D6: Types of childhood cancer* (website), http://www.epa.gov/ace/child_illness/d6-sources.html. Accessed November 15, 2011.

U.S. Environmental Protection Agency: *Essential principles for reform of chemicals management legislation* (website), www.epa.gov/oppt/existingchemicals/pubs/principles.html. Accessed June 14, 2010.

Vandenberg LN, Maffini MV, Sonnenschein C, et al: Bisphenol-A and the great divide: a review of controversies in the field of endocrine disruption, *Endocr Rev* 30(1):75–95, 2009.

vom Saal FS, Akingbemi BT, Belcher SM, et al: Chapel Hill bisphenol A expert panel consensus statement: integration of mechanisms, effects in animals and potential to impact human health at current levels of exposure, *Reprod Toxicol* 24(2):131–138, 2007.

Weinhold B: Epigenetics: the science of change, *Environ Health Perspect* 114(3):A160–A167, 2006.

Whorton D, Foliart D: DBCP: eleven years later, *Reprod Toxicol* 2(3-4):155–161, 1988.

Whorton D, Krauss R, Marshall S, Milby T: Infertility in male pesticide workers, *Lancet* 310(8051):1259–1261, 1977.

Wigle DT, Arbuckle TE, Turner MC, et al: Epidemiologic evidence of relationships between reproductive and child health outcomes and environmental chemical contaminants, *J Toxicol Environ Health B Crit Rev* 11(5-6):373–517, 2008.

Wigle DT, Turner MC, Krewski D: A systematic review and meta-analysis of childhood leukemia and parental occupational pesticide exposure, *Environ Health Perspect* 117(10):1505–1513, 2009.

Woodruff TJ, Carlson A, Schwartz JM, Giudice LC: Proceedings of the summit on environmental challenges to reproductive health and fertility: executive summary, *Fertil Steril* 89(2 Suppl):e1–e20, 2008.

Woodruff TJ, Giudice LC: Introduction. In Woodruff TJ, Janssen SJ, Guillette LJ Jr, Giudice LC, editors: *Environmental impacts on reproductive health and fertility*, Cambridge, 2010, Cambridge University Press, pp 1–7.

Woodruff TJ, Zeise L, Axelrad DA, Guyton KZ, et al: Meeting report: moving upstream—evaluating adverse upstream end points for improved risk assessment and decision-making, *Environ Health Perspect* 116(11):1568–1575, 2008.

Woodruff TJ, Burke TA, Zeise L: The need for better public health decisions on chemicals released into our environment, *Health Aff (Millwood)* 30(5):957–967, 2011 May. Review.

Woodruff TJ, Sutton P: Navigation Guide Work Group. An evidence-based medicine methodology to bridge the gap between clinical and environmental health sciences, *Health Aff (Millwood)* 30(5):931–937, 2011 May.

Woodruff TJ, Zota AR, Schwartz JM: Environmental chemicals in pregnant women in the United States: NHANES 2003-2004, *Environ Health Perspect* 119(6):878–885, 2011 Jun. Epub 2011 Jan 10.

References

Please go to expertconsult.com to view references.

Chapter 3

Pediatric and Adolescent Gynecology

ERICA BOIMAN JOHNSTONE

KEY UPDATES

1 Although timing of onset of puberty did not change significantly in the United States between the late 1960s and the early 1990s, the age of menarche decreased by 0.46 years in black girls, to 12.06, and by 0.34 years in white girls, to 12.55 years.

2 Increased linear growth can be attained in girls with Turner's syndrome on growth hormone therapy when low-dose estradiol is initiated and slowly increased, rather than starting with full maintenance dose.

3 Mutations in the GPR54 gene, a g-protein coupled receptor bound by the protein kisspeptin, are a novel cause of hypogonadotropic hypogonadism.

4 Continuous oral contraceptives are more effective than cyclic regimens in ameliorating pain due to endometriosis in adolescents, with resolution in 75% to 100%.

5 Use of the contraceptive patch results in increased ethinyl estradiol exposure compared with a 30-mcg ethinyl estradiol oral contraceptive or the vaginal contraceptive ring.

6 Use of depot medroxyprogesterone acetate for 3 years in women ages 16 to 24 is associated with significant bone loss, which is reversible upon discontinuation.

7 The quadrivalent human papilloma virus (HPV) vaccine, introduced in 2006, is recommended for girls beginning at age 11 or 12 and for all adolescent girls who have not yet received it.

8 Cervical cancer is rare among adolescents and young women; therefore, conservative therapy is recommended for cervical dysplasia.

9 Use of liquid-based cytology and performing two or more biopsies at colposcopy improves sensitivity for CIN-2 or greater.

10 Tdap (tetanus, diphtheria, acellular pertussis) vaccine is recommended to be given once to adolescents between age 11 and 18 to replace prior Td vaccine. MCV4 (meningococcal) vaccine is recommended to be given once prior to when a girl starts high school.

Normal Puberty and Menarche

- Typically, pubertal development proceeds in the following order:
  - Pubarche: median age 10.6 in white girls, 9.5 in black girls in the United States
  - Thelarche: median age 10.3 in white girls, 9.5 in black girls
  - Menarche: median age 12.55 in white girls, 12.06 in black girls, 12.25 in Hispanic girls; 2-3 years after thelarche (Herman-Giddens, 2005)
- The median age of menarche in the United States differs by ethnicity based on National Health and Nutrition Examination Survey (NHANES) data from 1988 to 1994 (Table 3-1).
- Irregular menses and anovulation are common after menarche, so a menstrual cycle length of 21 to 45 days should be considered normal in the first 2 years (5th percentile 23 days, 50th percentile 32 days, 95th 90 days).

- By 3 years after menarche, 60% to 80% of cycles are 21 to 34 days in length.
- By 4 years, the 95th percentile is 50 days.
- By 6 years, the 95th percentile is 38 days.
- Typical duration of flow is 2 to 7 days.
- Most adolescents use 3 to 6 pads or tampons per day.
- Early menarche associated is with early onset of ovulation: 50% of those with menarche before age 12 are ovulatory in the first year (American Academy of Pediatrics Committee on Adolescence, 2006).

UPDATE #1

The age of onset of female puberty decreased in the United States in the first half of the 20th century. However, there was no statistically significant change in the timing of the onset of puberty (Tanner stage II breasts or pubic hair) in black or white girls between the National Health Examination Survey III (NHES III,

TABLE 3-1 Racial Differences in Age of Menarche from NHANES

	10%	Fiducial Limits	25%	Fiducial Limits	50% Median	Fiducial Limits	75%	Fiducial Limits	90%	Fiducial Limits
Overall	11.11	10.95-11.25	11.73	11.62-11.84	12.43	12.33-12.53	13.13	13.01-13.25	13.75	13.61-13.92
By Race										
Non-Hispanic whites	11.32*	10.91-11.61	11.90*†	11.60-12.14	12.55*	12.31-12.79	13.20	12.95-13.52	13.78	13.47-14.22
Non-Hispanic blacks	10.52*	10.15-10.81	11.25*	10.98-11.48	12.06*	11.84-12.28	12.87	12.63-13.16	13.60	13.30-13.99
Mexican Americans	10.81	10.46-11.09	11.49†	11.23-11.71	12.25	12.04-12.46	13.01	12.78-13.29	13.69	13.40-14.07

*Significant racial difference, P value <.017 for each pair-wise comparison yielding a P value <.05 for the overall comparison-wise error rate. The fiducial limits for overall were based on 95% confidence limits.
†Race-specific fiducial limits were computed at 98.3% confidence limits so that the multiple (3) fiducial limits combined yielded a 95% confidence limit.
From Chumlea WE, Schubert CM, Roche AF, et al: Age at menarche and racial comparisons in US girls, *Pediatrics* 111:110-113, 2003.

1966 to 1970) and NHANES (1988-94). In Hispanic girls, the proportion having attained Tanner stage II breasts and pubic hair at age 10 or 11 increased between the Hispanic Health and Nutrition Examination Survey (HHANES, 1982-84) and NHANES (Sun et al, 2005). The median age at menarche decreased by 0.34 years in white girls, which was not statistically significant; however, in black girls the median age of menarche decreased by 0.46 years. The timing of menarche was associated with body mass index, with earlier menarche in heavier girls (Chumlea et al, 2003). Postulated reasons for earlier pubertal development include genetic differences between racial and ethnic groups, increased body weight, exposure to endocrine disrupting chemicals, estrogenic effects of soy-based infant formulas, dietary changes, exogenous hormone exposure, an increased prevalence of small-for-gestational age births, and psychosocial stress related to absent fathers and cultural hypersexualization (Herman-Giddens, 2005).

Primary Amenorrhea and Delayed Puberty

DEFINITIONS AND INDICATIONS FOR EVALUATION

- Although primary amenorrhea was traditionally defined as absence of menses by age 16, recent data about norms indicate that evaluation should begin in the absence of menses by age 15.
- Evaluation also indicated if menses do not occur within 5 years of thelarche.
- Absence of thelarche by age 13 warrants evaluation (American Society for Reproductive Medicine Practice Committee, 2004).

INITIAL EVALUATION

- Pregnancy test.
- Thyroid stimulating hormone (TSH), follicle stimulating hormone (FSH), prolactin (Figure 3-1).
- Breast examination.
- Examination of internal and external genitalia; pelvic ultrasound if inconclusive for the presence of a uterus.
- Causes of primary amenorrhea are detailed in Table 3-2.

BREAST DEVELOPMENT PRESENT, NORMAL FSH: 30%

- If examination shows uterus is absent, next step in evaluation is serum testosterone and karyotype.
- Testosterone in normal male range and 46,XY karyotype: androgen insensitivity syndrome. These patients typically have minimal pubic hair. Gonadectomy should be performed to prevent malignancy but may be delayed until adult height and complete breast development have been attained.
- If normal female range testosterone and 46,XX karyotype: Müllerian agenesis or outflow tract obstruction.
- If history reveals cyclic pelvic pain, evaluate with pelvic ultrasound; hematocolpos or hematometra indicates outflow obstruction, either imperforate hymen or tranverse vaginal septum.
- Imperforate hymen found in 1/2000 females. This is treated with an elliptical incision and drainage of material in vagina. One surgical technique involves a 0.5 cm central oval incision with placement of a 16F Foley catheter with 10 mL saline, left in place for 2 weeks with daily application of conjugated equine estrogen cream. This method leaves an intact hymenal ring, which may be culturally important (Acar et al, 2007).
- Transverse vaginal septum found in 1/80,000 females. Treatment involves resection and anastomosis of upper and lower vaginal segments. The complexity of this surgery is dependent on the location and thickness of the septum and may be facilitated by preoperative vaginal dilator use.
- Müllerian agenesis or Mayer-Rokitansky-Kuster-Hauser syndrome: congenital absence of any or all portions of the female genital tract. If the vagina is absent or inadequate, vaginal dilators are preferred first line therapy for adolescents and adult women. If unsuccessful, surgical neovagina creation may be undertaken. Both methods require maintenance dilator use, so ideal timing depends on individual psychosocial maturity.

NO BREAST DEVELOPMENT, HIGH FSH: 40%

- Next step in evaluation is karyotype.
- 45,X or mosaic including 45,X: Turner's syndrome.
  - Turner's syndrome found in 1/2500 to 1/3000 live births.

Suggested flow diagram aiding in the evaluation of women with amenorrhea.

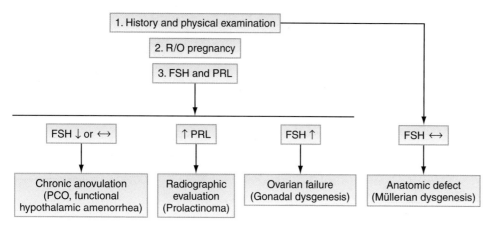

Figure 3-1. **Evaluation of amenorrhea.** (From American College for Reproductive Medicine Practice Committee: current evaluation of amenorrhea, *Fertil Steril* 82[1]: 266-272, 2004.)

TABLE 3-2 Causes of Primary Amenorrhea

Category	Approximate Frequency (%)
Breast Development	30
Müllerian agenesis	10
Androgen insensitivity	9
Vaginal septum	2
Imperforate hymen	1
Constitutional delay	8
No Breast Development: High FSH	40
46XX	15
46XY	5
Abnormal	20
No Breast Development: Low FSH	30
Constitutional delay	10
Prolactinomas	5
Kallmann syndrome	2
Other CNS	3
Stress, weight loss, anorexia	3
PCOS	3
Congenital adrenal hyperplasia	3
Other	1

From Current evaluation of amenorrhea. Practice Committee of the American Society for Reproductive Medicine, *Fertil Steril* 82(1): 266-272, 2004.

- Fifty percent have 45,X karyotype; the remainder either mosaicism of 45,X with other lineages or duplication of long arm of one X chromosome (46,X,i(Xq)).
- Phenotype varies depending on karyotype.
- Clinical features include the following:
  - Congenital lymphedema
  - Short stature
  - Gonadal dysgenesis (streak ovaries) in 90% of 45,X with absence of puberty because of premature depletion of primordial follicles; most will undergo normal adrenarche
  - Learning disabilities in 70%, usually perceptual motor and spatial processing skills

- Recurrent otitis media in childhood in >50%, caused by small eustachian tubes and palatal dysfunction
- Congenital cardiac defects in 17% to 45%, primarily coarctation of the aorta and bicuspid aortic valve
- Sensorineural hearing loss by adulthood in 44%
- Renal malformations in 40%, including horseshoe kidney and duplicated collecting system
- Ophthalmologic problems in 30%, including ptosis, strabismus, nystagmus, and cataracts
- Hypothyroidism in 15% to 30%, typically adult onset
- Skeletal dysplasias
- Melanocytic nevi
- Developmental delay in 10%, often with ring or marker chromosome
- Diabetes mellitus in 7%
- Inflammatory bowel disease is common in i(Xq) cell lineage
- Timing of ovarian failure is variable: while the majority with a 45,X karyotype will not initiate pubertal development, some girls will have pubertal arrest, and 40% of those with a 45,X/46,XX mosaicism will have spontaneous menarche.
- If diagnosis is strongly suspected but initial karyotype is 46,XX, karyotype should be performed on 100 lymphocytes; consider karyotyping of dermal fibroblasts.
- 46,XY with SRY deletion (46,X,del(Yp)) will present with Turner phenotype, but increased risk of gonadoblastoma, so gonadectomy should be performed (Sybert et al, 2004).
- Table 3-3 details recommended evaluations for those with Turner syndrome.
- Estrogen replacement should be initiated for pubertal induction at age 12 to 13 in girls without spontaneous pubertal development (Table 3-4).

UPDATE #2

Increased linear growth can be obtained in girls with Turner's syndrome using growth hormone when low-dose depot estradiol is initiated at age 12 or 14, rather than starting the treatment with full-dose estrogen supplementation (Rosenfield et al, 2005).

TABLE 3-3 Recommendations for Care of Girls and Women with Turner Syndrome

Procedure	At Diagnosis	Timing of Evaluation		
		Childhood	**Adolescence**	**Adulthood**
Physical examination*	Yes	As indicated by age	Yearly	Yearly
Echocardiography	Yes	Every 3-5 years[†]	Every 3-5 years[†]	Every 3-5 years[†]
Renal ultrasonography	Yes	—	—	—
Thyroid-function test	Yes	Repeat only if indicated by findings	Yearly	Yearly
Hearing test	Yes (baseline)	Optional	Optional	Yearly
Ophthalmic evaluation	Early referral to ophthalmologist if strabismus or ptosis is present	—	—	—
Lipid screening	—	—	—	Optional
Liver-function test	—	—	—	Optional
Screening for diabetes	Only if indicated by clinical findings	Only if indicated by clinical findings	Only if indicated by clinical findings	Optional
Evaluation for ovarian failure[‡]	Yes	—	Yes	Yes
Evaluation of growth issues[ʃ]	Yes	Yes	Yes	––
Evaluation for psychosocial issues[¶]	Yes	Yes	Yes	Yes
Weight-control measures	As needed	As needed	As needed	As needed

*Physical examination should include measurement of blood pressure, growth, weight, and vision, and an evaluation for scoliosis.
[†]Recommendations are current (best-guess) estimates with few data to support the use of this approach in patients without cardiac disease. If structural cardiac malformations are present, recommendations need to be individualized.
[‡]Measurement of gonadotropins may be helpful, as discussed in the text. Any discussion of gonadal dysgenesis, the need for hormone-replacement therapy, sexual function, and fertility should be age appropriate.
[ʃ]The use of recombinant human growth hormone should be discussed.
[¶]Schooling issues and the need for job and driver's training and other steps to independence should be discussed at appropriate ages.
From Sybert VP, McCauley E: Turner's syndrome, *N Engl J Med* 351(12):1227-1238, 2004.

TABLE 3-4 Ovarian Hormone Replacement in Turner Syndrome

Age (years)	Age-Specific Suggestions	Comments
10-11	Monitor for spontaneous puberty by Tanner staging and FSH level	Low-dose estrogen treatment may not inhibit GH-enhanced growth in stature
10-13	If no spontaneous development and FSH elevated, begin low-dose E2	Equivalent initial E2 doses: depot (im) E2, 0.2-0.4 mg/month; transdermal E2 6.25 µg daily;* micronized E2, 0.25 mg daily by mouth
12.5-15	Gradually increase E2 dose over about 2 years (e.g., 14, 25, 37, 50, 75, 100, 200 µg daily via patch to adult dose)	Usual adult daily dose is 100-200 µg transdermal E2, 2-4 mg micronized E2, 20 µg EE2, 1.25-2.5 mg CEE
14-16	Begin cyclic progesterone treatment after 2 years of estrogen or when breakthrough bleeding occurs	Oral micronized progesterone best option at present; usual adult dose is 200 mg/d on days 20-30 of monthly cycle or days 100-120 of 3-month cycle
14-30	Continue full dose at least until age 30 because normally estrogen levels are highest between age 15 and 30 years	Some women may prefer using oral or transdermal contraceptive for HRT; monitor endometrial thickness
30-50	The lowest estrogen dose providing full protection versus osteoporosis is 0.625 CEE or equivalent	Monitor osteoporosis risk factors, diet, exercise; obtain BMD and begin regular screening mammography by age 45 years
>50	Decision on estrogen based use on same considerations as other postmenopausal women	New HRT options are appearing, and these recommendations may need updating in near future

*The lowest-dose commercially available E2 transdermal patches deliver 14 and 25 µg daily; it is not established whether various means of dose fractionation (e.g., administering a quarter patch overnight or daily or administering whole patches for 7-10 days per month) are equivalent.
CEE, conjugated equine estrogens; E2, estradiol; EE2, ethinyl estradiol; HRT, hormone replacement treatment.
From Bondy CA: Clinical practice guideline: care of girls and women with Turner syndrome: a guideline of the Turner syndrome study group, *J Clin Endocrinol Metab* 92:10-25, 2007.

- 46,XY or mosaic including Y chromosomal material: Swyer's syndrome, 46,XY gonadal dysgenesis. Gonadectomy should be performed shortly after diagnosis because of a 25% risk of malignancy. In some cases, the uterus may be absent if testis was partially functional in utero and produced antimüllerian hormone. Female pubertal development should be induced using exogenous estrogen in the same manner as for Turner's syndrome.
- 46,XX karyotype: primary ovarian insufficiency. This is the most commonly idiopathic, but may be due to other rare causes:
  - Autoimmune primary ovarian insufficiency. This may be associated with other autoimmune endocrine dysfunction including Addison's disease with antiadrenal antibodies or autoimmune polyglandular syndrome, type I (APS I), caused by mutations in the AIRE gene.
  - Galactosemia.
  - FMR1 premutations (fragile X).
  - FOXL2 mutations, presenting with blepharophimosis, ptosis, and epicanthus inversus syndrome (BPES).
  - FSH receptor mutations.
  - Steroidogenic enzyme deficiencies including 17-hydroxylase and aromatase.

ELEVATED PROLACTIN

- Evaluate with brain magnetic resonance imaging (MRI); visible tumor in 50% to 60%.
- Microadenoma if <10 mm; macroadenoma if >10 mm.
- Primary therapy is dopamine agonist.
- Consider surgery if medical therapy fails.

NORMAL TO LOW FSH, NORMAL PROLACTIN

- Progestin challenge is no longer indicated due to poor sensitivity and specificity.
- If gonadotropins are very low to undetectable, may be due to congenital or acquired GnRH or gonadotropin deficiency. Brain MRI should be performed to assess for lesion affecting the hypothalamus or pituitary.
- Kallmann syndrome: gonadotropin deficiency and anosmia; may be caused by mutations in KAL1 gene or FGFR1.
- If low to normal FSH, assess for clinical hyperandrogenism (acne, hirsutism, or androgenic alopecia) or biochemical androgen abnormalities (elevated total testosterone, free testosterone, or dihydroepiandrostenedione sulfate); 17-hydroxyprogesterone should also be used to evaluate for nonclassic congenital adrenal hyperplasia.
- Amenorrhea plus clinical or biochemical hyperandrogenism: polycystic ovary syndrome (PCOS). It is difficult to make this diagnosis with certainty in the adolescent, as anovulation and acne are common in the early postmenarchal years. PCOS is often associated with obesity in the adolescent, and girls should be screened for type 2 diabetes and hyperlipidemia. Treatment may include oral contraceptives to prevent endometrial hyperplasia and decrease serum total and free androgens. Spironolactone can be used as an adjunct to oral contraceptives for treatment of clinical hyperandrogenism. Metformin may be used for

impaired fasting glucose or impaired glucose tolerance. Some patients will become ovulatory with metformin therapy. For overweight patients, a weight loss of 10% or greater may result in ovulation (Sanfilippo et al, 2009).
- If there is low-normal FSH and no clinical or biochemical hyperandrogenism, the likely diagnosis is functional hypothalamic amenorrhea, found in 3% of adolescents. This can be associated with anorexia, weight loss, extreme exercise, systemic illness, or high levels of psychosocial stress. Prevalence is threefold higher among competitive athletes.
- For all hypoestrogenic states, estrogen therapy is indicated to induce normal bone development. If normal breast development has been attained, oral contraceptives may be used. If pubertal development has not been initiated, estrogen should be slowly increased in the manner used to treat Turner's syndrome (discussed earlier).

UPDATE #3

Mutations in the GPR54 gene (g-protein coupled receptor) have been found in one consanguineous family and one additional proband with hypogonadotropic hypogonadism. The phenotype of hypogonadotropic hypogonadism has been confirmed in mouse studies. Kisspeptin is the ligand for this receptor; those with mutation show decreased intracellular inositol phosphate increase in response to kisspeptin. These patients show an exaggerated LH response to pulsatile GnRH in comparison with those with idiopathic hypogonadotropic hypogonadism without GPR54 mutations (Seminara et al, 2003).

Secondary Amenorrhea in the Adolescent

Evaluation should be initiated after 3 months of amenorrhea, or three normal menstrual cycles in a girl who has previously had regular menses. Evaluation should follow the algorithm for primary amenorrhea, including pregnancy test, FSH, and prolactin (Diaz et al, 2006).

Abnormal Uterine Bleeding in the Adolescent

CLINICAL HISTORY

- Anovulatory cycles are common for 2 to 5 years after menarche.
- Use of a menstrual calendar including days of bleeding and menstrual products used can assist in determining normal versus abnormal uterine bleeding.
- Normal menstrual bleeding is 30 mL per month; bleeding >80 mL is associated with anemia.
- Evaluation is recommended for adolescents with the following:
  - Menstrual periods that occurred monthly, then became increasingly irregular.
  - A menstrual cycle length that is persistently less than 21 days or greater than 45 days.
  - Menstrual bleeding lasting longer than 7 days (Diaz et al, 2006).
  - Menstrual bleeding saturating the pad or tampon per hour.
  - Passage of clots > 1 inch in size.

- Heavy bleeding at menarche leading to anemia (American College of Obstetricians and Gynecologists Committee on Adolescent Health Care, 2009).

CAUSES OF ABNORMAL VAGINAL BLEEDING IN ADOLESCENTS (ADAPTED FROM SANFILIPPO ET AL, 2009)

- Trauma.
- Foreign bodies.
- Infectious: Vaginitis or cervicitis due to sexually transmitted diseases, genital warts or dysplasia, endometritis, pelvic inflammatory disease.
- Tumors: Sarcoma botryoides (infants and children); endometrial polyps, ovarian neoplasms including mature teratoma, androgen-secreting, or granulosa-theca cell tumors, leiomyomata, and steroid-secreting adrenal tumors.
- Endometriosis.
- Congenital malformations of the uterus.
- Complications of pregnancy.
- Coagulopathies: von Willebrand's.
- Normal variation (midcycle bleeding or early postmenarchal menstrual irregularity)
- Breakthrough bleeding on hormonal contraception.
- Chronic anovulation.
- Systemic disease: hypo- or hyperthyroidism, Cushing's syndrome, liver disease, inflammatory bowel disease, autoimmune disease, hyperprolactinemia.
- Androgen excess: polycystic ovary syndrome, congenital adrenal hyperplasia, androgen-secreting neoplasm of the adrenal or ovary, exogenous androgens.
- Estrogen excess: granulosa-theca cell tumor of the ovary.
- Pituitary disorders.
- Hypothalamic dysfunction, including that induced by physical or psychological stress.
- Medications.
  - Endocrine medications: danazol, spironolactone.
  - Anticoagulants and platelet inhibitors.
  - Chemotherapeutic agents.
  - Herbal and natural supplements: DHEA, dong quai, yam extract.

EVALUATION

- History and physical examination, pelvic examination.
- If bleeding is irregular (oligomenorrhea or metromenorrhagia), begin with hormonal evaluation similar to that for amenorrhea.
- If bleeding is cyclic but heavy (menorrhagia), evaluate for abnormalities of coagulation.
  - CBC with differential.
  - Fibrinogen.
  - Prothrombin time.
  - Partial thromboplastin time.
  - Bleeding time.
  - This evaluation should be performed prior to estrogen therapy or transfusion.
  - For severe or prolonged bleeding at menarche, or abnormal initial testing, next steps include von Willebrand's factor antigen, factor VIII activity, factor XI antigen, ristocetin C cofactor, and platelet aggregation studies (Strickland et al, 2003).

- Von Willebrand's disease found in 1% of the population but 5% to 15% of Caucasian girls with menorrhagia, 1.3% of African-American girls.
- Other causes of menorrhagia include factor deficiencies, anatomic defects such as submucosal leiomyomata (rare in adolescence), hepatic failure, and malignancy.

THERAPY FOR MENORRHAGIA

- Mild anemia (Hb > 11 or Hct > 33%): oral iron supplementation, hormonal contraception (oral, transdermal, or vaginal) if indicated for contraceptive purposes.
- Moderate anemia (Hb 9-11 or Hct 27% to 33%): oral contraceptive pills (OCPs).
- Severe anemia (Hb <9 or Hct <27%): OCPs every 6 hours × 1 week with antiemetics, to be tapered overone1 pill pack, then cyclic OCPs.
- Can also consider cyclic or depot progestins (Sanfilippo et al, 2009).

Endometriosis in the Adolescent

PRESENTATION

- Endometriosis can be found in premenarcheal girls and shortly after menarche.
- The primary complaint of adolescents with endometriosis is dysmenorrhea (64% to 94%); approximately 60% will also report acyclic pelvic pain (Laufer et al, 2003).
- Müllerian anomalies with outflow obstruction are found in 6.5% to 40% of adolescents with endometriosis (Goldstein et al, 1979; Laufer et al, 1997; Schifrin et al, 1973); this almost universally resolves with treatment of outflow obstruction (Sanfilippo et al, 1986).
- Two thirds of adults diagnosed with endometriosis report symptoms began prior to age 20 (Laufer et al, 2003).

EVALUATION

- Initial evaluation includes history, symptom diary, abdominal and pelvic examination including bimanual, rectoabdominal, or ultrasound examination as tolerated (Figure 3-2).
- Laparoscopic evaluation and therapy are indicated if dysmenorrhea is refractory to oral contraceptives and NSAIDs.
- From 19% to 73% of adolescents with chronic pelvic pain have endometriosis at laparoscopy (American College of Obstetricians and Gynecologists, ACOG Committee Opinion No. 310, 2005).
- Sixty percent of adolescents with endometriosis have stage I disease at diagnosis (Goldstein et al, 1980).
- Endometriomata are rare in adolescents.
- Laparoscopic findings in adolescents are most likely to include clear and red endometriotic lesions and less likely to include black or white lesions or peritoneal windows (Laufer et al, 2003).
- All visible disease should be treated at laparoscopy.
- While an empiric trial of GnRH agonist is appropriate for adults with symptoms of endometriosis, this is controversial in adolescents because of the risk of bone loss.

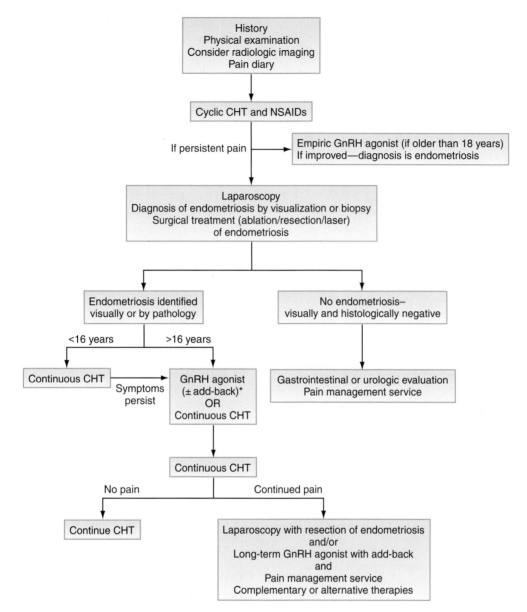

*Add-back indicates use of estrogen and progestin or norethindrone acetate alone.

Figure 3-2. Management of pelvic pain in the adolescent. CHT, combination hormone therapy (oral contraceptive pills, estrogen/progestin patch, estrogen/progestin vaginal ring, norethindrone acetate,medroxyprogesterone acetate); GnRH, gonadotropin-releasing hormone; NSAIDs, nonsteroidal antiinflammatory drugs. (Modified from Bandera CA, Brown LR, Laufer MR: Adolescents and endometriosis, *Clin Consult Obstet Gynecol* 7:206, 1995.)

TREATMENT

- Medical therapy must be continued after surgical treatment to prevent recurrence.
- First-line therapy is continuous oral contraceptives.

UPDATE #4

Continuous OCPs (20 to 30 mcg ethinyl estradiol) are more effective than cyclic in treatment of surgically confirmed endometriosis, with symptom improvement in 75% to 100% (Moghissi, 1999).

- Danazol is a therapeutic option, but adolescents often cannot tolerate the androgenic side effects.
- Progestin-only therapies (e.g. norethindrone, depot medroxyprogesterone acetate) are not ideal in adolescents because of the risk of bone loss.

- The GnRH agonist also causes bone loss; efficacy of add-back estrogen therapy has not been established in adolescents.
- Multidisciplinary management including educational and psychological resources is recommended (American College of Obstetricians and Gynecologists, ACOG Committee Opinion No. 310, 2005).

Contraception in the Adolescent

Sexual activity in adolescents in the United States (from the 2007 Youth Risk Behavior Survey):
- 48% of high school students reported having had sexual intercourse; 60% of 12th graders.
- 35% were sexually active within the past 3 months.

- 15% reported four or more total sexual partners.
- 61.5% reported condom use during last intercourse.
- Adolescents who perceive barriers to contraception are more likely to experience negative outcomes from sexual activity.

ORAL CONTRACEPTIVES (OCPS) (SANFILIPPO ET AL, 2009)

- May be used in cyclic or extended regimens with infrequent breaks.
- Breakthrough bleeding is increased in extended regimens.
- May start OCPs on date of clinic visit regardless of timing in menstrual cycle; this method leads to improved compliance in adolescents and is not associated with any known teratogenicity in the setting of early pregnancy (Lara-Torre et al, 2002).

VAGINAL OR TRANSDERMAL HORMONAL CONTRACEPTIVES

UPDATE #5

Higher area under the curve (AUC) for ethinyl estradiol (EE) is noted more with the birth control patch (Ortho Evra) than for a combined oral contraceptive (COC) containing 30 mcg EE or for the vaginal contraceptive ring (NuvaRing combined EE, and etonogestrel) when used according to manufacturer's instructions (van den Heuvel et al, 2005). This has raised concerns for increased risk of thromboembolic complications, although whether this is clinically relevant has not yet been determined.

PROGESTIN-ONLY ORAL CONTRACEPTIVES

- Increased failure rate because of short half-life.

DEPOT MEDROXYPROGESTERONE ACETATE (DMPA)

- Highly effective (>99% for perfect use, 95% for typical use).
- Side effects include weight gain (average 5 pounds in first year) and irregular bleeding.
- Use with 1200 to 1500 mg daily calcium intake recommended to minimize bone loss.

UPDATE #6

Three years of continuous DMPA use in women ages 16 to 24 was associated with 4.2% loss in bone mass density at spine, and 6% at femoral neck. Bone density was regained after stopping DMPA. A lesser degree of bone loss was seen in women using 20 mcg EE OCPs (Berenson et al, 2008).

INTRAUTERINE DEVICES

- Intrauterine devices, including both copper and levonorgestrel, are a safe and effective option, even for nulliparous adolescents.

BARRIER METHODS: MALE AND FEMALE CONDOM

- Recommended for all adolescents for prevention of sexually transmitted diseases, even when another contraceptive method is used.

EMERGENCY CONTRACEPTION

- "Plan B"—levonorgestrel 0.75 mg q 12 hours × 2 doses within 72 hours of unprotected intercourse has a 2.4% failure rate (American College of Obstetricians and Gynecologists, ACOG Practice Guideline no. 69, 2005).
- Equally effective when both pills taken together or at a 24-hour interval.
- Efficacy decreases with time since intercourse but can be used up to 120 hours postcoitus.
- Providing prescription in advance increases likelihood of use (Belzer et al, 2003).
- Alternative regimens involving combination OCPs are associated with more side effects.
- Adolescents understand key points of emergency contraception after reading OTC package label with 83% to 95% comprehension for all key points (Cremer et al, 2009).

Human Papilloma Virus (HPV) and Cervical Cancer Prevention in the Adolescent

EPIDEMIOLOGY OF HPV

- 6.2 million new HPV infections per year in United States; infection rate estimated 1.2% to 1.3% per month among young, sexually active women.
- 10,000 new cervical cancers per year, 3700 deaths.
- 15 genotypes associated with cervical cancer.
- 70% of cervical cancers associated with genotypes 16 and 18; 90% of genital warts associated with HPV genotypes 6 and 11.
- 40% of adolescents are infected within 16 months of onset of sexual activity (Steinbrook, 2006).
- HPV DNA detected in 60% of college students with biannual screening over a 3-year period (American College of Obstetricians and Gynecologists, ACOG Practice Bulletin no. 61, 2005).

NATURAL HISTORY OF HPV INFECTION

- Transmission is via sexual contact: genital skin, mucous membranes, or bodily fluids.
- 75% of those sexually exposed to genital warts will develop them.
- Number of sexual partners and age of initiation of sexual activity are key risk factors.
- Prevalence of HPV infection is highest among those ages 20 to 24, approximately 21%.
- However, only 1% to 3.6% have abnormal cervical cytology.
- Two thirds of those age 24 and younger will clear infection without developing cervical intraepithelial neoplasia (CIN); however, the proportion may be lower for high-risk subtypes.
- The average time to clear infection, based on DNA testing, is 8 months (American College of Obstetricians and Gynecologists, ACOG Practice Bulletin no. 61, 2005).
- The timeline for progression of HPV infection is shown in Figure 3-3.

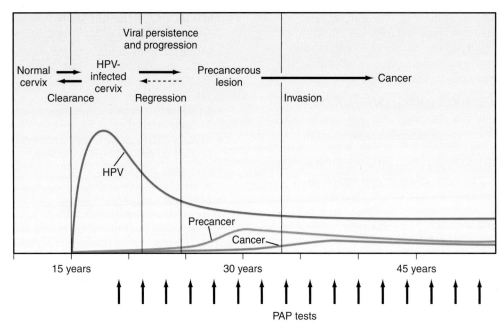

Figure 3-3. Timeline for HPV progression. (Adapted from Runowicz CD: Molecular screening for cervical cancer: time to give up PAP tests? *N Engl J Med* 357[16]:1650-1653, 2007.)

PREVENTION

- Risk decreased by limiting sexual partners, and selecting partners with few prior partners and a prolonged duration since last partner.
- Male circumcision decreases transmission to female partners.
- Condom use can decrease transmission but has not been shown to decrease CIN.
- HPV vaccine introduced in the United States in 2006.

UPDATE #7

In 2006, the Food and Drug Administration (FDA) approved the human papilloma virus (HPV) vaccine for females ages 9 to 26 in 2006. It protects against viral genotypes 6, 11,16, and 18. The vaccine is given in three doses over 6 months, with the second dose given 2 months after the first dose and the third dose given 4 months after the second dose. A bivalent vaccine, providing protection only against genotypes 16 and 18, is also available. Initial studies showed the vaccine to be 100% effective against CIN-2 and 3 and condylomata caused by these subtypes in women not previously infected. In women with prior infection, the vaccine does not promote clearance of the high risk HPV subtype but retains effectiveness against the other subtypes (Hildesheim et al, 2007). ACOG recommends offering the vaccine to all women in the appropriate age group who have not yet been vaccinated. Vaccination does not change recommendations for cervical cancer screening. HPV testing prior to vaccination is not indicated. The vaccine is class B in pregnancy and is appropriate for HIV-positive adolescents. It is not yet known whether a booster will be needed (Committee on Adolescent Care, 2006).

SCREENING

- Screening algorithms may include liquid-based or conventional PAPs, high-risk HPV (HR-HPV) DNA testing, or both.
- Sensitivity of PAP testing for CIN: liquid-based 65% to 95%, conventional 50% to 80%.

- HR-HPV testing improves sensitivity for CIN-2 and 3 but decreases specificity.
- Likelihood of detecting HR-HPV increases with severity of dysplasia: 66% in CIN-1, 95% in CIN-3.
- For adolescents, ACOG recommends pap testing within 3 years of initiation of intercourse or at age 21.
- HR-HPV testing is recommended only in the setting of abnormal cytology; when used with abnormal squamous cells of undetermined significance (ASCUS) PAPs, it decreases number of colposcopies performed.
- HR-HPV DNA testing can be used as a test of cure 6 months after treatment for CIN-2 or 3.
- However, approximately 5% are biopsy-proven CIN-3 negative for HR-HPV at the time of initial pap. The majority of these had an initial ASCUS pap (Castle et al, 2008).
- Management of abnormal cervical cytology and histology is shown in Table 3-5.

Colposcopy recommended in adolescents with low-grade squamous intraepithelial lesion (LSIL) or ASCUS only if persistent for 24 months.

UPDATE #8

Cervical cancer is rare in young women, with no cancers detected in evaluation of 622 abnormal paps in women ages 13 to 24. CIN-3 was found in 6.6% of all women with abnormal PAPs, and 27% of those with high grade squamous intraepithelial lesion (HSIL) (Moscicki et al, 2008).

UPDATE #9

An LSIL or ASCUS result on a liquid-based pap is more sensitive for CIN-2 or higher than the same result on conventional cytology. Sensitivities are similar for HSIL. Liquid-based pap results are less specific than conventional pap results (Arbyn et al, 2008). Performing two or more biopsies at colposcopy improves sensitivity for CIN-2 or greater, independent of provider type, and colposcopic impression (Gage et al, 2006).

TABLE 3-5 Recommendations for Abnormal Cervical Cytology and Histology in Adolescents

Diagnosis	Recommendation
ASC-US (no HPV testing)	Repeat cytology in 12 months
ASC-H	Colposcopy
LSIL (no HPV testing)	Repeat cytology in 12 months
HSIL	Colposcopy
AGC	Colposcopy (may need to refer to a specialist)
Cancer	Refer to specialist
Mild dysplasia	Repeat cytology in 1 year
Moderate dysplasia	Repeat colposcopy and cytology in 4-6 months
Severe dysplasia or CIS	Treat per ASCCP guidelines

ASC-US, atypical squamous cells of undetermined significance; HPV, human papillomavirus; ASC-H, atypical squamous cells cannot exclude high grade; LSIL, low-grade squamous intraepithelial lesion; HSIL, high-grade squamous intraepithelial lesion; AGC, atypical glandular cells; CIS, carcinoma in situ; ASCCP, American Society for Colposcopy and Cervical Pathology.
From Sanfilippo JS, Lara-Torre E : Adolescent gynecology, *Obstet Gynecol* 113(4):935-947, 2009.

TREATMENT OF CIN IN THE ADOLESCENT
(See Table 3-5) (Wright et al, 2007)

- CIN-1 on biopsy: repeat cytology at 12 months. Repeat colposcopy at 12 months for HSIL on repeat cytology; repeat colposcopy at 24 months for any cytologic abnormality.
- CIN-2: observation with cytology and colposcopy every 6 months for up to 24 months is preferred to immediate excisional treatment in the adolescent.
- CIN-3: excisional treatment is recommended.
- Follow-up after therapy should include cytology and HR-HPV DNA testing.

Sexually Transmitted Diseases in the Adolescent

HERPES SIMPLEX VIRUS (HSV)

- 26% of women over age 12 are positive for HSV-2 serology, 67% for HSV-1.
- Likelihood of infection is associated with age at first contact.
- Initial episode is associated with flulike symptoms (ACOG Committee on Practice Bulletins—Gynecology, 2004).

CHLAMYDIA TRACHOMATIS

- The most common bacterial sexually transmitted disease (STD) in the United States (>1 million cases/year, most younger than age 26).
- Prevalence is 2% overall, 4% in Hispanics, 13% in Native Americans, and 14% in African Americans.
- The Centers for Disease Control and Prevention (CDC) has recommended screening for all sexually active adolescents and women under age 25.
- However, only 16% of women ages 15 to 25 were screened at outpatient preventive care visits, and only 22% of those presenting with symptoms were screened (Hoover et al, 2008).

HUMAN IMMUNODEFICIENCY VIRUS (HIV)

- 25% of adolescent females have been screened.
- 20% to 25% of those diagnosed with HIV report no risk factors.
- Universal screening has not been demonstrated to prevent disease progression or death.
- Risk factors considered indications for screening in the asymptomatic adolescent include diagnosis of other sexually transmitted diseases, male homosexual contact, current or past injection drug use, exchange of sex for money or drugs, past or current sex partners with risk factors, or unprotected vaginal or anal intercourse with more than one partner (Chou et al, 2005).

Role of the Gynecologist in Adolescent Primary Care

- Routine assessments for adolescents shown in Table 3-6.
- ACOG recommends first gynecologic visit at age 13 to 15 to initiate education and preventive care (Committee on Adolescent Health, 2009).
- Pelvic examination may be deferred unless indicated because of the following:
  - Delayed or precocious puberty
  - Abnormal vaginal bleeding or discharge
  - Pelvic or abdominal pain
- Developmental staging may be evaluated by external visual examination.
- Confidentiality should be addressed with the patient and her parent(s) at the initial visit. State laws vary with regard to confidentiality and parental notification requirements; details can be found at www.guttmacher.org.
- In the sexually active adolescent, urine testing for gonorrheal and chlamydial infections may be performed.
- Initial pap and speculum examination recommended 3 years after the onset of sexual activity.
- The prevalence of overweight and obesity have been steadily increasing in adolescents since the 1980s. Weight, diet, and exercise should be addressed at every preventive care visit.
- Appropriateness of weight should be determined based on an age-specific body mass index (BMI) curve (Figure 3-4).
  - Adolescents at the 85th to 95th percentiles for BMI are considered "at-risk" for becoming overweight.
  - Adolescents at the 95th percentile or greater for BMI are considered overweight.
- The Surgeon General recommends 60 minutes of physical activity per day most days of the week for adolescents.

UPDATE #10

Rates of pertussis infection in people over age 10 have increased in the United States since the 1970s, resulting from loss of immunity. The Tdap (tetanus, diphtheria, acellular pertussis) vaccine has been demonstrated to be similar in safety and effectiveness to the Td vaccine for tetanus and diphtheria in adolescents (>99% with serum titers consistent with immunity). This vaccination is recommended in adolescents, to be given once between ages 11 and 18 (Pichichero et al, 2005).

TABLE 3-6   **Recommendations for Periodic Assessments in Adolescents**

Periodic Assessment: Ages 13-18 Years

Screening	Evaluation and Counseling	Skin Exposure to Ultraviolet Rays
History	*Sexuality*	*Tobacco, Alcohol, other Drug Use*
Reason for visit	Development	Immunizations
Health status: medical, menstrual, surgical, family	High-risk behaviors	Periodic
Dietary/nutrition assessment	Preventing unwanted/unintended pregnancy	Diphtheria and reduced tetanus toxoids and acellular pertussis vaccine booster (once between 11 and 18 years)ǀ
Physical activity	— Postponing sexual involvement	Hepatitis B vaccine (one series for those not previously immunized)
Use of complementary and alternative medicine	— Contraceptive options, including emergency contraception	Human papillomavirus vaccine (one series for those not previously immunized, ages 9-26 years)
Tobacco, alcohol, other drug use	Sexually transmitted diseases	Influenza vaccine (annually)
Abuse/neglect	— Partner selection	Measles—mumps—rubella vaccine (for those not previously immunized)
Sexual practices	— Barrier protection	Meningococcal conjugate vaccine (before entry into high school for those not previously immunized)
Physical Examination	*Fitness and Nutrition*	Varicella vaccine (one series for those without evidence of immunity)
Height	Exercise: discussion of program	
Weight	Dietary/nutrition assessment (including eating disorders)	*High-Risk Groups**
Body mass index (BMI)	Folic acid supplementation	Hepatitis A vaccine
Blood pressure	Calcium intake	Pneumococcal vaccine
Secondary sexual characteristics (Tanner staging)	*Psychosocial Evaluation*	*Leading Causes of Death*¶
Pelvic examination (when indicated by the medical history)	Suicide: depressive symptoms	1. Accidents (unintentional injuries)
Skin*	Interpersonal/family relationships	2. Malignant neoplasms
	Sexual orientation and gender identity	3. Intentional self harm (suicide)
Laboratory Testing	Personal goal development	4. Assault (homicide)
Periodic	Behavioral/learning disorders	5. Diseases of the heart
Chlamydia and gonorrhea testing (if sexually active)†	Abuse/neglect	6. Congenital malformations, deformations, and chromosomal abnormalities
Human immunodeficiency virus (HIV) testing (if sexually active)‡	Satisfactory school experience	7. Chronic lower respiratory diseases
High-risk groups*	Peer relationships	8. Cerebrovascular diseases
Colorectal cancer screening§	Date rape prevention	9. Influenza and pneumonia
Fasting glucose testing		10. In situ neoplasms, benign neoplasms, and neoplasms of unknown or uncertain behavior
Genetic testing/counseling	*Cardiovascular Risk Factors*	
Hemoglobin level assessment	Family history	
Hepatitis C virus testing	Hypertension	
Lipid profile assessment	Dyslipidemia	
Rubella titer assessment	Obesity	
Sexually transmitted disease testing	Diabetes mellitus	
Tuberculosis skin testing	*Health/Risk Behaviors*	
	Hygiene (including dental), fluoride supplementation*	
	Injury prevention	
	— Exercise and sports involvement	
	— Firearms	
	— Hearing	
	— Occupational hazards	
	— Recreational hazards	
	— Safe driving practices	

*See Table 3-1.

†Urine-based sexually transmitted disease screening is an efficient means for accomplishing such screening without a speculum examination.

‡Physicians should be aware of and follow their states' HIV screening requirements. For a more detailed discussion of HIV screening, see Branson BM, Handsfield HH, Lampe MA, et al: Revised recommendations for HIV testing for adults, adolescents, and pregnant women in health-care settings. Centers for Disease Control and Prevention (CDC), *MMWR Recomm Rep* 55(AR-14):1-17; quiz CE1-4, 2006. See also Routine human immunodeficiency virus screening: ACOG committee opinion no. 411, American College of Obstetricians and Gynecologists, *Obstet Gynecol* 112:401-403, 2008.

§Only for those with a family history of familial adenomatous polyposis or 8 years after the start of pancolitis. For a more detailed discussion of colorectal cancer screening, see Levin B, Lieberman DA, McFarland B, et al. Screening and surveillance for the early detection of colorectal cancer adenomatous polyps, 2008: a joint guideline from the American Cancer Society: US Multi-Society Task Force, American College of Radiology Colon Cancer Committee, *CA Cancer J Clin* 58:130-160, 2008.

ǀFor more information on the use of Td and Tdap, see Broder KR, Cortese MM, Iskander JK, et al. Preventing tetanus, diphtheria, and pertussis among adolescents: use of tetanus toxoid, reduced diphtheria toxoid and acellular pertussis vaccines recommendations of the Advisory Committee on Immunization Practices (ACIP), Advisory Committee on Immunization Practices (ACIP), *MMWR Recomm Rep* 55(RR-3):1-34, 2006.

¶Leading causes of mortality are provided by the Mortality Statistics Branch at the National Center for Health Statistics. Data are from 2004, the most recent year for which final data are available. The causes are ranked.

From American College of Obstetricians and Gynecologists: ACOG Committee opinion no> 452: Primary and preventive care: periodic assessments, *Obstet Gynecol* 114(6):1444-1451, 2009.

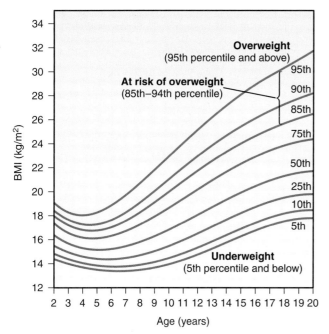

Figure 3-4. **Age-specific BMI percentiles.** (Adapted from American College of Obstetricians and Gynecologists: ACOG committee opinion no. 351: the overweight adolescent: prevention, treatment, and gynecologic implications, *Obstet Gynecol* 108:1337-1348, 2006.)

ACOG recommends the meningococcal conjugate vaccine (MCV4) for preadolescents at age 11 or 12 or prior to entry into high school. Pregnancy is not a contraindication to the MCV4 vaccine (American College of Obstetricians and Gynecologists, ACOG Committee Opinion no. 314, 2005).

Breast Concerns in the Adolescent

MASTALGIA (BREAST PAIN)

- May be associated with swelling and/or nodularity.
- Commonly in the upper outer quadrant.
- Typically worse premenstrually.
- Treatment: decreasing or eliminating nicotine and caffeine, use of supportive sports bras, and NSAIDs.
- OCPs may provide relief with fibrocystic breasts.

NIPPLE DISCHARGE

- Causes include local irritation, pregnancy, and medications including OCPs.
- Galactorrhea (milky white discharge) may be seen in hypothyroidism or hyperprolactinemia. Evaluate with TSH and prolactin.
- Brown or bloody discharge should be evaluated with ultrasound to assess for ductal ectasia, intraductal papilloma, or papillomatosis.

BREAST MASS

- May be reported by parent with development of breast buds at age 8 to 10.
- Breast asymmetry is common in adolescence and may persist into adulthood; this may be reported as a mass but rarely is associated with abnormality.
- Breast masses in the adolescent should be evaluated with ultrasound, not mammography.

- 67% of masses in adolescents are fibroadenomata. The majority will decrease in size or resolve spontaneously within 10 years.
- 15% of masses are due to fibrocystic changes.
- 3% are due to infectious etiologies: mastitis or abscess.
- Primary breast malignancy occurs in less than 1/100,000 women under age 20.
- Therefore, biopsy should be performed only in cases of rapid enlargement, skin changes, or in adolescents with a prior history of malignancy.

BREAST HYPERTROPHY

- "Juvenile" or "virginal" breast hypertrophy is typically seen in females with normal pubertal breast development followed by ongoing rapid growth. This may be unilateral or bilateral.
- Breast hypertrophy is associated with significant distress and social dysfunction as well as back and shoulder pain.
- Reduction mammoplasty is associated with high satisfaction (75% to 94%) and improvement in self-esteem when performed at age 15 to 17.
- Potential complications of surgery include pain, scar formation, and occasionally difficulty breast-feeding.
- Exact timing is somewhat controversial. Some surgeons wait until breasts stop growing for 6 months or until age 18, but in some cases mammoplasty is performed sooner because of the severity of symptoms and associated distress.

BREAST AUGMENTATION

- The American Society for Plastic Surgery recommends breast augmentation for aesthetic reasons should be limited to those age 18 and older.

BREAST SELF-EXAMINATION (BSE)

- There are no data to support routine teaching for breast self-examination in the adolescent population as an effective screening technique.
- BSE in the adolescent may lead to unnecessary invasive procedures.
- Teaching BSE may be appropriate in adolescents at high risk for breast cancer, including daughters of women with BRCA1 or BRCA2, those with prior malignancy, or those with a history of chest radiotherapy (ACOG Committee on Adolescent Health Care, ACOG Committee Opinion no. 350, 2006).

SUGGESTED READINGS

Normal Puberty

American Academy of Pediatrics Committee on Adolescence, et al: Menstruation in girls and adolescents: using the menstrual cycle as a vital sign, *Pediatrics* 118(5):2245–2250, 2006.

Chumlea WE, Schubert CM, Roche AF, et al: Age at menarche and racial comparisons in US girls, *Pediatrics* 111(1):110–113, 2003.

Herman-Giddens M: Recent data on pubertal milestones in United States children: the secular trend toward earlier development, *Int J Androl* 29(1):241–246, 2005.

Sun SS, Schubert CM, Liang R, et al: Is sexual maturity occurring earlier among U.S. children? *J Adolesc Health* 37(5):345–355, 2005.

Abnormal Puberty and Amenorrhea

Acar A, Balci O, Karatayli R, et al: The treatment of 65 women with imperforate hymen by a central incision and application of Foley catheter, *BJOG* 114(11):1376–1379, 2007.

American Society for Reproductive Medicine Practice Committee: Current evaluation of amenorrhea, *Fertil Steril* 82(1):266–272, 2004.

Bondy CA, and the Turner Syndrome Consensus Study Group: Care of girls and women with Turner syndrome: a guideline of the Turner syndrome study group, *J Clin Endocrinol Metab* 92(1):10–25, 2007.

Rosenfield RL, Devine N, Hunold JJ, et al: Salutary effects of combining early very low-dose systemic estradiol with growth hormone therapy in girls with Turner syndrome, *J Clin Endocrinol Metab* 90(12):6424–6430, 2005.

Sanfilippo JS, Lara-Torre E: Adolescent gynecology, *Obstet Gynecol* 113(4):935–947, 2009.

Seminara SB, Messager S, Chatzidaki EE, et al: The GPR54 gene as a regulator of puberty, *N Engl J Med* 349(17):1614–1627, 2003.

Sybert VP, McCauley E: Turner's syndrome, *N Engl J Med* 351(12):1227–1238, 2004.

Abnormal Uterine Bleeding

American College of Obstetricians and Gynecologists Committee on Adolescent Health Care, et al: ACOG committee opinion no. 451: Von Willebrand disease in women, *Obstet Gynecol* 114(6):1439–1443, 2009.

Strickland J, Wall J: Abnormal uterine bleeding in adolescents, *Obstet Gynecol Clin North Am* 30(2):321–335, 2003.

Endometriosis

American College of Obstetricians and Gynecologists: ACOG committee opinion no. 310. Endometriosis in adolescents, *Obstet Gynecol* 105(4):921–927, 2005.

Goldstein DP, deCholnoky C, Leventhal JM, Emans SJ: New insights into the old problem of chronic pelvic pain, *J Pediatr Surg* 14(6):675–680, 1979.

Goldstein DP, de Cholnoky C, Emans SJ: Adolescent endometriosis, *J Adolesc Health Care* 1(1):37–41,1980.

Laufer MR, Goitein L, Bush M, et al: Prevalence of endometriosis in adolescent girls with chronic pelvic pain not responding to conventional therapy, *J Pediatr Adolesc Gynecol* 10(4):199–202, 1997.

Laufer MR, Sanfilippo J, Rose G: Adolescent endometriosis: diagnosis and treatment approaches, *J Pediatr Adolesc Gynecol* 16(Suppl 3):S3–S11, 2003.

Moghissi K: Medical treatment of endometriosis, *Clin Obstet Gynecol* 42(3):620–632, 1999.

Sanfilippo JS, Wakim NG, Schikler KN, Yussman MA: Endometriosis in association with uterine anomaly, *Am J Obstet Gynecol* 154(1):39–43, 1986.

Schifrin BS, Erez S, Moore JC: Teen-age endometriosis, *Am J Obstet Gynecol* 116(7):973–980, 1973.

Contraception

American College of Obstetricians and Gynecologists: ACOG practice bulletin: clinical management guidelines for obstetrician-gynecologists no. 69 (replaces practice bulletin no. 25, March 2001): emergency contraception, *Obstet Gynecol* 106(6):1443–1452, 2005.

American College of Obstetricians and Gynecologists Committee on Adolescent Health Care: ACOG committee opinion No. 351: the overweight adolescent: prevention, treatment, and gynecologic implications, *Obstet Gynecol* 108(5):1337–1348, 2006.

Belzer M, Yoshida E, Tejirian T, et al: Advanced supply of emergency contraception for adolescent mothers increased utilization without reducing condom or primary contraception use, *J Adolesc Health* 32(2):122–123, 2003.

Berenson AB, Rahman M: Radecki Breitkopf C, Bi LX: Effects of depot medroxyprogesterone acetate and 20-microgram oral contraceptives on bone mineral density, *Obstet Gynecol* 112(4):788–799, 2008.

Cremer M, Holland E, Adams B, et al: Adolescent comprehension of emergency contraception in New York City, *Obstet Gynecol* 113(4):840–844, 2009.

Gavin L, MacKay AP, Brown K, et al: Sexual and reproductive health of persons aged 10-24 years—United States, 2002-2007, *MMWR Surveill Summ* 58(6):1–58, 2009.

Lara-Torre E, Schroeder B: Adolescent compliance and side effects with Quick Start initiation of oral contraceptive pills, *Contraception* 66(2):81–85, 2002.

van den Heuvel MW, van Bragt AJ, Alnabawy AK, Kaptein MC: Comparison of ethinylestradiol pharmacokinetics in three hormonal contraceptive formulations: the vaginal ring, the transdermal patch and an oral contraceptive, *Contraception* 72(3):168–174, 2005.

HPV

American College of Obstetricians and Gynecologists: ACOG practice bulletin: clinical management guidelines for obstetrician-gynecologists no. 61: human papillomavirus, *Obstet Gynecol* 105(4):905–918, 2005.

Arbyn M, Bergeron C, Klinkhamer P, et al: Liquid compared with conventional cervical cytology: a systematic review and meta-analysis, *Obstet Gynecol* 111(1):167–177, 2008.

Castle PE, Cox JT, Jeronimo J, et al: An analysis of high-risk human papillomavirus DNA-negative cervical precancers in the ASCUS-LSIL Triage Study (ALTS), *Obstet Gynecol* 111(4):847–856, 2008.

Committee on Adolescent Care, et al: ACOG Committee opinion no. 344: human papillomavirus vaccination, *Obstet Gynecol* 108(3 Pt 1):699–705, 2006.

Gage JC, Hanson VW, Abbey K, et al: Number of cervical biopsies and sensitivity of colposcopy, *Obstet Gynecol* 108(2):264–272, 2006.

Hildesheim A, Herrero R, Wacholder S, et al: Effect of human papillomavirus 16/18 L1 viruslike particle vaccine among young women with preexisting infection: a randomized trial, *JAMA* 298(7):743–753, 2007.

Moscicki AB, Ma Y, Wibbelsman C, et al: Risks for cervical intraepithelial neoplasia 3 among adolescents and young women with abnormal cytology, *Obstet Gynecol* 112(6):1335–1342, 2008.

Runowicz CD: Molecular screening for cervical cancer—time to give up Pap tests? *N Engl J Med* 357(16):1650–1653, 2007.

Steinbrook R: The potential of human papillomavirus vaccines, *N Engl J Med* 354(11):1109–1112, 2006.

Wright TC Jr, Massad LS, Dunton CJ, et al: 2006 consensus guidelines for the management of women with abnormal cervical cancer screening tests, *Am J Obstet Gynecol* 197(4):346–355, 2007.

Sexually Transmitted Diseases

American College of Obstetricians and Gynecologists Committee on Practice Bulletins—Gynecology: clinical management guidelines for obstetrician-gynecologists no. 57: gynecologic herpes simplex virus infections, *Obstet Gynecol* 104(5 Pt 1):1111–1117, 2004.

Chou R, Huffman LH, Fu R, et al: Screening for HIV: a review of the evidence for the U.S. Preventive Services Task Force, *Ann Intern Med* 143(1):55–73, 2005.

Hoover K, Tao G, Kent C: Low rates of both asymptomatic chlamydia screening and diagnostic testing of women in US outpatient clinics, *Obstet Gynecol* 112(4):891–898, 2008.

Primary and Preventive Care

American College of Obstetricians and Gynecologists: ACOG committee opinion no. 314: meningococcal vaccination for adolescents, *Obstet Gynecol* 108(3):667–669, 2005.

American College of Obstetricians and Gynecologists Committee on Adolescent Health: ACOG committee opinion no. 335: the initial reproductive health visit, *Obstet Gynecol* 107(5):1215–1219, 2006.

American College of Obstetricians and Gynecologists Committee on Adolescent Health Care: ACOG committee opinion no. 350: breast concerns in the adolescent, *Obstet Gynecol* 108(5):1329–1336, 2006.

American College of Obstetricians and Gynecologists Committee on Gynecologic Practice: ACOG committee opinion no. 452: primary and preventive care: periodic assessments, *Obstet Gynecol* 114(6):1444–1451, 2009.

Pichichero ME, Rennels MB, Edwards KM, et al: Combined tetanus, diphtheria, and 5-component pertussis vaccine for use in adolescents and adults, *JAMA* 293(24):3003–3011, 2005.

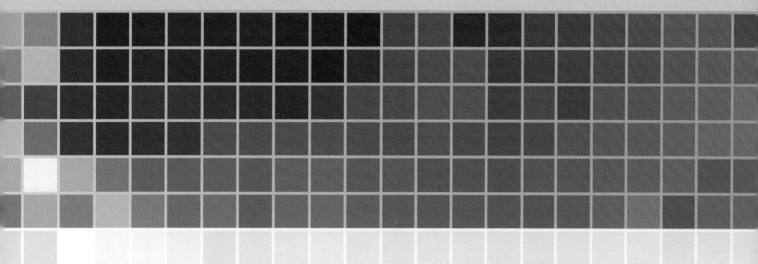

Pregnancy: The First Trimester

Chapter 4

Prenatal Care

THOMAS R. MOORE

KEY UPDATES

1. All pregnant women should be tested for syphilis at their first prenatal visit. For women in high-risk groups, many organizations recommend repeated serologic testing in the third trimester and at delivery.

2. All pregnant women and their partners should be asked about past genital and orolabial herpes simplex virus (HSV) infection. Women with recurrent genital herpes should be offered suppressive antiviral therapy in the late third trimester.

3. All pregnant or preconceptional women in high-risk groups should be screened for hemoglobinopathies.

4. The American College of Obstetricians and Gynecologists (ACOG) recommends offering carrier screening for *four* diseases (cystic fibrosis, Tay Sachs, Canavan disease, and familial dysautonomia) to couples with one or both parents of Ashkenazi background.

5. A *psychosocial screening tool should be used in at-risk women early in pregnancy and at the postpartum visit.*

6. Use the 5 A's for smoking cessation.

7. Women who have undergone bariatric surgery or who are vegans should be evaluated for nutritional deficiencies and vitamin supplementation where indicated.

8. The Institute of Medicine has recently changed the recommendations for total weight gain based on the prepregnant or initial pregnant body mass index (BMI). In obese women the recommended weight gain has been reduced to 11 to 20 pounds.

9. ACOG recommends psychosocial screening at least once per trimester to increase the likelihood of identifying important issues and reducing poor birth outcomes.

The Prenatal Care Record

- Because of the complexity of contemporary antepartum surveillance, and also because of increased medicolegal scrutiny, the prenatal chart has assumed a position of extreme importance.
- The completeness and accuracy of the prenatal record frequently determines the effectiveness of management. Sloppy or incomplete prenatal data increases medicolegal exposure.
- Use of an electronic health record (EHR) enhances completeness, accuracy, and availability of the pregnant woman's prenatal issues.

First Prenatal Visit

HISTORY

- Date of last menstrual period, cycle length
- Determination of estimated delivery date (EDD)
- Race, ethnicity, country of origin, primary language,
- Relationship status, education, occupation
- Medical history
- Surgical history
- Family history
- Psychiatric history
- Genetic history
- Medication allergies
- Previous pregnancies and outcomes
- Gynecologic history including sexually transmitted infections

PHYSICAL EXAMINATION

- Vital signs, height and weight
- Calculation of body mass index (BMI)
- Thyroid
- Heart, lungs
- Back, spine
- Abdomen
- Extremities
- Pelvic examination

41

- Ultrasound evaluation for dating (crown rump length) and viability.

SCREENING

All pregnant women should undergo or be offered screening for the following at the first prenatal visit:

- Hemoglobin/hematocrit
- Blood type and antibody screen
- Rubella if immunity not previously documented
- Syphilis

UPDATE #1

The U.S. Preventive Services Task Force has reaffirmed its recommendation that all pregnant women should be tested for syphilis at their first prenatal visit. For women in high-risk groups, many organizations recommend repeated serologic testing in the third trimester and at delivery (U.S. Preventive Services Task Force, 2009).

- HIV
- Hepatitis B surface antigen
- Herpes simplex virus (HSV)

UPDATE #2

All pregnant women and their partners should be asked about past genital and orolabial herpes simplex virus (HSV) infection. Active HSV infection during vaginal delivery or after prolonged rupture of membranes poses a risk of vertical transmission of 30% to 60% for a primary infection and 3% for a recurrent HSV infection. Women with recurrent genital herpes should be offered suppressive antiviral therapy, because the rate of HSV shedding at delivery is reduced by 75% and the rate of cesarean delivery reduced by 40% (Centers for Disease Control, 2006).

- Infection screening for at-risk populations
  - Hepatitis C (if at-risk)
  - Chlamydia and gonorrhea (at-risk populations)
  - Tuberculosis (at-risk populations.)
- History of disease or prior immunity or obtain antibody status for
  - Varicella
  - Tetanus
- Urine culture
- Urine dipstick for protein and glucose determination as indicated
- Pap smear with reflex human papillomavirus (HPV) testing (if not normal within previous 3 months)
- Genetic screening questionnaire
- Aneuploidy screening via first trimester serum or serum + ultrasound (10 to 14 weeks)
- Specific genetic screening for at-risk populations:
  - Hemoglobinopathies

UPDATE #3

All pregnant or preconceptional women in high-risk groups should be screened for hemoglobinopathies.
   High risk: African, Southeast Asian, and Mediterranean ancestry.
   Low risk: northern Europeans, Japanese, Native Americans, Inuit, and Koreans.

Tests to perform:
   For Southeast Asian or Mediterranean descent: CBC and MCV. If anemia with reduced MCV is found with normal iron studies, a hemoglobin electrophoresis should be obtained. If this is normal and the individual is not Southeast Asian, no further workup is needed. If the patient is Southeast Asian, consider evaluation for alpha-thalassemia using DNA-based testing.
   In African descent, a CBC and hemoglobin electrophoresis will be diagnostic (American College of Obstetricians and Gynecologists, ACOG Practice Bulletin No. 78, 2007).

- Cystic fibrosis
- Ashkenazi Jewish screening

UPDATE #4

ACOG recommends offering carrier screening for *four* diseases (cystic fibrosis, Tay Sachs, Canavan disease, and familial dysautonomia) to couples with one or both parents with Ashkenazi background. ACOG added familial dysautonomia as a recommendation in 2007.

Offer carrier testing for other diseases increased among Ashkenazi Jews if family history indicates (e.g., Bloom, Fanconi, Gaucher, Niemann-Pick, Mucolipidosis IV). Offer invasive fetal testing if both parents are carriers for any of these diseases (American College of Obstetricians and Gynecologists, Opinion No. 442, 2009).

- Gestational diabetes. High-risk should be screened in the first trimester:
  - Marked obesity (BMI greater than 27 kg/m2)
  - Diabetes in a first-degree relative
  - History of glucose intolerance
  - Previous infant greater than 4500 grams
  - Current glycosuria
  - Previous impaired fasting glucose with fasting 110 to 125 mg/dL
  - Previous gestational diabetes mellitus
  - Screening for these patients should occur at the initial antepartum visit or as soon as possible
- Psychosocial questionnaire

UPDATE #5

Psychosocial Screening Tool

1. Do you have any problems (job, transportation, etc.) that prevent you from keeping your health care appointments?
2. Do you feel unsafe where you live?
3. In the past 2 months have you used any form of tobacco?
4. In the past 2 months have you used drugs or alcohol (including beer, wine, or mixed drinks)?
5. Has anyone forced you to perform any sexual act that you did not want to do?
6. On a 1 to 5 scale, how do you rate your current stress level?
7. How many times have you moved in the past 12 months?
8. If you could change the timing of this pregnancy, would you want it earlier, later, not at all, no change?

(American College of Obstetricians and Gynecologists, Committee Opinion No. 316, 2005)

- Medication use (illicit, prescribed, over the counter, dietary/herbal supplements)
- Nicotine use
- Alcohol use
- Environmental exposures: smoke, seafood.
- Exercise

- Household pets
- Dietary habits or restrictions
- Universal prenatal screening *not* recommended:
  - Maternal lead exposure
  - Maternal periodontal disease
  - Maternal bacterial vaginosis

EDUCATION

- Avoid tobacco, alcohol, illicit drugs
  - Fetal alcohol syndrome (FAS) is a preventable cause of mental disability, with an incidence of 9 per 1000 births. Among reproductive-age women, 10% are heavy drinkers and 34% binge drink. Screening for maternal alcohol use has been shown to result in reduced alcohol consumption (American College of Obstetricians and Gynecologists, Opinion No. 422, 2008).
  - Smoking cessation should be discussed at each visit. Prenatal tobacco cessation programs are effective in reducing smoking rates and the frequency of low-birth-weight infants.

UPDATE #6

Use the 5 A's for smoking cessation:
- *Ask*—about smoking status
- *Advise*—to stop smoking with clear message of benefits
- *Assess*—willingness to attempt to quit in next 30 days
- *Assist*—by providing pregnancy-specific self-help materials
- *Arrange*—follow-up visits to track progress
(American College of Obstetricians and Gynecologists, Opinion No. 316, 2005; U.S. Preventive Services Task Force, 2009)

- Prenatal vitamins, folic acid, and nutritional supplements
  - All women should take a prenatal vitamin with 400 to 1000 mcg folic acid and at least 30 mg iron daily. Other nutritional supplements have not been demonstrated to improve outcome in unselected populations.

UPDATE #7

Women who have undergone bariatric surgery or who are vegans may have deficiencies in iron, vitamin B_{12}, folate, and calcium. Patients should be evaluated for nutritional deficiencies and vitamin supplementation where indicated (American College of Obstetricians and Gynecologists, Opinion No. 315, 2005).

- The requirements for omega-3 fatty acids during pregnancy have not been established. Omega-3 fatty acids are critical for fetal neurodevelopment and may be important for the timing of gestation and birth weight. For pregnant women to obtain adequate omega-3 fatty acids, a variety of sources must be consumed: vegetable oils, two low-mercury fish servings a week, and supplements (fish oil or algae-based docosahexaenoic acid).
- Calcium supplementation is recommended for pregnant women with poor dietary calcium intake.
- Vitamin D supplementation in pregnancy is recommended for women who are complete vegetarians and those who lack vitamin D–fortified milk in their diet. These women should receive 400 IU or 10 micrograms of vitamin D daily.
- There is no demonstrated benefit for universal prenatal supplementation of the following:
  - Multivitamins
  - Magnesium
  - Amino acids/protein supplements
  - Pyridoxine (vitamin B_6)
  - Zinc
  - High doses of vitamin A and molybdenum are contraindicated in pregnancy
- Gestational weight gain goals based on patient's BMI
  - Obesity or underweight
  - The patient's BMI should be calculated at the first prenatal visit, and weight gain during pregnancy should be monitored at each subsequent prenatal visit.

UPDATE #8

The Institute of Medicine has recently changed the recommendations for total weight gain based on the prepregnant or initial pregnant BMI. In obese women, the recommended weight gain has been reduced to 11 to 20 pounds (Table 4-1) (Rasmussen et al, 2009).

- Safe physical activities
- Using seat belts
- Benefits of breast-feeding for infant and mother
- Risk factors for sexually transmitted infections including HIV
- Value of seasonal and H1N1 influenza immunization
- Environmental exposures
  - Cat feces
  - Raw meats
  - High temperatures (saunas/hot tubs, etc.)
  - Secondhand smoke

TABLE 4-1   **New Recommendations for Total and Rate of Weight Gain during Pregnancy, by Pregnancy BMI**

Prepregnancy BMI	Total Weight Gain		Rates of Weight Gain* Second and Third Trimester	
	Range in kg	Range in lbs	Mean (range) in kg/week	Mean (range) in lbs/week
Underweight (< 18.5 kg/m²)	12.5-18	28-40	0.51 (0.44-0.58)	1 (1-1.3)
Normal weight (18.5–24.9 kg/m²)	11.5-16	25-35	0.42 (0.35-0.50)	1 (0.8-1)
Overweight (25.0–29.9 kg/m²)	7-11.5	15-25	0.28 (0.23-0.33)	0.6 (0.5-0.7)
Obese (≥ 30.0 kg/m²)	5-9	11-20	0.22 (0.17-0.27)	0.5 (0.4-0.6)

*Calculations assume a 0.5-2 kg (1.1-4.4 lbs) weight gain in the first trimester (based on Siega-Riz et al., 1994; Abrams et al., 1995; Carmichael et al., 1997).
From Institute of Medicine (US) and National Research Council (US) Committee to Reexamine Institute of Medicine Pregnancy Weight Guidelines: *weight gain during pregnancy: reexamining the guidelines*, Washington, DC, May 2009, National Academic Press.

- Registering for childbirth, breast-feeding, and infant cardiopulmonary resuscitation (CPR) education classes

At Each Prenatal Visit

SCREENING

- Gestational age, maternal vital signs, and weight
- Uterine fundal height (20 to 36 weeks)
- Urinary protein and glucose
- Fetal cardiac activity
- Fetal movements (after 20 weeks)
- Maternal stress, depression, physical abuse, and pain
- Contractions, bleeding, leaking fluid

Second Trimester (14 to 27 weeks)

SCREENING

- Multiple marker aneuploidy screen blood test for aneuploidy and neural tube defects (16 to 20 weeks)
- Fetal anatomy ultrasound for gestational age, growth, structural anomalies, and markers of aneuploidy (18 to 20 weeks)
- Gestational diabetes (24 to 28 weeks)

EDUCATION

- Signs and symptoms of preterm labor
- Plans for urgent medical transportation to hospital, child care
- Childbirth options and preferences
- Benefits of breast-feeding
- Registration for childbirth, breast-feeding, infant CPR classes
- Postpartum living arrangements

Third Trimester (28 to 40 weeks)

SCREENING

- Antibody testing for Rh-negative patients (28 weeks)
- Administer Rh immune globulin as indicated (28 weeks)
- Repeat screening for HIV, syphilis, chlamydia, gonorrhea, other sexually transmitted infections (if high risk) (28 to 32 weeks)
- Repeat screening for depression
- The prevalence of depression in pregnant women and new mothers is 5% to 25%; untreated depression is associated with poor prenatal clinic attendance, substance misuse, poor weight gain, and fetal growth restriction

> **UPDATE #9**
> ACOG recommends psychosocial screening at least once per trimester to increase the likelihood of identifying important issues and reducing poor birth outcomes (American College of Obstetricians and Gynecologists, Opinion No. 343, 2006).

- Group B streptococcus rectovaginal culture (35 to 37 weeks)

EDUCATION

- Maternal
  - Signs and symptoms of preeclampsia
  - Travel restrictions
  - Family planning after delivery
  - Returning to work or other activities and related issues, including mental/physical health and disability
  - Signs and symptoms of postpartum depression
- Fetal
  - Instruct in fetal movement counting
- Birthing
  - Signs and symptoms of labor
  - Risk factors for preterm labor
    - Pathologic distention of the uterus
    - Low socioeconomic status
    - Cervical cerclage
    - Low BMI
    - Prior cone biopsy or loop electrosurgical excision procedure (LEEP)
    - Prior myomectomy
    - Prior preterm delivery
    - Three or more first-trimester losses
    - Cocaine, marijuana, benzodiazepine, or other street drug use
    - Domestic violence or life stress
    - Intrauterine growth retardation
    - Tobacco use
    - Periodontal disease
    - Pyelonephritis or urinary tract infection
    - Vaginal bleeding after 12 weeks
    - Polyhydramnios
    - Uterine anomalies
  - Birth planning (preferences and concerns about birthing, pain control, others to be present)
  - Anesthesia and analgesia options
  - Episiotomy
  - Postdates management
- Infant
  - Circumcision
  - Benefits of breast-feeding
  - Attending infant CPR class
  - Obtaining a car seat for the baby
  - Choosing a clinician for the baby and scheduling a prenatal visit, if desired

Post Due Date (40 to 42 weeks)

SCREENING

- Antenatal biophysical testing (nonstress test [NST] with amniotic fluid index [AFI] or biophysical profile [BPP])
- Cervical exam
- Review fetal movement counting

EDUCATION

- Stillbirth risks
- Methods of labor induction

Postpartum Visit

INTERVAL HISTORY

- Breast issues: mastitis, milk supply
- Surgical site complications: perineal, abdominal
- Uterine bleeding
- Incontinence: bowel or bowel

- Medical complications: hypertension, diabetes
- Mood disturbances
- Immunizations: rubella, tetanus, diphtheria, and pertussis vaccine (Tdap)
- Coitus
- Infant

PHYSICAL EXAMINATION

- Thyroid
- Breasts including nipples and axillae
- Abdomen including cesarean scar if present
- Perineum including episiotomy or laceration repairs
- Vagina and cervix
- Uterus and adnexae
- Pelvic support musculature

SCREENING

- Pap smear if indicated
- Screen for postpartum depression and psychosocial assessment
- Diabetes

EDUCATION

- Breast-feeding plans: emphasize American College of Obstetricians and Gynecologists (ACOG)/American Academy of Pediatrics (AAP)/American Academy of Family Practice (AAFP) recommendation of exclusive breast-feeding for at least 6 months
- Returning to work, maintaining milk supply, safe medications for breast-feeding, and so on
- Losing weight gained during pregnancy, plus additional weight loss if initial BMI >25
- Family planning and birth control
- Resuming sexual activity
- Preconception counseling and risk factors for future pregnancies
- Plans to address other health issues identified during pregnancy; link patient with primary care provider as needed

SUGGESTED READINGS

Practice Guidelines Relevant to Prenatal Care

Abrams B, Selvin S: Maternal weight gain pattern and birth weight, *Obstet Gynecol* 86(2):163–169, 1995 Aug.

American Academy of Pediatrics, The American College of Obstetricians and Gynecologists: *Guidelines for perinatal care*, ed 6, Washington, DC, 2007.

American College of Obstetricians and Gynecologists: ACOG committee opinion no. 315: obesity in pregnancy, *Obstet Gynecol* 106(3):671–675, 2005.

American College of Obstetricians and Gynecologists: ACOG committee opinion no. 316: smoking cessation during pregnancy, *Obstet Gynecol* 106(4):883–888, 2005.

American College of Obstetricians and Gynecologists: ACOG committee opinion no. 419: use of progesterone to reduce preterm birth, *Obstet Gynecol* 112(4):963–965, 2008.

American College of Obstetricians and Gynecologists: ACOG committee opinion no. 438: update on immunization and pregnancy: tetanus, diphtheria, and pertussis vaccination, *Obstet Gynecol* 114(2 Pt 1):398–400, 2009.

American College of Obstetricians and Gynecologists: ACOG practice bulletin no. 55: management of postterm pregnancy, *Obstet Gynecol* 104(3):639–646, 2004.

American College of Obstetricians and Gynecologists: ACOG practice bulletin no. 60: pregestational diabetes mellitus, *Obstet Gynecol* 105(3):675–685, 2005.

American College of Obstetricians and Gynecologists: ACOG practice bulletin no. 78: Hemoglobinopathies in pregnancy, *Obstet Gynecol* 109(1):229–237, 2007.

American College of Obstetricians and Gynecologists: ACOG practice bulletin no. 115: vaginal birth after previous cesarean delivery, *Obstet Gynecol* 116:450–463, 2010.

Carmichael S, Abrams B, Selvin S: The pattern of maternal weight gain in women with good pregnancy outcomes, *Am J Public Health* 87(12):1984–1988, 1997 Dec.

Duhl AJ, Paidas MJ, Ural SH, et al: Antithrombotic therapy and pregnancy: consensus report and recommendations for prevention and treatment of venous thromboembolism and adverse pregnancy outcomes, *Am J Obstet Gynecol* 197(5):457, e1–e21, 2007.

Institute of Medicine (US) and National Research Council (US) Committee to Reexamine IOM Pregnancy Weight Guidelines: *Weight gain during pregnancy: reexamining the guidelines*, Washington, DC, 2009, National Academies Press.

National High Blood Pressure Education Program Working Group on High Blood Pressure in Pregnancy: Report of the national high blood pressure education program working group on high blood pressure in pregnancy, *Am J Obstet Gynecol* 183(1):S1–S22, 2000.

Siega-Riz AM, Adair LS, Hobel CJ: Institute of Medicine maternal weight gain recommendations and pregnancy outcome in a predominantly Hispanic population, *Obstet Gynecol* 84(4):565–573, 1994 Oct.

Tita ATN, Landon MB, Spong CY, et al: Timing of elective repeat cesarean delivery at term and neonatal outcomes, *N Engl J Med* 360(2):111–120, 2009.

Screening Tests in Prenatal Care

American College of Obstetricians and Gynecologists: ACOG committee opinion no. 325: update on carrier screening for cystic fibrosis, *Obstet Gynecol* 106(6):1465–1468, 2005.

American College of Obstetricians and Gynecologists: ACOG committee opinion no. 442: preconception and prenatal carrier screening for genetic disease of Eastern European Jewish descent, *Obstet Gynecol* 114(4):950–953, 2009.

American College of Obstetricians and Gynecologists: ACOG committee opinion no. 453: screening for depression during and after pregnancy, *Obstet Gynecol* 115(2 Pt 1):394–395, 2010.

American College of Obstetricians and Gynecologists: ACOG practice bulletin no. 58: ultrasonography in pregnancy, *Obstet Gynecol* 104(6):1449–1458, 2004.

American College of Obstetricians and Gynecologists: ACOG practice bulletin no. 77: screening for fetal chromosomal abnormalities, *Obstet Gynecol* 109(1):217–227, 2007.

Infections in Pregnancy

American College of Obstetricians and Gynecologists: ACOG committee opinion no. 411: routine human immunodeficiency virus screening, *Obstet Gynecol* 111(6):1495–1502, 2008.

American College of Obstetricians and Gynecologists: ACOG practice bulletin no. 82: management of herpes in pregnancy, *Obstet Gynecol* 109(6):1489–1498, 2007.

American College of Obstetricians and Gynecologists: ACOG practice bulletin no. 86: viral hepatitis in pregnancy, *Obstet Gynecol* 110(4):941–956, 2007.

American College of Obstetricians and Gynecologists Committee on Obstetric Practice: ACOG Committee Opinion No. 485: Prevention of early-onset group B streptococcal disease in newborns, *Obstet Gynecol* 117(4):1019–1027, 2011 Apr.

Centers for Disease Control: *Pregnant women and novel influenza A (H1N1) considerations for clinicians* (website). www.dcd.gov.h1n1flu/clinical pregnant.htm. Accessed 2009.

U.S. Preventive Services Task Force: Screening for bacterial vaginosis in pregnancy: recommendations and rationale, *Am J Prev Med* 20 (Suppl 3):59–61, 2001.

U.S. Preventive Services Task Force: Screening for chlamydial infection: U.S. prevention services force recommendation statement, *Ann Intern Med* 147(2):128–134, 2007.

U.S. Preventive Services Task Force: Screening for syphilis infection in pregnancy: U.S. preventive services task force reaffirmation recommendation statement, *Ann Intern Med* 150(10):705–709, 2009.

References

Please go to expertconsult.com to view references.

Chapter 5

Ectopic Pregnancy: Diagnosis and Management

DEIRDRE A. CONWAY • MOUSA I. SHAMONKI

KEY UPDATES

1 Timely diagnosis of ectopic pregnancy (EP) is imperative to early intervention. New diagnostic algorithms integrating transvaginal ultrasound and serum human chorionic gonadotropin (hCG) measurements have assisted in this process.

2 Undiagnosed EP increases the risk of rupture, maternal morbidity, and mortality.

3 Using a "discriminatory zone" serum hCG level of 1500 to 2000 mIU/mL, above which an intrauterine pregnancy should be seen on transvaginal ultrasound, helps to raise suspicion of EP.

4 The risk of a failing medical treatment with methotrexate (MTX) rises with rising serum hCG levels.

5 With a rising number of women conceiving through infertility treatment, the incidence of heterotopic pregnancy has risen markedly. Thus, clinicians should have a high index of suspicion in women who conceive through the use of infertility treatment.

Ectopic pregnancy (EP) is defined as any pregnancy that implants outside the uterine cavity.

Background

INCIDENCE AND EPIDEMIOLOGY

- The most common site of EP is in the fallopian tube, accounting for over 95% of all EPs
  - Tubal sites: ampullary (55%), isthmic (25%), fimbrial (17%)
  - Other sites (3%): abdominal cavity, ovary, and cervix
- Incidence of EP has increased from approximately 0.5% of pregnancies in 1970 to 2% of pregnancies by 1992
- Rising incidence is thought to be associated with increased incidence of pelvic inflammatory disease leading to damaged fallopian tubes
- Recent noninvasive diagnostic methods and algorithims have led to earlier diagnosis and therefore a greater use of conservative treatment modalities
- However, ruptured EP still accounts for approximately 10% of all pregnancy-related deaths, despite improved diagnostic tools

UPDATE #1

Timely diagnosis is imperative. Studies have demonstrated the utility of noninvasive diagnostic algorithms integrating transvaginal ultrasound and serum human chorionic gonadotropin (hCG) measurement. The use of these diagnostic tools has been integrated into prediction models aiding with diagnosis and early intervention (Condous et al, 2004).

Risk Factors

HIGH-RISK FACTORS

- Prior ectopic pregnancy: approximately 15% risk for recurrence
- Known tubal pathology from infection or congenital anomalies
- Tubal reconstructive surgery or sterilization: one third of pregnancies following sterilization are ectopic
- In utero diethylstilbestrol (DES) exposure: ninefold increased risk of EP
- Intrauterine contraception: although overall ectopic risk is reduced, if pregnancy occurs there is a much higher risk that it will be an EP

MODERATE TO LOW-RISK FACTORS

- Prior pelvic infections such as chlamydia, gonorrhea, or nonspecific peritonitis
- Multiple sexual partners: likely related to an increased risk of acquiring pelvic infections
- Infertility: could reflect increased prevalence of tubal disease in this population

- Tobacco use: possibly reflecting an effect of tobacco use on tubal motility
- In-vitro fertilization (IVF): overall rate of EP in pregnancies conceived through IVF is 2% to 3%, only slightly higher than the overall rate of EP in the United States

Diagnosis

UPDATE #2

Undiagnosed tubal ectopic pregnancy increases the risk for rupture and maternal morbidity and mortality. When ectopic pregnancy was suspected, four factors increased the risk of rupture: (1) never having used contraception, (2) a history of tubal damage and infertility, (3) induction of ovulation, and (4) a high level of hCG (>10,000 IU/L) (Job-Spira et al, 1999).

DIFFERENTIAL DIAGNOSIS

- Appendicitis
- Endometriosis
- Leiomyomas, particularly degenerating
- Pelvic infections
- Ovarian neoplasms
- Ovarian torsion
- Abnormal or normal intrauterine pregnancy
- Urinary tract abnormalities
- Small or large bowel abnormalities

SYMPTOMS

- Any sexually active woman of reproductive age with abdominal pain or vaginal bleeding should be screened for pregnancy
- High suspicion for EP aids in early diagnosis, preventing ruptured EP
- Classic symptoms of ruptured or unruptured EP:
  - Abdominal pain (99%)
  - Amenorrhea (74%)
  - Vaginal bleeding (56%)

SERUM MARKERS: hCG

- Most intrauterine pregnancies are visible by high-resolution transvaginal ultrasound (TVUS) with an hCG level of ≥1500 IU/L to 2000 mIU/mL, referred to as the "discriminatory zone"
- Absence of an intrauterine gestational sac visualized on TVUS, above the discriminatory zone, is highly suspicious for an EP or abnormal intrauterine pregnancy
- At hCG levels below the discriminatory zone, serial hCG measurements every 48 hours can be particularly useful in determining pregnancy location
- Mean serum hCG doubling time is approximately 2 days for viable intrauterine pregnancies, ranging from 1.4 to 2.1 days
- Abnormally rising serum hCG levels raise suspicion for EP:
  - An increase in serum hCG of under 53% over 48 hours is 99% sensitive at confirming an early, abnormal pregnancy
  - An increase in serum hCG of under 66% over 48 hours is 85% sensitive at confirming an early, abnormal pregnancy

UPDATE #3

Although initially reported to be between 1500 and 2000 mIU/mL, the discriminatory hCG value has been suggested to range between 1500 and 3000 nIU/mL, depending on the ultrasound, examiner, and anatomic factors. It should be kept in mind that using a value at the lower threshold of the range will increase the sensitivity for diagnosing an ectopic, but it will also increase the rate of false positives. Conversely, using a higher discriminatory value will increase specificity but will increase the rate of false negatives (Barnhart, 2009).

TRANSVAGINAL ULTRASOUND (TVUS)

- TVUS should be used routinely to detect the presence, or absence, of a pregnancy within the uterus
- A gestational sac containing a yolk sac with or without an embryo within the uterine cavity confirms an intrauterine pregnancy
- When the exact gestational age is known, if no gestational sac is visualized at or beyond 24 days following conception, abnormal pregnancy is highly likely
- When the exact gestational age is not known, the "discriminatory zone" for serum hCG is used in conjunction with TVUS to gauge suspicion for EP, as described under Serum markers: hCG
- If no intrauterine pregnancy is visualized below the hCG discriminatory zone and the patient is stable and asymptomatic, serum hCG should be repeated in 48 hours
- If no intrauterine pregnancy is visualized above the hCG discriminatory zone, suspicion for EP should be high and treatment should be considered
- The most common ultrasonographic finding in tubal pregnancy is an extraovarian adnexal mass; therefore, the space between the uterus and the ovary should be carefully inspected
- Sonographic adnexal findings in the case of an EP can vary, but confirmation is made when an extrauterine sac with a yolk sac or an embryo with cardiac activity is visualized
- An adnexal finding suggestive of an early ectopic pregnancy is a highly echogenic "tubal ring" with no yolk sac; however, this is not entirely diagnostic and should be discriminated from a corpus luteum when in or near the ovary
- A small amount of free fluid in the cul-de-sac is normal; however, larger quantities of free fluid is likely pathologic, particularly if it is echogenic or complex, suggesting hemoperitoneum
- Small, centrally located collections of fluid in the endometrial cavity called "pseudosacs" can be seen in up to 20% of EPs and can sometimes be confused with an intrauterine pregnancy

SERUM MARKERS: PROGESTERONE

- Serum progesterone levels over 20 ng/mL are typically associated with viable intrauterine pregnancies
- Thus, abnormal progesterone levels can raise suspicion of an abnormally developing pregnancy (either ectopic or failed intrauterine pregnancy)
  - Levels under 5 ng/mL have a specificity of 100% in confirming an abnormal pregnancy
  - Levels between 5 and 20 ng/mL are considered equivocal

- The majority of ectopic pregnancies are associated with progesterone levels ranging from 10 to 20 ng/mL, limiting the clinical utility of progesterone in discriminating between viable, nonviable, and ectopic pregnancies

SUCTION OR SHARP INTRAUTERINE CURETTAGE

- Trophoblastic tissue obtained by curettage confirms the presence of an intrauterine pregnancy
- Although this option is most often used when discriminating between a failed intrauterine pregnancy and an EP, clinical application is limited by the small chance of disrupting a normal intrauterine pregnancy
- Furthermore, false negatives can occur; in up to 20% of pathology specimens from elective terminations, chorionic villi are not detected
- If there is remaining uncertainty, a decrease in the hCG level of 20% or more 12 to 24 hours after intrauterine curettage suggests that the trophoblastic cells were probably removed from the uterus
- Overall, the option of intrauterine curettage is currently used in low frequency because of the less invasive diagnostic modality of serum markers and TVUS

Treatment Options

OBSERVATION

- Generally recommended only when serum hCG levels are low (<200 IU/L) and decreasing, and the patient is asymptomatic and stable

WHEN LEVELS ARE UNDER 200 IU/L, 88% OF PATIENTS HAVE SPONTANEOUS RESOLUTION WITH METHOTREXATE (MTX)

- Mechanism of action
  - Initially used to treat gestational trophoblastic disease; used to treat ectopic pregnancies since 1982
  - Folic acid antagonist that inhibits DNA synthesis and cell turnover, particularly in rapidly dividing cells such as fetal cells
  - Rapidly cleared by the kidneys
  - Some protocols incorporate adjunctive treatment with reduced folates such as leucovorin, in order to spare other normally dividing cells in the body from toxicity
- Absolute contraindications (American College of Obstetricians and Gynecologists, 2008; Practice Committee of American Society for Reproductive Medicine, 2008)
  - Hemodynamic instability
  - Unrelenting or severe abdominal pain
  - Breast-feeding
  - Immune, hepatic, or renal dysfunction
  - Blood dyscrasia such as thrombocytopenia, bone marrow hypoplasia, leucopenia, or significant anemia
  - Heterotopic pregnancy with desired continuation of intrauterine pregnancy
  - Noncompliance or difficult access to a medical institution
  - Peptic ulcer disease
- Relative contraindications (ACOG Practice Bulletin No. 94; ASRM Practice Committee)
  - Embryonic cardiac activity
  - Gestational sac size of 3.5 cm or greater
  - Serum hCG level over 5,000 IU/L

UPDATE #4

The risk of failing MTX increases with increasing serum hCG levels. A level between 5000 and 10,000 IU/L leads to a 14% failure rate and if >10,000 IU/L; the rate of failure is 18% (Menon et al, 2007).

- Precautions during treatment
  - Avoid sun exposure to limit dermatitis
  - Avoid vitamins and foods with folic acid
  - Avoid nonsteroidal anti-inflammatory drugs
  - Avoid vaginal intercourse
- Single-dose MTX
  - Initial dose of 50 mg/m^2 IM on day 1
  - hCG levels are measured on days 4 and 7 post MTX administration
  - Levels from day 1 to day 4 can rise, but levels from day 4 to day 7 should drop by at least 15%
  - If levels do not drop appropriately on day 7, the patient should be reevaluated and a second MTX dose 50 mg/m^2 or a surgical approach should be considered
  - Approximately 15% to 20% of patients will require a second dose; however, less than 1% will need more than two doses
  - If a second dose is administered, the same algorithm is applied as noted previously
  - hCG levels should be checked weekly until undetectable
  - If hCG levels plateau during follow-up, a repeat dose of MTX should be considered
  - A recent meta-analysis showed a success rate of 88% for single-dose therapy; however, cumulative treatment success of single-dose MTX with repeat dosing as needed has been shown to be as high as 94% in different study
  - This treatment regimen is optimal in patients with a low initial hCG level
- Multiple-dose MTX with leucovorin rescue
  - MTX is administered 1 mg/kg IM on days 1, 3, 5, and 7
  - Leucovorin is given on alternating days (days 2, 4, 6, 8) at a dose of 0.1 mg/kg
  - hCG levels should be checked on days 1, 3, 5, and 7, and if the hCG level drops more than 15% from the prior measurement, treatment should be stopped
  - After treatment has stopped, hCG levels should be checked weekly; if levels drop less than 15% from the prior week, an additional dose of MTX 1 mg/kg IM should be given (and one dose of leucovorin on the following day)
  - hCG levels should be followed until undetectable
  - Efficacy is slightly higher than single-dose MTX: a recent meta-analysis of patients treated with the multiple-dose regimen found a 93% success rate
  - The same meta-analysis showed that the multiple-dose regimen was more effective at treating more advanced gestations and those with cardiac activity
- Two-dose MTX
  - Initial dose of 50 mg/m^2 IM on day 0, with repeat dose of 50 mg/m^2 IM on day 4
  - Measure hCG levels on days 4 and 7
  - If levels drop over 15% from day 4 to 7, measure hCG levels weekly until undetectable

- If levels drop less than 15% from day 4 to 7, give additional dose 50 mg/m^2 on days 7 and 11, measuring hCG levels
- Repeat algorithm, and if decrease is less than 15% during the second round, the patient should be reevaluated and surgical intervention considered
- The two-dose MTX regimen has 87% treatment success and high patient satisfaction; however, it has not been directly compared to the single- and multiple-dose regimens
- This regimen may be optimal for patients presenting with hCG values of over 5000
- MTX side effects
  - Typically mild and self-limited
  - Mild abdominal pain is common several days after receiving MTX, possibly related to tubal distention or abortion, and can be treated with acetaminophen
  - Occasionally pain can be severe; if hemodynamically stable, often these patients do not require surgical intervention
  - Other common side effects: stomatitis and conjunctivitis
  - Rare side effects: gastritis, enteritis, dermatitis, pneumonitis, alopecia

SURGICAL TREATMENTS

- Indications
  - Hemodynamic instability
  - Impending or ongoing rupture of ectopic mass
  - Contraindications to MTX
  - Heterotopic pregnancy
  - Noncompliance or lack of easy access to medical facility
  - Failed medical management
  - Desire for permanent contraception or plan to undergo IVF
- In a stable patient, surgery should be considered only if ultrasound is highly suggestive of a tubal ectopic pregnancy or adnexal mass; if no abnormality is visualized, the patient should ideally be followed with medical or expectant management and the ultrasound repeated in 2 to 7 days (Barnhart, 2009)
- Laparotomy
  - Reserved for hemodynamically unstable patients, patients with extensive bleeding, or laparoscopics with poor visualization
- Laparoscopy
  - The preferred surgical approach to a hemodynamically stable patient with an EP
  - Benefits of laparoscopy include shorter operation time, less perioperative blood loss, a shorter hospital stay, and, thus, lower costs
- Laparoscopic salpingostomy
  - Was traditionally the standard approach in women who desired fertility preservation
  - Can be considered in women who appear to have salvageable fallopian tubes on inspection during laparoscopy
  - However, salpingostomy is associated with a significantly higher rate of persistent or recurrent ectopic pregnancy when compared to laparoscopic salpingectomy
  - Furthermore, the chance of intrauterine conception has not been consistently shown to be higher following salpingostomy compared to salpingectomy
  - Salpingectomy is often the preferred option, because of a higher risk of recurrent ectopic with salpingostomy without clear benefit in subsequent intrauterine pregnancy rates
- Laparoscopic salpingectomy
  - Good candidates are patients that have a low probability of having normal tubal function in the future, and thus higher risk of recurrent EP, including patients with the following conditions:
    - Significantly damaged tubes
    - Large tubal diameter
    - Lack of hemostasis
    - History of more than one prior EP
    - Women who do not desire future childbearing or who plan to proceed with IVF
  - With no clear compromise to subsequent intrauterine pregnancy rates, along with a reduced risk of recurrent ectopic pregnancy compared to salpingostomy, salpingectomy is often the preferred surgical approach

Other Types of EP

OVARIAN EP

- Has become more common over the years, occurring in approximately 0.5% to 3% of EPs
- Appears to be a random event not associated with a history of infertility or tubal disease
- Diagnosing an ovarian EP on ultrasound can be challenging; therefore, the diagnosis is often confirmed intraoperatively
- Treatment typically involves surgical excision of the involved organ, although several case reports have shown that medical management with MTX can be successful

CERVICAL EP

- Pregnancy that implants in the endocervical canal
- Accounts for less than 1% of EPs and may be slightly more likely in pregnancies conceived through IVF
- Sonographic criteria include the following:
  - Gestational sac or placenta within the cervix
  - Normal endometrial stripe
  - Hourglass-shaped uterus with ballooned cervical canal
- Hemodynamically stable women are typically treated with a trial of multidose methotrexate, with intraamniotic or intrafetal injection of potassium chloride if fetal cardiac activity is present
- In patients who are hemodynamically unstable or who opt for surgical treatment, dilation and evacuation is the preferred approach; however, the risk of hemorrhage and need for a hysterectomy are high
- Preoperative uterine artery embolization has been suggested as a measure to prevent hemorrhage following dilation and evacuation

ABDOMINAL EP

- Pregnancy that has implanted in the peritoneal cavity
- Estimated to account for approximately 1.4% of EPs
- Risk factors include tubal disease, pelvic inflammatory disease, endometriosis, IVF, and multiparity
- If diagnosed early, laparoscopic removal is an option; preoperative selective arterial embrolization can minimize the risk of hemorrhage when removing the placenta

- Methotrexate therapy has been largely unsuccessful in treating early abdominal pregnancies
- Treatment of advanced abdominal pregnancies is primarily surgical, although the optimal approach is undetermined, and laparoscopy should be avoided when implantation on a vascular surface is suspected

HYSTEROTOMY SCAR EP

- Occurs in approximately 6% of EPs in women with a prior cesarean sections
- There is little evidence to support one treatment modality over another because reports of EP at this location are overall rare
- Medical management with systemic MTX with or without local injection of MTX or potassium chloride (if fetal cardiac activity is present) is an option; however, rupture, hemorrhage, and need for a hysterectomy are possible risks
- Surgical treatment options include wedge resection of the EP via laparotomy or laparoscopy if possible, or hysterectomy
- Uterine artery embolization has been used to reduce the risk of hemorrhage with surgery or MTX injection

INTERSTITIAL (CORNUAL) EP

- Pregnancy that occurs in the proximal end of the fallopian tube, which is embedded in the uterine myometrium
- Accounts for approximately 2% of all EPs
- Can be confused with intrauterine pregnancies because of its close proximity to the uterine cavity; thus uterine rupture is a more common presentation as a result of delayed diagnosis
- Diagnostic clues on ultrasound include an eccentric location and thin myometrium surrounding the gestational sac
- If diagnosed early, these patients can be treated medically similar to hysterotomy scar EP (discussed previously)
- If the patient is unstable or requires surgical intervention, cornual resection via laparotomy or laparoscopy is a viable alternative to hysterectomy, depending on the clinical scenario and the surgeon's expertise

---

UPDATE #5

With a rising number of women conceiving through infertility treatment, the incidence of heterotopic pregnancy has risen markedly. What was once thought to occur with an incidence of only 1 in 30,000 pregnancies has now increased to an incidence of approximately 1 in 3900 pregnancies. Thus, clinicians should have a high index of suspicion in women who conceive through the use of infertility treatment (Cheng et al, 2004).

HETEROTOPIC EP

- Concurrent pregnancies at two different sites, most often an intrauterine along with a tubal ectopic pregnancy
- With a rising number of women conceiving through infertility treatment, the incidence of heterotopic pregnancy has increased to approximately 1 in 3900 pregnancies
- The presence of a viable intrauterine prevents the use of MTX as a treatment option
- The standard approach for a simultaneous tubal EP is a laparoscopic salpingectomy if the patient is hemodynamically stable

SUGGESTED READINGS

Incidence and Epidemiology

Centers for Disease Control and Prevention (CDC): Ectopic pregnancy—United States, 1990-1992, *MMWR Morb Mortal Wkly Rep* 44(3):46–48, 1995.

Condous G, Okaro E, Khalid A, et al: The use of a new logistic regression model for predicting the outcome of pregnancies of unknown location, *Hum Reprod* 19:1900–1910, 2004.

Risk Factors

Job-Spira N, Fernandez H, Bouyer J, et al: Ruptured tubal ectopic pregnancy: risk factors and reproductive outcome: results of a population-based study in France, *Am J Obstet Gynecol* 180(4):938–944, 1999.

Yao M, Tulandi T: Current status of surgical and nonsurgical management of ectopic pregnancy, *Fertil Steril* 67(3):421–433, 1997.

Diagnosis

Barnhart KT: Clinical practice: ectopic pregnancy, *N Eng J Med* 361(4):379–387, 2009.

Condous G, Kirk E, Lu C, et al: Diagnostic accuracy of varying discriminatory zones for the prediction of ectopic pregnancy in women with a pregnancy of unknown location, *Ultrasound Obstet Gynecol* 26(7):770–775, 2005.

Kadar N, Bohrer M, Kemmann E, et al: The discriminatory human chorionic gonadotropin zone for endovaginal sonography: a prospective, randomized study, *Fertil Steril* 61(6):1016–1020, 1994.

Silva C, Sammel MD, Zhou L, et al: Human chorionic gonadotropin profile for women with ectopic pregnancy, *Obstet Gynecol* 107(3):605–610, 2006.

Treatment

American College of Obstetricians and Gynecologists: ACOG practice bulletin no. 94: medical management of ectopic pregnancy, *Obstet Gynecol* 111(6):1479–1485, 2008.

Barnhart KT, Gosman G, Ashby R, et al: The medical management of ectopic pregnancy: a meta-analysis comparing "single dose" and "multidose" regimens, *Obstet Gynecol* 101:778–784, 2003.

Dubuisson JM, Morice P, Chapron C, et al: Salpingectomy: the laparoscopic surgical choice for ectopic pregnancy, *Hum Reprod* 11(6):1199–1203, 1996.

Hajenius PJ, Mol F, Mol BW, et al: Interventions for tubal ectopic pregnancy, *Cochrane Database Syst Rev* 24(1):CD000324, 2007.

Menon S, Colins J, Barnhart KT: Establishing a human chorionic gonadotropin cutoff to guide methotrexate treatment of ectopic pregnancy: a systematic review, *Fertil Steril* 87(3):481, 2007.

Mol F, Mol BW, Ankum WM, et al: Current evidence on surgery, systemic methotrexate and expectant management in the treatment of tubal ectopic pregnancy: a systematic review and meta-analysis, *Hum Reprod Update* 14(4):309–319, 2008.

Practice Committee of American Society for Reproductive Medicine: Medical treatment of ectopic pregnancy, *Fertil Steril* 90(Suppl 5):S206–S212, 2008.

Other Types of EP

Atrash HK, Friede A, Hogue CJ: Abdominal pregnancy in the United States: frequency and maternal mortality, *Obstet Gynecol* 69(3 Pt 1):333–337, 1987.

Bouyer J, Coste J, Fernandez H, et al: Sites of ectopic pregnancy: a 10 year population-based study of 1800 cases, *Hum Reprod* 17(12):3224–3230, 2002.

Cheng PJ, Chueh HY, Qiu JT: Heterotopic pregnancy in natural conception cycle presenting as hematometra, *Obstet Gynecol* 104(5 Pt 2):1195, 2004.

Gaudoin MR, Coulter KL, Robins AM, et al: Is the incidence of ovarian ectopic pregnancy increasing? *Eur J Obstet Gynecol Reprod Biol* 70(2):141–143, 1996.

Hofman HM, Urdl W, Hofler H, et al: Cervical pregnancy: case reports and current concepts in diagnosis and treatment, *Arch Gynecol Obstet* 241(1):63–69, 1987.

Moawad NS, Mahajan ST, Moniz MH, et al: Current diagnosis and treatment of interstitial pregnancy, *Am J Obstet Gynecol* 202(1):15–29, 2010.

Rotas MA, Haberman S, Levgur M: Cesarean scar ectopic pregnancies: etiology, diagnosis, and management, *Obstet Gynecol* 107(6):1373–1381, 2006.

Yao M, Tulandi T: Practical and current management of tubal and non-tubal ectopic pregnancies, *Curr Probl Obstet Gynecol Fertil* 23:89, 2000.

References

Please go to expertconsult.com to view references.

Chapter 6

Gestational Trophoblastic Disease

SUSANNAH MAY MOURTON • ANNE O. RODRIGUEZ

KEY UPDATES

1 Cytogenetic studies of familial recurrent complete hydatidiform mole (CHM) show a biparental origin, and genetic mapping has identified causative genes on chromosome 19q13.4.

2 CHM are now diagnosed earlier and classic pathologic findings are often not present. The absence of P53 (KIP2) staining can help to differentiate this from a partial mole or hydropic abortion.

3 The likelihood of developing postmolar gestational trophoblastic disease (GTN) after one normal human chorionic gonadotropin (hCG) appears low, which may simplify surveillance after molar pregnancy.

4 In 2000, the International Federation of Gynecology and Obstetrics (FIGO) published a staging and risk factor scoring system for gestational trophoblastic diseases, which combines FIGO anatomic staging with a modified World Health Organization prognostic score.

5 Actinomycin-D may be associated with higher cure rates compared with methotrexate in low-risk GTN.

6 Quiescent GTN is a clinical entity of low hCG levels not responsive to chemotherapy in which the hyperglycosylated hCG is very low or absent. Close monitoring is required as some cases progress to invasive GTN and require treatment.

Overview of Gestational Trophoblastic Disease

- Spectrum of diseases: partial hydatidiform mole (PHM), complete hydatidiform mole (CHM); persistent, invasive, or metastatic mole; placental-site trophoblastic tumor (PSTT); gestational choriocarcinoma
- Gestational trophoblastic neoplasia (GTN) represents the malignant end of the spectrum (persistent, invasive, or metastatic mole; PSTT; and gestational choriocarcinoma)
- Incidence of molar pregnancies in the United States and Europe is approximately 1 in 1000, with higher rates in some parts of Asia and the Middle East (100 to 1000 per 100,000 pregnancies); the variation in worldwide incidence is likely related to differences in reporting (hospital versus population-based data)
- CHM: increased rates with decreased dietary carotene and animal fat, advanced maternal age, prior spontaneous abortion, and infertility
- PHM: diet and maternal age not risk factors
- Human chorionic gonadotrophin (hCG): highly sensitive and specific tumor marker used in diagnosis and treatment monitoring
- Highly chemosensitive: high cure rates even in the presence of metastatic disease
- Fertility-sparing treatment and subsequent pregnancy is possible in the majority of cases

Molar Pregnancy

CYTOGENETICS

- CHM: diploid androgenetic (46XX or 46XY), occurs from fertilization of an anuclear ovum by a haploid sperm (23X) with subsequent duplication (90%), or by two sperm (46XX or 46XY) (10%)
- PHM: triploid biparental (69XXY, 69XXX, or 69XYY) occurs from fertilization of a normal haploid (23X) ovum by two sperm

UPDATE #1

Recent studies in families with inherited CHM (autosomal recessive inheritance) have shown diploid biparental origin (compared with diploid androgenetic) and are associated with the *NALP7* gene located on chromosome 19q13.4 (Murdoch et al, 2006). Other genes have also been implicated showing genetic heterogeneity.

PRESENTATION AND DIAGNOSIS

- Signs/symptoms:
  - Vaginal bleeding
  - Size larger than dates

- Absent fetal heart sounds
- Markedly elevated hCG (hCG >100,000 mIU/mL in 40% to 50% of CHM, rare with PHM)
- Hyperemesis gravidarum
- Cystic enlargement of the ovaries
- Vaginal bleeding is still the most common presenting symptom of a CHM (90%); uterine size greater than dates, anemia, preeclampsia, hyperthyroidism, and hyperemesis are seen less frequently with the widespread use of hCG assay and first trimester ultrasound
- Ultrasound findings
  - Vesicular sonographic pattern is observed as a result of swelling of the chorionic villi
  - Early CHM can look similar to degenerating chorionic tissue (correlate with hCG level)
  - PHM: focal cystic changes and a ratio of >1.5 of the transverse to anteroposterior diameter of the gestational sac, fetus with features of triploidy (growth restricted, multiple congenital abnormalities)
- Most CHM have clinical or ultrasonographic findings; PHM is usually diagnosed after pathology review of a missed or spontaneous abortion
- Pathology:
  - CHM: trophoblastic proliferation, hydropic degeneration and absence of vasculature, fetal or placental tissue.
  - PHM: both a placenta and fetus may be seen (the fetus usually dies prior to 9 weeks); focal villous swelling and trophoblastic hyperplasia is usually only seen in the syncytial layer

UPDATE #2

With earlier diagnosis, CHM may have smaller villi, less trophoblastic hyperplasia, and less global necrosis, making it difficult to distinguish from a PHM or hydropic abortion. P53 (KIP2) is paternally imprinted and maternally expressed; consequently, absence of nuclear immunostaining confirms complete androgenic chromosomes and therefore the diagnosis of CHM (Popiolek et al, 2006)

MANAGEMENT OF MOLAR PREGNANCY

- Preoperative workup: history and physical; complete blood count; electrolytes; coagulation profile; renal, hepatic, and thyroid function tests; and chest x-ray
- Stabilization of medical problems (anemia, preeclampsia, hyperthyroidism) prior to evacuation; perioperative beta-blockade reduces the risk of thyroid storm
- CHM is usually managed by suction evacuation followed by sharp curettage; preparation for anticipated blood loss should include blood products and oxytocin (start after cervical dilation); anticipate laparotomy in patients with large uteri; oxytocin use is not associated with increased risk of trophoblastic embolization
- Complications of suction curettage include uterine perforation, hemorrhage, trophoblastic emboli with associated acute respiratory distress syndrome (ARDS); ARDS is managed with invasive hemodynamic monitoring and ventilatory support
- Hysterectomy can be considered in those who have completed childbearing, as it decreases the risk of malignant sequelae from 20% to 4%; hysterectomy

should be considered in women >40 years who have an increased risk of postmolar GTN
- Rh immune globulin should be given to Rh-negative women (Rh D factor is expressed on the trophoblast)
- Surveillance: baseline hCG within 48 hours of evacuation, weekly hCG monitoring until normal then monthly for 6 months, reliable birth control during surveillance
- Subsequent pregnancy: there is a 10-fold increased risk (1% to 2%) of subsequent molar pregnancy in patients with prior PHM or CHM; early obstetrical ultrasound is recommended

UPDATE #3

Recent evidence may simplify the follow-up of patients with molar pregnancy. Feltmate and colleagues studied 400 randomly selected patients at the New England Trophoblastic Center; 63% of patients that did not develop GTN completed recommended follow-up; of the 320 patients that achieved at least 1 undetectable hCG level, there were no subsequent cases of GTN (Feltmate et al, 2003). Lavie and colleagues also showed that none of the 74 patients that had one undetectable hCG level after PHM developed GTN (Lavie et al, 2005). As most cases of GTN occur within 6 months of evacuation, the American College of Obstetricians and Gynecologists (ACOG) currently recommends 6 months surveillance (American College of Obstetricians and Gynecologists, 2004).

PROPHYLACTIC CHEMOTHERAPY

- High-risk CHM (hCG >100,000, excessive uterine enlargement, and theca lutein cysts >6 cm), risk of local invasion and metastases 31% and 9%, respectively
- Chemoprophylaxis reduces the risk of GTN; however, anecdotal reports of chemotherapy-related deaths exist and when GTN develops, more chemotherapy is often required; chemoprophylaxis does not alleviate the need for surveillance
- Chemoprophylaxis at the time of evacuation of CHM is controversial and currently not recommended by ACOG, but it can be considered in high-risk patients if follow-up is unavailable or unreliable

Postmolar Gestational Trophoblastic Neoplasia (GTN) (Table 6-1)

PRESENTATION AND WORKUP OF GTN

- Malignant sequelae occur in 15% to 20% of CHM and 4% of PHM. After CHM, 15% develop local uterine invasion, 4% metastases; after PHM, most are nonmetastatic persistent/invasive disease
- Increased risk of malignant sequelae is seen in those patients with advanced maternal age, hCG >100,000, large uterine size, and theca lutein cysts > 6 cm
- Evaluate the extent of disease: history and physical; hCG level; complete blood count; hepatic, renal, and thyroid function tests; pelvic ultrasound; chest x-ray
- There is a 40% chance of detecting lung metastases on computed tomography (CT) chest after a negative chest x-ray
- Magnetic resonance imaging (MRI) brain in those with vaginal or lung metastases, or choriocarcinoma on pathology; most patients with cerebral metastases

TABLE 6-1 FIGO Criteria for Diagnosis of Postmolar Gestational Trophoblastic Disease

Four values or more of plateau of hCG over at least 3 weeks (i.e., days 1, 7, 14, and 21)
A rise in hCG of 10% or greater for 3 values or longer over at least 2 weeks (i.e., days 1, 7, and 14)
Persistence of hCG 6 months after molar evacuation
The presence of histologic choriocarcinoma

Adapted from Kohorn EI: The new FIGO 2000 staging and risk factor scoring system for gestational trophoblastic disease: description and critical assessment, *Int J Gynecol Cancer* 11(1):73-77, 2001.

are symptomatic (from raised intracranial pressure or hemorrhage)
- Biopsy of vaginal lesions should be absolutely avoided, as they are highly vascular and there is a significant risk of hemorrhage
- Locally invasive disease can perforate the myometrium and lead to intraperitoneal bleeding; secondary infection can occur with a large necrotic tumor
- Choriocarcinoma
  - 1 in 20,000 to 40,000 pregnancies
  - Can occur after any pregnancy: 50% term pregnancy, 25% after molar pregnancy, 25% from other gestational event
  - Absence of villi, mononuclear cytotrophoblasts and multinucleated syncytiotrophoblasts
  - Metastatic lesions are hemorrhagic, occurring most commonly in the lung followed by the genital tract, brain, liver, kidney, and gastrointestinal tract

STAGING AND PROGNOSTIC SCORE

- FIGO currently uses a combined anatomic staging score along with a prognostic score; prognostic score predicts the response to single-agent chemotherapy
- Generally, stage I disease has a low prognostic score and stage IV a high prognostic score; prognostic score is most commonly used in stage II/III disease
- The clinical classification system separates metastatic disease into good-prognosis or bad-prognosis based on the duration from pregnancy, hCG level, presence of brain or liver metastases, antecedent pregnancy type, and prior chemotherapy

UPDATE #4

In 2000, the FIGO staging and risk factor scoring system for gestational trophoblastic diseases was published using the FIGO anatomic staging and a modified World Health Organization (WHO) prognostic score. The modifications to the WHO prognostic score included removing the ABO blood group, moving liver metastases to the high-risk group, and expressing the score as either low or high risk (eliminating the middle risk group) (Kohorn, 2001) (Tables 6-2, 6-3, and 6-4).

MANAGEMENT OF NONMETASTATIC AND LOW-RISK GTN

- Modified WHO prognostic score of 0 to 6
- Hysterectomy with one dose of adjuvant single-agent chemotherapy is appropriate in those who have completed childbearing

TABLE 6-2 The 1982 International Federation of Gynecology and Obstetrics Anatomic System for Gestational Trophoblastic Disease

Stage	Definition
I	Disease confined to the uterus
II	Disease outside of the uterus but limited to the genital structures
III	Disease extends to the lungs with or without known genital tract involvement
IV	Distant metastases

Adapted from Kohorn EI: The new FIGO 2000 staging and risk factor scoring system for gestational trophoblastic disease: description and critical assessment, *Int J Gynecol Cancer* 11(1):73-77, 2001.

- Single-agent methotrexate or actinomycin-D, or sequential single-agent chemotherapy (Table 6-5)
- Methotrexate less short-term toxicity (mucositis most common side effect), most common first agent, with or without folinic acid rescue
- Salvage treatment: most patients who are resistant to single-agent chemotherapy will respond to combination chemotherapy; either methotrexate, actinomycin-D, and cyclophosphamide (MAC) or etoposide, methotrexate, actinomycin-D, cyclophosphamide, and vincristine (EMA-CO); MAC is frequently used because etoposide is associated with an increased risk of secondary malignancies; surgical resection or hysterectomy can be considered if there is resistance to combination chemotherapy

UPDATE #5

Methotrexate is associated with fewer side effects than actinomycin-D and is the most commonly used first agent. However, there is increasing evidence that response rates are higher with actinomycin-D. The Gynecologic Oncology Group (GOG) recently presented (in abstract form) the results of a randomized control trial comparing weekly methotrexate with biweekly actinomycin-D for treatment of low-risk GTN. The remission rate was 69% with actinomycin-D compared with 53% with methotrexate (Osborne et al, 2008). A phase 2 GOG study showed a 74% (28/38) complete response to biweekly actinomycin-D (1.25 mg/m2) in patients with low-risk disease who had failed methotrexate. The median number of cycles to complete response was 4 (range 2 to 10). No patients stopped therapy because of toxicity. All patients that failed actinomycin-D achieved a complete response to subsequent chemotherapy (Covens et al, 2006). There is also evidence that the daily actinomycin-D regimen is more efficacious and better tolerated than the pulsed/biweekly regimen, with four out of five patients who did not respond to the biweekly regimen showing a response to the daily regimen (Kohorn, 2002).

MANAGEMENT OF HIGH-RISK GTN, STAGES II AND III

- All patients should be treated with EMA-CO (Table 6-6); MAC only leads to remission in 50% of cases and is inadequate primary treatment
- Complete remission in 76% to 86% with EMA-CO

TABLE 6-3   The Modified World Health Organization Prognostic Scoring System

Prognostic Factor	Score			
	0	1	2	4
Age (years)	≤39	>39		
Antecedent Pregnancy	Hydatidiform mole	Abortion	Term pregnancy	
Interval (months) from Index Pregnancy	<4	4-6	7-12	>12
Pretreatment hCG (IU/l)#	<10*3	10*3-10*4	10*4-10*5	>10*5
Largest Tumor Size Including Uterus	3-4 cm	5 cm		
Site of Metastases	Lung	Spleen, kidney	Gastrointestinal tract	Brain, liver
Number of Metastases Identified	0	1-4	5-8	>8
Previous Failed Chemotherapy			Single drug	Two or more drugs

The International Federation of Gynecology and Obstetrics modified this system in 2000. The total score is obtained by adding the individual scores for each prognostic factor. Placental-site trophoblastic tumors are excluded from this scoring system. A score of 0 to 6 indicates low risk and ≥ 7 indicates high risk

Adapted from Kohorn EI: The new FIGO 2000 staging and risk factor scoring system for gestational trophoblastic disease: description and critical assessment, *Int J Gynecol Cancer* 11(1):73-77, 2001.

TABLE 6-4   Clinical Classification System for Patients with Malignant Gestational Trophoblastic Disease

Category	Criteria
Nonmetastatic gestational trophoblastic disease	No evidence of metastases; not assigned to a prognostic category
Metastatic gestational trophoblastic disease	Any extrauterine metastases
—Good-prognosis metastatic gestational trophoblastic disease	No risk factors —Short duration (<4 mo) —Pretherapy hCG level <40,000 mIU/mL —No brain or liver metastases —No antecedent term pregnancy —No prior chemotherapy
—Poor-prognosis metastatic gestational trophoblastic disease	Any risk factor —Long duration (≥4 mo since last pregnancy) —Pretherapy hCG level ≥ 40,000 mIU/mL —Brain or liver metastases —Antecedent term pregnancy —Prior chemotherapy

Adapted from Hammond CB, Borchert LG, Tyrey L, et al: Treatment of metastatic trophoblastic disease: good and poor prognosis, *Am J Obstet Gynecol* 115(4):451-457, 1973; and Soper JT, Evans AC, Conaway MR, et al: Evaluation of prognostic factors and staging in gestational trophoblastic tumor, *Obstet Gynecol* 84(6):969-973, 1994.

TABLE 6-5   Methotrexate and Actinomycin Regimens

Methotrexate Regimens

Weekly	30 to 40 mg/m2 weekly IM (can dose escalate to 50 mg/m2) until hCG normal × 3 weeks
Daily	0.4 mg/kg/day IM × 5 days, repeat every 14 days until hCG normal × 3 weeks
Alternate day	1 mg/kg IM days 1, 3, 5, and 7, folinic acid 0.1 mg/kg IM days 2, 4, 6, and 8 (30 hrs after the methotrexate) Folinic acid can be given orally 7.5-15 mg; one course given, additional course at double dose if hCG decline is inadequate
	Methotrexate 50 mg IM days 1, 3, 5, and 7 Folinic acid 6 mg IM or 7.5-15 mg orally days 2, 4, 6, and 8 (30 hrs after the methotrexate dose) Repeat every 14 days until hCG normal × 6-8 weeks
Continuous infusion	Methotrexate 100 mg/m2 IV bolus followed by 12 hr infusion 200 mg/m^2 day 1 Folinic acid IM or oral 15 mg/12 hrs days 2 and 3 Additional course if inadequate hCG decline

Actinomycin Regimens

Daily	0.1-0 .5 mg/day IV daily × 5 days Repeat every 14 days
Biweekly	40 μg/kg IV × 1 Or 1.25 mg/m^2 IV × 1 Repeat every 14 days

TABLE 6-6 EMA-CO Regimen

Time	Treatment
Day 1	Etoposide 100 mg/m2 IV infusion over 30 min
	Actinomycin-D 0.5 mg IV push
	Methotrexate 300 mg/m2 IV infusion over 12 hrs
Day 2	Etoposide 100 mg/m2 by IV infusion over 30 min
	Actinomycin-D 0.5 mg IV push
	Folinic acid 15 mg IM or PO every 12 hrs for four doses beginning 24 hrs after starting methotrexate
Day 8	Cyclophosphamide 600 mg/m2 IV push
	Oncovin (vincristine) 0.8 mg/m2 (maximum dose 2 mg) IV push

EMACO is repeated every 14 days until hCG normal and then for a further 2 to 4 additional courses

Adapted from Newlands ES, Bagshawe KD, Begent RH, et al: Developments in chemotherapy for medium and high-risk patients with gestational trophoblastic tumours, *Br J Obstet Gynaecol* 93:63-69, 1986.

- Common short-term toxicities include nausea, alopecia, myelosuppression, and neurotoxicity
- Rare late toxicities include second malignancies, most commonly AML
- Failed response to EMA-CO should be treated with EMA-EP; EMA-EP differs from EMA-CO in that etoposide 150 mg/m2 and cisplatin 75 mg/m2 are given on day 8

MANAGEMENT OF STAGE IV GTN

- Treated with primary chemotherapy with EMA-CO with selective radiation and surgical treatment
- If there is resistance to EMA-CO, EMA-EP should be tried; cisplatin, vinblastine, and bleomycin (PVB) have also been used effectively
- In the presence of cerebral metastases, whole-brain irradiation should be started as soon as possible to reduce the risk of cerebral hemorrhage
- Surgery can be indicated to excise foci of resistant disease, and hysterectomy may be necessary to control uterine bleeding, sepsis, or to remove resistant disease

PLACENTAL SITE TROPHOBLASTIC TUMOR

- Rare variant of choriocarcinoma
- Absence of villi, composed of mononuclear intermediate trophoblasts
- Usually occurs after a term pregnancy (average 3.4 years)
- Tendency for chemoresistance
- Hysterectomy recommended for disease confined to the uterus
- Excretes low levels of hCG (usually <250 mIU/mL) and significant tumor may be present before the hCG elevation is detected; serum human placental lactogen can also be used to monitor PSTT

SURVEILLANCE AFTER TREATMENT OF GTN

- Stages I, II, III: weekly hCG until normal, monthly for 12 months
- Stage IV: weekly hCG until normal, monthly for 24 months

PERSISTENT LOW-LEVEL hCG

- Need to exclude false-positive hCG/phantom hCG
  - Caused by heterophilic antibodies or nonspecific protein interference
  - If appropriate, confirm the hCG result
    - Urine hCG (heterophilic antibodies not found in urine)
    - Serial dilutions
    - Use of different immunoassays or hCG reference laboratory (heterophilic antibodies removed from sera)
- Pituitary hCG: occurs in perimenopausal and postmenopausal women, result of uncontrolled gonadotrophin-releasing hormone (GnRH) stimulation that leads to hCG production by pituitary gonadotrope cells; high dose combined oral contraception pills will suppress pituitary hCG production and confirm the diagnosis
- Quiescent GTN: syndrome of inactive GTN, not responsive to chemotherapy; hyperglycosylated hCG (hCG-H) is produced by invasive cytotrophoblasts and is a marker of invasive disease; therefore the absence of hCG-H confirms this diagnosis

UPDATE #6

Quiescent GTN was first described by the USA hCG Reference Service in 2003 and is a syndrome of inactive GTN composed of highly differentiated syncytiotrophoblastic cells. Most cases resolve spontaneously within 6 months, but there is a reported 15% risk of progression to active invasive disease, which is preceded by an increase in the hCG-H, prior to a significant rise in the total hCG (Cole et al, 2010). Therefore, these patients need close monitoring with reliable contraception until the hCG is undetectable for at least 6 months.

SUGGESTED READINGS

Molar Pregnancy

American College of Obstetricians and Gynecologists: ACOG practice bulletin no. 53: diagnosis and treatment of gestational trophoblastic disease, *Obstet Gynecol* 103(6):1365–1377, 2004.

Epidemiology and Cytogenetics

Fisher RA, Hodges MD, Newlands ES: Familial recurrent hydatidiform mole: a review, *J Reprod Med* 49(8):595–601, 2004.
Murdoch S, Djuric U, Mazhar B, et al: Mutations in NALP7 cause recurrent hydatidiform moles and reproductive wastage in humans, *Nat Genet* 38(3):300–302, 2006.
Popiolek DA, Yee H, Mittal K, et al: Multiplex short tandem repeat DNA analysis confirms the accuracy of p57(KIP2) immunostaining in the diagnosis of complete hydatidiform mole, *Hum Pathol* 37(1):1426–1434, 2006.

Surveillance

Feltmate CM, Batorfi J, Fulop V, et al: Human chorionic gonadotropin follow-up in patients with molar pregnancy: a time for reevaluation, *Obstet Gynecol* 101(4):732–736, 2003.
Lavie I, Rao G, Castillon DH, et al: Duration of human chorionic gonadotrophin surveillance for partial hydatidiform moles, *Amer J Obstet Gynecol* 192(5):1362–1364, 2005.

Staging and Prognostic Score

Kohorn EI: The new FIGO 2000 staging and risk factor scoring system for gestational trophoblastic disease: description and critical assessment, *Int J Gynecol Cancer* 11(1):73–77, 2001.

Management of Low-Risk GTN

Covens A, Filiaci VL, Burger RA, et al: Phase II trial of pulsed dactinomycin as salvage therapy for low-risk gestational trophoblastic neoplasia, *Cancer* 107(6):1280–1286, 2006.

Foulmann K, Guastalla JP, Caminet N, et al: What is the best protocol of single-agent methotrexate chemotherapy in nonmetastatic or low-risk metastatic gestational trophoblastic tumors? A review of the evidence, *Gynecol Oncol* 102(1):103–110, 2006.

Kohorn EI: Is the lack of response to single-agent chemotherapy in gestational trophoblastic disease associated with dose scheduling or chemotherapy resistance? *Gynecol Oncol* 85(1):36–39, 2002.

Osborne R, Filiaci V, Schink J, et al: A randomized phase III trial comparing weekly parenteral methotrexate and pulsed dactinomycin as primary management of low risk gestational trophoblastic neoplasia, *Gynecol Oncol* 108:s2, 2008.

Management of High-Risk GTN

Xue Y, Zhang J, Wu TX, An RF: Combination chemotherapy for high-risk gestational trophoblastic tumour, *Cochrane Database Syst Rev* 3:CD005196, 2009.

Persistent Low-Level hCG

American College of Obstetricians and Gynecologists Committee on Gynecologic Practice: ACOG opinion no. 278: avoiding inappropriate clinical decisions based on false-positive human chorionic gonadotropin test results, *Obstet Gynecol* 100(5 Pt 1):1057–1059, 2002.

Cole LA, Butler SA, Khanlian SA, et al: Gestational trophoblastic diseases: 2. hyperglycosylated hCG as a reliable marker of active neoplasia, *Gynecol Oncol* 102(2):151–159, 2006.

Cole LA, Muller CY: Hyperglycosylated hCG in the management of quiescent and chemorefractory gestational trophoblastic diseases, *Gynecol Oncol* 116(1):3–9, 2010.

Chapter 7

Aneuploidy Screening

ESTHER FRIEDRICH • MANUAL PORTO

KEY UPDATES

1 First-trimester ultrasound (US) for early pregnancy assessment with nuchal translucency (NT) measurement: part of a comprehensive approach to genetic screening.

2 Combined first-trimester NT and maternal serum markers perform better in aneuploidy screening than second-trimester triple or quad screening.

3 Additional first-trimester screening markers: ductus venosus Doppler, nasal bone measurement, tricuspid regurgitation; not standard of care yet.

4 Second-trimester quad screening still beneficial: patient without NT measurement or late prenatal care; screening for structural anomalies such as neural tube defects (NTDs).

5 Integrated screening (NT ultrasound and first- and second-trimester maternal serum markers): new gold standard of noninvasive aneuploidy screening.

6 Second-trimester genetic ultrasound is a valuable component of aneuploidy screening and detection of structural fetal anomalies.

7 Invasive diagnostic procedures (chorionic villus sampling [CVS], amniocentesis): offered to *all* pregnant women regardless of US findings or screening results or age.

8 Diagnostic testing—more than karyotype: prenatal microarray, other new genetic technologies and noninvasive prenatal diagnosis; enlarged NT associated with cardiac defects, genetic syndromes; genetic counseling integral.

9 Aneuploidy screening detects obstetric complications: serum marker anomalies indicate risk for adverse pregnancy outcome.

Background

- Screening for fetal aneuploidy integral part of modern prenatal pregnancy assessment
- Chromosomal aneuploidy (trisomy, monosomy, triploidy) most common genetic abnormality detected by prenatal diagnosis; ~90% involve chromosomes 21, 18, 13, X, Y
- Down syndrome most common, prevalence ~1 in 660 births; risk increases with increasing maternal age, but highest number of births in age group <35 years old
- Maternal age of 35 as "threshold" for invasive testing has been replaced
- Ethnicity-based screening for single gene disorders part of a comprehensive screening approach (e.g., cystic fibrosis, Tay Sachs disease, hemoglobinopathies)
- Aneuploidy screening by different modalities possible throughout pregnancy

First-Trimester Nuchal Translucency Ultrasound

- Fetal nuchal translucency (NT) thickness in first trimester increased in most fetuses with Down syndrome; established marker for T21
- NT performance as screening marker declines with advancing gestational age (GA) between 10 and 13 weeks

TECHNIQUE

- 11⁵⁄₇ to 13⁵⁄₇ weeks' gestational age, crown-rump length (CRL) 45 to 84 mm
- Sagittal view, fetus in neutral position (Figure 7-1)
- Zoom as large as possible (e.g., 75% of screen), reduce gain
- Place calipers on lines forming the NT, not into empty space (Figure 7-2)
- Measure NT clearly distinct from amnion; three measurements at least; use largest
- Assess remaining early anatomy (Figure 7-3)
- Quality assurance: sufficient training and ongoing quality assessment essential for screening programs utilizing NT measurement (operator experience and equipment known cause for inconsistent results in early studies); for example:
  - Nuchal Translucency Quality Review Program (www.ntqr.org)
  - Fetal Medicine Foundation USA (www.fetalmedicine.com/fmf/)
- NT up to 2.5 mm considered normal; up to 3.4 mm may benefit from addition of serum markers; ≥3.5 mm and septated cystic hygroma both associated with significant

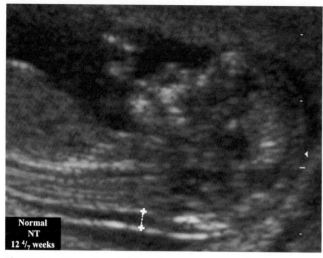

Figure 7-1. Normal nuchal translucency measurement at 12⁵/₇ weeks' gestational age in optimal sagittal cut and zoom. (Image courtesy of Dr. E. Friedrich.)

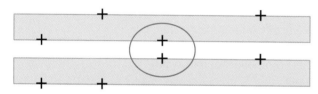

Figure 7-2. Schematic drawing of optimal caliper placement in nuchal translucency measurement. Correct placement is shown in the red circle.

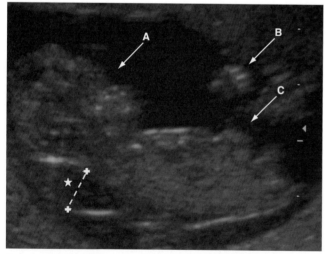

Figure 7-3. Abnormal nuchal translucency measurement of 7.2 mm at 12⁵/₇ weeks, marked by (x); additional findings pictured and marked by arrows: midline facial defect with proboscis, small omphalocele, polydactyly; findings not pictured: holoprosencephaly, cardiac defect, single umbilical artery. Karyotype after CVS: 47, XY+13. (Image courtesy of Dr. E. Friedrich.)

risk for aneuploidy, up to 17% and 50%, respectively; justifies immediate diagnostic assessment without serum analytes (Figure 7-4)

- NT assessment best aneuploidy screening strategy in high-order multiples for individual risk assessment (triplets, quads); serum screening not valid; invasive procedure associated with higher risk

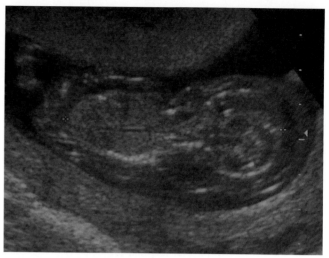

Figure 7-4. Severe cystic hygroma and fetal hydrops at 12²/₇ weeks; karyotype after CVS: 45,X. (Image courtesy of Dr. E. Friedrich.)

UPDATE #1

Aneuploidy screening has developed into comprehensive prenatal screening and diagnostic testing for all pregnant women (Norton, 2008; Ram et al, 2010). First-trimester ultrasound assessment allows for early aneuploidy screening with benefits to the couple, including time for decision making and earlier pregnancy termination if desired. Multiple landmark studies have established fetal nuchal translucency measurement as a sensitive marker for Down syndrome and other aneuploidies (Malone et al, 2003; Nicolaides et al, 1992; 2004). A major benefit of routine early ultrasound screening is accurate pregnancy dating reducing the misdiagnosis of preterm and postdates pregnancies (Neilson et al, 2000), reliable identification of twin pregnancies, and early detection of major structural anomalies (D'Alton et al, 2005), A number of recent studies reported a 52% to 100% detection rate of major fetal anomalies in the first trimester, dependent on type of anomaly (Syngelaki et al, 2011; Timor-Trisch et al, 2009), with first-trimester detection rates (DR) for severe structural defects such as NTDs approaching higher numbers: anencephaly 90%, encephalocele 80%, and open NTD 44% (Cameron et al, 2009). Improvements in ultrasound technology allow increasing assessment, even of fetal cardiac anatomy, in the first trimester by trained specialists (Lombardi et al, 2007).

First-Trimester Serum Analytes and Combined First-Trimester Screening

PAPP-A

- Pregnancy associated plasma protein A (PAPP-A)
- Measured between 9 and 13⁵/₇ weeks' gestational age (GA)
- Performance as marker declines with increasing GA
- Complex, high-molecular-weight glycoprotein

FREE BETA- hCG AND TOTAL BETA-hCG

- Free beta human chorionic gonadotropin (hCG)
  - Measured between 9 and 13⁵/₇ weeks
  - Performance as marker best if assayed at 9 to 13 weeks of gestation; improves with increasing GA within the interval

- Total beta hCG
  - Measured between 11 and 13⁶⁄₇ weeks
  - Total beta-hCG not effective before 11 weeks GA; if first-trimester serum screening performed before 11 weeks, use *free* beta-hCG

COMBINED FIRST-TRIMESTER SCREENING

- Typically done between 11 to 13 weeks' GA
- Three components:
  - PAPP-A, hCG, NT ultrasound (US) measurement
  - Maternal age, maternal characteristics (ethnicity, body weight, diabetes mellitus, smoking, multiple gestation, in vitro fertilization [IVF]) and crown-rump length (CRL) considered by computer software calculating individual risk
- One composite numeric result for trisomy 21 (T21) and trisomy 18 (T18)
- Typical cutoff for elevated risk 1:100; varies in different screening programs
- Typical serum analyte pattern in T21: low PAPP-A, high beta-hCG (+ increased NT)
- Typical serum analyte pattern in T18: very low beta-hCG, very low PAPP-A (+ increased NT)
- T13, NTD and ventral wall defect (VWD), Smith-Lemli-Opiz syndrome (SLOS) not assessed
- Can be utilized in twins:
  - Serum concentrations of markers about twice as high as in singleton pregnancies
  - Individual contributions cannot be assessed except for NT measurement
  - Serum screening not as efficient in twins when compared to singletons, but still offers benefit over NT alone
  - Serum screening in high-order multiple pregnancies (>twins) cannot be interpreted; NT assessment for each fetus should be offered
- Don't offer first-trimester *combined* screening if:
  - High-order multiple gestation: offer NT only
  - Fetal demise ("vanishing twin"): offer NT only
  - Multifetal pregnancy reduction: offer NT only
- Abnormal first-trimester maternal serum analytes associated with obstetric complications (see Update #9)

UPDATE #2

Combined first-trimester screening performs better than second-trimester quad screening with a higher detection rate (DR) of about 85% = sensitivity and a lower false positive rate (FPR) of 5% for Down syndrome (when compared to 81% of quad screening alone). The FASTER, SURUSS, and BUN trials evaluating first-trimester screening all had similar results (Malone et al, 2005; Wald et al, 2003; Wapner, 2005). Additionally, most of these trials showed the cost effectiveness of the combined test. In the FASTER trial, 60% of trisomy 18 cases were identified at a 0.1% FPR, and 78% of all non-T21 aneuploidies were detected, with an overall FPR of 6%, similarly outperforming the quad screening detection rate for both (Breathnach et al, 2007). PAPP-A levels can be influenced by the presence of an early vanishing twin, and NT only should be performed. If an empty gestational sac only present, analysis of serum markers showed no significant difference (Spencer et al, 2010).

DETAILED FIRST-TRIMESTER ULTRASOUND

- Additional ultrasound markers for assessment of risk: part of early anatomy assessment; may be used in specialized centers
  - Nasal bone assessment
  - Ductus venosus Doppler
  - Tricuspid regurgitation

UPDATE #3

Absence or hypoplasia of the nasal bone is associated with Down syndrome. In a review of nine studies totaling over 35,000 nasal bone measurements, evaluation of the fetal profile in a sagittal view for the presence or absence of the line of the nasal bone was possible during NT ultrasound in 94.3%. An average of 65% of fetuses with T21 were found to have an absent nasal bone (Rosen et al, 2007). If nasal bone assessment is incorporated into calculations of risk for trisomy 21, an increase in DR of up to 92% at an FPR rate of 2.9% has been reported (Kagan et al, 2009).

Abnormal (reverse) flow in the ductus venosus has been found in aneuploid fetuses and is also associated with cardiac defects. In a report on almost 20,000 assessed fetuses, reversed a-wave was observed in 3.2% of the euploid fetuses, and in 66.4%, 58.3%, 55.0%, and 75.0% of fetuses with trisomies 21, 18, and 13, and Turner syndrome, respectively. Including DV Doppler into the calculation of risk improved DRs to 96%, 92%, 100%, and 100% of trisomies 21, 18, and 13, and Turner syndrome, respectively, at a false-positive rate of 3% (Maiz et al, 2009). The same group evaluated the finding of tricuspid regurgitation, which was observed in 0.9% of the euploid fetuses and 55.7%, 33.3%, and 30% of the fetuses with trisomies 21, 18, and 13, respectively, and in 37.5% of those with Turner syndrome. Improvement of risk assessment was in a similar range (Kagan et al, 2009). The clinical application of these findings should remain limited to specialized centers (Borell, 2009).

Second-Trimester Maternal Serum Screening

- Should be offered to all women
  - As part of integrated aneuploidy screening (see the Integrated Aneuploidy Screening section, presented later in the chapter)
  - Women presenting for prenatal care after completed first trimester
  - Women with completed first-trimester diagnostic procedures (CVS) as isolated NTD/VWD/SLOS screening
- Screening time frame 15 to 22 weeks' GA (laboratory dependent)
- Optimal frame 16 to 18 weeks' GA

QUAD SCREENING (FORMERLY TRIPLE SCREEN)

- Alpha fetoprotein: AFP (MSAFP = maternal serum AFP)
  - Fetal specific globulin produced in yolk sac, gastrointestinal (GI) tract, fetal liver
- Human chorionic gonadotropin: beta-hCG
- Unconjugated estriol: uE3
- Inhibin A: InhA (added to triple screening for improved DR, lower FPR)

- Composite result for four conditions, dependent on screening program: Down syndrome (T21), trisomy 18 (T18), neural tube and ventral wall defects (NTD/VWD), Smith-Lemli-Opitz syndrome (SLOS)
- Maternal age, maternal characteristics (ethnicity, body weight, diabetes mellitus, smoking, multiple gestation, IVF), and gestational age alter risk calculation
- Typical serum analyte pattern in T21: low AFP, low uE3, high hCG, high InhA
- Typical serum analyte pattern in T18: low AFP, low uE3, low hCG, low InhA
- No consistent pattern in T13: slightly lower uE3
- Can be used in twins; higher-order multiples cannot be interpreted
- Typical midtrimester cutoff for elevated risk 1:250 to 1:300.
- Do not offer second-trimester maternal serum analyte analysis if:
  - High-order multiple gestation: NT in first trimester, second-trimester genetic US only
  - Fetal demise after 8 weeks' GA: NT in first trimester, second-trimester genetic US only
  - Multifetal pregnancy reduction: NT in first trimester, second-trimester genetic US only
  - As *independent* risk assessment after completed combined first-trimester screening
- Abnormal second-trimester serum analytes associated with obstetric complications (see Update #9)

DETECTION OF OPEN NEURAL TUBE DEFECTS AND VENTRAL WALL DEFECTS

- Typical serum analyte pattern in NTD/VWD: AFP >2.5 MoM (singleton pregnancy)
- Risk for NTD at >2.5 Multiples of the Median (MoM) = 4.5%; increases with level of MoM
- Prenatal DR through screening 88%; coupled with US higher: 92% to 100%
- Elevated MSAFP also associated with the following:
  - Advanced GA (requiring redating and recalculation if possible)
  - Undetected multiple gestation
  - Fetal omphalocele, gastroschisis = VWD
  - Fetal teratomas, cystic hygromas, obstructive uropathy
  - Congenital nephrosis (Finnish type): recessive disease associated with very high MSAFP (>5 MoM); suspect if no US detection of NTD, negative acetylcholinesterase enzyme activity (AchE) on amniocentesis

SMITH-LEMLI-OPITZ SYNDROME

- Rare autosomal recessive defect in cholesterol metabolism; associated with growth failure, intellectual disability, dysmorphic features; birth prevalence is low, ~1 in 20,000 to 100,000
- Typical analyte pattern in SLOS: very low uE3 due to deficient steroid/estriol synthesis, AFP, hCG slightly reduced
- Diagnosis by amniocentesis: test for cholesterol, cholesterol precursors; mutation analysis

Integrated Aneuploidy Screening

- Uses markers of both first and second trimester to calculate single risk estimate for Down syndrome; different approaches described in the literature as follows:
  - Serum integrated screening: PAPP-A, beta-hCG, AFP, uE3, InhA
    - Highest DR, lowest FPR if *no* NT US is available
  - Fully integrated screening: PAPP-A, beta-hCG, AFP, uE3, InhA, *and* first-trimester NT measurement
    - Highest DR, lowest FPR of all screening approaches
    - Cutoff for screen positive midtrimester risk usually higher (e.g., >1:100 risk for T21) because of lower FPR
- Table 7-1a: Detection rates of recognized Down syndrome screening strategies
- Table 7-1b: Combined and integrated first-trimester screening study outcomes
- Main remaining difference lies in timing of disclosure of abnormal results
  - Stepwise sequential screening
    - Combined first-trimester screening results only disclosed to women at very high risk
    - Cutoff depends on screening program (e.g., >1:50 for T21)
    - Genetic counseling and CVS offered if abnormal
    - All others proceed with second-trimester serum analyte analysis, one final composite risk disclosed
    - Genetic counseling, amniocentesis offered if abnormal
  - Modified stepwise sequential screening
    - Combined first-trimester screening results disclosed to all women
    - Final composite screening result disclosed to all women
    - Genetic counseling, diagnostic testing offered based on risk

TABLE 7-1a **Down Syndrome Screening Tests and Detection Rates of Available and Historic Aneuploidy Screening Models**

Screening Test	Detection Rate (%)
First Trimester	
NT measurement	64-70*
NT measurement, PAPP-A, free or total β-hCG†	82-87*
Second Trimester	
Triple screen (MSAFP, hCG, unconjugated estriol)	69*
Quadruple screen (MSAFP, hCG, unconjugated estriol, inhibin A)	81*
First Plus Second Trimester	
Integrated (NT, PAPP-A, quad screen)	94-96*
Serum integrated (PAPP-A, quad screen)	85-88*
Stepwise sequential	95*
First-trimester test result:	
• Positive: diagnostic test offered	
• Negative: second-trimester test offered	
• Final: risk assessment incorporates first and second results	
Contingent sequential	88-94‡
First-trimester test result:	
• Positive: diagnostic test offered	
• Negative: no further testing	
• Intermediate: second-trimester test offered	
• Final: risk assessment incorporates first and second results	

*From the FASTER trial (Malone F, Canick JA, Ball RH, et al: First-trimester or second-trimester screening, or both, for Down's syndrome: First- and Second-Trimester Evaluation of Risk (FASTER) Research Consortium, *N Engl J Med* 353:2001-2011, 2005).
†Also referred to as combined first-trimester screen.
‡Modeled predicted detection dates (Cuckle H, Benn P, Wright D: Down syndrome screening in the first and/or second trimester: model predicted performance using meta-analysis parameters, *Semin Perinatol* 29:252-257, 2005).
Abbreviations: hCG, human chorionic gonadotropin; MSAFP, maternal serum alpha-fetoprotein; NT, nuchal translucency; PAPP-A, pregnancy associated plasma protein-A; quad, quadruple.

- Contingent screening: relies on definition of the following three risk cutoffs:
  - Women at very high risk after first-trimester screening: offer CVS
  - Women at very low risk after first-trimester screening: no further screening necessary
  - Women at intermediate risk: perform second-trimester portion with maternal serum analytes
- Integrated screening offers one composite result for T21, T18, NTD/VWD, and SLOS
- Multiple studies have assessed DR, average: 85% DR at 1% FPR, or 90% DR, at 2% FPR
  - Table 7-2a and Table 7-2b: current detection rates for T21 (a), T18 (b) utilized by the State of California Prenatal Screening Program; modified stepwise sequential screening implemented in 2009

TABLE 7-1b **Combined and Integrated Screening Prospective Study Outcomes***

Study	Patients	Down Syndrome Cases	Detection Rate† (%)
BUN‡	8,216	61	79
FASTER§	33,557	84	83
SURUSS¶	47,053	101	83
OSCAR[a]	15,030	82	90
Total	103,856	328	84

*First-trimester detection rate (DR) at 5% of false-positive rate (FPR).
†95% CI:79.7-87%
‡Wapner RJ, Thom EA, Simpson JL, et al: First-trimester screening for trisomies 21 and 18: First Trimester Maternal Serum Biochemistry and Fetal Nuchal Translucency Screening (BUN) Study Group, *New Engl J Med* 349:1405-1413, 2003.
§Malone FD, Wald NJ, Canick JA, et al: First- and second trimester evaluation of risk (FASTER) trial: principal results of the NICHD multicenter Down syndrome screening study [abstract], *Am J Obstet Gynecol* 189: (suppl 1): s56, 2003.
¶Wald NJ, Rodeck C, Hackshaw AK, et al: First- and second trimester antenatal screening for Down's syndrome: the results of the Serum, Urine, and Ultrasound Screening Study (SURUSS) [published erratum appears in *J Med Screen* 13:51-52, 2006], *J Med Screen* 10:56-104, 2003.
[a]Spencer K, Spencer CE, Power M, et al: Screening for chromosomal abnormalities in the first trimester using ultrasound and maternal serum biochemistry in a one-stop clinic: a review of three years prospective experience, *BJOG* 110:281-286, 2003.
Reprinted from Wapner RJ: First trimester screening: the BUN study, *Semin Perinatol* 29:236-239, 2005. With permission from Elsevier.

LIMITATIONS

- Remains screening test, does *not* detect 100% of aneuploidies
- Requires coordination of lab, practitioner, skills, resources; NT US and CVS not yet available in all states and counties

UPDATE #5

SURUSS (S) and FASTER (F) trials (Malone et al, 2005; Wald et al, 2003) evaluated Down syndrome screening strategies in both first and second trimesters, evaluating more than 47,000 and 38,000 singleton pregnancies, respectively. At a DR of 85%, the FPRs were as follows:
- First-trimester combined screening: 6.1 (S), 4.8 (F) %
- First and second-trimester serum integrated screening: 2.7 (S), 4.4 (F) %
- First and second-trimester fully integrated screening: 1.3 (S), 0.8 (F) %
- Second-trimester quad screening: 6.2 (S), 7.3 (F) %

  Stepwise sequential screening achieved a DR for T21 of 95% with an FPR of 5% (2.5% first trimester, 2.5% second-trimester portion). The high DR and significantly decreased FPR suggests fully integrated or modified stepwise sequential screening as the most efficient screening test for Down syndrome, significantly reducing subsequent procedure-related unaffected fetal loss rates (9 per 100,000 versus 45 per 100,000). The availability of first-trimester screening and improved sensitivity for T21 detection has begun to cause a steady decline in invasive testing in women of advanced maternal age at a rate of 3% to 4% per year with a recent increase in acceptance of CVS procedures (Nakata et al, 2010).

TABLE 7-2a   California State Genetic Disease Screening Program Estimated Detection Rates for Down Syndrome in Relation to Maternal Age

| Age | Quad | | Serum Integrated | | (Full) Integrated | | | |
| | | | | | First Trimester | | Total after Second Trimester* | |
	Positive Rate	Detection Rate	Positive Rate	Detection Rate	Positive Rate	Detection Rate	Positive Rate	Detection Rate
18	2%	61%	2%	71%	1%	55%	2%	81%
19	2%	61%	2%	72%	1%	55%	2%	81%
20	2%	61%	2%	73%	1%	55%	2%	81%
21	2%	61%	2%	72%	1%	55%	2%	81%
22	2%	62%	2%	72%	1%	55%	2%	81%
23	2%	62%	2%	72%	1%	55%	2%	81%
24	2%	62%	2%	73%	1%	56%	2%	81%
25	2%	63%	2%	73%	1%	57%	2%	82%
26	2%	63%	2%	73%	1%	58%	2%	83%
27	2%	64%	2%	74%	1%	58%	2%	83%
28	2%	65%	3%	74%	1%	59%	3%	83%
29	3%	67%	3%	76%	1%	61%	3%	84%
30	3%	68%	3%	77%	1%	61%	3%	84%
31	3%	69%	4%	78%	2%	64%	4%	86%
32	4%	72%	4%	80%	2%	66%	4%	87%
33	5%	74%	5%	82%	3%	69%	5%	88%
34	7%	78%	6%	84%	3%	72%	6%	89%
35	8%	81%	7%	86%	5%	75%	8%	91%
36	10%	84%	10%	88%	6%	79%	9%	92%
37	12%	86%	12%	90%	8%	81%	12%	93%
38	16%	89%	15%	92%	10%	84%	14%	94%
39	19%	91%	18%	94%	13%	86%	18%	94%
40	23%	93%	21%	94%	16%	89%	21%	96%
41	26%	94%	25%	95%	20%	90%	25%	96%
42	29%	95%	28%	96%	22%	92%	27%	97%
43	32%	95%	31%	96%	26%	93%	31%	97%
44	34%	96%	33%	97%	28%	94%	33%	97%
45	37%	96%	35%	97%	30%	94%	36%	97%
46	38%	97%	37%	97%	32%	94%	38%	98%
47	40%	97%	39%	98%	35%	95%	39%	98%
48	41%	97%	40%	98%	35%	95%	40%	98%
49	42%	97%	40%	98%	36%	95%	41%	98%
50	43%	97%	41%	98%	37%	95%	42%	98%
<35	3%	68%	3%	77%	1%	62%	3%	85%
≥35	15%	90%	14%	93%	10%	86%	14%	94%
All ages	4.5%	80%	4.5%	85%	2.5%	75%	4.5%	90%

*Second trimester rates assume that patients with positive results in the first trimester accept referral and all patients with preliminary (negative) risk assessments return for second-trimester screening.

Reproduced with permission from the Genetic Disease Screening Program of the California Department of Health at www.cdph.ca.gov/programs/GDSP.

SUMMARY OF RECOMMENDATIONS

Algorithm I: optimal prenatal screening strategy for low-risk women with normal screening results. (Figure 7-5)

Algorithm II: optimal treatment strategy in low- and high-risk women with normal and abnormal screening results and diagnostic testing. (Figure 7-6)

Genetic Ultrasound

- ACOG guidelines: ultrasound (US) has benefits and limitations; reasonable in patients who request it; US is recommended, but not required in pregnancy
- Detailed second-trimester screening for fetal malformations commonly referred to as genetic sonogram

TABLE 7-2b California State Genetic Disease Screening Program Estimated Detection Rates for Trisomy 18 in Relation to Maternal Age

Age	Quad Positive Rate	Quad Detection Rate	Serum Integrated Positive Rate	Serum Integrated Detection Rate	(Full) Integrated First Trimester Positive Rate	(Full) Integrated First Trimester Detection Rate	(Full) Integrated Total after Second Trimester* Positive Rate	(Full) Integrated Total after Second Trimester* Detection Rate
18	0.08%	50%	0.06%	74%	<0.1%	28%	0.08%	68%
19	0.12%	50%	0.07%	74%	<0.1%	29%	0.05%	68%
20	0.07%	51%	0.06%	74%	<0.1%	29%	0.10%	68%
21	0.08%	51%	0.08%	74%	<0.1%	29%	0.07%	68%
22	0.05%	51%	0.10%	74%	<0.1%	29%	0.08%	69%
23	0.10%	51%	0.10%	75%	<0.1%	29%	0.06%	69%
24	0.10%	51%	0.08%	75%	<0.1%	27%	0.10%	69%
25	0.10%	52%	0.10%	75%	<0.1%	27%	0.09%	70%
26	0.11%	52%	0.08%	75%	<0.1%	27%	0.07%	71%
27	0.06%	53%	0.09%	76%	<0.1%	27%	0.09%	71%
28	0.10%	53%	0.09%	75%	0.05%	32%	0.10%	71%
29	0.12%	55%	0.09%	77%	0.10%	33%	0.07%	73%
30	0.13%	55%	0.10%	78%	0.07%	36%	0.19%	74%
31	0.16%	56%	0.12%	78%	0.08%	38%	0.21%	76%
32	0.20%	58%	0.14%	80%	0.11%	40%	0.22%	77%
33	0.30%	62%	0.18%	81%	0.12%	43%	0.25%	79%
34	0.37%	63%	0.31%	83%	0.16%	48%	0.27%	82%
35	0.36%	67%	0.35%	85%	0.23%	57%	0.51%	84%
36	0.78%	69%	0.37%	86%	0.39%	61%	0.81%	86%
37	0.97%	73%	0.65%	88%	0.45%	66%	0.95%	89%
38	1.39%	75%	0.84%	90%	0.72%	70%	1.27%	91%
39	1.70%	78%	1.12%	91%	1.13%	74%	1.92%	92%
40	2.44%	79%	1.27%	92%	1.40%	77%	2.29%	93%
41	2.90%	81%	1.62%	93%	1.65%	79%	2.78%	94%
42	3.94%	83%	1.80%	94%	2.77%	81%	4.12%	95%
43	4.45%	83%	2.17%	95%	2.84%	83%	4.17%	95%
44	5.12%	85%	2.33%	95%	3.78%	84%	5.15%	96%
45	5.89%	85%	2.49%	95%	4.15%	85%	5.54%	96%
46	5.43%	86%	3.07%	95%	4.50%	86%	6.07%	96%
47	6.07%	86%	3.12%	95%	4.75%	86%	6.50%	97%
48	7.24%	87%	3.05%	96%	4.77%	87%	6.62%	97%
49	7.24%	86%	2.95%	96%	5.03%	87%	6.82%	97%
50	7.24%	87%	3.13%	95%	5.06%	87%	6.70%	97%
<35	0.13%	55%	0.11%	75%	0.05%	36%	0.12%	76%
≥ 35	1.38%	77%	0.80%	91%	0.82%	72%	1.41%	91%
All ages	0.31%	67%	0.21%	79%	0.16%	59%	0.31%	81%

*Second trimester rates assume that patients with positive results in the first trimester accept referral and all patients with preliminary (negative) risk assessments return for second-trimester screening.
Reproduced with permission from the Genetic Disease Screening Program of the California Department of Health at www.cdph.ca.gov/programs/GDSP.

- Optimal timing: 18 to 20 weeks of GA
  - Good visualization of anatomy: higher DR of anomalies
  - Diagnostic procedure can be performed at same time (amniocentesis)
  - Adjunct studies can be performed (fetal echocardiogram, magnetic resonance imaging [MRI])
- Pregnancy dating can be adjusted if necessary
- Legal termination remains option if desired
- Detection of fetal anomalies by second-trimester screening US controversial, based on older studies
- RADIUS trial
  - Largest US trial, 15,000 women, randomized
    - 15 to 22 weeks for screening US

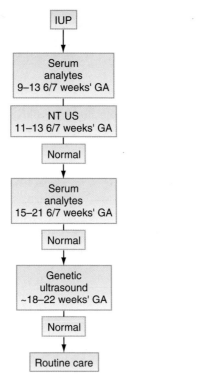

Figure 7-5. Algorithm for optimal aneuploidy screening strategy in low-risk women with normal results.

- 31 to 35 weeks for screening US
  - US only for indication: 45% received US
- Increased DR of anomalies, no improvement in perinatal outcomes
- DR 34.8%, higher in tertiary care centers
- Helsinki trial
  - 1986-1987; 4691 women, screening US 16 to 20 weeks
  - 4619 controls, US only for indication: 77% received US
  - Reduction in perinatal mortality, increased DR of anomalies
  - DR community 36%, tertiary care center 77%
- Eurofetus trial
  - 1999, 61 European centers, 18 to 22 weeks
  - Overall DR 56.2% for anomalies
  - Major anomalies 73.7%, minor 45.7%, (cardiac 38.8% and 20.8%)
  - Fewer live births in anomalous group
- Components of standard second-trimester screening US shown in Table 7-3 (American Institute of Ultrasound in Medicine, 2010; see also ACOG Practice Bulletin No. 101, 2009)
- Fetuses with sonographically detected anomaly at increased risk of chromosomal anomalies; background risk for any major or minor anomaly in population ~2% to 3.5%

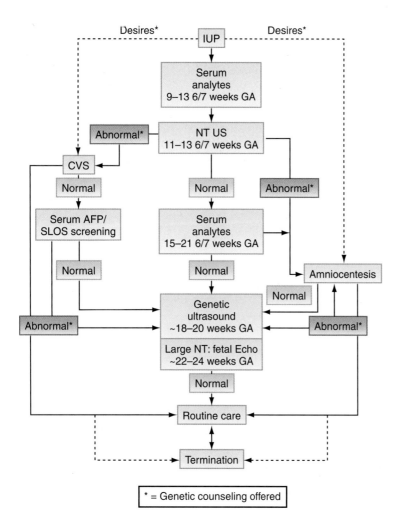

Figure 7-6. Algorithm for optimal treatment strategy in low- and high-risk women with normal and abnormal screening results and diagnostic testing.

TABLE 7-3   Components of a Standard Obstertic Fetal Anatomic Survey

Head, face, and neck
- Cerebellum
- Choroid plexus
- Cisterna magna
- Lateral cerebral ventricles
- Midline falx
- Cavum septi pellucid
- Upper lip
- Nuchal translucency*

Chest
- Cardiac four-chamber view
- Outflow tracts if technically feasible

Abdomen
- Stomach—presence, size, situs
- Kidneys
- Bladder
- Umbilical cord insertion site
- Umbilical cord vessel number

Spine
- Cervical
- Thoracic
- Lumbar
- Sacral

Extremities
- Legs—presence/absence
- Arms—presence/absence

Sex
- Indicated in low-risk pregnancies only in multiple gestations

*May be helpful during a specific age interval as assessment of increased risk aneuploidy.
Adapted from the AIUM Practice Guideline for the Performance of Obstetric Ultrasound Examinations, October 1, 2007 (website). www.aium.org/publications/guidelines/obstetric.pdf; same as American College of Radiology practice guidelines for the performance of obstetrical ultrasound.

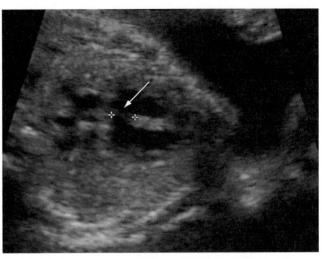

Figure 7-8. Atrioventricular (AV) canal defect of heart in a fetus with Down syndrome; arrow illustrates defect at level of AV valves and septum. (Image courtesy of Chris Norton, RDMS.)

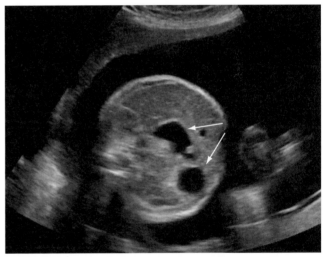

Figure 7-9. Classic US finding of "double bubble" resulting from duodenal atresia in a fetus with Down syndrome. Arrows illustrate fetal stomach and dilated duodenum adjacent to stomach bubble. (Image courtesy of Chris Norton, RDMS.)

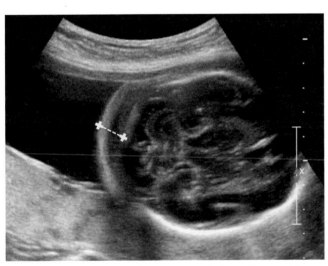

Figure 7-7. Enlarged second-trimester nuchal translucency of 12 mm, correct measurement shown. (Image courtesy of Chris Norton, Registered Diagnostic Medical Sonographer [RDMS].)

- For aneuploidies like T18, T13—associated with multiple structural anomalies—second-trimester US shows high DR, average >90%
- Modification of calculated risk for T21 based on first, second, or integrated screening based on genetic ultrasound results controversial, but practiced in some countries (UK); increase or decrease of risk possible

- Increase in risk depends on nature of anomaly
  - US hard markers: structural anomalies strongly associated with aneuploidy
    - Second-trimester increased NT (Figure 7-7)
    - Cystic hygroma
    - Cardiac defect (Figure 7-8)
    - "Double bubble" = duodenal atresia (Figure 7-9), rarely seen before 20 weeks' gestational age
    - Intrauterine growth restriction (IUGR) *and* structural defect
  - US soft markers: common finding of uncertain significance, sometimes transient or resolving, often found in euploid fetuses (11% to 17%), more commonly in aneuploid fetuses with increased likelihood of aneuploidy the more are found in single fetus
  - Table 7-4: likelihood ratios of aneuploidy associated with specific markers
    - Echogenic bowel

TABLE 7-4   **Likelihood Ratios for Fetal Aneuploidy Associated with Sonographic Soft Markers**

Sonographic Marker	Trisomy 21	Normal	Positive LR	Negative LR	LR for Isolated Marker
Nuchal fold	107/319 (33.5%)	59/9331 (0.6%)	53.05	0.67	9.8
Short humerus	102/305 (33.4%)	136/9254 (1.5%)	22.76	0.68	4.1
Short femur	132/319 (41.4%)	486/9331 (5.2%)	7.94	0.62	1.6
Hydronephrosis	56/319 (17.6%)	242/9331 (2.6%)	6.77	0.85	1.0
Echogenic focus	75/266 (28.2%)	401/9199 (4.4%)	6.41	0.75	1.1
Echogenic bowel	39/293 (13.3%)	58/9227 (0.6%)	21.17	0.87	3.0
Major defect	75/350 (21.4%)	61/9384 (0.65%)	32.96	0.79	5.2

From Nicolaides, KH: Screening for chromosomal defects, *Ultrasound Obstet Gynecol* 21:313-321, 2003.

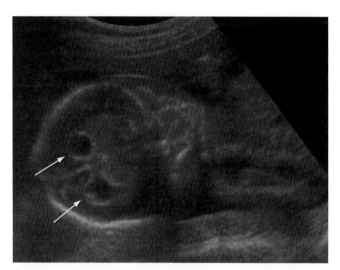

Figure 7-10. Arrows illustrate bilateral large choroid plexus cysts in a fetus with trisomy 18. (Image courtesy of Dr. E. Friedrich).

- Pyelectasis
- Ventriculomegaly
- Single umbilical artery
- Shortened long bones
- Choroid plexus cyst (Figure 7-10)
- Absent nasal bone
- Others: sandal gap toe, short ear length, clinodactyly (Figures 7-11, *A* and *B*), widened pelvic angle, multiple echogenic intracardiac foci
- Detectable anomalies without significant increase for aneuploidy—but possibility of other genetic disorders
  - Diaphragmatic hernia
  - Intestinal anomalies (e.g., gastroschisis)
  - Isolated renal anomalies (e.g., multicystic dysplastic kidneys)
  - Isolated cleft lip or cleft palate
- Limitations
  - Operator experience
  - Late gestational age unsuitable as primary screening tool
  - Intellectual disabilities, many single gene disorders not associated with structural defects
  - 40% to 50% of T21 fetuses show no detectable anomalies
- Adjunct benefits of second-trimester US
  - Improved pregnancy dating reduces incidence of postterm pregnancies, incidence of inductions

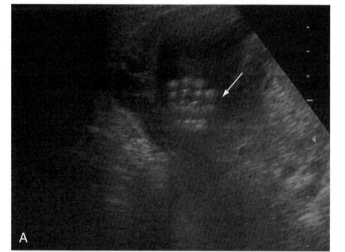

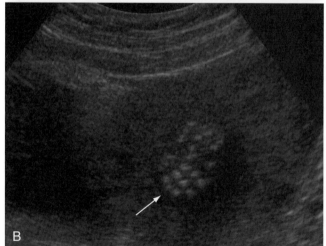

Figure 7-11. A, Ultrasound finding of hypoplasia/aplasia of middle-phalanx of digit V; arrow illustrates absent visualization of bone; fetus karyotypically normal. **B,** Ultrasound finding of very mild hypoplasia of middle phalanx of digit V, resulting in clinodactyly; fetus with Down syndrome. (**A,** Image courtesy of Dr. E. Friedrich. **B,** Image courtesy of Dr. E. Friedrich.)

  - Improved neonatal outcomes with higher 5-minute Apgar scores, less positive pressure ventilation (see comments in Update #1)
- New technologies
  - 3/4D US utilized by trained specialist to further characterize recognized fetal structural anomalies (Figure 7-12)

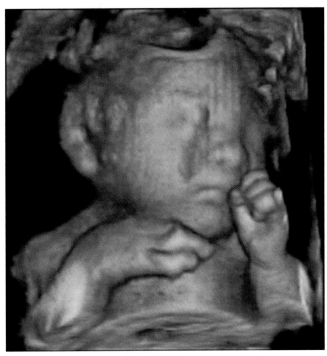

Figure 7-12. Three-dimensional US image of a fetus with multiple structural anomalies depicting the mild facial feature of Down syndrome. (Image courtesy of Chris Norton, RDMS.)

- ACOG advises against use of US in pregnancy for nonmedical indications (boutique or "mall" US)
- Fetal fast MRI useful and accurate in select cases to further characterize severe structural anomalies (neural tube defects, cranial and brain malformations, fetal tumors)

UPDATE #6

Despite the results of RADIUS and Helsinki trials, the use of the second-trimester sonography in aneuploidy screening is increasingly accepted (Fang et al, 2008). Multiple large studies have established the use of sonographic markers in the detection of aneuploidies, potentially responsible for a substantial modification of risk when used with serum markers (Nyberg et al, 1995). In older studies, an average decrease in T21 risk by four- to fivefold was expected with a negative screening US in the low-risk general obstetric population. If more (greater than one) US markers for T21 are found, risk for T21 increases six- to sevenfold (Benacerraf et al, 1992). Similar results are found in newer studies, where the genetic sonogram has been reported to have a sensitivity ranging from 59% to 87%, positive likelihood ratios ranging from 3 to 20, and negative likelihood ratios ranging from 0.1 to 0.4 in the detection of Down syndrome (Breathnach et al, 2007). Depending on a woman's assigned risk (by age or quad screening), US can change from a screen-negative to a screen-positive result. In high-risk women with increased risk for T21, overall DR of T21 with one or more markers was 79%, FPR 12%. The remaining 21% of cases originally classified as high risk would be missed if only negative US findings were used (Smith-Bindmann et al, 2007). More recently, the addition of second-trimester genetic sonography to first-trimester screening increased the DR of T21 to 90% and higher (Aagaard-Tillery et al, 2009; Wax et al, 2009).

Three-dimensional ultrasound can be a helpful adjunct in the diagnosis of fetal facial anomalies, neural tube defects, and skeletal anomalies (Goncalves et al, 2005). Recent studies

suggest that fetal MRI as an adjunct study to US can add significantly to the diagnosis and management of more than NTD-associated malformations (Mitchell et al, 2004), such as fetal tumors and abnormalities of placentation for both fetal and maternal indications (Laifer-Narin et al, 2007).

Diagnostic Testing

- Abnormal screening results should prompt offer of genetic counseling
- Diagnostic testing available to the patient:
  - Chorionic villus sampling (CVS)
  - Amniocentesis
  - Rarely: Percutaneous umbilical (fetal cord) blood sampling (PUBS)
  - IVF associated: preimplantation genetic diagnosis (PGD)/preimplantation genetic screening (PGS)
- Only *definitive* diagnostic test for aneuploidies: fetal karyotype or similar genetic test (e.g., array-comparative genomic hybridization [CGH]; see Update #8)

CVS

- Preferred GA 11 to 13 weeks; if >14 weeks = "placental biopsy" (e.g., in anhydramnios)
- Technique
  - Sterile field
  - Transabdominal (TA): 18- to 20-gauge needle
    - Procedure-related loss rates similar to midtrimester amniocentesis ~1/1-200
    - Recommended technique for early diagnosis
  - Transcervical (TC): catheter or forceps
    - Requires steep learning curve
    - Indicated: posterior placental implantations unsuitable for TA CVS
    - Procedure-related loss rate slightly higher 1 to 2/100; increases with number of passes
- Chorionic villi analysis for the following:
  - Fetal karyotype and genetic analysis by direct preparation or culture
  - Higher incidence of mosaicism encountered than amniocentesis, genetic counseling advised
    - Follow-up amniocentesis necessary in 1% to 10% for ambiguous results
    - Confined placental mosaicism in ~1%
- Early procedures <10 weeks' GA associated with limb defects, obsolete
- Common complications
  - Vaginal spotting/bleeding, up to 30% if TC CVS
  - Fluid leakage, chorioamnionitis <0.5%
- CVS in twins and multiple gestations
  - Loss rate increased, particularly in TC CVS
  - Less in experienced hands
  - Requires clear identification of placental area and border ("lambda" sign)
  - Limited data in pregnancies greater than twins

AMNIOCENTESIS

- Performed in the second trimester to obtain amniocytes for cytogenetic analysis
- Preferred GA 15 to 20 weeks, technically feasible to term

- Greater than 99% cytogenetic accuracy
- Amniocentesis technique
  - Continuous ultrasound guidance; perpendicular approach to control third dimension
  - Sterile field, no sterile sleeve necessary
  - Local anesthesia not indicated, not effective in pain control
  - A 20- or 22-gauge needle, no difference in outcome
  - 20 to 30 ccs of fluid removed, discard first 2 ccs for maternal contamination or use for amniotic fluid AFP analysis
- Amniotic fluid can be analyzed for the following:
  - Enzymes
  - Proteins
  - Hormones
  - Infectious agents (e.g., cytomegalovirus DNA by polymerase chain reaction [PCR])
  - Delta OD450 (Rh-disease)
  - Lung maturity
  - Fetal cells for cell culture and genetic analysis
- Procedure-related loss rate <0.5/100
- Common complications
  - Fluid leakage in 1% to 2%, almost 80% to 90% resealing rate
  - Transient vaginal spotting
  - Fetal injury, chorioamnionitis negligible at <1:1000
  - Transplacental passage does *not* increase loss rate
- Early amniocentesis (13 to 15 weeks) higher procedure-related loss risk (~1.7%); more often associated with technical difficulties; abandoned
- Amniocentesis in twins and multiple gestations
  - Loss rates are higher
  - Use indigo carmine to map amniotic cavity; single puncture trans-membranous approach utilized by some
  - Limited data in pregnancies greater than twins

PERCUTANEOUS UMBILICAL BLOOD SAMPLING

- Preferred GA >18 to 20 weeks
- Rarely done for genetic purposes: does not require cell culture, fast results from direct analysis; largely replaced by fluorescent in situ hybridization (FISH) and array-CGH technologies
- Procedure-related loss rate ~2/100
- Usually performed with therapeutic intent (transfusion, medication application)

PREIMPLANTATION GENETIC DIAGNOSIS (PGD) OR SCREENING (PGS)

- Tests for cytogenetic and mendelian disorders after in vitro fertilization (IVF) prior to implantation
- Biopsy of one to two cells from embryo at 6 to 8 cell stage (blastomere), day 5 to 6 embryo (blastocyst) or polar body
- PGD if testing performed to identify known heritable abnormalities or mutation in family
  - Single gene disorders detectable—if familiar mutation known—by PCR or targeted mutation analysis
  - HLA typing possible to, for example, select HLA-compatible offspring for bone marrow transplantation ethically controversial
  - Sex determination in X-linked disease

- PGS if procedure performed to screen for aneuploidy before embryo transfer; value and accuracy of PGS controversial
  - Fluorescent in situ hybridization (FISH) with chromosome-specific probes used to exclude most common aneuploidies and unbalanced chromosome rearrangements
  - Misses ~10% of chromosomal aneuploidies; postimplantation diagnostic procedures *still* indicated
    - Does not account for trisomic rescue
    - Does not result in full karyotype (common probes: chromosomes 21, 18, 13, X, Y, and chromosomes 16, 17, 22, 14)
    - Postzygotic events may lead to aneuploidy such as T21 despite normal PGS
  - Does not improve implantation rates in IVF pregnancies

UPDATE #7

In 2007, the American College of Obstetricians and Gynecologists (ACOG) Practice Bulletin No. 77 recommended the following:
- All women should be offered aneuploidy screening before 20 weeks' GA
- All women have the option of invasive testing regardless of maternal age
- Prenatal diagnostic procedures (rather than screening) should be considered in women of any age at high risk of Down syndrome (or other aneuploidies), such as the following:
  - After a prior pregnancy with a fetal trisomy
  - One major or two minor fetal structural anomalies
  - Known parental chromosomal rearrangement

Procedure-related loss rates of both amniocentesis and CVS in experienced hands appear to be low without evidence of a statistically significant difference in loss rate between the two (Caughey et al, 2006). The number of procedures has a significant effect on risk of loss in a study reporting on <500, 500 to 1000, 1001 to 1500, and >1500 procedures during an 11-year period, Particularly in CVS, risk of loss was 40% increased in departments with lower procedure numbers (Tabor et al, 2009). The FASTER trial showed 1% spontaneous loss after midtrimester amniocentesis and 0.94% spontaneous loss in the control group, not statistically significantly different. Resulting procedure-related loss rate from amniocentesis was 0.06% for all or 0.15% for screen-negative women (Eddleman et al, 2006). A recent 16-year retrospective cohort evaluating amniocentesis and CVS in twins found an attributable risk of pregnancy loss after midtrimester amniocentesis in twins of 1.8% (Cahill et al, 2009). A smaller cohort did not show a significant difference in loss rates or preterm premature rupture of membranes (PPROM) <34 weeks when comparing CVS and amniocentesis single versus double puncture techniques (Simonazzi et al, 2010).

PGS does not improve reproductive outcome in patients with advanced maternal age (Debrock et al, 2010); in a recent randomized controlled trial, lower pregnancy rates (8.9% in PGS, 24.5% in control group) were found (Hardarson et al, 2008).

Adjunct Benefits of Aneuploidy Screening

ENLARGED NT AND NORMAL KARYOTYPE

- Associated with significantly increased risk for congenital heart defects (CHD)
- Second-trimester targeted US and fetal echocardiography recommended

- NT ≥99th percentile associated with significantly increased risk of spontaneous fetal loss ≤24 weeks
- NT alone is a marker of various chromosome abnormalities and genetic syndromes resulting from single gene defects
  - Approximately 50% of fetuses with enlarged NT *and* chromosome abnormalities have a chromosomal abnormality other than T21
  - If karyotype is normal, genetic malformations cannot be ruled out; may be found on a submicroscopic level
    - Genetic counseling advised
    - Consider additional genetic studies such as array CGH or targeted mutation analysis

NEW TECHNOLOGIES

- Fetal Rh genotyping in maternal blood commercially available
- Fetal sex determination in maternal blood possible by PCR of Y chromosome–specific targets; useful in cases of X-linked or sex-specific disorders (e.g., congenital adrenal hyperplasia)
- Aneuploidy screening by noninvasive prenatal diagnosis (NIPD) not clinically validated at this time

UPDATE #8

Follow-up data from the FASTER trial in more than 34,000 fetuses showed a likelihood ratio for a major CHD of 22.5 with an NT of >2.5 MoM. Though sensitivity was low, specificity was high for the detection of CHD; screening in an unselected population is not recommended, but fetal echocardiography is indicated in fetuses with elevated NT >99th percentile (2.5 MoM) (Simpson et al, 2007). Cases of cystic hygroma show an increased incidence of CHD (Sananes et al, 2010).

Continued efforts are placed in the development of NIPD. Particularly, Rh-genotyping utilizing fetal DNA from maternal blood shows an accuracy of 94% to 100% and has been made commercially available worldwide, promising a significant reduction in use of anti-D immunoglobulin (Daniels et al, 2009; Gautier et al, 2005). Aneuploidy detection by examination of fetal cells, cell-free DNA, and mRNA in maternal blood proves more difficult, but new technologies such as high throughput shotgun sequencing and the differentiation of maternally and paternally inherited single nucleotide polymorphisms (SNPs) are promising; investigation into these technologies is ongoing (Avent et al, 2009; Dhallan et al, 2007; Ehrich et al, 2011).

Chromosomal microarrays (array CGH) utilize thousands to millions of FISH probes over the entire genome with significantly greater resolution than microscopic karyotyping. Previously unrecognized microdeletions, microduplications, and other subtle submicroscopic rearrangements can now easily be identified. However, benign polymorphisms will be detected in up to 20% of cases, which can make it challenging to interpret results (Van den Veyver et al, 2009). Being increasingly used prenatally and technically feasible at a cost similar to that of a karyotype, smaller studies have supported array CGH use, especially in cases of fetal anomalies with a normal conventional karyotype. Up to an additional 5% to 10% of genetic anomalies may be detected by use of array technology (American College of Obstetricians and Gynecologists, ACOG Committee Opinion No. 446, 2009). Ethically, caution is advised: inadvertently presymptomatic testing for adult-onset conditions such as Huntington disease or BRCA mutations may be performed prenatally (Greifman-Holtzman et al, 2009).

ABNORMAL SERUM MARKERS AND ADVERSE PREGNANCY OUTCOME

- Abnormal first- and second-trimester maternal serum values associated with obstetrical complications
- Intervention protocols and monitoring controversial
  - No clear improvement of pregnancy outcome
  - No documented cost effectiveness
- Conditions associated with abnormal maternal serum analytes
  - Preeclampsia
  - Fetal growth restriction
  - Preterm birth
  - Fetal death
  - Sudden infant death syndrome
  - Placental abnormalities
  - Placental abruption
  - Oligohydramnios
- Risk increases as number and level of abnormal serum markers increase

UPDATE #9

First-trimester serum analytes were analyzed for secondary outcomes in the FASTER and many other trials. PAPP-A levels ≤ fifth percentile were associated with significantly higher rates of spontaneous fetal loss ≤24 weeks, low birth weight, preeclampsia, and preterm birth. NT ≥ ninety-ninth percentile or free beta-hCG ≤ first percentile were also associated with a significantly increased risk of spontaneous fetal loss ≤24 weeks (Dugoff et al, 2004). Low PAPP-A levels in absence of an abnormal karyotype showed an association with preterm delivery in a report of almost 55,000 women. At the fifth percentile of normal, the odds ratio for delivery before 34 weeks was 2.35. Similarly, low PAPP-A levels were associated with IUGR, though detection rates for small for gestational age (SGA) were low at 12% to 16% (Spencer et al, 2008).

In the second trimester, numerous associations between abnormal markers and adverse outcome have been described, but with low sensitivity and positive predictive value. The risk increased if more than one marker was abnormal (Dugoff et al, 2005). Elevated MSAFP levels as late as 28 weeks have been reported as predictive of preterm birth (Moawad et al, 2002). Unexplained elevated second-trimester hCG levels >5 to 8 MoM have shown an association with SGA newborns in 40% to 80% of newborns, respectively, and increased surveillance is recommended (Ganapathy et al, 2007).

The risk of sudden infant death syndrome (SIDS) appears to increase in women who have high MSAFP levels. In a preliminary population-based study, SIDS occurred significantly more often in infants of women in the fourth and fifth quintiles of AFP concentration than in those in the first (lowest) quintile (odds ratio 2.2, 95% confidence interval 1.1 to 4.4) (Smith et al, 2004).

SUGGESTED READINGS

First-Trimester Ultrasound and General Approach to Genetic Screening

D'Alton ME, Cleary-Goldman J: Additional benefits of first trimester screening, *Semin Perinatol* 29(6):405–411, 2005.

Nicolaides KH: Nuchal translucency and other first trimester sonographic markers of chromosomal abnormalities, *Am J Obstet Gynecol* 191(1):45–67, 2004.

Timor-Tritsch IE, Fuchs KM, Monteagudo A, D'Alton ME: Performing a fetal anatomy scan at the time of first-trimester screening, *Obstet Gynecol* 113(2 Pt 1):402–407, 2009.

First-Trimester Screening

American College of Obstetricians and Gynecologists: ACOG committee opinion no. 296: first-trimester screening for fetal aneuploidy, *Obstet Gynecol* 104(1):215–217, 2004.

Malone FD, Canick JA, Ball RH, et al: First-trimester or second-trimester screening, or both, for Down's syndrome, *N Engl J Med* 353(19):2001–2011, 2005.

Wapner RJ: First trimester screening: the BUN study, *Semin Perinatol* 29(4):236–239, 2005.

Wapner RJ, Thom E, Simpson JL, et al: First-trimester screening for trisomies 21 and 18, *N Engl J Med* 349(15):1405–1413, 2003.

First-Trimester Ultrasound Markers

Kagan KO, Valencia C, Livanos P, et al: Tricuspid regurgitation in screening for trisomies 21, 18 and 13 and Turner syndrome at 11+0 to 13+6 weeks of gestation, *Ultrasound Obstet Gynecol* 33(1):18–22, 2009.

Maiz N, Valencia C, Kagan KO, et al: Ductus venosus Doppler in screening for trisomies 21, 18 and 13 and Turner syndrome at 11-13 weeks of gestation, *Ultrasound Obstet Gynecol* 33(5):512–517, 2009.

Rosen T, D'Alton ME, Platt LD, Wapner R: First-trimester ultrasound assessment of the nasal bone to screen for aneuploidy, *Obstet Gynecol* 110(2 Pt 1):399–404, 2007.

Second-Trimester Screening

Ball RH, Caughey AB, Malone FD, et al: First- and second-trimester evaluation of risk for Down syndrome, *Obstet Gynecol* 110(1):10–17, 2007.

Berkowitz RL, Cuckle HS, Wapner R, D'Alton ME: Aneuploidy screening: what test should I use? *Obstet Gynecol* 107(3):715–718, 2006.

Norem CT, Schoen EJ, Walton DL, et al: Routine ultrasonography compared with maternal serum alpha-fetoprotein for neural tube defect screening, *Obstet Gynecol* 106(4):747–752, 2005.

Integrated Screening

American College of Obstetricians and Gynecologists: ACOG practice bulletin no. 101: ultrasonography in pregnancy, *Obstet Gynecol* 113(2 Pt 1):451–461, 2009.

American College of Obstetricians and Gynecologists Committee on Practice Bulletins: ACOG practice bulletin no. 77: screening for fetal chromosomal abnormalities, *Obstet Gynecol* 109(1):217–227, 2007.

Breathnach FM, Malone FD, Lambert-Messerlian G, et al: First- and second-trimester screening: detection of aneuploidies other than Down syndrome, *Obstet Gynecol* 110(3):651–657, 2007.

Wald NJ, Rodeck C, Hackshaw AK, et al: First and second trimester antenatal screening for Down's syndrome; the results of the Serum, Urine and Ultrasound Screening Study (SURUSS), *J Med Screen* 10(2):56–104, 2003.

Second-Trimester Ultrasound

Aagaard-Tillery KM, Malone FD, Nyberg DA, et al: Role of second-trimester genetic sonography after Down syndrome screening, *Obstet Gynecol* 114(6):1189–1196, 2009.

American Institute of Ultrasound in Medicine: AIUM practice guidelines for the performance of obstetric ultrasound examinations, *J Ultrasound Med* 29(1):157–166, 2010.

LeFevre ML, Bain RP, Ewigman BG, et al: A randomized trial of prenatal ultrasonographic screening: impact on maternal management and outcome, *Am J Obstet Gynecol* 169(3):483–489, 1993.

Diagnostic Testing

American College of Obstetricians and Gynecologists: ACOG committee opinion no. 430: preimplantation genetic screening for aneuploidy, *Obstet Gynecol* 113(3):766–767, 2009.

American College of Obstetricians and Gynecologists: ACOG practice bulletin no. 88, December 2007. Invasive prenatal testing for aneuploidy, *Obstet Gynecol* 110(6):1459–1467, 2007.

Tabor A, Vestergaard CHF, Lidegaard O: Fetal loss rate after chorionic villus sampling and amniocentesis: an 11-year national registry study, *Ultrasound Obstet Gynecol* 34(1):19–24, 2009.

Additional Benefits of Screening and New Technologies

American College of Obstetricians and Gynecologists: ACOG committee opinion no. 446: array comparative genomic hybridization in prenatal diagnosis, *Obstet Gynecol* 114(5):1161–1163, 2009.

Daniels G, Finning K, Martin P, Massey E: Noninvasive prenatal diagnosis of fetal blood group phenotypes: current practice and future prospect, *Prenat Diagn* 29(2):101–107, 2009.

Simpson LL, Malone FD, Bianchi DW, et al: Nuchal translucency and the risk of congenital heart disease, *Obstet Gynecol* 109(2 Pt 1):376–383, 2007.

Van den Veyver IB, Patel A, Shaw CA, et al: Clinical use of array comparative genomic hybridization (aCGH) for prenatal diagnosis in 300 cases, *Prenat Diagn* 29(1):29–39, 2009.

Adverse Pregnancy Outcome

Dugoff L, Hobbins JC, Malone FD, et al: First-trimester maternal serum PAPP-A and free-beta subunit human chorionic gonadotropin concentrations and nuchal translucency are associated with obstetric complications: a population-based screening study (The FASTER Trial), *Am J Obstet Gynecol* 191(4):1446–1451, 2004.

Dugoff L, Hobbins JC, Malone FD, et al: Quad screen as a predictor of adverse pregnancy outcome, *Obstet Gynecol* 106(2):260–267, 2005.

References

Please go to expertconsult.com to view references.

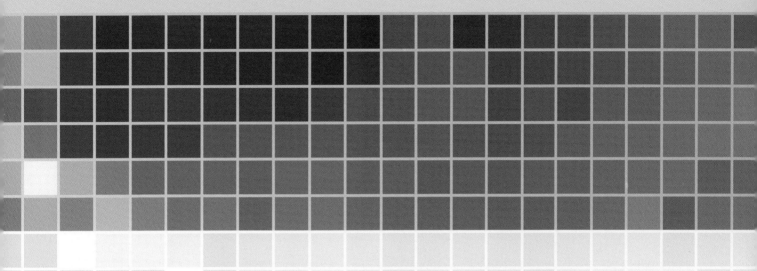

SECTION 3

Second-Trimester Complications

Chapter 8

Cervical Insufficiency

JENNIFER A. JOLLEY • MANUEL PORTO

KEY UPDATES

1 Intraamniotic inflammation may be present in the majority of cases of acute cervical insufficiency.

2 *Ureaplasma urealyticum* and *Mycoplasma hominis* are the microorganisms isolated most frequently from women with cervical insufficiency and short cervix.

3 Data showing an association between excisional procedures for cervical dysplasia and subsequent future pregnancy complications are increasing.

4 Cerclage may be beneficial for decreasing preterm birth in certain populations with short cervical length.

5 Cerclage may prevent preterm birth <35 weeks in women with a prior spontaneous preterm birth <34 weeks and cervical length <15 mm.

6 In women with a short cervix, treatment with progesterone reduces the rate of spontaneous early preterm delivery.

Background

- Inability of the uterine cervix to retain a pregnancy to term in the absence of contractions or labor (American College of Obstetricians and Gynecologists, Practice Bulletin No. 48, 2003)
- Previously termed "cervical incompetence"; now preferred terminology is cervical insufficiency
- Presumed physical weakness that leads to loss of otherwise normal pregnancy
- Continuum of cervical function that may be expressed differently in subsequent pregnancies, as opposed to either functional or nonfunctional
- Difficult to distinguish between cervical insufficiency and other etiologies of early spontaneous preterm birth as history, symptoms, and physical findings can be the same
- May result in second trimester spontaneous abortion, periviable delivery, preterm delivery, and preterm premature rupture of membranes (PPROM)
- Difficult to ascertain incidence because of a lack of clear diagnostic criteria (Figure 8-1)

Etiology

- Probable spectrum of disease with congenital and acquired etiologies
  - Structural
  - Inflammatory
  - Hormonal
  - Histologic
  - Multifactorial

Risk Factors

- Most women have no identifiable risk factors
- Cervical surgery
  - Excisional
    - Conization
    - Loop electrosurgical excision procedure (LEEP)
  - Ablative
    - Laser ablation
    - Cryotherapy
- Cervical trauma
  - Laceration with vaginal or cesarean delivery
  - During dilation and curettage or evacuation
- Congenital
  - Inherent short cervix
  - Collagen synthesis defects
    - Ehlers-Danlos
  - Müllerian anomalies
  - In utero DES exposure
    - No studies have proved that cervical insufficiency is more frequent in DES-exposed women
- Uterine overdistension
  - Multiple gestations
  - Polyhydramnios

Inflammation and Infection

UPDATE #1

Intraamniotic inflammation may be present in the majority of patients with acute cervical insufficiency. Elevated matrix metalloproteinase-8 concentration, a marker for inflammation, was present in approximately 80% of patients with acute

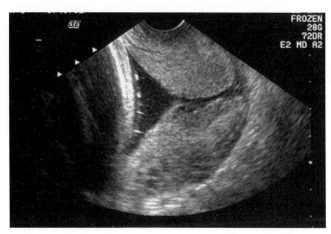

Figure 8-1. Endovaginal ultrasound image of the cervix in a woman with preterm labor. (Courtesy of Jay D. Iams, MD.)

cervical insufficiency, whereas only 8% of the same patients had a positive amniotic fluid culture (Lee et al, 2008). Intraamniotic inflammation was a risk factor for impending preterm delivery and poor neonatal outcome, therefore assessment of the state of inflammation of the amniotic cavity may have prognostic value in patients with cervical insufficiency.

- There appears to be a correlation between severe cervical shortening and intraamniotic inflammation
- Cervical length ≤ 5 mm is associated with significant increases in amniotic fluid inflammatory cytokines even in absence of infection or labor (Kiefer et al, 2009)

UPDATE #2

Genital mycoplasmas (*Ureaplasma urealyticum* and *Mycoplasma hominis)* are the microorganisms isolated most frequently from women with cervical insufficiency (Romero et al, 1992) and short cervix (Hassan et al, 2006).

- Genital mycoplasmas are found frequently in the lower genital tract of sexually active women and normal pregnant women (Romero et al, 2008)
- Intrauterine presence of mycoplasmas is associated with increased production of inflammatory cytokines, prostaglandins, and matrix metalloproteinases (Yoon et al, 1998)
- Ultrasound visualization of intraamniotic debris or sludge suggests subclinical infection and is a poor prognostic sign (Kusanovic et al, 2007)
- *Ureaplasma urealyticum* is the most common microorganism isolated from amniotic fluid of women with preterm labor and intact membranes (Gomez et al, 2005)
- Forty-three percent of patients with cervical length <15 mm and gestational age ≤ 30 weeks had microbial invasion of the amniotic cavity, significantly higher than those with cervical length ≥15 mm (Gomez et al, 2005)
- Positive *U. urealyticum* and *M. hominis* cord blood cultures are more common in those delivering at earlier gestational ages (Goldenberg et al, 2008)
  - 44% of infants born at 23 to 24 weeks' gestational age had cord blood cultures positive for *U. urealyticum* and/ or *M. hominis* (Goldenberg et al, 2008)

- Identification of infection as the cause of cervical insufficiency may allow targeted interventions for certain patients

Cervical Surgery

UPDATE #3

Data showing an association between excisional procedures for cervical dysplasia and subsequent future pregnancy complications are increasing (Jakobsson et al, 2007, 2009; Kyrgiou et al, 2006; Nøhr et al, 2007, 2009; Sadler et al, 2004; Samson et al, 2005).

- Starting in the 1980s, researchers have generally found an increase in preterm birth after cold knife conization
- The risk of very preterm (28 to 31 weeks) and extremely preterm (<28 weeks) delivery increase after cervical conization (RR 1.99, 95% CI 1.81 to 2.20; RR 2.86, 95% CI 2.22 to 3.70; RR 2.10, 95% CI 1.30 to 2.32, respectively) (Jakobsson et al, 2007)
- A large meta-analysis found a significant association between cold knife conization and preterm delivery (RR 2.59, 95% CI 1.80 to 3.72, eight studies, n = 28,378), and low birth weight (RR 2.53, 95% CI 1.19 to 5.36, four studies, n = 13,490) (Kyrgiou et al, 2006)
- Many practitioners have used early studies that did not show an association with obstetric morbidity to counsel patients prior to undergoing loop electrosurgical excision procedure (LEEP)
- More recently, authors have found that LEEP is significantly associated with preterm delivery, low birth weight, and PPROM (Jakobsson et al, 2009; Kyrgiou et al, 2006; Nøhr et al, 2007, 2009; Sadler et al, 2004; Samson et al, 2005)
- Increasing depth of LEEP is associated with a significant increase in the risk of preterm delivery, with an estimated 6% increase in risk per each additional millimeter of tissue excised (Noehr et al, 2009)
- There are several mechanisms by which excisional cervical procedures may increase the risk of early delivery and PPROM
  - Decreased mechanical support and length of the cervix
  - Increased susceptibility to infection after loss of cervical mucus production
- Surprisingly, the length of the cervix does not appear to be permanently altered in all patients who have undergone excisional cervical procedures
  - Ultrasonographic measurement of the cervix after LEEP was not different from the measurement before the procedure (Gentry et al, 2000)
  - Only 28% of women with prior cone biopsy, LEEP, or laser conization had a short cervix (Berghella et al, 2004)
- Because the cervical length is not necessarily distorted after excisional surgery, measuring or observing a change in the length during pregnancy may be of value
- Berghella et al. showed that cervical length is predictive of preterm birth in women with prior excisional cervical surgery (Berghella et al, 2004)

Diagnosis

- There is no objective diagnostic test for cervical insufficiency
- Although highest risk is with short cervical length <10th percentile, there is no threshold value below which a patient always presents with cervical insufficiency
- Methods proposed for diagnosis in the nonpregnant state do not predict subsequent pregnancy outcomes
  - Balloon elastance test (Kiwi et al, 1988)
  - Passage of Hegar or Pratt dilators through the internal cervical os
  - Hysterosalpingography with balloon traction on the cervix (Zlatnick et al, 1989)
- History
  - Recurrent painless dilation of cervix prior to preterm birth in second trimester
- Symptoms
  - Vaginal pressure
  - Copious vaginal discharge
  - Vaginal bleeding/spotting
  - Asymptomatic
- Physical examination
  - Sterile speculum exam with visualization of prolapsed fetal membranes
- Ultrasound examination
  - Transvaginal sonographic measurement of cervical length (Table 8-1)

Cervical Length

- Transvaginal sonography after 16 weeks provides most accurate and consistent measurement
- Between 22 and 30 weeks, length of cervix described by normal bell-shaped curve (Iams et al, 1996)
  - 5th percentile: 20 mm
  - 10th percentile: 25 mm
  - 50th percentile: 35 mm
  - 90th percentile: 45 mm
- "Short cervix" variously defined as ≤25 mm and ≤15 mm
- Cervical length used as surrogate for cervical insufficiency but length that predicts cervical insufficiency is not defined

Please see Figure 8-2.

Cervical Length in Prediction of Preterm Birth

- Short cervical length on transvaginal ultrasonography has been shown to be one of the best predictors of preterm birth (Berghella et al, 2007; Iams et al, 1996)
- Relative risk of preterm delivery increases with decreasing cervical length
- Not predictive of preterm birth risk when cervix dilated ≥2 cm
- Transvaginal ultrasonographic measurement of cervical length has highest sensitivity and positive predictive value (both >60%) in women with a prior preterm birth and a singleton pregnancy (Owen et al, 2001)

TABLE 8-1 Technique of Transvaginal Cervical Length

Empty bladder

Condom-covered probe

Let patient insert probe

Guide probe into anterior fornix

Obtain sagittal sonographic view of cervix with echogenic endocervical mucosa along the length of the canal

Withdraw probe until blurred, then reinsert making sure to avoid excessive pressure

Enlarge image (at least two thirds of screen)

Obtain symmetric image of entire endocervical canal, with internal os at flat or isosceles angle, and symmetric view of external os (anterior lip diameter should be equal to posterior lip diameter)

Measure from internal os to external os along entire cervical canal

Obtain three measurements, use shortest best

Apply transfundal pressure for at least 15 seconds

Total examination duration: at least 5 minutes

Modified from Berghella V: Novel developments on cervical length screening and progesterone for preventing preterm birth, *BJOG* 116:182-187, 2008.[7]

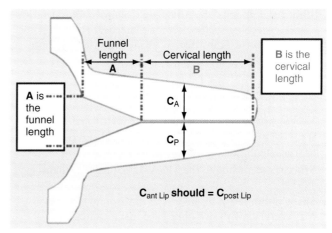

Figure 8-2. **Measurement of the cervix.** (From Johnson J, Iams J: *Prediction of prematurity by transvaginal ultrasound assessment of the cervix* [website]. UpToDate.com. Last updated February 3, 2010.)

- Women with prior birth <24 weeks significantly more likely to experience cervical shortening <25 mm and at earlier gestational age than women with prior birth at 24 to 33⁶⁄₇ weeks (Szychowski et al, 2009)
- Systematic review showed that in asymptomatic women at increased risk of preterm birth, measurement of <25 mm before 20 weeks' gestation predicted preterm delivery prior to 35 weeks' gestation (LR 4.31, 95% CI: 3.08 to 6.01, 14 studies, n = 2258) (Crane et al, 2008)
- Risk of spontaneous preterm birth increases as length of cervix decreases and as gestational age decreases (Berghella et al, 2007)
- Predictive value of cervical length measurement at <20 weeks' gestation is greater than measurement after 20 weeks of gestation (Crane et al, 2008)

TABLE 8-2   Key Points for Interpretation of Transvaginal Cervical Length for Prediction of Preterm Birth

Best gestational age for screening is 16-24 weeks

Normal CL: 15-50 mm

CL <25 mm is below the 10th percentile at 16-24 weeks

CL <15 mm is below the second percentile at 21-25 weeks

Not very helpful before 14 weeks (CL usually normal even if later PTB)

Not very helpful after 28 weeks (CL may be physiologically short)

The shorter the CL, the higher the risk of PTB

The earlier the short CL is detected, the higher the risk of PTB

Sensitivity, specificity, and positive and negative predictive values vary widely depending on population

Best (blinded) studies have mostly used TVU CL screening at 16-24 weeks, with a cutoff of <25 mm and an outcome of PTB <35 weeks

From Berghella V: Novel developments on cervical length screening and progesterone for preventing preterm birth, *BJOG* 116:182-187, 2008.

- Sensitivity for prediction of preterm birth lower in low-risk women
  - Routine cervical length screening in low-risk populations not recommended by American College of Obstetricians and Gynecologists (Society for Maternal Fetal Medicine Publications Committee, ACOG Committee Opinion No. 419, 2008) (Table 8-2)

Cervical Funneling

- Visible separation of sidewalls of the internal os
- If funnel present, length of residual closed cervix recorded as true length
- Proceeds according to the T-Y-V-U sequence (Zilianti et al, 1995)
- Shape of funnel on midtrimester ultrasound evaluation may correlate with risk of cervical insufficiency and preterm birth
- Progression over time from a T- to a V- to a U-shaped funnel associated with earlier gestational age at delivery (Berghella et al, 2007)
- Resolution of V-shaped funnel associated with term delivery (Berghella et al, 2007)
- Similar gestational age at delivery with or without funneling if cervical length <25 mm (30.6+/−8.0 weeks compared with 31.9+/−6.6 weeks; P = 0.59) (Berghella et al, 2007)
- Funneling predictive of early gestational age at delivery but does not add significantly to the prediction obtained by an accurate cervical length measurement in women with prior preterm birth (Figure 8-3)

Management of Cervical Insufficiency

- Interventions to treat cervical insufficiency have had mixed results, likely because of the inability to differentiate multiple etiologies of short cervix

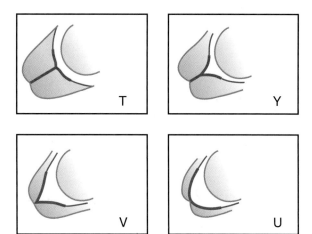

Progression of cervical effacement at the internal cervical os from completely uneffaced (T) to completely effaced (U).

Figure 8-3. Diagram of cervical effacement. (Adapted from Zilianti M, Azuaga A, Calderon F, et al: Monitoring the effacement of the uterine cervix by transperineal sonography: a new perspective, *J Ultrasound Med* 14:719-724, 1995.)

Cerclage

- Mechanism by which cerclage confers benefit is unknown
- Rationale is that cerclage compensates for inherent weakness of the cervix
- Significant controversy remains regarding appropriate candidate selection
- Randomized controlled trials have had mixed results reflecting disparity in patient populations
  - All studies target women with short cervical length
  - Studies showing benefit of cerclage use maternal history consistent with cervical insufficiency in selection criteria

HISTORY INDICATED

- Women with three or more second-trimester spontaneous abortions or preterm births may benefit from prophylactic cerclage Medical Research Council/Royal College of Obstetricians, 1993)
- Women with one or two second-trimester spontaneous abortions or preterm births can be followed with cervical length measurement (Althuisius et al, 2000)

ULTRASOUND INDICATED

UPDATE #4

Cerclage should be reserved for certain groups with short cervical length on transvaginal ultrasound. A meta-analysis suggested that cerclage may decrease preterm birth at less than 35 weeks in certain subgroups with short cervical length: singleton gestations with prior preterm birth, singleton gestations with prior second-trimester loss, and singleton gestations with cervical length <25 mm (Berghella et al, 2005).

UPDATE #5

Cerclage prevents preterm birth <35 weeks in women with a prior spontaneous preterm birth <34 weeks and cervical length <15 mm (Owen et al, 2009).

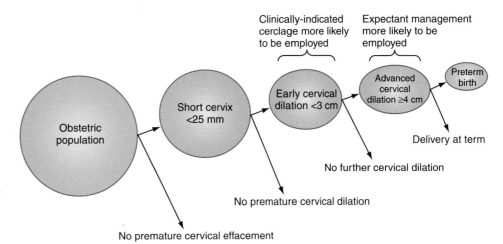

Figure 8-4. Inherent bias of cerclage procedures. (Adapted from Pereira L, Cotter A, Gomez R, et al: Expectant management compared with physical examination-indicated cerclage (EM-PEC) in selected women with a dilated cervix at 14⁶⁄₇ to 25⁶⁄₇ weeks: results from the EM-PEC international cohort study, *AJOG* 197:483.e1-483.e8, 2007.)

This figure demonstrates the source of bias inherent when clinicians perform cerclage procedures earlier in the continuum of cervical change because only a proportion of the population will naturally progress to the next stage.

- Only one third of women with prior preterm birth manifest a short cervix in subsequent pregnancy
- There is an interaction between cerclage efficacy and cervical length
- In women with previous preterm birth <34 weeks and cervical length <25 mm, cerclage decreased birth <24 weeks and perinatal mortality (Owen et al, 2009)
- In women with CL<15 mm there is a significant benefit from cerclage assignment in decreasing recurrent preterm birth <35 weeks (OR 0.23, 95% CI 0.08 to 0.66) (Owen et al, 2009)
- Cerclage placement in some women may increase the risk of preterm birth
- A retrospective study suggested that cerclage may be harmful in patients with a short cervix and elevated levels of cervical IL-8, a marker for inflammation (Sakai et al, 2006)

PHYSICAL EXAMINATION INDICATED

- Cerclage placed because of second trimester cervical dilation or prolapsed membranes
- Rate of preterm delivery >90% with expectant management in these patients
- Historical cohort study in patients between 14⁶⁄₇ and 25⁶⁄₇ weeks dilated ≥1 cm suggested that cerclage was associated with longer interval between presentation and delivery and improved neonatal survival (Pereira et al, 2007)
  - Patients who had cerclage were more likely to have had previous second-trimester miscarriage
- Contraindicated if clinical evidence of chorioamnionitis, preterm contractions, PPROM
- Clinical signs are late markers of intraamniotic infection, thus consideration should be given to performing amniocentesis prior to cerclage placement
- Further study of the risks and benefits of physical examination indicated cerclage needed

- Further study of methods to evaluate for presence of intraamniotic inflammation and infection ongoing (Figure 8-4)

Cervical Pessary

- Some practitioners have used ringlike pessaries to provide support similar to that of a cerclage in patients with sonographically short cervix
- Small trials in patients with CL <15 mm in the midtrimester have shown that pessary placement decreased rate of preterm delivery (Arabin et al, 2003) and increased the average gestational age at delivery (Ludmir et al, 2002)
- Two randomized trials ongoing in Europe

Progesterone

UPDATE #6

In women with a short cervix, treatment with progesterone reduces the rate of spontaneous early preterm delivery (DeFranco et al, 2007; Fonseca et al, 2007).

- Progesterone appears to have anti-inflammatory properties and may act by preventing cervical ripening (Xu et al, 2008)
- In women with a cervical length ≤15 mm measured between 20 and 25 weeks, spontaneous preterm delivery before 34 weeks was significantly less frequent with administration of vaginal progesterone 200 mg daily versus placebo (19.2% versus 34.4%, RR 0.56, 95% CI 0.36 to 0.86) (Fonseca et al, 2007)
- The overall reduction in preterm birth in women with cervical length ≤15 mm was 44% (Fonseca et al, 2007)
- In women with a previous preterm birth who also had a short cervical length <28 mm in the midtrimester, daily supplementation with 90 mg of vaginal progesterone gel significantly reduced the frequency of preterm birth ≤32 weeks' gestation (0% versus 29.6%, p = 0.014) (DeFranco et al, 2007)

- Thus, progesterone may be effective for a larger subset of women with short cervical length, as frequency of midtrimester cervical length ≤ 15 mm is only 1.7% (Fonseca et al, 2007), but <28 mm is approximately 9% (DeFranco et al, 2007)
- In women with a previous spontaneous preterm birth between 20 and 36 weeks 6 days gestation, weekly injections of 250 mg of 17 alpha-hydroxyprogesterone caproate (17P) significantly decreased risk of recurrent preterm delivery (Meis et al, 2003)
  - Less than 37 weeks (36.3% versus 54.9%, RR 0.66, 95% CI 0.54 to 0.81)
  - Less than 35 weeks (20.6% versus 30.7%, RR 0.67, 95% CI 0.48 to 0.93)
  - Less than 32 weeks (11.4% versus 19.6%, RR 0.58, 95% CI 0.37 to 0.91)
- Given that a large proportion of patients diagnosed with cervical insufficiency will either have a history of preterm birth or a short cervical length, progesterone supplementation may be appropriate in this population

Bed Rest

- There is no evidence to support or refute use of bed rest to prevent preterm delivery

Tocolysis

- No studies of second trimester tocolysis in women with diagnosis of cervical insufficiency
- One meta-analysis found indomethacin therapy for short cervix <25 mm at 14 to 27 weeks without cerclage did not prevent spontaneous preterm birth <35 weeks but did prevent preterm birth <24 weeks (Berghella et al, 2006)
- Currently, insufficient evidence to assess if women with cerclage for short cervix benefit from indomethacin or other tocolysis
- The standard indications for tocolysis may apply for patients with cervical insufficiency and threatened periviable or preterm delivery

Hospitalization

- Inpatient management may be appropriate when the limit of viability has been reached
- Evidence suggests improved outcomes with the administration of corticosteroids at viability

Antibiotic Administration

- Some administer prophylactic broad-spectrum antibiotics prior to cerclage placement to attempt to reduce incidence of infection and preterm birth
- No randomized controlled trials evaluating the efficacy of antibiotic therapy for prevention of preterm birth in women with short cervix <25 mm
- No proven benefit of latency antibiotics in setting of intact membranes

Special Considerations

MULTIPLE GESTATIONS

- Mechanism of preterm birth in multiples may be uterine overdistension leading to preterm labor, rather than cervical insufficiency
- In twins with short cervix <25 mm, cerclage was associated with a *higher* incidence of preterm birth <35 weeks compared to controls (RR 2.15, 95% CI 1.15 to 4.01) (Berghella et al, 2005)
- Progesterone supplementation does *not* decrease risk of preterm delivery in twins (Rouse et al, 2007)

Future Directions

- Define different pathways to cervical insufficiency
- Develop methods to differentiate between women with and without intraamniotic inflammation and infection
- Define etiology-specific therapies that target different causes of cervical shortening
- Tailored management of women at risk for second trimester spontaneous abortion, periviable and preterm delivery (Figure 8-5)

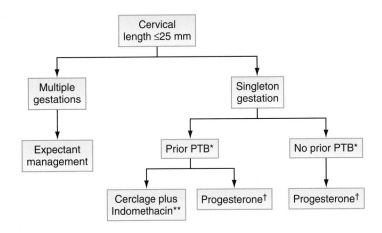

*Fetal fibronectin and interleukin-8 may further stratify women to prevent unnecessary cerclages.
**Indomethacin was used in studies that were originally designed to study the utility of cerclage in asymptomatic women with short cervical length.
†Available evidence supports the use of progesterone to women with cervical length ≤15 mm. PTB, preterm birth.

Figure 8-5. Algorithm for evaluation and management of cervical insufficiency. (Adapted from Sinno A, Usta I, Nassar A: A short cervical length in pregnancy: management options, *Am J Perinatol* 26:761-770, 2009.)

SUGGESTED READINGS

Inflammation and Infection

Goldenberg RL, Andrews WW, Goepfert AR, et al: The Alabama Preterm Birth Study: umbilical cord blood *Ureaplasma urealyticum* and *Mycoplasma hominis* cultures in very preterm newborn infants, *Am J Obstet Gynecol* 198(1):43.e1-e5, 2008.

Gomez R, Romero R, Nien JK, et al: A short cervix in women with preterm labor and intact membranes: a risk factor for microbial invasion of the amniotic cavity, *Am J Obstet Gynecol* 192(3):678–689, 2005.

Kiefer DG, Keeler SM, Rust OA, et al: Is midtrimester short cervix a sign of intraamniotic inflammation?, *Am J Obstet Gynecol* 200(4):374.e1-e5, 2009.

Lee SE, Romero R, Park CW, et al: The frequency and significance of intraamniotic inflammation in patients with cervical insufficiency, *Am J Obstet Gynecol* 198(6):633.e1-e8, 2008.

Cervical Surgery

Jakobsson M, Gissler M, Paavonen J, Tapper AM: Loop electrosurgical excision procedure and the risk of preterm birth, *Obstet Gynecol* 114(3):504–510, 2009.

Kyrgiou M, Koliopoulos G, Martin-Hirsch P, et al: Obstetric outcomes after conservative treatment for intraepithelial or early invasive cervical lesions: systematic review and meta analysis, *Lancet* 367(9509):489–498, 2006.

Noehr B, Jensen A, Frederiksen K, et al: Loop electrosurgical excision of the cervix and subsequent risk for spontaneous preterm delivery: a population-based study of singleton deliveries during a 9-year period, *Am J Obstet Gynecol* 201(1):33.e1-e6, 2009.

Cervical Length in Prediction of Preterm Birth

Berghella V, Roman A, Daskalakis C, et al: Gestational age at cervical length measurement and incidence of preterm birth, *Obstet Gynecol* 110(2 Pt 1):311–317, 2007.

Iams JD, Goldenberg RL, Meis PJ, et al: The length of the cervix and the risk of spontaneous preterm delivery: National Institute of Child Health and Human Development Maternal Fetal Medicine Unit Network, *N Engl J Med* 334(9):567–572, 1996.

Cerclage

Berghella V, Odibo A, To M, et al: Cerclage for short cervix on ultrasonography: meta-analysis of trials using individual patient-level data, *Obstet Gynecol* 106(1):181–189, 2005.

Owen J, Hankins G, Iams J, et al: Multicenter randomized trial of cerclage for preterm birth prevention in high-risk women with shortened midtrimester cervical length, *Am J Obstet Gynecol* 201(4):375.e1-e8, 2009.

Progesterone

DeFranco EA, O'Brien JM, Adair CD, et al: Vaginal progesterone is associated with a decrease in risk for early preterm birth and improved neonatal outcome in women with a short cervix: a secondary analysis from a randomized, double-blind, placebo-controlled trial, *Ultrasound Obstet Gynecol* 30(5):697–705, 2007.

Fonseca EB, Celik E, Parra M, et al: Progesterone and the risk of preterm birth among women with a short cervix, *N Engl J Med* 357(5):462–469, 2007.

Meis PJ, Klebanoff M, Thom E, et al: Prevention of recurrent preterm delivery by 17 alpha-hydroxyprogesterone caproate, *N Engl J Med* 348(24):2379–2385, 2003.

Rouse DJ, Caritis SN, Peaceman AM, et al: A trial of 17 alpha-hydroxyprogesterone caproate to prevent prematurity in twins, *N Engl J Med* 357(5):454–461, 2007.

References

Please go to expertconsult.com to view references.

Chapter 9

Multifetal Pregnancy

LYNLEE M. WOLFE • DAVID B. SCHRIMMER

KEY UPDATES

1 Complete pregnancy loss rate with multifetal pregnancy reduction (MPR) has remained stable at approximately 5% and is unlikely to be lower as this is the background loss rate for twins after cardiac activity is documented. Also of note, the mean gestational age at delivery was later and birth weights were larger with reduction to singleton versus twins.

2 Serum analyte screening for aneuploidy in multiples must be interpreted with caution. Altered serum levels of an affected twin can be "normalized" by the other twin.

3 The decision to deliver discordant twins prematurely is based on the combination of fetal and maternal status, gestational age, fetal growth patterns, Doppler studies, and, ultimately, the fetal heart rate tracing.

4 The Eurofetus study comparing twin-twin transfusion syndrome (TTTS) treatment options of laser versus serial amnioreduction strongly suggested that selective laser photocoagulation (SLPC) is the treatment of choice for TTTS. It should be noted that even with SLPC, surviving TTTS twins have a 5% risk of cerebral palsy.

5 Modification of TTTS staging using a cardiovascular scoring profile clearly identifies a subset of TTTS patients with more advanced disease than what would be appreciated by Quintero scoring alone. Thus, fetal echocardiogram is recommended as part of TTTS staging.

6 Cervical cerclage has not been shown to have benefit in twins when used either prophylactically or in conjunction with a sonographically shortened cervix and may be associated with an increase in preterm birth rate in twins.

7 Fetal fibronectin can be used in multiple gestations with symptoms of labor and has a negative predictive value of 97% for delivery within 2 weeks of testing.

8 There is no benefit for the use of 17 alpha-hydroxyprogesterone caproate or vaginal progesterone in twins when used to prevent preterm birth of <35 weeks.

Multiple Gestations

- Incidence
- 3% of all live births
- Natural (spontaneous) incidence of the following:
  - Twins: 1 in 90 births
  - Triplets: 1 in 8000 births
  - Quadruplets: 1 in 600,000 births
- In the United States since 1980, the twin birth rate has risen 65% and the triplet and higher-order multiple births has quadrupled largely secondary to advanced maternal age and assisted reproductive therapies (Malone et al, 2009)
- In 2008 there were 32.6 twins per 1000 live births and 147.6 triplets and higher-order multiples per 100,000 live births (Martin et al, 2010)
- Assisted reproductive therapy (ART) has affected the natural incidence of multiples in developed countries, as greater than 50% of multiples are a result of ART

- Since 2004, the incidence of twin deliveries has been relatively stable and the rate of higher-order multiples (triplets or more) has decreased
- Of naturally occurring twins, approximately 33% are monozygotic whereas approximately 67% are dizygotic
  - Monozygotic twins (MZT): a single fertilized ovum splits into two genetically identical embryos
  - MZT occurs in approximately 4 per 1000 births; the birth rate of MZT is relatively constant worldwide and does not vary by race
  - Dizygotic twins (DZT): two separate ova are fertilized by two different sperm resulting in genetically different embryos
  - The natural rate of DZT is variable depending on race
    - Highest in blacks (10 to 40 per 1000 births)
    - Whites (7 to 10 per 1000 births)
    - Lowest in Asians (3 per 1000 births)
    - U.S. average: 1 in 90 births

- The DZT rate is also affected by advancing maternal age, parity, and the use of assisted reproductive therapy (ART)
- Types of monozygotic twins (Figure 9-1)
  - Dependent on timing of splitting of the zygote:
    - Dichorionic/diamniotic (Di/Di)
    - Monochorionic/diamniotic/(Mo/Di)
    - Monochorionic/monoamniotic (Mo/Mo)
    - Conjoined twins
- Diagnosis
  - Knowledge of chorionicity and amnionicity are critical for counseling and pregnancy management
  - Accuracy of diagnosis of amnionicity and chorionicity is best in the first trimester and early second trimester
  - May require serial early exams to accurately identify the presence and type of membrane structure
  - Ultrasound characteristics useful in the diagnosis of amnionicity and chorionicity in the first trimester and early to mid second trimester:
    - Number of fetuses
    - Number of gestational sacs
    - Number of amnions
    - Number of yolk sacs
    - Membrane pattern:
      - Dichorionic-diamniotic (DC/DA)
        - Two visible distinct chorionic sacs should be seen by the seventh week
        - Lambda sign by 10 to 14 weeks' gestation (Figure 9-2)
        - "Thick membrane," containing four total layers, two amnions, two chorions
    - Monochorionic-diamniotic (MC/DA)
      - A single chorionic sac seen with two visible yolk sacs
      - Sufficient amniotic fluid should be present by the eighth week for distinct amnions to be visible
      - T sign by 10 to 14 weeks' gestation (Figure 9-3)
      - "Thin membrane," containing two layers (amnion) only
    - Monochorionic-monoamniotic (MC/MA)
      - Single amniotic cavity is the major diagnostic criterion
      - Thin dividing membrane is absent between the twins
      - Cord entanglement may be visible early in the pregnancy
      - May see a single yolk sac, but this is not definitive as the yolk sac may be divided or there may be two
      - Monoamnionicity is often overcalled and requires two to three follow-up scans for confirmation of an absent dividing membrane
- Gender
  - Different genders → likely dichorionic but 50% of dichorionic twins are same gender
  - Rare fetal genetic or structural abnormalities may confuse gender even with monozygotic twinning
- Placental location
  - Two distinct placental masses seen → dichorionic
- Membrane characteristics (visible on ultrasound):
  - Membrane thickness 2 mm or more is suggestive of dichorionicity 95% of the time (Winn et al, 1989)
- "Counting" the layers of the membrane
  - With ultrasound magnification, you can often see a thick membrane composed of four layers (amnion-chorion-chorion-amnion), which is diagnostic of a DC/DA gestation; membranes less than 2-mm thick are likely only two layers (amnion-amnion) and representative of MC/DA

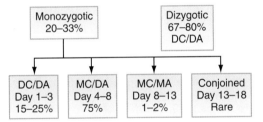

Figure 9-1. Types and frequency of spontaneous twinning correlated with timing of splitting.

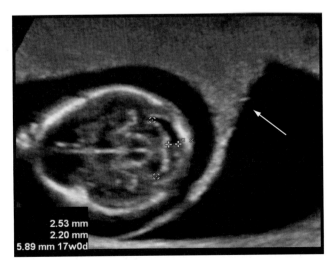

Figure 9-2. Ultrasonographic appearance of twin peak or lambda sign representative of dichorionic diamnionic twins.

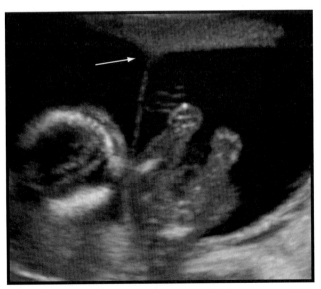

Figure 9-3. Ultrasonographic appearance of T sign representative of monochorionic diamnionic twins.

- Membrane insertion onto the chorionic plate or fetal surface of the placenta
  - Twin peak sign or lambda sign (see Figure 9-2):
    - Triangular projection of tissue with same echogenicity as the placenta→ likely DC/DA
    - 97% positive predictive value (Carrol et al, 2002)
    - Best if determined between 10 and 16 weeks
  - T sign (see Figure 9-3):
    - Thin wispy membrane inserts onto chorionic plate at 90-degree angle→ likely MC/DA
- Other diagnostic considerations
  - Vanishing twin
    - Early loss of one twin, most commonly prior to 8 weeks' gestation
      - Estimated as high as 20% to 50% of twins, 53% of triplets, and 65% of quadruplets (Dickey et al, 2002)
- First trimester management
  - Risk of miscarriage
    - Occurs in as high as 50% of twins diagnosed in the first trimester
    - Typically does not affect the remaining pregnancy
    - If loss is prior to 8 weeks' gestation, prenatal genetic screening tests are typically not affected and can accurately be performed
    - Loss greater than 8 weeks invalidates serum screening tests; thus, they should not be performed (Gjerris et al, 2009)
  - Genetic screening
    - An important consideration in that multiples are associated with both advanced maternal age (AMA) and assisted reproductive technologies (ART)
    - Serum screening is invalidated by fetal losses as noted previously
    - Serum screening is not accurate with higher-order multiples (triplets and above)
    - The age-related risk for each fetus is the same as for singletons; therefore, it has been proposed with two fetuses that the age cutoff for AMA should be lowered to somewhere between 31 and 33 because the midtrimester risk of having one fetus with Down syndrome is similar to that of a 35-year-old (American College of Obstetricians and Gynecologists, 2001)
    - In contrast to serum analyte screening, nuchal translucency screening can be done for any number of fetuses
      - Equally sensitive for multiples as for singletons—88% detection rate for trisomy 21 with 7.3% screen positive rate (Sebire et al, 1996)
    - Chorionic villi sampling (CVS) can be done by skilled practitioners in multiples, generally between 11 and 13 weeks
      - Loss rates generally quoted as 1 in 200 after adjustment for first-trimester spontaneous losses
      - Both transvaginal and transabdominal approaches are used
      - Monochorionic twins need only one sample, as they share placentas
      - Dichorionic twins will need two separate samples

UPDATE #1

Complete pregnancy loss rate with multifetal pregnancy reduction (MPR) has remained stable at 5% since the introduction and is unlikely to be lower as this is the background loss rate for twins after cardiac activity is documented (Stone et al, 2008).

- Multifetal pregnancy reduction (MPR; nonselective reduction)
  - Should be offered for triplets and higher-order multiples to reduce pregnancy complications
  - Can be offered for twins
  - Must know exact chorionicity of each fetus and avoid attempt at reduction of one fetus in a monochorionic-diamniotic pair because of placental vascular anastomosis
  - With dichorionic triamniotic triplets, reduction to a singleton is often suggested to avoid the complications of monochorionic twins
  - Loss rate after reduction is approximately 5% (in the first trimester) when reduced to twins and was less if singleton and more for triplets or higher (Stone et al, 2008)
- Selective reduction of anomalous fetus
  - Typically performed after diagnosis of anomalous fetus, thus may be done in the late first trimester through the second trimester
  - Suggested if anomaly is associated with polyhydramnios and preterm birth such as anencephaly
  - If DC/DA usually performed through KCl or digoxin injection
  - If MC/DA injection is not possible due to placental vascular anastomosis, umbilical cord occlusion is the preferred method (laser, radiofrequency ablation)
- Maternal nutrition
  - Caloric recommendations: 2700 to 4000 kcal/day depending on body mass index (BMI)
  - Weight gain: 25 to 54 pounds depending on BMI (Goodnight et al, 2009)*
    - BMI < 18.5 kg/m² (underweight): > 50 lbs.
    - BMI 18.5 to 24.9 kg/m² (normal weight): weight gain 37 to 54 lbs (16.8 to 24.5 kg)
    - BMI 25 to 29.9 kg/m² (overweight): weight gain 31 to 50 lbs (14.1 to 22.7 kg)
    - BMI >30 kg/m² (obese): weight gain 25 to 42 lbs (11.4 to 19.1 kg)
  - Additional supplements
    - Multivitamins: one daily in first trimester, two in second and third trimester
    - Folate: ≥1 mg/day
    - Iron: 60 mg/day, which may be included in the multivitamins
    - Calcium: 1500 mg/day in first trimester, 2000 mg/day in second and third trimester
    - Vitamin D: 1000 IU/day
- Second/third trimester management
  - Spontaneous losses may still occur (D'Alton et al, 1995)
    - Estimated in twins: 2% to 5%

---

*These thresholds represent the 25th through 75th percentile weight gains in women who gave birth to twins weighing at least 2500 g.

- Estimated in triplets: 14% to 17%
- Second-trimester genetic screening
  - Quad screen (serum alpha-fetoprotein [AFP], human chorionic gonadotropin [hCG], unconjugated estriol, and inhibin-A) can be performed in twins but not higher-order multiples
  - On average, serum analytes are twice as high in twins as they are in singletons of the same gestational age
  - Quad screen alone in twins has a 47% detection rate for Down syndrome with a 5% false-positive rate compared to 77% detection rate with singletons (Cuckle, 1995)
  - Integrated screening for T-21 has a 93% detection rate for MC twins and a 78% detection rate for DC twins versus a 95% detection rate for singletons (Wald et al, 2005)
  - Maternal serum AFP alone can be used to detect open neural tube defects using a cutoff of 4.5 MoM with detection rate of 50% to 85% and with a 5% false-positive rate (Wapner, 1995)

UPDATE #2

Serum analyte screening for aneuploidy in multiples must be interpreted with caution. Altered serum levels of an affected twin can be "normalized" by the other twin, making test performance poorer than in singletons. In addition, assisted reproductive technology (ART) may alter serum screening in an unpredictable fashion. Lastly, a twin demise later than 8 weeks and zero days invalidates all serum screening. Serum screening is never valid in high-order (triplet or more) multiples (ACOG Committee on Practice Bulletins, 2007; Gjerris et al 2009).

- Amniocentesis
  - Is done between 15 and 20 weeks' gestation similar to singleton gestations
  - With dichorionic twins, typically both sacs are sampled
  - Separate needle insertions are generally recommended, with instillation of indigo carmine after the first fluid withdrawal as a marker of the first sampled sac
  - Possible increased loss rate; 1.8% attributable risk (Cahill et al, 2009)
- Congenital anomalies
  - Incidence is increased in MZT as compared to DZT
  - Most have a normal co-twin
  - Concordant rate for any one anomaly is only 3.6% to 18.8% depending on the anomaly (Little et al, 1986)
- Growth
  - Growth patterns for twins are similar to singletons until 30 to 32 weeks, at which time growth begins to slow
  - Average birth weights for multiples are as follows (Martin et al, 2006):
    - 2333 g for twins
    - 1700 g for triplets
    - 1276 g for quadruplets
    - 1103 g for quintuplets
  - Growth sonograms are recommended approximately every 4 weeks if the pregnancy is progressing normally in dichorionic twins; monochorionic twins may require more frequent assessment
    - Discordancy equation: (estimated fetal weight [EFW] larger twin − EFW smaller twin) ÷ EFW larger twin

- Concordant growth: EFW of each twin within 20% of the other
- Discordant growth: EFW difference > 20%
  - Discordant growth is an indication for closer surveillance and not necessarily immediate delivery
  - Antenatal testing
  - Doppler velocimetry
  - Possible hospitalization for continuous monitoring

UPDATE # 3

The decision to deliver discordant twins prematurely is based on the combination of fetal and maternal status, gestational age, fetal growth patterns, Doppler studies, and, ultimately, the fetal heart rate tracing.

It should also be noted that monochorionic diamniotic twins have a 3- to 10-fold higher rate of perinatal morbidity and mortality secondary to common placental vasculature, high rates of discordant fetal growth, intrauterine growth restriction (IUGR), and congenital fetal abnormalities (Pasquini et al, 2004)

- Maternal complications of multiple gestations:
  - Preeclampsia
    - Fourfold increase with twins independent of maternal race or parity (Coonrod et al, 1995)
  - Gestational diabetes
    - Early diabetic screening is recommended with repeat screening at 24 to 28 weeks if negative
  - Maternal anemia
  - Operative delivery
  - Maternal hemorrhage
  - Preterm labor
    - Average gestational age at delivery:
      - Twins: 36 weeks
      - Triplets: 32 to 33 weeks
      - Quadruplets: 28 to 29 weeks
    - Incidence of premature delivery is 40% twins and 75% for triplets (Kovacs et al, 1989)
  - Mortality rate is increased threefold in twins; in a Swedish population study, the fetal and infant mortality rate was 4.1 and 5 per 1000 for singletons versus 12 and 16 per 1000 for twins (Rydhstroem et al, 2001)
- Specific complications of monochorionic-diamniotic twin gestations:
  - Twin-twin transfusion syndrome (TTTS)
    - Occurs in 10% to 15% of monochorionic pregnancies
    - Result of abnormal placental vascular anastomosis resulting in overperfusion and volume overload of the recipient twin and underperfusion and severe anemia of the donor twin
    - Diagnosis of TTTS is classically based on ultrasound findings of discordant twins, with the donor twin demonstrating severe IUGR and oligohydramnios, whereas the recipient twin is typically appropriate for gestational age (AGA) and has polyhydramnios
      - Polyhydramnios is defined as a maximum vertical pocket (MVP) of > 8 cm
      - Oligohydramnios is defined as a MVP of <2 cm
        - Severe oligohydramnios results in the finding of a "stuck" twin on ultrasound; thus, the donor

twin may be trapped against the uterine wall by its collapsed amniotic sac

- Severity of TTTS is graded based on a staging system; the first such system proposed was described by Rubin Quintero
  - Quintero staging (Quintero et al, 1999)
    - Stage 1: oligohydramnios is present in the sac of the donor twin and polyhydramnios is present in the sac of the recipient twin; a visible bladder is present in both twins
    - Stage 2: bladder is not visible in donor twin
    - Stage 3: abnormal Doppler studies
    - Stage 4: hydrops in one or both twins
    - Stage 5: death of one twin
  - Recent proposed modifications to Quintero staging use fetal cardiac abnormalities as another indicator of stage 3 TTTS (Harkness et al, 2005; Rychik et al, 2007)
- Severe TTTS has a very poor prognosis if untreated, with mortality rates greater than 90%
- Treatment options
  - Selective laser photocoagulation of anastomotic vessels (SLPC)
  - Serial amnioreduction
  - Amniotic septostomy
- Death of one twin in utero places the surviving twin at high risk for either fetal death or neurologic sequelae

---

UPDATE #4

The Eurofetus study, comparing TTTS treatment options of laser versus serial amnioreduction, strongly suggested that SLPC is the treatment of choice for TTTS. It should be noted that even with SLPC, surviving TTTS twins have a 5% risk of cerebral palsy (Senate et al, 2004).

UPDATE #5

Modification of TTTS staging using a cardiovascular scoring profile clearly identifies a subset of TTTS patients with more advanced disease than what would be appreciated by Quintero scoring alone. Thus, a fetal echocardiogram is recommended as part of TTTS staging (Harkness et al, 2005; Rychik et al, 2007).

- Monochorionic-monoamniotic twin gestations
  - 1% of monozygotic twins
  - Single amniotic sac
  - Risk of cord entanglement: 70% to 100%
  - Up to 50% mortality rate
  - Aggressive management at viability is recommended; inpatient management with frequent monitoring has been proved to decrease the risk for intrauterine fetal demise as well as improve birth weights, gestational age at delivery, and neonatal morbidity (Heyborne et al, 2005)
  - Continuous fetal monitoring is extremely difficult if not impossible to achieve
  - Delivery by cesarean section is recommended
  - Delivery by 34 weeks is recommended for improved infant survival with a decreased risk of stillbirth
- Conjoined twins
  - 1 in 50,000 pregnancies
  - Classified according to shared anatomy

- Thoracopagus—thorax
- Omphalopagus—abdominal wall
- Pygopagus—sacrum
- Ischiopagus
- Craniopagus
- Parapagus (pelvis and variable trunk)
- Detailed ultrasound and echocardiogram should be performed at diagnosis
- Recommend delivery by cesarean section
- Twin reversed arterial perfusion (TRAP): acardiac twin
  - Occurs in about 1% of monozygotic twins with resultant birth of only 1 in 35,000 to 1 in 150,000 births
  - Commonly diagnosed in early second trimester
  - Caused by the early development of a direct arterial-to-arterial anastomoses between the umbilical arteries of monochorionic twins
  - Involves a normal *pump twin,* which perfuses itself and the recipient or *perfused twin*
  - Causes reversal of flow in the umbilical artery of the perfused twin
    - Perfused twin receives deoxygenated blood from the pump twin
    - There is hypoperfusion to the upper portion of the perfused twin, causing severe anomalies
      - The perfused twin may have a trunk and lower limbs, but typically there is an absent or rudimentary heart and poor or underdeveloped upper body
  - The pump twin is at risk of developing cardiac failure
    - Prognosis is correlated with the ratio of the weight of the acardiac perfused twin to that of the pump twin (Moore et al, 1990)
      - Ratio > 0.70, 30% to 50% chance of congestive failure in the pump twin
      - Ratio < 0.70, 10% risk of congestive failure of in the pump twin
      - Other predictors of congestive failure include hydramnios (MVP >8 cm), severely abnormal Doppler studies, cardiac enlargement, or tricuspid regurgitation in the pump twin
  - 35% to 55% mortality rate with conservative (untreated) management because of high output cardiac failure and hydramnios leading to premature delivery
  - Treatment of high-risk pump twins requires separation of the circulation; this can be accomplished by the following methods:
    - Laser photocoagulation of the acardiac cord
    - Radiofrequency ablation (RFA) of the acardiac cord
  - If the acardiac twin is <50% of the weight of the pump twin, then conservative management is a safe and potential option (Jelin et al, 2010)
- Other considerations in the management of multiple gestation pregnancies:
  - Cerclage placement
    - No proven benefit in twins, even if cervical length is less than 2.5 cm (Berghella et al, 2005; Newman et al, 2002)
    - Would consider only if history of cervical insufficiency

---

UPDATE #6

Cervical cerclage may be associated with an increase in preterm birth rate in twins (Berghella et al, 2005).

- Intrauterine fetal demise (IUFD) of one twin
  - Demise in monochorionic twins can have serious sequelae
    - Death of one twin leads to a loss of vascular tone and hypotension in the dead fetus; as a result, the viable twin may exsanguinate back into the demise twin, causing either death or severe hypotension in the surviving twin; resultant neurologic impairment is common
    - 10% to 20% risk of demise to surviving co-twin
    - 20% to 25% risk of neurologic complications, including cerebral palsy, to surviving co-twin
    - Rapid delivery following IUFD may not prevent neurologic injuries; risk of injury must be compared to the risk of a premature delivery
  - Maternal risks
    - Previously believed that maternal risk of disseminated intravascular coagulation (because of retained dead fetus) was as high as 25%; more recent reviews have not supported this seemingly rare complication
- Preterm premature rupture of membranes
  - Management with in-hospital observation, fetal monitoring, antenatal steroids, and antibiotics as singletons
  - Tocolytic medications should be avoided
  - Delivery at 34 weeks if spontaneous labor, evidence of infection, or fetal distress does not force delivery earlier
- Preterm labor
  - Incidence of premature delivery is 40% for twins and 75% for triplets (Kovacs et al, 1989)
  - Mean age at delivery:
    - 38.8 weeks for singleton gestations
    - 35.3 weeks for twins
    - 32.2 weeks for triplets
    - 29.9 weeks for quadruplets
  - Incidence for very premature delivery (<32 weeks) is 1.6% for singletons, 11.6% for twins, and 38.5% triplets (Martin et al, 2010)

UPDATE #7

Fetal fibronectin can be used in multiple gestations with symptoms of labor and has a negative predictive value of 97% for delivery within 2 weeks of testing (Singer et al, 2007).

- Fetal fibronectin (fFN) as a predictor of preterm labor in twins
  - Can be used in twins with labor symptoms to predict delivery within 14 days; when used in twins, sensitivity, specificity, as well as positive and negative predictive values were 71%, 74%, 19%, and 97%, respectively (Singer et al, 2007)
  - fFN has some utility in the prediction of preterm delivery but is not currently recommended as a screening tool for asymptomatic multiple pregnancies
  - Recent studies have shown that using routine fFN screening in conjunction with cervical length screening may have utility in the predication of preterm birth
    - Cervical length <2 cm with a positive fFN was reported to have a 50% delivery rate at <32 weeks (Fox et al, 2009)
- Cervical length screening

- Recommended screening varies from every 2 weeks if risk factors are present to every 4 weeks in the absence of risk factors
- Shortened cervix <2.5 cm at 24 weeks is a predictor of preterm delivery; the Maternal Fetal Medicine Network noted that a transvaginal cervical length of 2.5 cm or less at 24 weeks had a 6.9-fold increase in delivery before 32 weeks (Goldenburg et al, 1996)
- Tocolytics
  - No demonstrated long-term efficacy in the prevention of preterm birth in multiples
  - Because of intravascular volume expansion, women with multiples are at significant risk for pulmonary edema; therefore, intravenous hydration, magnesium sulfate, and beta-adrenergic agonists must be used with extreme caution

UPDATE #8

Currently, studies have not demonstrated a benefit in the use of 17 alpha hydroxyprogesterone caproate or vaginal progesterone in twins when used to prevent preterm birth (Norman et al, 2009; Rouse et al, 2007).

- Progesterone
  - 17 hydroxy progesterone caproate and vaginal progesterone have been shown to reduce the risk of preterm birth in singletons with a history of preterm birth or shortened cervix; trials involving multiples have not shown this benefit, possibly because of differing mechanisms of preterm labor for singletons compared to multiples (Norman et al, 2009; Rouse et al, 2007)
- Intrauterine infection
  - If suspected, amniocentesis should be performed on the presenting fetus (baby A) because infections usually ascend from the vagina; if Gram stain/cultures return negative and there is still strong suspicion, then baby B can sampled
- Discordant fetal growth
  - Occurs in 15% of twins
  - Risk factors
    - Monochorionicity
    - Velamentous placental cord insertion
    - Abnormal serum analytes
    - Underlying maternal medical condition
      - Chronic hypertension, lupus
      - Abnormal serum analytes
  - Antepartum management:
    - Ultrasound surveillance for fetal growth every 2 weeks or as indicated
    - Doppler studies
    - Antenatal testing
    - Antenatal steroids if premature delivery appears likely in the next 14 days
    - Magnesium sulfate exposure for 12 to 24 hours for fetal neuroprotection if delivery is imminent
- Peripartum management
  - Antepartum testing
    - Routine antenatal testing in uncomplicated, AGA, concordant, multiple gestations is not indicated
    - Complicated pregnancies should be followed with antenatal testing including non-stress test (NST), biophysical profile (BPP), amniotic fluid index (AFI), or Doppler studies as indicated

- Delivery
  - Route of delivery
    - Vertex/vertex twins occur in approximately 35% to 40% of twin pregnancies
      - Vaginal delivery should be anticipated in the absence of complicating maternal or obstetric complications
      - With appropriate external or internal fetal monitoring, there is not an absolute time limit for delivery of the second twin
    - Vertex/nonvertex presenting twins occur in approximately 35% to 40% of twin pregnancies
      - A vaginal delivery may be offered with either a version or breech delivery if
        - Twins are not discordant (<25% difference in EFW)
        - Fetal weight is greater than 1500 gm
        - Gestational age >28 weeks
        - Fetal head is not hyperextended
        - Available obstetric staff members are comfortable and skilled with a vaginal breech delivery
      - Version is a risk factor for abruption, cord prolapse, and emergent cesarean section
    - Nonvertex presenting twins occur in 15% to 20% of twin pregnancies
      - Delivery by cesarean section is generally recommended, though the risk of interlocking fetal heads in the breech-vertex presentation is extremely low
  - Timing of delivery
    - Optimal time for delivery is between 37 and 38 weeks and should not go beyond 39 weeks, as perinatal mortality rate increases (Hartley et al, 2001)
    - American College of Obstetricians and Gynecologists (ACOG) guidelines recommend amniocentesis for elective delivery of twins prior to 38 weeks and 0 days gestation
      - Amniocentesis of one twin is generally adequate for lung maturity
      - Sampling of the twin less likely to be mature is recommended (example: male fetus) (Whitworth et al, 1999)
  - Delayed interval delivery
    - Delivery of one fetus that is not followed immediately by the delivery of the second fetus
    - Acceptable only under extreme circumstances such as a previable gestational age of the remaining fetus or high risk for severe complications of prematurity
    - Contraindicated in the following cases:
      - Monochorionicity, chorioamnionitis, suspected abruption, and preeclampsia

SUGGESTED READINGS

Prenatal Diagnosis

Carrol SG, Soothill PW, Abdel-Fattah SA, et al: Prediction of chorionicity in twin pregnancies at 10-14 weeks of gestation, *Br J Obstet Gyn* 109(2):182–186, 2002.

Selective Fetal Reduction

Stone J, Ferrara L, Kamrath J, et al: Contemporary outcomes of the latest 1000 cases of Multifetal pregnancy reduction (MPR), *Am J of Obstet Gynecol* 199(4):406.e1-e4, 2008.

Nutrition in Multiples

Goodnight W, Newman R: Optimal nutrition for improved twin pregnancy outcome, *Obstet Gynecol* 114(5):1121–1134, 2009.

Genetic Screening in Twins

Cahill AG, Macones GA, Stamilio DA, et al: Pregnancy loss rate after midtrimester amniocentesis in twin pregnancies, *Amer J Obstet Gynecol* 200(3):257.e1-e6, 2009.

Wald NJ, Rish S: Prenatal screening for Down syndrome and neural tube defects in twin pregnancies, *Prenat Diagn* 25(9):740–745, 2005.

Twin-Twin Transfusion Syndrome

Fisk N, Galea P: Twin-twin transfusion—as good as it gets? *N Engl J Med* 351(2):182–184, 2004.

Rychik J, Tian Z, Bebbington M, et al: The twin-twin transfusion syndrome: spectrum of cardiovascular abnormality and development of a cardiovascular score to assess severity of disease, *Am J Obstet Gynecol* 197(4):392.e1-e8, 2007.

Senate MV, Deprest J, Boulvain M, et al: Endoscopic laser surgery versus serial amnioreduction for severe twin-to-twin transfusion syndrome, *N Engl J Med* 351(2):136–144, 2004.

Cerclage in Twins

Berghella V, Odibo AO, Rust OA, et al: Cerclage for short cervix on ultrasonography: meta-analysis of trials using individual patient-level data, *Obstet Gynecol* 106(1):181–189, 2005.

Romero R, Espinoza J, Erez O, et al: The role of cervical cerclage in obstetric practice: can the patient who could benefit from this procedure be identified? *Am J Obstet Gynecol* 194(1):1–9, 2006.

Prevention and Prediction of Preterm Labor

Fox NS, Saltzman DH, Klauser CK, et al: Prediction of spontaneous preterm birth in asymptomatic twin pregnancies with the use of combined fetal fibronectin and cervical length, *Am J Obstet Gynecol* 201(3):313.e1-e5, 2009.

Norman J, Mackenzie F, Owen P, et al: Progesterone for the prevention of preterm birth in twin pregnancy (STOPPIT): a randomized, double-blind, placebo-controlled study and meta-analysis, *Lancet* 373(9680):2034–2040, 2009.

Rouse D, Caritis S, Peaceman A, et al: A trial of 17 alpha-hydroxyprogesterone caproate to prevent prematurity in twins, *N Engl J Med* 357(5):454–461, 2007.

Delivery in Twins

D'Alton M: Delivery of the second twin: revisiting the age-old dilemma, *Obstet Gynecol* 115(2 Pt 1):221–222, 2010.

References

Please go to expertconsult.com to view references.

Chapter 10

Fetal Therapy

DAVID B. SCHRIMMER

KEY UPDATES

1 Increasingly sophisticated ultrasound techniques (Doppler, three-dimensional imaging) have played a major role in the advancement of fetal therapy.

2 Magnetic resonance imaging (MRI) is considered safe for advanced evaluation of the fetus.

3 Fetoscopy has largely replaced open fetal surgery for most invasive procedures. The exception is in the treatment of myelomeningocele, where the recently completed Management of Myelomeningocele Study (MOMS) trial demonstrated improved outcomes in fetuses treated prior to birth.

4 The twin anemia-polycythemia sequence (TAPS) is a variant of the twin-twin transfusion syndrome (TTTS) and may present without the typical findings associated with TTTS.

5 Radio frequency ablation (RFA) using a small needle is a minimally invasive method of cord occlusion.

6 Twin-twin transfusion staging should include fetal echocardiography evaluation in addition to traditional (Quintero) staging.

7 Many congenital cystic adenomatoid malformations (CCAMs) will appear to resolve with pregnancy. Pediatric follow-up after delivery is essential.

History of Fetal Therapy

- Fetal manipulations in the animal model began to occur in the 1930s and 1940s (Jancelewicz et al, 2009; Jost, 1946)
- First human fetus treatment was in 1960
  - Sir William Liley, intra-abdominal transfusion of blood for fetal hydrops fetalis secondary to Rh sensitization (Liley, 1963)
    - Involved a blind needle insertion in the fetal abdomen
- Direct access to the fetal circulation was attempted through uterine incisions in 1966 with poor success; however, this was the beginning of fetal surgery beyond a blind needle insertion (Adamsons, 1966)
- Surfactant deficiency identified as the cause of respiratory distress syndrome (RDS) leading to antenatal steroid administration in 1972; first direct pharmacologic application with regard to fetal therapy (Liggins et al, 1972)
- The development of the medical application of ultrasound imaging in obstetrics and gynecology opened the door to prenatal diagnosis and, ultimately, fetal therapy (Woo, 2011)
  - First article on ultrasound use in obstetrics and gynecology published in 1958 (Donald et al, 1958)
  - First successful fetal therapy was done on a fetus with bladder outlet obstruction resulting from posterior urethral valves; a double pigtail shunt was placed with a successful outcome (Harrison et al, 1982)
- First ultrasound-directed fetal transfusion not done until 1982 when image quality was sufficient (Bang et al, 1982)

Imaging

ULTRASOUND

- Plays a critical primary role in the accurate diagnosis of an existing fetal condition and subsequent selection of fetal therapy candidates
- Used for selecting both incision site and trocar insertion site for open and closed fetal therapy
  - Used intraoperatively for the following:
    - Fetal cardiac monitoring during a procedure
    - Monitoring amniotic fluid volume
    - Orientation of fetal position, especially with multiples
    - Used as a tool to look for intra-amniotic bleeding (streaming)
- Used for direct procedural guidance for the following:
  - Shunt placement (Wilson, 2003)
  - Umbilical cord sampling or fetal transfusion
  - Insertion of radio frequency ablation (RFA) needles with tines (Lee et al, 2007)
- Used during EX Utero Intrapartum Treatment (EXIT) procedures, especially for placental site, incision site selection (Hopkins et al, 2009)

- Postfetal intervention (surgical or pharmacologic) ultrasound is used for fetal monitoring to assess fetal well-being and the need for further intervention

UPDATE #1

Sophisticated, high-resolution ultrasound imaging, including Doppler velocimetry, three-dimensional imaging, and volume estimation, is playing an increasingly important role in the accurate diagnosis, treatment, and follow-up of conditions amenable to fetal therapy (Glenn et al, 2006; Kunisaki et al, 2008).

FETAL ECHOCARDIOGRAPHY

- Increasingly important for fetal therapy for the following reasons:
  - Identification of primary cardiac anomalies (Gottliebson et al, 2006)
  - Identification and treatment of fetal arrhythmias (Simpson et al, 1998)
  - Serial cardiac studies have helped delineate the natural progression of fetal disease states in utero (Trines et al, 2004)
    - Can be used to assist in the decision as to whether or not to proceed with fetal surgery (i.e., deterioration of fetal condition)
      - Congenital cystic adenomatoid malformation (CCAM) (Klam et al, 2005)
      - Congenital diaphragmatic hernia (CDH) (Harrison et al, 1997)
    - Used to assist with staging of fetal disease as in twin-twin transfusion syndrome (Kunisaki et al, 2008)
  - Postprocedure monitoring of fetal status

MAGNETIC RESONANCE IMAGING

- Magnetic resonance imaging (MRI) is also increasingly being used to evaluate the fetus as an adjunct to fetal ultrasound (Coakley et al, 2004); especially useful for evaluating the following:
  - Fetal brain (Raybaud et al, 2003; Glenn et al, 2006)
    - Ventriculomegaly
    - Suspected absent corpus callosum
    - Destructive parenchymal lesions
    - Intracerebral hemorrhage
  - Fetal body abnormalities (Adzick et al, 1998; Hill et al, 2005)
    - Congenital high airway obstruction syndrome (CHAOS) (Shimabukuro et al, 2007)
    - Pulmonary sequestration (Dhingsa et al, 2003)
    - Congenital cystic adenomatoid malformation (CCAM) (Hubbard et al, 1999)
    - Congenital diaphragmatic hernia (CDH) (Leung et al, 2000)
    - Abdominal masses (Hill et al, 2005)
    - Neck masses (Knox et al, 2005)
    - Obstructive urogenital malformations (Caire et al, 2003)
  - Pre- and postfetal surgery screening and evaluation
  - Pregnancy involving oligohydramnios
  - Severe maternal obesity
- Ultrafast MRI imaging techniques are increasingly available and improving to combat fetal movement
  - Single-shot rapid acquisition with refocused echoes is used
    - By compiling a series of single images, the loss of image clarity by fetal movement is diminished

- Higher tissue contrast resolution than ultrasound may help with the distinction between normal and abnormal tissue (Coakley et al, 2004)
  - May separate destructive lesions from developmental abnormalities—for example, in the fetal brain
- Safety of MRI
  - No known fetal side effects when MRI strengths of 1.5 tesla or lower are used (Chew et al, 2001; Clements et al, 2000; Kok et al, 2004)
  - Use of MRI for fetal evaluation has been endorsed by the American College of Radiology in any trimester when deemed appropriate (Kanal et al, 2002, 2007)
  - Ideal gestational age is about 20 weeks if possible
  - Maternal or fetal sedation is not recommended to avoid fetal exposure
  - Limitations to MRI fetal size, especially in early gestations
- Excessive
  - Small fetal movement

UPDATE #2

MRI is considered safe for use in evaluating the developing fetus. Rapid acquisition sequences can be useful for evaluating the fetus, especially fetal brain abnormalities (Kanal et al, 2002).

Invasive Fetal Therapy

FETAL TRANSFUSION

- Ultrasound-guided needle placement directly into the umbilical cord, most commonly the umbilical vein
- Primarily used for transfusion of packed red blood cells for fetal anemia
  - Hemolytic disease
    - Rh sensitization
      - Anti Rh-D; most common
      - Anti Rh-c; less common than Rh-D, but can also cause severe hemolytic disease
    - Atypical blood group antibodies
      - Kell antibodies: associated with severe hemolytic disease
      - Duffy, Kidd: both associated with mild to moderate hemolytic disease
  - Parvovirus
    - Causes a temporary aplastic anemia in the fetus (Markenson et al, 1998)
    - Fetal surveillance with weekly Doppler studies for approximately 10 weeks after documented exposure
  - Monitoring and prediction of fetal anemia is routinely done using middle cerebral artery Doppler studies (Divakaran et al, 2001; Mari, 2000; Zimmerman et al, 2002)
    - This methodology has replaced serial amniocentesis and delta OD450 measurements

OPEN FETAL THERAPY

- Involves a hysterotomy with either removal or partial removal of the fetus for surgical repair
- When completed, the fetus is replaced into the uterus, continuing the pregnancy

- Key elements to open fetal therapy (Harrison et al, 1991, 1993)
  - Maternal general anesthesia using halogenated anesthetics to enhance uterine relaxation
  - Careful maternal fluid management so as to avoid hypotension as well as fluid overload leading to pulmonary edema
  - Maternal laparotomy
  - Requires careful ultrasound localization of the fetus and placenta to the direct uterine incision site
  - Hysterotomy with resorbable lactomer staples around the (uterine) incision edges to prevent maternal hemorrhage
  - Fetal analgesia during the procedure
  - Uterine incision is closed in layers postprocedure
  - Delivery will require an elective cesarean section because of the risk of uterine rupture
- Severe complications from open fetal surgery include the following:
  - Preterm labor
  - Premature rupture of membranes
  - Infection
  - Maternal pulmonary edema from attempts at tocolysis, mirror syndrome

CURRENTLY INDICATED FOR AN EXTREMELY LIMITED NUMBER OF FETAL CONDITIONS

- Myelomeningocele repair (Adzick et al, 2011; Hirose et al, 2009)
- Recently completed Management of Myelomeningocele Study (MOMS) trial (Adzick et al, 2011) demonstrated that fetuses treated prior to birth had the following traits:
  - Decreased rate of death by age 12 months
  - Decreased need for shunting to relieve hydrocephaly
  - Improved outcome with regard to walking, nerve function
- Large thoracic masses causing pulmonary hypoplasia; for example, large congenital cystic adenomatoid malformation (CCAM) (Adzick et al, 1998)
- Large fetal masses causing high output cardiac failure; for example, large sacrococcygeal teratoma (Langer et al, 1989)
- Exit procedure
  - Generally used to establish fetal airway control
    - Large fetal neck masses
    - Severe micrognathia
  - The fetus is partially delivered through a hysterotomy incision while it remains attached to the uteroplacental circulation (Hedrick et al, 2005)
  - Rapidly becoming the most frequent "open" procedure
    - Indicated for congenital airway obstruction, large head, neck, facial tumors and malformations, and more recently CCAM resection

UPDATE #3

With the exception of myelomeningocele repair (Adzick et al, 2011), the role of open fetal surgery has been declining because of maternal morbidity and significant pregnancy complications (premature rupture of membranes, preterm delivery) (Golombeck et al, 2006). At the same time, minimally invasive procedures such as fetoscopy and ultrasound-guided techniques (radio frequency ablation, cardiac balloon dilatation) are steadily increasing with less fetal and maternal morbidity.

CLOSED FETAL THERAPY (FETOSCOPY)

- Minimally invasive, using 3- to 3.8-mm fetoscopes
- Generally used in concert with ultrasound observations/guidance
- Dual channel operating scopes allow both visualization and the passage of microinstruments such as a laser fiber or microscissors (De Lia et al, 1995)
- Can be used for the following:
  - Twin-twin transfusion syndrome (TTTS)
    - Selective laser photocoagulation of anastomotic vessels
  - Twin anemia-polycythemia sequence (TAPS)
    - Selective laser photocoagulation of anastomotic vessels
- Cord ligation
  - Twin reversed arterial perfusion (TRAP)
  - Severe TTTS
  - Severe complications of monochorionic twins
    - Discordant anomalies
    - Severe growth discordance from unequal placental sharing
  - Amniotic band syndrome
  - Tracheal balloon occlusion for congenital diaphragmatic hernia
- Complications
  - Premature membranes
  - Infection (rarely)
  - Membrane separation or placental abruption (rarely)
  - Septostomy
  - Radio frequency ablation (Lee et al, 2007; Livingston et al, 2007)
- Uses high-frequency alternating currents
  - Smaller diameter than a fetoscope (17-gauge needle versus a 3- to 3.8-mm scope)
  - Single needle or needle with extendable tines (umbrella shape) for larger lesions
  - Placement is guided by ultrasound
  - Slowly generates local heat (to approximately 105° C) causing coagulation and tissue desiccation
- Uses
  - Cord ligation for TRAP sequence or severely anomalous twin
  - Severe TTTS
- Complications
  - Premature rupture of membranes
  - Thermal injury to surrounding tissue such as the uterine wall
  - Infection
  - Potential neurologic injury to surviving twin as a result of the intravascular release of tissue thromboplastins during the coagulation procedure and prior to complete cord occlusion

UPDATE #4

Twin anemia/polycythemia sequence (TAPS) represents a variant of the classic twin-twin transfusion syndrome (TTTS) (Lopriore et al, 2007). Like TTTS, one twin is severely anemic and one is plethoric. Unlike TTTS, hydramnios and oligohydramnios may be absent and Doppler studies may be inconsistent and confusing. TAPS is present in 1% to 2% of monochorionic twins and is more often created by TTTS laser therapy.

Specific Fetal Conditions

TWIN-TWIN TRANSFUSION SYNDROME (TTTS)

- Occurs in 10% to 15% of chorionic twins
- Classically identified by the presence of twin oligohydramnios-polyhydramnios sequence (TOPS) (Acosta-Rojas et al, 2007)
- Results from unbalanced placental vascular anastomosis (De Lia et al, 2000)
  - Arterioarterial (AA) anastomosis
  - Venovenous (VV) anastomosis
  - Arteriovenous (AV) anastomosis

- AA and VV anastomosis tend to be balanced with bidirectional flow
- AA anastomosis thought to be protective against TTTS
- AV has unidirectional flow and can lead to the anemia-polycythemia imbalance characteristic of TTTS
- Staging of TTTS: four staging systems have been described
  - Quintero staging system (Table 10-1) (Quintero et al, 1999)
    - First staging system described for TTTS
    - Based on ultrasound findings only, but does not include fetal echocardiogram findings
  - Cincinnati staging system (Table 10-2) (Harkness et al, 2005)
    - Modifies the Quintero staging to include fetal echocardiogram findings
  - Cardiovascular profile scoring system (Table 10-3) (Hofstaetter et al, 2006)
    - Based on fetal echocardiographic findings
  - Children's Hospital of Philadelphia (CHOP) system (Rychik et al, 2007)
    - Based on fetal echocardiographic findings

TABLE 10-1   Summary of Quintero Staging

Stage	Oligohydramnios/ Polyhydramnios (Donor/Recipient)	Bladder Visualization/ Filling (Donor/Recipient)	Abnormal Doppler Studies	Fetal Hydrops	Fetal Death
Stage I	Poly–recipient Oligo–donor	Present–recipient Absent–donor	None	None	No
Stage II	Poly–recipient Oligo – donor	Present, may be enlarged–recipient Absent–donor	None	None	No
Stage III	Poly–recipient Oligo – donor	Present, may be enlarged–recipient Absent–donor	Present in either donor or recipient	None	No
Stage IV	Poly–recipient Oligo–donor	Present, may be enlarged–recipient Absent–donor	Present in either donor or recipient	Hydrops in donor or recipient	No
Stage V	Poly–recipient Oligo–donor	Present, may be enlarged–recipient Absent–donor	Present in either donor or recipient	Hydrops in donor or recipient	Demise in donor or recipient

Adapted from Quintero RA: Twin-twin transfusion syndrome, *Clin Perinatol* 30(3):591-600, 2003.

TABLE 10-2   Summary of Cincinnati Staging System

Stage	Donor	Recipient	Recipient Cardiomyopathy
Stage I	Oligohydramnios	Polyhydramnios	No
Stage II	Bladder not visible	Bladder visible	No
Stage III	Abnormal Doppler	Abnormal Doppler	None
—Stage IIIA			Mild
—Stage IIIB			Moderate
—Stage IIIC			Severe
Stage IV	Hydrops	Hydrops	
Stage V	Death	Death	
Variables			
—Cardiomyopathy	Mild	Moderate	Severe
—AV regurgitation	Mild	Moderate	Severe
—RV/LV thickness	>2 + Z score	>3 + Z score	>4 + Z score
— Myocardial Performance Index TEI	>2 + Z score	>3 + Z score	Severe biventricular dysfunction

Modified from Harkness UF, Crombleholme TM: Twin-twin transfusion syndrome: where do we go from here? *Semin Perinatol* 29:296-304, 2005.

- Advantages and disadvantages of the various staging methods
  - Quintero staging
    - Easy to use, requires only basic ultrasound skills
    - Weighted toward the status of the donor fetus
    - Does not consider the basic cardiovascular changes that occur with TTTS (Michelfelder et al, 2007)
    - Does not predict progression of disease
  - Cincinnati staging
    - Simple modification of an already familiar (Quintero) system
    - Requires fetal echocardiography and the myocardial performance index (Tei index)
    - Echo findings relate to survival, treatment, and progression of disease
    - Best predictor of recipient survival (Shah et al, 2008)
  - Cardiovascular profile scoring system
    - Requires fetal echocardiography (Hofstaetter et al, 2006)
  - CHOP system
    - Requires advanced fetal echocardiography assessment (Rychik et al, 2007)
    - Not well correlated yet with fetal prognosis (Habli et al, 2009)

UPDATE #6

TTTS staging should include some method of cardiac evaluation (fetal echocardiography), as well as the traditional components found in Quintero staging (Habli et al, 2009). This is important in order to avoid missing more severe fetal disease than what would be suggested by Quintero staging alone. The optimal modification of Quintero staging is still under investigation, as are the most advantageous staging criteria for laser intervention.

- Treatment options for TTTS
  - Amnioreduction
    - Treatment of choice prior to laser
    - Involves the simple removal of amniotic fluid via amniocentesis
    - Thought to improve uteroplacental blood flow by reducing pressure in the amniotic space and on placental vasculature
    - Overall survival rates of 49% (range 39% to 83%) (Elliott et al, 1991; Moise, 1993; Reisner et al, 1993)
    - Higher incidence of neurologic sequelae than those treated with laser therapy (De Lia et al, 1990; Ville et al, 1995)

- Septostomy
  - Technique involves creating a septostomy in the intertwin membrane to allow equalization of amniotic fluid in each sac (Saade et al, 1998)
  - Controlled studies did not show an improvement in outcome as compared to amnioreduction (Johnson et al, 2001; Moise et al, 2005)
  - Largely abandoned because of the risk of creating a monoamniotic gestation (Ross et al, 2006) as well as the improved outcomes reported with laser therapy (Senat et al, 2004)
- Selective laser photocoagulation
  - Initial attempts involved laser photocoagulation of all placental vessels that crossed the intertwin membrane
  - Technique evolved to selective photocoagulation of only vessels that directly connected the two placental sides (AA, VV, AV anastomosis) or an unpaired artery to a placental cotyledon, which in turn is drained by an unpaired vein going to the opposite placental side
  - Further refinement incorporates selective photocoagulation with stage-based treatment
  - Laser outcomes
    - Eurofetus trial (Senat et al, 2004)
      - Prospective, randomized trial compared laser to serial amnioreduction
      - Used Quintero staging
      - Enrollment halted at interim analysis
        - Significantly higher survival of at least one twin with laser group versus amnioreduction group
        - Overall survival reported as 53% for laser versus 39% for amnioreduction
    - National Institutes of Health (NIH) TTTS trial (Crombleholme et al, 2007)
      - Prospective, randomized U.S. trial again comparing amnioreduction to laser
      - Stopped after only 42 patients because of adverse outcomes (decreased survival) noted in the recipient twin group treated with laser
      - No statistically different rate of overall neonatal survival for laser versus amnioreduction group
      - Importantly, study design for the NIH trial was markedly different than the Eurofetus trial, and thus the two studies are difficult to compare

TABLE 10-3   **Cardiovascular Profile 10-Point Scoring System**

Findings	Normal (2 points each)	A 1-Point Deduction	A 2-Point Deduction
Hydrops fetalis	None	Ascites; pleural and pericardial effusion	Skin edema
Venous Doppler	Normal	Ductus venosus atrial systolic reversal	Umbilical venous pulsation
Cardiothoracic ratio	<0.35	>0.35 and <0.50	>0.5
Cardiac function	Ventricular shortening fraction >0.28 and valve regurgitation	Shortening fraction <0.28 or tricuspid regurgitation or semilunar valve regurgitation	Tricuspid regurgitation plus dysfunction or any mitral regurgitation
Arterial Doppler	Normal	Absent end-diastolic flow in the umbilical artery	Reverse end-diastolic flow in the umbilical artery

Modified from Hofstaetter C, Hansmann M, Eik-Nes SH, et al: A cardiovascular profile score in the surveillance of fetal hydrops, *J Matern Fetal Neonatal Med* 19(7):407-413, 2006; and Shah AD, Border WL, Crombleholme TM, et al: Initial fetal cardiovascular profile score predicts recipient twin outcome in twin-twin transfusion syndrome, *J Am Soc Echocardiogr* 21(10):1105-1108, 2008.

- Generally, the studies for selective laser photocoagulation (SLPC) show marked improvement in survival as compared to studies looking at amnioreduction, and thus laser is typically considered the treatment of choice for TTTS
  - Survival of both twins: 76% Quintero stage I, 61% stage II, 54% stage III, 50% stage IV
  - Survival of one twin: 93% stage I, 83% stage II, 83% stage III, 70% stage IV (Huber et al, 2005)
  - Neurologic outcomes are still being investigated following laser therapy; studies thus far show rates of cerebral palsy as high as 9% (Sutcliffe et al, 2001) and of other neurologic abnormalities from 7% to 17% (delayed motor development, abnormal speech, strabismus, hemiparesis, and spastic quadriplegia) (Banek et al, 2003)
  - The optimal TTTS stage for intervention via laser therapy remains under investigation (Stamillo et al, 2010)
- Cord ligation
  - Has been used in some institutions for severe TTTS (stage IV) or when it is thought that neurologic injury has already occurred
  - Can be accomplished via laser, bipolar cautery, and radio frequency ablation (RFA)
    - Using laser beyond 20 weeks is of concern because of cord thickness and incomplete vessel occlusion
    - RFA is of concern because of slow thermal coagulation and the possibility of tissue thromboplastin release into the bloodstream of the surviving twin
- Can also present as twin anemia-polycythemia sequence (TAPS)
  - Less severe form of vascular anastomosis; may result from a very small vessel connection
  - Severe anemia in the donor twin is present, and there is polycythemia in the recipient twin
  - Classic TTTS polyhydramnios/oligohydramnios sequence is not present
  - May occur in 1% to 2% of monochorionic twin gestations
  - May occur in 5% to 10% of postlaser correction TTTS cases

Twin Reversed Arterial Perfusion (TRAP)

- One percent of monochorionic twin gestations
- Fundamental pathology is that of an arterial-arterial anastomosis with the death of one twin and reversal of vascular flow in the demised twin
- Definitive therapy (if required) is cord ligation of the acardiac or demised twin
  - Laser cord coagulation and RFA have both been used; the RFA needle is smaller and therefore potentially less likely to cause the preterm premature rupture of membranes (Lee et al, 2007)
  - Cord ligation recommended if evidence of cardiac failure in the surviving, "pump" twin, or early, rapid growth of the acardiac twin with a volume estimate of >50% to 70% of the viable twin (Moore et al, 1990)

Congenital Diaphragmatic Hernia (CDH)

- One in 2500 to 5000 pregnancies (Butler et al, 1962)
  - Most are left sided (85%)
  - Thirteen percent: right sided
  - Two percent: complete agenesis
  - Forty percent of affected fetuses have associated anomalies
- Prognosis correlates with the lung area to head circumference ratio; observed (O) values are compared against expected (E) values to create O/E ratios (Jani et al, 2006)
- With O/E ratio of >1.0, postdelivery repair is recommended
- An O/E ratio of <1.0 is correlated with severe to extreme pulmonary hypoplasia and thus a poor outcome; the prognosis improves with increasing O/E ratio and the presence of the liver in the abdominal cavity (not chest)
- In those with a poor prognosis (O/E ratio <1.0), attempts have been made to repair the CDH prior to birth
  - Results of CDH repair with open fetal surgery were poor and have been abandoned (Harrison et al, 1997)
  - Temporary tracheal occlusion is being actively studied in Europe and San Francisco (Deprest et al, 2004; Harrison et al, 2001)
    - Tracheal occlusion using a fetoscopically placed tracheal balloon is done at 26 weeks' gestation
      - Backpressure into the lung by accumulating fluid stimulates alveolar growth
    - The balloon is removed at 34 weeks to assist with type II pneumocyte development

Thoracic Lesions

- Most common lesion is the congenital cystic adenomatoid malformation (CCAM)
  - One in 3000 to 5000 pregnancies
    - Type I
      - Fifty percent of CCAM lesions
      - Characteristic large, cystic pattern
        - Cysts may be up to 10 cm in size
    - Type II
      - Forty percent of CCAM lesions
      - Small cystic lesions
        - Cysts range from 3 to 10 mm
    - Type III
      - Appear solid on ultrasound
      - Only 10% of CCAM lesions
      - Most lethal condition
- Prognosis varies by type, with type I carrying the greatest survival rate
- In utero treatment is conservative unless hydrops is present (Wilson et al, 2003)
- Up to 20% of CCAMs will resolve spontaneously
- Clinical trials are currently in progress at the University of California, San Francisco; they are looking at the efficacy of steroid use in the treatment of large, type III lesions
- If hydrops is present, treatment options include open fetal surgery with CCAM resection or, more commonly, placement of a pleuroamniotic shunt (Wilson et al, 2003)

- Bronchopulmonary sequestration
  - Lung mass with no connection to the trachea
  - Extremely rare
  - Has its own anomalous blood supply
  - Repair is done postdelivery unless there is fetal hydrops, which carries a poor prognosis
- Fetal hydrothorax
  - Pleuroamniotic shunting has been effective in preventing pulmonary hypoplasia
  - High association with other fetal anomalies

Myelomeningocele

- One in 2000 births
  - The basis for in utero closure has been the "two hit theory" (Heffez et al, 1990; Hutchins et al, 1996)
  - First hit is the original developmental defect
  - Second hit is thought to be due to exposure to amniotic fluid and direct trauma to the exposed neural elements both in utero and at the time of delivery
  - Attempts at fetal repair
    - Fetoscopic attempts were largely unsuccessful (Farmer et al, 2003)
    - Open fetal surgery has been successfully completed (Bruner et al, 2000), and the recently completed Management of Myelomeningocele Study (MOMS) trial is highly encouraging as an in utero treatment option (Adzick et al, 2011); the study results demonstrated that fetuses treated prior to birth had the following characteristics:
      - Decreased rate of death by age 12 months
      - Decreased need for shunting to relieve hydrocephaly
      - Improved outcome with regard to walking, nerve function

Lower Urinary Tract Obstructions

- Vesicoamniotic shunts
  - Placed to relieve obstructive uropathy
  - Save or salvage fetal renal function
  - Potentially prevent pulmonary hypoplasia
  - Candidate selection has been based on urinary electrolytes
- Results have been variable
  - Up to one third have normal renal function
  - Up to one third ultimately required dialysis and renal transplant
- Evidence to support shunting has been questioned and a randomized multicenter trial has been proposed (Clark et al, 2003)

Sacrococcygeal Teratoma

- Treatment is generally done postdelivery unless the teratoma is causing fetal cardiac failure or hydrops
  - RFA has been successfully used to decrease tumor mass and blood flow

Cardiac Anomalies

- Most frequent fetal anomaly
- Fetal arrhythmia, especially supraventricular tachycardia, has been successfully treated by transplacental transfer of traditional cardiac medications (digoxin, flecainide, amiodarone) (Kleinman et al, 2004)
- Requires careful maternal monitoring for evidence of maternal toxicity
- Corrective (surgical) therapy of structural cardiac anomalies has traditionally been done postdelivery
- Given the frequency of cardiac anomalies, as well as the improved prenatal diagnostic imaging techniques, fetal correction to improve function is on the horizon
  - Therapy thus far has focused on the potential treatment of stenotic or atretic lesions (valves), as well as hypoplastic ventricles (Matsui et al, 2007)
    - Aortic and pulmonic valve lesions have been treated with balloon valvuloplasty
    - Treatment must be attempted before permanent cardiac damage has already occurred

Amniotic Bands

- Amniotic bands have been successfully "released" with fetoscopy
  - Amputation-like defects may potentially be prevented if the bands are released prior to permanent limb damage

Discordant Fetal Anomalies

- Severe anomalies in one twin (or multiple) raise the issue of selective reduction of the anomalous fetus
  - Selective reduction via potassium chloride injection has been used
    - 5% loss rate of the pregnancy when done in the first trimester
    - 10% loss rate when done in the second trimester
    - Risk of disseminated intravascular coagulation (DIC) to the mother is extremely rare and has been overemphasized in the past
  - Cord ligation

Future Fetal Therapy

STEM CELL TRANSPLANTATION

- Animal research for metabolic storage diseases

GENE THERAPY

- Animal models for hemophilia, muscular dystrophy, cystic fibrosis

SUGGESTED READINGS

History of Fetal Therapy

Jancelewicz T, Marrison M: A history of fetal surgery, *Clin Perinatol* 36(2):vii, 227–236, 2009.

Ultrasound Imaging; Development and Use in Fetal Therapy

Bang J, Bock JE, Trolle D, et al: Ultrasound-guided fetal intravascular transfusion for severe Rheusus haemolytic disease, *Br Med J (Clin Res Ed)* 284(6313):373–374, 1982.

Hopkins LM, Feldstein VA: The use of ultrasound in fetal surgery, *Clin Perinatol* 36(2):255–272, 2009.

Kunisaki SM, Jennings RW: Fetal surgery, *J Intensive Care Med* 23(1):33–51, 2008.

Trines J, Hornberger LK: Evolution of heart disease in utero, *Pediatr Cardiol* 25(3):287–298, 2004.

Magnetic Resonance Imaging in the Evaluation of the Fetus

Glenn OA, Barkovich AJ: Magnetic resonance imaging of the fetal brain and spine: an increasingly important tool in prenatal diagnosis, part 1, *Am J Neuroradiol* 27(8):1604–1611, 2006.

Kanal E, Barkovich AJ, Bell C, et al: ACR guidance document for safe MR practices: 2007, *Am J Roentgenol* 188(6):1447–1474, 2007.

Doppler Use in Fetal Therapy

Mari G, Deter RL, Carpenter RL, et al: Noninvasive diagnosis by Doppler ultrasonography of fetal anemia due to maternal red-cell alloimmunization, *N Engl J Med* 342(1):9–14, 2000.

Invasive Fetal Therapy and Surgery

Acosta-Rojas R, Becker J, Muñoz-Abellaña B, et al: Twin chorionicity and the risk of adverse perinatal outcome, *Int J Gynaecol Obstet* 96(2):98–102, 2007.

Golombeck K, Ball RH, Lee H, et al: Maternal morbidity after maternal-fetal surgery, *Am J Obstet Gynecol* 194(3):834–839, 2006.

Hedrick HL, Flake AW, Crombleholme TM, et al: The ex utero intrapartum therapy procedure for high-risk fetal lung lesions, *J Pediatr Surg* 40(6):1038–1043, 2005.

Lee H, Wagner AJ, Sy E, et al: Efficacy of radiofrequency ablation for twin-reversed arterial perfusion sequence, *Am J Obstet Gynecol* 196(5):459.e1–e4, 2007.

Lopriore E, Middeldrop JM, Oepkes D, et al: Twin anemia-polycythemia sequence in two monochorionic twin pairs without oligo-polyhydramnios sequence, *Placenta* 28(1):47–51, 2007.

Fetal Therapy in Twin-Twin Transfusion Syndrome

Crombleholme TM, Shera D, Lee H, et al: A prospective randomized, multicenter trial of amnioreduction vs selective fetoscopic laser photocoagulation for the treatment of severe twin-twin transfusion syndrome, *Am J Obstet Gynecol* 197(4):396.e1–e9, 2007.

Habli M, Wagner AJ, Sy E, et al: Twin-to-twin transfusion syndrome: a comprehensive update, *Clin Perinatol* 36(2):x, 391–416, 2009.

Harkness UF, Lim FY, Crombleholme T, Crombleholme TM: Twin-twin transfusion syndrome: where do we go from here? *Semin Perinatol* 29(5):296–304, 2005.

Hofstaetter C, Hansmann M, Eik-Nes SH, et al: A cardiovascular profile score in the surveillance of fetal hydrops, *J Matern Fetal Neonatal Med* 19(7):407–413, 2006.

Huber A, Diehl W, Bregenzer T, et al: Stage-related outcome in twin-twin transfusion syndrome treated by fetoscopic laser coagulation, *Obstet Gynecol* 108:333–337, 2006.

Rychik J, Tian Z, Bebbington M, et al: The twin-twin transfusion syndrome: spectrum of cardiovascular abnormality and development of a cardiovascular score to assess severity of disease, *Am J Obstet Gynecol* 197(4):392.e1–e8, 2007.

Senat MV, Deprest J, Boulvain M, et al: Endoscopic laser surgery versus serial amnioreduction for severe twin-to-twin transfusion syndrome, *N Engl J Med* 351(2):136–144, 2004.

Stamilio DM, Fraser WD, Moore TR: Twin-twin transfusion syndrome: an ethics-based and evidence-based argument for clinical research, *Am J Obstet Gynecol* 203(1):3–16, 2010.

Treatment of Other Fetal Conditions

Adzick NS, Thom Ea, Spong CY, et al: A randomized trial of prenatal versus postnatal repair of myelomeningocele, *N Engl J Med* 364(11):993–1004, 2011.

Clark TJ, Martin WL, Divakaran TG, et al: Prenatal bladder drainage in the management of fetal lower urinary tract obstruction, *Obstet Gynecol* 102(2):367–382, 2003.

Deprest J, Gratacos E, Nicolaides KH, et al: Fetoscopic tracheal occlusion (FETO) for severe congenital diaphragmatic hernia: evolution of a technique and preliminary results, *Ultrasound Obstet Gynecol* 24(2):121–126, 2004.

Laberge JM, Flageole H, Pugash D, et al: Outcome of the prenatally diagnosed congenital cystic adenomatoid lung malformation: a Canadian experience, *Fetal Diagn Ther* 16(3):178–186, 2001.

Matsui H, Gradiner H, et al: Fetal intervention for cardiac disease: the cutting edge of perinatal care, *Semin Fetal Neonatal Med* 12(6):482–489, 2007.

References

Please go to expertconsult.com to view references.

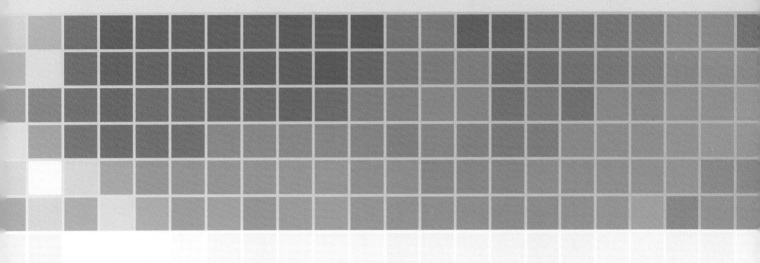

The Third Trimester and Late Pregnancy Complications

Chapter 11

Fetal Growth Disorders

TATIANA STANISIC CHOU • JULIANNE S. TOOHEY

KEY UPDATES

1 Thrombophilias may be associated with intrauterine growth restriction (IUGR).

2 Multiple-dose steroids have been associated with growth restriction.

3 Customized growth curves should be employed when possible to allay bias in the population.

4 Doppler velocimetry has been found to be a predictor of adverse perinatal outcome.

5 In an attempt to identify a fetus in distress prior to the severe consequences of hypoxemia or acidemia, the ductus venosus has been investigated because of its rapid blood flow.

6 Several studies of long-term outcomes in IUGR infants reveal an association between lower IQ and an increase in emotional and behavioral issues. Long-term outcomes of IUGR fetuses are associated with decreased IQ as well as emotional and behavioral issues.

7 An increased incidence of the metabolic syndrome with type 2 diabetes, obesity, cardiovascular disease, and hypertension in adult life has been associated with IUGR.

Intrauterine Growth Restriction

BACKGROUND

- Intrauterine growth restriction (IUGR) refers to the condition of a fetus unable to achieve its genetically determined potential size. This definition would exclude constitutionally small fetuses that would not be at risk for adverse outcome; however, often this cannot be determined absolutely until after delivery. In addition, there is a subset of fetuses that are intrinsically small and for whom intervention will not affect outcome such as in Trisomy 18. The clinical challenge is to identify a fetus that is at risk for poor outcome with the hope that modification of risk factors and appropriate interventions will improve such outcomes. We also would like to identify small but otherwise healthy fetuses in order to avoid unnecessary and inadvisable interventions.
  - Incidence rate of IUGR in singleton fetuses is 3% to 7% (Romo et al, 2009) and 15% to 25% in twins (McCormick et al, 1985).
  - Correct diagnosis requires accurate dating, which can be difficult and is frequently inaccurate.
  - Ethnicity and racial considerations affect the expected growth rate of a fetus, which complicates population-based growth curves.

DEFINITION

- Estimated fetal weight measured as less than 10th percentile for the gestational age (small for gestational age, or SGA) with the understanding that not all SGA infants are pathologically growth restricted and may in fact be constitutionally small. Similarly, not all fetuses that have failed to achieve their growth potential fall under the 10th percentile for the gestational age.
- Can be associated with maternal, fetal, or placental causes.

SYMMETRICAL AND ASYMMETRICAL

- Symmetrical IUGR occurs during the first few months of gestation and is caused by the failure of one or more cell cycles leaving all organ systems equally smaller in size.
- Asymmetrical IUGR occurs in the second half of the pregnancy and is associated with malnutrition and hypoxemia of the fetus.

CLASSIFICATIONS

- Constitutionally small fetus measurements are symmetrical with normal amniotic fluid.
- Chromosomal and structural abnormalities, often symmetrical measurements with aberrations of the amniotic fluid volume.
- Substrate deficiencies and placental insufficiency, usually asymmetrical growth restriction with associated oligohydramnios.

ETIOLOGIES

- *Fetal causes.* Include genetic disorders such as chromosomal and structural abnormalities.

- *Maternal causes.* Include conditions such as hypertension, renal disease, restrictive lung disease, Class F or greater diabetes, cyanotic heart disease, antiphospholipid syndrome, collagen-vascular disease, and hemoglobinopathies, which could lead to fetal hypoxemia, vasoconstriction, or decreased fetal perfusion leading to IUGR. Clinical maternal vascular disease and the presumed decrease in uteroplacental perfusion can account for 30% of growth-restricted infants.

UPDATE #1

Thrombophilias have shown some correlation with IUGR. Meta-analysis (Howley et al, 2005) found an association with factor V Leiden and prothrombin gene mutation; however, more recent studies show no relationship.

- *Other possible causes.* Exposure to teratogens, malnutrition (less than 1500 kcal/day), smoking, or substance abuse (fetal alcohol syndrome strongly correlates with IUGR). Maternal cigarette smoking decreases birth weight approximately 135 to 300 gm, the fetus being symmetrically smaller. If smoking is discontinued prior to the third trimester, the deleterious effect on birth weight is reduced. Prolonged use of some medications, including steroids, Dilantin and Coumadin, has also been associated with growth restriction in the fetus. Uterine abnormalities such as fibroids or bicornuate or separated uteri are also a cause of IUGR as is prolonged exposure to high altitudes.

UPDATE #2

Steroids have been used to improve fetal morbidity and mortality by advancing fetal lung maturity in preterm births. The practice of repeated dosing became commonplace in the United States despite a lack of evidence for its necessity. Studies have shown that the group receiving repeat courses of beta-methasone, specifically four or more doses, had a birth weight reduction of 95 g (Wapner et al, 2006), which was not seen in the group receiving zero to three doses. Repeated steroid dosing more commonly resulted in birth weight below the 5th and 10th percentiles for gestational age. This study also failed to show any benefit to repeated dosing compared to placebo. A single rescue course of steroids given prior to 33 weeks was shown to improve outcome without increased short-term risk (Garite et al, 2009).

- *Infections* including viruses such as fetal rubella, Cytomegalovirus, and varicella are a cause for intrauterine growth restriction. Additionally protozoal infections such as *Toxoplasma gondii* and *Toxoplasma cruzi* as well as syphilis are other possible causes. Bacterial infections are not shown to cause IUGR.
- *Multiple gestations* are associated with an increased risk for intrauterine growth restriction as well as a progressive decrease in fetal and placental weight as the number of offspring increases. IUGR can be seen in both monochorionic and dichorionic twins. Twins are considered discordant when there is greater than 20% difference in growth. There is no established standard for what amount of discordance is significant.

Studies have shown that compared to symmetric twins, asymmetric discordant twins are at higher risk for adverse outcomes (Dashe et al, 2000). However, each dichorionic twin must be assessed individually, as each fetus follows its own growth velocity curve. Normal growth velocity in each twin is of greater importance than a discordant measurement between the two fetuses. Monochorionic twins must be evaluated in light of possible vascular anastomoses. Severe IUGR can be seen as part of the twin-twin transfusion syndrome. Early diagnosis is essential in order to manage complications related to this condition.
- *Primary placental disease* can also be related to IUGR often leading to impaired perfusion because of conditions such as placenta previa, hemangiomas, abruption, or infarcts. IUGR without other abnormalities is usually associated with a small placenta with diminished diffusing capacity. Abnormal cord insertions such as velamentous and marginal cord insertions are other causes of IUGR.

SCREENING

- Lagging fundal height noted during prenatal exam is typically the first indication but is often inaccurate and should only be used for screening.
- Essentially, all pregnant women will be screened by measuring fundal height when receiving prenatal care, which at 32 to 34 weeks' gestational age provides 96% specificity and 70% to 85% sensitivity (Leeson et al, 1997).
- Those women with previous IUGR pregnancies should be screened by ultrasound because of their increased risk. The recurrence rate for IUGR in a previous pregnancy is nearly 20% (Berghella et al, 2007).

UPDATE #3

The use of population-based growth curves has been the standard. However, there is currently much discussion of customized growth curves to allay bias in the population. Some portion of the variability in fetal birth weight can be attributed to fetal and maternal factors including gender of the fetus, ethnicity, maternal body habitus, age, and education. Studies (Gardosi et al, 2009) have found that 33% of the babies identified as IUGR by the customized curve were not recognized by the population-based curve, and 26% of those were born prematurely. Additionally, 17.2% of those found to be IUGR by the population-based curve were within normal growth patterns by the customized standards and were born without any of the studied adverse outcomes. Multicenter investigations sponsored by the National Institute of Child Health and Development (NICHD) and the World Health Organization (WHO) are under way to address these issues sonographically.

DIAGNOSIS

- Estimated fetal weight by ultrasound
- Head-to-abdomen or femur-to-abdomen ratios
- Growth velocity tracked over time
- Evaluation of amniotic fluid

EVALUATION

- Detailed anatomic survey
- Consideration for fetal karyotyping
- TORCH titers if viral infection is suspected

- Consider amniotic viral DNA testing
- Consider a thrombophilia workup, though this is controversial

FETAL EVALUATION

- Nonstress testing (NST)
- Biophysical profile (BPP)
- Contraction stress test
- Serial ultrasound exams for growth velocity every 2 to 4 weeks
- Doppler velocimetry

UPDATE #4

Doppler velocimetry was found to be the best predictor of adverse perinatal outcome in IUGR (Gonzalez et al, 2007). Indices used for Doppler evaluation include systolic/diastolic ratio, the resistance index (systolic velocity—diastolic velocity/systolic velocity) and the pulsatility index (systolic velocity—diastolic velocity/mean velocity) (Hoffman et al, 2009).

- *Umbilical artery.* Providing an early sign of IUGR, umbilical artery Doppler indicates vascular blockage at the placenta by measuring the systolic/diastolic ratio. As more of the vasculature is affected, the end diastolic flow decreases until it is eventually absent or reversed, which is an indication of fetal vascular distress with a potentially fatal outcome (Hoffman et al, 2009).
- *Middle cerebral artery.* Once umbilical artery blood flow is found to be abnormal, the middle cerebral artery is examined to look for brain sparing resulting from blood shunting to the brain in the condition of hypoxemia or hypercapnia. In 2008, Mari and Hanif found that the middle cerebral artery peak systolic velocity consistently showed an increase in blood velocity and then a decrease immediately prior to fetal demise.

UPDATE #5

In an attempt to identify a fetus in distress prior to the severe consequences of hypoxemia or acidemia, the ductus venosus has been investigated because of its rapid blood flow. Using color and duplex Doppler to identify abnormal blood flow or reversed or absent end-diastolic flow has been suggested as an indicator for delivery; however, this remains in debate (Mari et al, 2008). Mari and Picconi have argued against using ductus venosus reverse flow (DVRF) for delivery indications prior to 32 weeks' gestation, noting that acidemia is uncommon in DVRF fetuses and each week of gestation between 25 and 29 weeks significantly decreases mortality.

- Staging (Mari et al, 2008).
  - Stage I: Normal NST and umbilical artery Doppler show no hypoxemia or fetal acidosis.
  - Stage II: Normal NST and abnormal umbilical artery Doppler found 5% rate of hypoxia or acidosis.
  - Stage III: Abnormal NST and umbilical artery Doppler found a rate of 60% hypoxia or acidosis.

TREATMENT

- There has been limited success in treating fetal growth restriction. Gulmezoglu and colleagues reported a meta-analysis in 1997 that found three interventions improving fetal growth. These included strategies to decrease smoking, providing nutritional supplements for undernourished women, and treating malaria when this was found to be the etiology for the growth restriction.
- Pollack and colleagues reported in 1997 on in-hospital bed rest and found no improvement in fetal condition.
- The only treatment that has improved neonatal outcome is administration of steroids when premature delivery is anticipated. Bernstein reported similar benefits in the growth-restricted infant compared to its normally grown counterpart.
- Recent reports have noted that there may be a subset of particularly at-risk fetuses. In 2004, Simchen et al. noted that after administration of steroids in a group of chromosomally normal IUGR fetuses with either absent or reverse diastolic flow, 45% had a transient improvement in the Doppler waveform. This group had significantly better outcomes than the group that had no improvement.
- Despite the theoretic benefits of aspirin to treat or prevent IUGR, studies are conflicting, and as such the role of aspirin is undetermined.

MANAGEMENT

- Once IUGR is diagnosed, serial exams should be conducted including non-stress test (NST), biophysical profile (BPP), and ultrasound to follow the development of the fetus and track its condition. Steroids are given when preterm delivery is anticipated.
- Timing of delivery depends on several factors:
  - *Abnormal fetus.* Timing depends on etiology and desire to intervene.
  - *Placental insufficiency.* Depends on growth velocity, gestational age, fetal status, and lung maturity.
  - *Term or near term.* Deliver for preeclampsia, for no growth over 2 to 4 weeks, for BPP of 6 or less, and for absent end or reverse diastolic blood flow.
  - *Remote from term.* Individualization is made based on gestational age and fetal status.
  - *Constitutionally small fetus.* If a fetus has normal growth velocity on serial ultrasounds, symmetrical measurements, no abnormalities, and normal amniotic fluid volume, expectant management can be employed.

OUTCOME

- IUGR is associated with an increase in fetal morbidity and mortality, including the need for induction, fetal compromise during labor, cesarean section, iatrogenic prematurity, and stillbirth. Gardiosi and colleagues noted in 1998 that nearly 40% of stillbirths with no abnormalities were small for gestational age.
- Morbidity for neonates with IUGR includes increased rates of thrombocytopenia, temperature instability, necrotizing enterocolitis, and renal failure.
- Considerations for long-term outcome of these infants include developmental, academic and physical growth.

UPDATE #6

Evaluating several published studies of long-term outcomes of IUGR infants, the *Perinatal Outcome and Later Implications of Intrauterine Growth Restriction* publication (Pallotto et al, 2006) noted several long-term complications for these children. Studies of the IQ of IUGR infants and their average-sized controls have generally found an association between IQ and IUGR resulting in a four- to eight-point decrease in IUGR infants. Abnormal Doppler studies in IUGR have also been associated with impaired cognitive function (Tideman et al, 2007). Additionally, greater emotional and behavioral issues have been reported in IUGR infants.

UPDATE #7

Several articles have reported an increased incidence of the metabolic syndrome with type 2 diabetes, obesity, cardiovascular disease, and hypertension in adult life associated with IUGR (Barker et al, 1993). The pathophysiology is not completely understood; however, it is thought that intrauterine malnutrition results in insulin resistance and a predisposition to type 2 diabetes.

SUGGESTED READINGS

IUGR Etiologies

Dashe JS, McIntire DD, Santos-Ramos R, Leveno KJ: Impact of head-to-abdominal circumference asymmetry on outcomes in growth-discordant twins, *Am J Obstet Gynecol* 183(5):1082–1087, 2000.

Garite T: Impact of a "rescue course" of antenatal steroids: a multicenter randomized placebo-controlled trial, *Am J Obstet Gynecol* 200(3), 248.e1–e9, 2009.

Howley H, Walker M, Rodger M: A systematic review of the association between factor V Leiden or prothrombin gene variant and intrauterine growth restriction, *Am J Obstet Gyn* 192:694–708, 2005.

McCormick MC, Richardson DK: Access to neonatal intensive care, *Future Child* 5(1):162–175, 1995.

Romo A, Carceller R, Tobajas J: Intrauterine growth retardation (IUGR): epidemiology and etiology, *Pediatr Endocrinol* 6(Suppl 3):332–336, 2009.

Wapner R, Sorokin Y, Thom E, et al: Single versus weekly courses of antenatal corticosteriods: evaluation of safety and efficacy, *Am J Obstet Gyn* 195(3):633–642, 2006.

IUGR Screening

Berghella V: Prevention of recurrent fetal growth restriction, *Obstet Gynecol* 110(4):904–912, 2007.

Leeson S, Aziz N: Customised fetal growth assessment, *Br J Obstet Gynaecol* 104(6): 648–651, 1997.

IUGR Fetal Evaluation

Gardosi J, Francis A: Adverse pregnancy outcome and association with small for gestational age birthweight by customized and population-based percentiles, *Am J Obstet Gynecol* 201(1), 2009. 28.e1–8.

Gonzalez J, Stamilio D, Ural S, et al: Relationship between abnormal fetal testing and adverse perinatal outcomes in intrauterine growth restriction, *Am J Obstet Gynecol* 196(5):e48–e51, 2007.

Hoffman C, Galan H: Assessing the at-risk fetus: Doppler ultrasound, *Curr Opin Obstet Gynecol* 21(2):161–166, 2009.

Mari G, Hanif F: Fetal Doppler: umbilical artery, middle cerebral artery, and venous system, *Semin Perinatol* 32(4):253–257, 2008.

Mari G, Picconi J: Doppler vascular changes in intrauterine growth restriction, *Semin Perinatol* 32(3):182–189, 2008.

IUGR Treatment and Management

Bernstein IM, Horbar JD, Badger GJ, et al: Morbidity and mortality among very-low-birth-weight neonates with intrauterine growth restriction. The Vermont Oxford Network, *Am J Obstet Gynecol* 182(1 Pt 1):198–206, 2000.

Gülmezoglu M, de Onis M, Villar J: Effectiveness of interventions to prevent or treat impaired fetal growth, *Obstet Gynecol Surv* 52(2):139–149, 1997.

Pollack RN, Yaffe H, Divon MY: Therapy for intrauterine growth restriction: current options and future directions, *Clin Obstet Gynecol* 40(4):824–842, 1997.

Simchen MJ, Alkazaleh F, Adamson SL, et al: The fetal cardiovascular response to antenatal steroids in severe early-onset intrauterine growth restriction, *Am J Obstet Gynecol* 190(2):296–304, 2004.

IUGR Outcome

Barker D, Gluckman P, Godfrey K, et al: Fetal nutrition and cardiovascular disease in adult life, *Lancet* 341(8850):938–941, 1993.

Gardosi J, Mul T, Mongelli M, Fagan D: Analysis of birthweight and gestational age in antepartum stillbirths, *Br J Obstet Gynaecol* 105(5): 524–530, 1998.

Pallotto E, Kilbride H: Perinatal outcome and later implications of intrauterine growth restriction, *Clin Obstet Gynecol* 49(2):257–269, 2006.

Tideman E, Marsál K, Ley D: Cognitive function in young adults following intrauterine growth restriction with abnormal fetal aortic blood flow, *Ultrasound Obstet Gynecol* 29(6):614–618, 2007.

Chapter 12

Premature Rupture of Membranes

ROBERT M. EHSANIPOOR • CAROL A. MAJOR

KEY UPDATES

1. The administration of 17 hydroxyprogesterone caproate in the second and third trimester to patients with a prior spontaneous preterm birth reduces the risk of a subsequent preterm birth.
2. Antioxidants have been shown to be ineffective in the prevention of preterm premature rupture of membranes (PPROM) and may actually increase risk of PROM.
3. AmniSure is a new product that may be helpful with the diagnosis of ruptured membranes.
4. The use of broad spectrum latency antibiotics has been demonstrated to improve outcomes.
5. Peripartum administration of magnesium sulfate prior to preterm delivery improves long term neurologic outcomes of infants born prematurely.
6. Misoprostol can be used as a cervical ripening agent in the setting of PROM with an unfavorable cervix.
7. Limited data suggest that expectant management of patients with PPROM at early gestational ages and active recurrent genital herpes is appropriate.
8. Limited data suggest that expectant management of patients with HIV and PPROM at early gestational ages is appropriate. Antiretroviral therapy should be given.

Background

DEFINITION

- Premature rupture of membranes (PROM) refers to membrane rupture prior to the onset of labor
- Preterm premature rupture of membranes (PPROM) is PROM prior to 37 weeks' gestation

INCIDENCE

- PROM occurs in 8% of pregnancies at term
- PPROM complicates 3% of pregnancies
- Associated with one third of preterm births

PROM at Term

NATURAL COURSE

- With expectant management, the median time to active labor is 17.3 hours and median time to delivery is 33.3 hours; chorioamnionitis risk is directly correlated with length of membrane rupture

MANAGEMENT

- Induction of labor with oxytocin reduces the median time to active labor to 5 hours and median time to delivery to 17.2 hours
- Induction of labor is associated with lower rates of infection
- Induction of labor is associated with patient satisfaction (Hannah et al, 1996)

Etiology and Risk Factors for PPROM

PATHOPHYSIOLOGY

- The etiology of PPROM is likely multifactorial, and one or more factors may contribute in each case
- Choriodecidual inflammation and infection play an important role, particularly at early gestational ages
- Abnormalities of the connective tissues such as decreased collagen content and alterations in the regulation of matrix metalloproteases
- Uterine overdistention
- Amniocentesis: the membranes most often reseal in patients with PPROM related to amniocentesis

RISK FACTORS

- Most cases of PPROM occur in women without identifiable risk factors
- PPROM has a recurrence risk of 13.5% to 32%
- Genital tract infection
- Antepartum bleeding
- Smoking
- Low socioeconomic status
- Low body mass index (BMI) or nutritional deficiencies
- Signs or symptoms of preterm
- Prior cervical procedures

PREVENTION OF PPROM

> **UPDATE #1**
>
> The use of progesterone in patients with a history of a spontaneous preterm birth or shortened cervix has been associated with reduced rates of spontaneous preterm birth (Tita et al, 2009).

> **UPDATE #2**
>
> The use of antioxidants during pregnancy is not associated with reduced rates of PPROM and may be associated with increased rates of PROM (Spinnato et al, 2008).

Natural Course of PPROM

COMPLICATIONS

- Abruption (4% to 12%)
- Chorioamnionitis (13% to 60%)
- Endometritis (2% to 13%)
- Abnormal lie
- Umbilical cord prolapse
- Neonatal complications related to prematurity
- Pulmonary hypoplasia and skeletal deformities related to oligohydramnios in the second trimester

LATENCY

- Without antibiotics >50% deliver within 48 hours
- Typically 50% will deliver within 1 week
- Latency period is inversely proportional to gestational age

MEMBRANES RESEAL AND FLUID REACCUMULATES IN 2.8% TO 13% OF CASES

Diagnosis of PROM

HISTORY

- Classically reports a "gush" of clear yellow fluid
- Intermittent or slow constant leaking is not uncommon (Table 12-1)

PHYSICAL EXAM

- Sterile speculum exam and the observation of amniotic fluid passing through the cervical canal or the direct visualization of large amounts of amniotic fluid in the vagina are the best methods of diagnosing PPROM

NITRAZINE

- Vaginal pH is typically acidic (pH <6) and the pH of amniotic fluid is typically >7
- The presence of blood, semen, alkaline antiseptics, or bacterial vaginosis can result in false positive tests (Figure 12-1 and Table 12-1)

FERNING

- Fluid from the posterior fornix of the vagina is placed on a slide and allowed to dry; it is then viewed under a microscope and when amniotic fluid is present a delicate ferning pattern should be seen
- See Figure 12-2 and Table 12-1

OLIGOHYDRAMNIOS

- Decreased amniotic fluid volume is common after PPROM, and this can aid in the diagnosis when combined with the history and other findings

FETAL FIBRONECTIN

- Is positive in >90% of patients with ruptured membranes and can in some cases aid in excluding the diagnosis

TABLE 12-1 **Methods of Diagnosing Ruptured Membranes**

Method	Sensitivity	Specificity	PPV	NPV	Accuracy
Ferning	93	95	97	89	94
Nitrazine	89	84	83	90	87
Patient History	90	89	88	90	89

Modified from Canavan TP, Simhan HN, Caritis S: An evidence-based approach to the evaluation and treatment of premature rupture of membranes: Part I, *Obstet Gynecol Surv* 59(9):669-677, 2004.

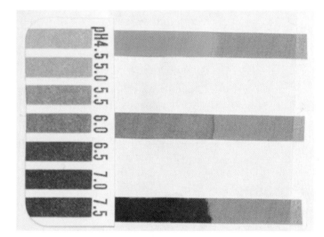

Figure 12-1. **Nitrazine paper for pH testing.** (From Aron Schuftan, MD. Copyright © Aron Schuftan, MD.)

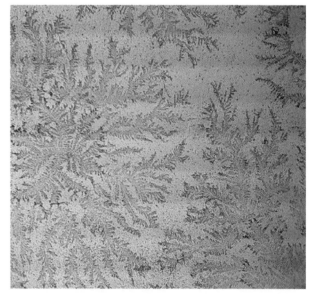

Figure 12-2. **Ferning.** (Obtained from http://upload.wikimedia.org/wikipedia/commons/b/ba/Positive_Fern_Test.jpg. Accessed March 15, 2010.)

INDIGO CARMINE

- In equivocal cases, 1 mL of indigo carmine can be diluted with 9 mL of normal saline and instilled into the amniotic fluid via amniocentesis; a tampon is placed into the vagina and subsequently examined for the presence of blue dye

PLACENTAL ALPHA MICROGLOBULIN-1 (AmniSure)

UPDATE #3

AmniSure is a rapid test to detect the presence of placental alpha microglobulin-1 protein in vaginal secretions. A few studies have been conducted, and it appears to be sensitive, but positive results in patients with intact membranes have been reported, especially in patient with symptoms of labor (Cousins et al, 2005; Lee et al, 2007, 2009).

Initial Evaluation and Management

ESSENTIAL TO CONFIRM GESTATIONAL AGE

EVALUATE FOR EVIDENCE OF INFECTION

CONDUCT ULTRASOUND AND FETAL MONITORING TO DETERMINE FETAL PRESENTATION AND FETAL STATUS

EVALUATE THE CERVICAL STATUS BY SPECULUM EXAM

- Avoid digital until the diagnosis of PPROM is excluded unless the patient is in active labor or immediate delivery is planned; digital exams have been associated with shortened latency period

CONSIDER TESTING FOR GROUP B STREPTOCOCCUS COLONIZATION

CONSIDER TRANSFER TO A TERTIARY CENTER IF INDICATED

Management Considerations for PPROM

LATENCY ANTIBIOTICS

- Infection can be an etiology of PPROM or a consequence of PPROM

UPDATE #4

Multiple placebo-controlled, randomized controlled studies have demonstrated longer latency periods, improved neonatal outcomes, and lower rates of maternal infection with the use of broad-spectrum antibiotics

- The optimal regimen is controversial and may vary based on resistance patterns. The inclusion of erythromycin in the antibiotic regimen appears to be strongly supported. The use of amoxicillin-clavulanate has been associated with necrotizing enterocolitis (Kenyon et al, 2001).
- Parenteral ampicillin with erythromycin for 48 hours followed by oral amoxicillin with erythromycin for 5 days demonstrated benefit in one of the largest trials and is a recommended regimen (Mercer et al, 1997).

CORTICOSTEROIDS

- The administration of corticosteroids in cases of PPROM prior to 32 weeks' gestation is associated with improved neonatal outcomes
- The use of corticosteroids between 32 to 34 weeks in the setting of PPROM is controversial; some recommend the routine use of corticosteroids at this gestational age, whereas others limit the use to cases with documented pulmonary immaturity

TOCOLYSIS

- The use of tocolysis in the setting of PPROM is controversial
- Small trials evaluating the use of tocolysis have not been adequate to either support or refute any recommendation regarding tocolysis
- See the discussion that follows regarding the use of magnesium sulfate for neuroprotection

PROGESTERONE SUPPLEMENTATION

- There are inadequate data to support the use of progesterone in patients with ruptured membranes

HOSPITALIZATION

- Inpatient management is recommended
- Limited data suggest no difference in outcomes between inpatient and outpatient management, but the number studied is small and only a minority of patients would meet the criteria needed for outpatient management

FETAL MONITORING

- The optimal regimen for monitoring the fetus has not been clearly established and each case should be managed as deemed clinically appropriate based on factors unique to the case

TISSUE SEALANTS

- Variant treatments to repair ruptured membranes, but there is inadequate evidence to support their routine clinical use

Timing of Delivery

TERM OR NEAR TERM (>34 WEEKS' GESTATION)

- Proceed to delivery due to the relatively low risk of complications with expectant management
- Induction of labor is typically recommended and cesarean section is reserved for the usual indications
- If the cervix is unfavorable, misoprostol can be used for cervical ripening
- Antibiotic prophylaxis for group B Streptococcus as indicated

PRETERM (32 TO 33⁵⁷ WEEKS' GESTATION)

- Consider amniocentesis to evaluate for the presence of fetal lung maturity or infection, and proceed with delivery if either is present
- If unable to perform amniocentesis, collect a sample of amniotic fluid from the vagina to test for the presence of phosphatidyl glycerol and deliver if present

- If unable to demonstrate fetal lung maturity, proceed with expectant management until 34 weeks and then proceed with delivery

PRETERM (<32 WEEKS' GESTATION)

- The risks of prematurity outweigh the risks of expectant management in appropriate cases; outcomes can be improved with the administration of latency antibiotics and corticosteroids as discussed earlier
- Consider evaluation for fetal lung maturity between 32 to 34 weeks or delivery at 34 weeks (Figure 12-3 provides an algorithm for the evaluation and management of PPROM between 24 and 37 weeks)

Previable PPROM (14 to 24 weeks)

COMPLICATES 4/1000 PREGNANCIES

STABLE PATIENTS

- Counseled regarding termination of pregnancy versus conservative management
- Consider amniocentesis

NATURAL COURSE

- Approximately 40% to 50% deliver within 1 week
- Approximately 70% to 75% deliver within 2 weeks
- If amniocentesis was the cause, then the majority reseal and have favorable outcomes

PULMONARY HYPOPLASIA AND SKELETAL DEFORMITIES

- Pulmonary hypoplasia complicates 9% to 20% of cases
- Skeletal deformities present
- More likely with PPROM <20 weeks, oligohydramnios, and longer latency periods

INFECTION

- 38% develop chorioamnionitis
- 11% develop endometritis
- 1% develop sepsis

SURVIVAL

- Likely overestimated in the literature because of selection bias
- Risk of intrauterine death is 31%
- Survival in PPROM <22 weeks is approximately 14.4%
- Survival with PPROM >22 weeks is approximately 57.7%

MANAGEMENT

- In stable patients, consider outpatient management until viability and then admission
- Limited evidence suggests improved outcomes with the administration of antibiotics
- Limited evidence suggests improved outcomes with the administration of corticosteroids at viability
- There is no evidence to support the use of tocolysis in this setting
- See Figure 12-4 for an algorithm for the management of previable PPROM

PPROM and Neurologic Outcomes

A. Pregnancies complicated by PPROM are at high risk for developing chorioamnionitis
B. Chorioamnionitis has been associated with subsequent development of cerebral palsy
- This includes both preterm and term pregnancies (Wu et al, 2003)

UPDATE #5

Randomized controlled trials treating women at high risk for pre-term delivery have shown that treatment with intravenous magnesium sulfate prior to delivery reduces the rate of cerebral palsy. In the Beneficial effects of antenatal magnesium sulfate (BEAM) trial, 87% of the patients had PPROM (Rouse et al, 2008).
- The number needed to treat with magnesium sulfate to prevent one case of cerebral palsy is 63 (Doyle et al, 2009).

Delivery Considerations

A. Cesarean section reserved for usual indications
B. Cervical ripening

UPDATE #6

The use of prostaglandins in the setting of ruptured membranes at term appears to be safe and effective (Dare et al, 2006)

C. GBS prophylaxis should be initiated as indicated
D. Consider magnesium sulfate for neuroprotection if <34 weeks (see Section VIII)

Unique Considerations

CERCLAGE

- There are no prospective studies evaluating the optimal management if a cerclage is in place
- Some evidence suggests increased infectious morbidity with retention of the cerclage
- Some evidence suggests a possible brief prolongation of pregnancy

HERPES SIMPLEX VIRUS

UPDATE #7

A recent review of 29 patients expectantly managed prior to 32 weeks' gestation revealed no cases of neonatal HSV (Major et al, 2003).

- Consider prophylactic treatment with antiviral agents
- Cesarean section is recommended if active lesions are present

HUMAN IMMUNODEFICIENCY VIRUS

UPDATE #8

Very limited data suggest that expectant management is appropriate in pregnancies complicated by PPROM at <30 to 34 weeks.
- Antiretroviral therapy should be initiated or continued (Alvarez et al, 2007).

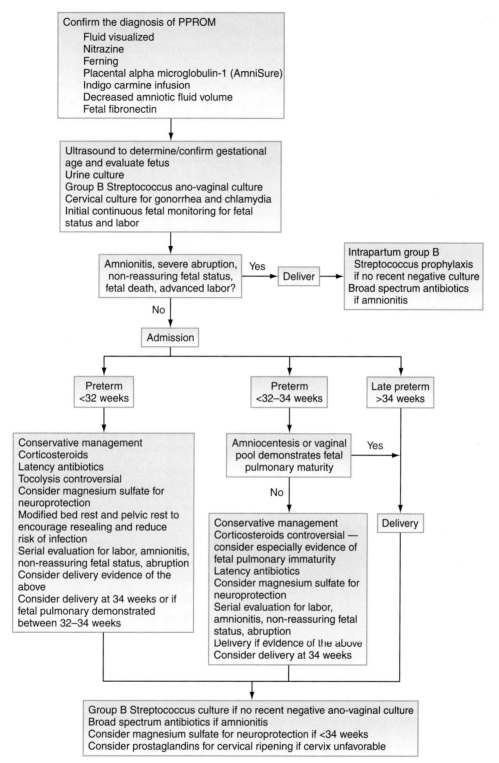

Figure 12-3. An algorithm for the evaluation and management of PPROM 24 to 37 weeks. (Adapted from Mercer BM: Preterm premature rupture of the membranes, *Obstet Gynecol* 101[1]:178-193, 2003.)

TWINS

- PPROM complicates 7.5% of twin pregnancies
- Some evidence suggests that infection is less common in twins
- There are no prospect trials evaluating management in twins; therefore, the recommended management is similar to that for singletons

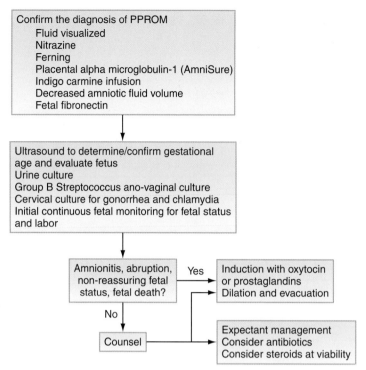

Figure 12-4. An algorithm for the management of previable PPROM. (Adapted from Waters TP, Mercer BM: The management of preterm premature rupture of the membranes near the limit of fetal viability, *Am J Obstet Gynecol* 201(3):230-240, 2009.)

SUGGESTED READINGS

General Review

American College of Obstetricians and Gynecologists Committee on Practice Bulletins—Obstetrics: ACOG practice bulletin no. 80: premature rupture of membranes: clinical management guidelines for obstetrician-gynecologists, *Obstet Gynecol* 109(4):1007–1019, 2007.

Canavan TP, Simhan HN, Caritis S: An evidence-based approach to the evaluation and treatment of premature rupture of membranes: Part I, *Obstet Gynecol Surv* 59(9):669–677, 2004.

Canavan TP, Simhan HN, Caritis S: An evidence-based approach to the evaluation and treatment of premature rupture of membranes: Part II, *Obstet Gynecol Surv* 59(9):678–689, 2004.

Mercer BM: Preterm premature rupture of the membranes, *Obstet Gynecol* 101(1):178–193, 2003.

Term PROM

Hannah ME, Ohlsson A, Farine D, et al: Induction of labor compared with expectant management for prelabor rupture of the membranes at term: TERMPROM study group, *N Engl J Med* 334(16):1005–1010, 1996.

Prevention of PPROM and Preterm Delivery

Spinnato JA 2nd, Freire S, Pinto e Silva JL, et al: Antioxidant supplementation and premature rupture of the membranes: a planned secondary analysis, *Am J Obstet Gynecol* 199(4):433.e1–433.e8, 2008.

Tita AT, Rouse DJ: Progesterone for preterm birth prevention: an evolving intervention, *Am J Obstet Gynecol* 200(3):219–224, 2009.

AmniSure to Diagnose Ruptured Membranes

Cousins LM, Smok DP, Lovett SM, Poeltler DM: AmniSure placental alpha microglobulin-1 rapid immunoassay versus standard diagnostic methods for detection of rupture of membranes, *Am J Perinatol* 22(6):317–320, 2005.

Lee SE, Park JS, Norwitz ER, et al: Measurement of placental alpha-microglobulin-1 in cervicovaginal discharge to diagnose rupture of membranes, *Obstet Gynecol* 109(3):634–640, 2007.

Lee SM, Lee J, Seong HS, et al: The clinical significance of a positive AmniSure test in women with term labor with intact membranes, *J Matern Fetal Neonatal Med* 22(4):305–310, 2009.

Latency Antibiotics

Kenyon S, Boulvain M, Neilson J: Antibiotics for preterm premature rupture of membranes, *Cochrane Database Syst Rev* (4):CD001058, 2001.

Kenyon SL, Taylor DJ, Tarnow-Mordi W: Broad-spectrum antibiotics for preterm, prelabour rupture of fetal membranes: the ORACLE I randomised trial. ORACLE Collaborative Group, *Lancet* 357(9261):979–988, 2001.

Mercer BM, Miodovnik M, Thurnau GR, et al: Antibiotic therapy for reduction of infant morbidity after preterm premature rupture of the membranes: a randomized controlled trial. National Institute of Child Health and Human Development Maternal-Fetal Medicine Units Network, *JAMA* 278(12):989–995, 1997.

Corticosteroids

American College of Obstetricians and Gynecologists Committee on Obstetric Practice: ACOG committee opinion no. 402: antenatal corticosteroid therapy for fetal maturation, *Obstet Gynecol* 111(3):805–807, 2008.

Effect of corticosteroids for fetal maturation on perinatal outcomes, *NIH Consens Statement* 12(2):1–24, 1994.

Timing of Delivery

Lieman JM, Brumfield CG, Carlo W, Ramsey PS: Preterm premature rupture of membranes: is there an optimal gestational age for delivery? *Obstet Gynecol* 105(1):12–17, 2005.

Periviable PPROM

Waters TP, Mercer BM: The management of preterm premature rupture of the membranes near the limit of fetal viability, *Am J Obstet Gynecol* 201(3):230–240, 2009.

Magnesium Sulfate and Neurologic Outcomes

Doyle LW, Crowther CA, Middleton P, et al: Magnesium sulphate for women at risk of preterm birth for neuroprotection of the fetus, *Cochrane Database Syst Rev* (1):CD004661, 2009.

Rouse DJ, Hirtz DG, Thom E, et al: A randomized, controlled trial of magnesium sulfate for the prevention of cerebral palsy, *N Engl J Med* 359(9):895–905, 2008.

Wu YW, Escobar GJ, Grether JK, et al: Chorioamnionitis and cerebral palsy in term and near-term infants, *JAMA* 290(20):2677–2684, 2003.

Prostaglandins for Induction of Labor with Ruptured Membranes

Dare MR, Middleton P, Crowther CA, et al: Planned early birth versus expectant management (waiting) for prelabour rupture of membranes at term (37 weeks or more), *Cochrane Database Syst Rev* (1):CD005302, 2006.

Herpes Simplex Virus

Major CA, Towers CV, Lewis DF, Garite TJ: Expectant management of preterm premature rupture of membranes complicated by active recurrent genital herpes, *Am J Obstet Gynecol* 188(6):1551–1554, 2003: discussion 1554-1555.

Human Immunodeficiency Virus

Alvarez JR, Bardeguez A, Iffy L, Apuzzio JJ: Preterm premature rupture of membranes in pregnancies complicated by human immunodeficiency virus infection: a single center's five-year experience, *J Matern Fetal Neonatal Med* 20(12):853–857, 2007.

Chapter 13

Preterm Labor and Delivery

TAMERA J. HATFIELD • JUDITH H. CHUNG

KEY UPDATES

1 Nonsurgical treatment of periodontal disease was not effective in reducing preterm births.

2 Late preterm birth is associated with increased rates of infant mortality, need for resuscitation, respiratory distress, infection, and longer hospital stay.

3 A single rescue course of antenatal glucocorticoids has been shown to reduce neonatal morbidity if given for the recurrent threat of preterm delivery, 2 weeks after the first course and prior to 33 weeks' gestation.

4 Use of magnesium sulfate appears to confer neuroprotective benefits when administered to infants born prematurely.

5 Long-term follow-up data on women with intact membranes treated with erythromycin had an increased risk of functional impairment. Exposure to erythromycin or amoxicillin-clavulanate was associated with an increased risk of cerebral palsy.

6 17-OH progesterone caproate (250 mg IM weekly) starting at 16 to 20 weeks significantly reduced the rate of preterm delivery and neonatal morbidity in women with a history of prior preterm delivery among women with singleton gestations.

7 Multiple gestations (twins and triplets) do not benefit from administration of 250 mg weekly of 17-OH progesterone caproate; there was no reduction in the rate of preterm birth.

8 Women with a prior history of spontaneous preterm birth may benefit from cerclage placement if the cervical length is <15 mm at < 23 weeks' gestation.

Introduction

- Preterm birth is defined as any birth occurring before 37 weeks' gestation
- Preterm birth can be further subdivided into:
  - Late preterm birth (34 to 36 weeks)
  - Early preterm (<34 weeks)
  - Very preterm (<32 weeks)
  - Extremely preterm (<28 weeks)
- In the United States, preliminary data from the Center for Disease Control/National Center for Health Statistics, National Vital Statistics System for 2008 shows a slight decline in the rates of preterm birth (12.3%) and early preterm birth (3.6%) as compared to 2007 (Matthews et al, 2011)
- Up to the year 2006, the U.S. preterm birth rate had been steadily rising for more than two decades (Figure 13-1) (Matthews et al, 2011)
- In the United States, prematurity is the leading cause of infant death, accounting for approximately 36% of infant deaths in 2005 (Matthews et al, 2011)

- Preterm infants are more likely to suffer neurologic impairment, chronic lung disease, cerebral palsy, and developmental delay
- Despite the morbidity and mortality associated with prematurity, neonatal mortality rates have declined

Risk Factors

- A previous history of preterm birth is the strongest risk factor associated with future preterm delivery (Esplin et al, 2008).
  - One large series showed the risk to be 14% to 22% after one spontaneous preterm birth, 28% to 42% after two preterm births, and 75% after three preterm births (McManemy et al, 2007)
  - A term birth decreases the risk of preterm birth in subsequent pregnancies
- Short interpregnancy interval appears to be a risk factor for preterm birth
- Assisted reproduction appears to confer approximately a twofold increased risk for spontaneous preterm birth in singleton gestations (Jackson et al, 2004)

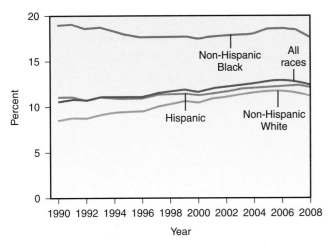

Figure 13-1. Preterm birth rates in the United States. (From Hamilton BE, Martin JA, Ventura SJ: Births: preliminary data for 2008. National Vital Statistics Reports, volume 58, number 16. Hyattsville, MD, National Center for Health Statistics. Released April 6, 2010.)

- Multifetal gestations account for 17% of births <37 weeks and 23% of births <32 weeks (American College of Obstetricians and Gynecologists Committee on Practice Bulletins—Obstetrics, ACOG Practice Bulletin No. 56, 2004)
- Decidual hemorrhage, which clinically presents as first and second trimester bleeding, increases the risk of preterm birth; however, persistent vaginal bleeding incurs an even higher risk of preterm labor when compared to an isolated incident (Harger et al, 1990; Salafia et al, 1995; Williams et al, 1991)
- Infection and inflammation play a large role in the etiology of preterm labor, particularly among early preterm births
- Asymptomatic bacteriuria is a notable risk factor for preterm labor/birth such that treatment of asymptomatic bacteriuria has been shown to significantly reduce the rate of preterm births (Villar et al, 1998)
- Maternal periodontal disease has been shown to be associated with increased risk of preterm labor and low birth weight (Offenbacher et al, 2001)
  - Proposed mechanisms to explain the association of periodontal disease and preterm birth include seeding of the placenta or amniotic fluid by oral pathogens and systemic inflammation
  - Oral bacteria associated with an increased risk of preterm delivery and low birth weight include *Bacteroides forsythus, Porphyromonas gingivalis, Actinobacillus actinomycetemcomitans, Treponema denticola,* and *Fusobacterium nucleatum* (Offenbacher et al, 1998)

UPDATE #1

Nonsurgical treatment of periodontal disease was not effective in reducing preterm births, low birth weight, or growth restriction. Treatment of periodontal disease did, however, improve periodontitis in the treated group (Michalowicz et al, 2006).

- Genital infections have been found to be associated with preterm birth; however, causality has not been proved (Table 13-1)
- Although treatment for genital infections is often indicated, it has not been shown to reduce the risk of preterm birth

TABLE 13-1   Risk of Preterm Birth with Preterm Genitourinary Infection

Risk of Preterm Birth with Selected Infections

Infection	Odds Ratio (95% confidence interval)
Bacterial vaginosis before 16 weeks	7.55 (1.8-31.7)
N. gonorrhoae	5.31 (1.57-17.9)
Asymptomatic bacteriuria	2.08 (1.45-3.03)
Chlamydia trachomatis	
—at 24 weeks	2.2 (1.03-4.78)
—at 28 weeks	0.95 (0.36-2.47)
Trichomonas vaginalis	1.3 (1.1-1.4)
U. urealyticum	1.0 (0.8-1.2)

Adapted from Klein LL, Gibbs RS: Use of microbial cultures and antibiotics in the prevention of infection associated- preterm birth. *Am J Obstet Gynecol* 190:1493, 2004.

- Other risk factors for preterm birth include the following:
  - Tobacco use; there is a dose-dependent increase in the risk of preterm birth (Kyrklund-Blomberg et al, 1998)
  - Substance abuse
  - Short cervix
  - Cervical surgery
  - Uterine malformation
  - Large uterine leiomyomas >5 cm
  - Moderate to severe anemia in the first trimester
  - Fetal factors such as growth restriction, congenital anomalies, and male gender

Etiology

- Approximately 80% of preterm deliveries are spontaneous and occur as a result of preterm labor or preterm, premature rupture of membranes
- Four primary pathologic processes are thought to lead to preterm labor and delivery:
  - Premature activation of the maternal or fetal hypothalamic-pituitary-adrenal axis
    - Increased release of corticotropin releasing factor (CRH), leading to the release of prostaglandins and to further activation of the fetal and maternal hypothalamic-pituitary-adrenal (HPA) axis (Korebrits et al, 1998)
    - Increased release of fetal pituitary adrenocorticotropic hormone, which may stimulate placental estrogens related to myometrial activation and labor (Challis et al, 1989)
    - In one study, serum levels of CRH (measured between 17 to 30 weeks) were two multiples of the median higher in women who delivered prior to 37 weeks (McLean et al, 1999)
    - Increased fetal adrenal zone size correlates with enhanced adrenal activity, and fetal adrenal gland volume may be a future predictor of prematurity (Buhimschi et al, 2008)
  - Inflammation/infection (Figure 13-2)
    - Both systemic infection and ascending genital tract infections are linked to spontaneous preterm birth (Goldenberg et al, 2000)
    - Chorioamnionitis (clinical and subclinical) is more common in preterm compared to term deliveries and may account for up to 50% of preterm births prior to 30 weeks (Gravett et al, 2004)

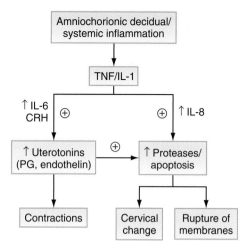

CRH, Corticotropin releasing hormone; IL, interleukin; PG, prostaglandins; TNF, tumor necrosis factor.

Figure 13-2. Inflammation/infection as an etiology for preterm labor. (Courtesy of Charles Lockwood, MD.)

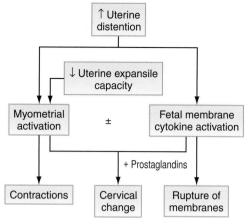

Figure 13-3. Uterine overdistention as an etiology for preterm labor. (Courtesy of Charles Lockwood, MD.)

- Maternal and fetal inflammatory responses mediated by interleukins, tumor necrosis factor, granulocyte colony stimulating factor, and matrix metalloproteinases enhance prostaglandin production, which degrades the extracellular matrix of the fetal membranes and cervix (Fortunato et al, 2002; So et al, 1992)
- Amniotic fluid cultures are positive in approximately 13% of patients with preterm labor and intact membranes compared to 32% in patients with preterm premature rupture of membranes (Romero et al, 2002)
  - Earlier gestational ages at preterm birth are more likely to be associated with amniotic fluid infection (Watts et al, 1992)
  - The most common organisms found in amniotic fluid cultures are genital mycoplasmas and *U. urealyticum*
- Decidual hemorrhage
  - Vaginal bleeding from decidual hemorrhage is associated with a high risk of preterm labor and preterm premature rupture of membranes (Harger et al, 1990; Salafia et al, 1995; Williams et al, 1991)
  - Pathogenesis may be related to high concentrations of tissue factor which mediates hemostasis (Lam et al, 1999; MacKenzie et al, 2004; Rosen et al, 2002)
- Pathologic uterine distention (Figure 13-3)
  - Multifetal gestations and polyhydramnios are the most common causes of uterine distention
  - Myometrial distention leads to the formation of gap junctions, up-regulation of oxytocin receptors, and production of prostaglandins, which all contribute to uterine contractions and cervical dilatation

Diagnosis

- Identifying women with true preterm labor has been fraught with difficulty
- Up to half of women hospitalized for preterm labor deliver at term
- Although exceedingly nonspecific, signs and symptoms of preterm labor include cramping, back pain, contractions, and bloody show
- The diagnosis is based on the criteria of regular painful uterine contractions with cervical dilatation or effacement at a preterm gestational age

Clinical Evaluation

- Tocodynamometry to evaluate for the presence of uterine contractions
- Speculum exam to assess for ruptured membranes or bleeding
- Initial laboratory evaluation should include urinalysis with culture, urine toxicology screening, and group B strep culture
- Analysis of cervicovaginal fetal fibronectin (fFN) may be useful when the diagnosis of preterm labor is uncertain
  - The utility of fFN lies in its high negative predictive value
  - In one study, over 99% of symptomatic patients with a negative fFN did not deliver within 14 days
  - Cannot be performed in the presence of vaginal bleeding, ruptured membranes, or after recent intercourse, vaginal examination, or transvaginal ultrasound (within the past 24 hours)
- Transvaginal ultrasound for cervical length
  - Women with cervical length >30 mm are low risk for preterm birth (Leitich et al, 1999)
  - Women with a cervical length of less than 20 mm should be considered high risk for preterm delivery
- Use of fFN combined with transvaginal ultrasound
  - Women with a cervical length >30 mm are unlikely to deliver preterm
    - One study showed the addition to fFN did not enhance the predictive value of cervical ultrasound (Gomez et al, 2005)
  - fFN should be considered in symptomatic women with a cervical length of 20 to 30 mm
    - A combination of fFN and cervical ultrasound was found to predict preterm delivery with a higher sensitivity and negative predictive value than either method alone (Hincz et al, 2002)
- Amniocentesis may be considered to rule out intra-amniotic infection as source of preterm labor

TABLE 13-2 **Rates of Preterm Birth and Late Preterm Birth in the United States by Year**

Percentage of Preterm Births: United States, Final, 1990, 2000, 2005, and 2006 Preliminary 2007*

Year	Total preterm†	Late preterm‡	32-33 weeks	Less than 32 weeks
2007	12.66	9.03	1.59	2.04
2006	12.80	9.14	1.62	2.04
2005	12.73	9.09	1.60	2.03
2000	11.64	8.22	1.49	1.93
1990	10.61	7.30	1.40	1.92

*Data for 2007 are based on a continuous file of records received from the states.
†Preterm is less than 37 completed weeks of gestation.
‡Late preterm is 34 to 36 completed weeks of gestation.
Reproduced from Hamilton BE, Martin JA, Ventura SJ: Births: Preliminary data for 2007. *Natl Vital Stat Rep* 57:14, 2009.

Late Preterm Birth

- Late preterm birth is defined as a preterm birth between 34 to 37 weeks' gestation
- The rate of late preterm birth has been rising since 1990, although recent years show a slight drop in rates from 9% in 2007 to 8.8% in 2008 (Table 13-2) (Hamilton et al, 2009; Matthews et al, 2011; Martin et al, 2010)
- The overall rise in preterm births has been largely attributed to the increasing late preterm birth rate (7.3% in 1990 to 9.1% in 2006), even though more recent numbers show a slight decline in late preterm births (Hamilton et al, 2009; Matthews et al, 2011)
- Factors that may result in late preterm births:
  - Increased surveillance for maternal and fetal conditions resulting in medically indicated preterm births
    - Medically indicated preterm births rose from 29% in 1992 to 41% in 2002
  - Assisted reproductive technology and multiple gestations has also contributed to the risk in late preterm births
    - Mean gestational age for twin delivery is 35 weeks
    - Mean gestational age for triplet delivery is 32 weeks
  - Increasing average maternal age and obesity rates may also play a role, as these patients tend to have increased risk for medical comorbidities
- Recent trends indicate that late preterm neonates are managed more like term neonates
- However, late preterm birth is associated with increased morbidity when compared to the term birth population

UPDATE #2

A review of British Columbia registry data indicates that late preterm birth was significantly associated with increased rates of infant mortality, need for resuscitation, respiratory distress, infection, and longer hospital stays (Khashu et al, 2009).

- In another large population-based study, neonatal morbidity was seven times higher in late preterm births as compared to term births (Shapiro-Mendoza et al, 2008)
  - The morbidity rate doubled for each week prior to 38 weeks

- The morbidity rate increased 10 to 14 times when maternal risk factors such as hypertension, diabetes, infection, and hemorrhage were considered
- Late preterm infants are more likely to be diagnosed with hypothermia, hypoglycemia, respiratory distress, apnea, hyperbilirubinemia, and feeding difficulties
- Long-term outcomes of late preterm infants suggests increased risk for neurodevelopmental morbidity (Morse et al, 2009; Petrini et al, 2009)
- Maternal complications such as preterm premature rupture of membranes and chorioamnionitis were also found to be more common among late preterm births compared to term deliveries (Khashu et al, 2009)
- One step in the prevention of late preterm births is to ensure that no elective deliveries take place prior to 39 weeks' gestation

Management

ANTENATAL CORTICOSTEROIDS

- Administration of antenatal glucocorticoids to reduce the morbidity and mortality associated with preterm birth has been documented in several randomized placebo-controlled trials
- Antenatal glucocorticoids enhance neonatal lung function by inducing maturational changes in lung architecture as well as enzymes necessary for biochemical maturation (Ballard et al, 1995)
  - As an example, they accelerate development of type 1 and type 2 pneumocytes as well as regulate enzymes in type 2 pneumocytes necessary for surfactant release
- Improved morbidities include decreased rates of respiratory distress syndrome, intraventricular hemorrhage, necrotizing enterocolitis, sepsis, and death (Roberts et al, 2006)
- The current recommendation is to administer a course of antenatal glucocorticoids to patients at risk for preterm delivery within the next 7 days
- All fetuses between 24 to 34 weeks at risk for delivery with intact membranes should be considered candidates for antenatal corticosteroids
  - Meta-analysis has shown decreased rates of respiratory distress syndrome (RDS), intraventricular hemorrhage (IVH), and neonatal death when antenatal glucocorticoids are administered at 26 weeks or greater; however, there are limited data on their use prior to 26 weeks (Roberts et al, 2006)
  - Although few primitive alveoli are present prior to 24 weeks, suggesting a theoretic lack of efficacy, one study showed a decreased risk of death in neonates exposed to betamethasone between 23{0/7} and 23{6/7 }weeks (Hayes et al, 2008)
- Patients with preterm premature rupture of membranes (PPROM) should receive antenatal glucocorticoids prior to 32 weeks unless there is evidence of chorioamnionitis necessitating delivery (U.S. Department of Health and Human Services)
  - Studies have failed to show improved neonatal benefit from 32 to 34 weeks, and further exposure appeared to increase the risk chorioamnionitis (Guinn et al, 2001; Lee et al, 2004)

- Consideration may be given to antenatal glucocorticoids in the setting of PPROM after 32 weeks with documented pulmonary immaturity (American College of Obstetricians and Gynecologists Committee Opinion 402, 2008, U.S. Department of Health and Human Services)
- Dosing regimens found to improve outcomes include either betamethasone 12 mg intramuscularly every 24 hours × 2 doses or dexamethasone 6 mg intramuscularly every 12 hours × 4 doses (U.S. Department of Health and Human Services)
  - Increased drug dose or frequency of dosing has not been found to confer additional benefit
- Optimal benefit occurs after 24 hours of administration and lasts up to 7 days
- Treatment should not be withheld unless delivery is imminent, as treatment even less than 24 hours has been show to incur some benefit (U.S. Department of Health and Human Services, 1994)
- Transient hyperglycemia may occur beginning 12 hours and up to 5 days post administration of antenatal glucocorticoids
  - Diabetic patients may require additional insulin therapy during this period
- There is no association between a single course of antenatal glucocorticoids and adverse neonatal events including poor neurologic outcome or clinically significant adrenal suppression (Roberts et al, 2006; U.S. Department of Health and Human Services, 1994)

UPDATE #3

A multicenter randomized placebo-control trial demonstrated a significant decrease in composite morbidity (and in particular respiratory morbidity) after administration of a single rescue course of betamethasone. Patients included those with singletons or twins who presented with a recurring threat of preterm delivery 14 days after an initial steroid course but prior to 33 weeks' gestation (Garite et al, 2009).

TOCOLYSIS

- Goal is to delay delivery until antenatal glucocorticoids can be administered or to allow for maternal transport to a facility with the appropriate level of neonatal care, should delivery ensue
- Contraindications
  - Intrauterine fetal demise
  - Chorioamnionitis
  - Severe preeclampsia or eclampsia
  - Maternal hemorrhage with hemodynamic instability
  - Nonreassuring fetal status
  - Severe intrauterine growth restriction
- Selection of tocolytic should be based on safety and efficacy for mother and fetus
- A meta-analysis of 58 randomized controlled trials (RCTs) concluded that commonly used tocolytics were more effective than placebo or no treatment to delay delivery for 48 hours and even 7 days; however, no neonatal reductions in RDS or neonatal death were observed (Haas et al, 2009)

- Beta-adrenergic receptor agonists
  - Cause myometrial relaxation by interacting with beta-2-adrenergic receptors, triggering intracellular second messenger systems to decrease intracellular calcium interfering with activity of myosin and ultimately myometrial contractility
  - Cochrane review of 11 RCTs demonstrated efficacy in delay of preterm delivery for 48 hours (Anotayanonth et al, 2004)
  - Maternal side effects
    - Increased heart rate and stroke volume
    - Peripheral vasodilation, diastolic hypotension, bronchial relaxation leading to tachycardia, palpitations, and hypotension
    - Tremor
    - Shortness of breath
    - Chest discomfort
    - Pulmonary edema is uncommon but may occur with compounding risks factors such as infection
    - Increased risk for hypokalemia and hyperglycemia
  - Contraindications
    - Maternal cardiac disease resulting from chronotropic effects on the heart
    - Poorly controlled hyperthyroidism
    - Poorly controlled diabetes
      - Women with well-controlled diabetes are candidates for beta-adrenergic therapy but require close monitoring of glucose and potassium
  - Terbutaline was the most commonly used medication in this class
    - Food and Drug Administration (FDA) "Black Box" warning issued February 17, 2011
  - Terbutaline dosing
    - Intravenous (IV) infusion of 2.5 to 5 mcg/min can be increased every 20 min to a maximum of 25 mcg/min until uterine quiescence is achieved
      - FDA warned that injectable terbutaline should *not* be used beyond 48 to 72 hours, because of potential serious maternal cardiac complications including death with prolonged treatment
    - Subcutaneous dosing: 0.25 mg limit doses after FDA warning
      - Monitor glucose and potassium during parenteral use
      - Monitor for pulmonary edema during parenteral use
      - Hold for adverse maternal symptoms or tachycardia greater than 120 beats/min
- Magnesium sulfate
  - Mechanism not completely understood but thought to compete with calcium at voltage-gated receptors interfering with myosin and myometrial contractility
  - A systematic review of RCTs demonstrated no reduction in delivery within 48 hours, 7 days, or prior to 37 weeks when compared to placebo or no tocolysis (RR = 0.75[0.54 to 1.03]); in addition, no observed improvements in neonatal outcomes (Mercer et al, 2009)
  - Maternal side effects
    - Diaphoresis and flushing
    - Pulmonary edema
    - Magnesium sulfate toxicity related to serum levels
    - Magnesium sulfate is contraindicated in women with myasthenia gravis
    - Avoid use in women with myocardial compromise

- Caution is advised in patients with impaired renal function because of renal clearance and increased risk for magnesium toxicity
- Dosing
  - 6 g load followed by continuous infusion of approximately 2 g/hr, titrating to serum levels and uterine quiescence
  - Avoid continuous infusion or use lower dosing in women with renal insufficiency
  - Serum levels may be monitored every 6 hours until steady state is achieved or as clinically indicated
  - Use of magnesium sulfate appears to confer neuroprotective benefits

UPDATE #4

A recent meta-analysis of randomized control trials evaluating the use of magnesium sulfate for neuroprotection demonstrated reduced occurrence of cerebral palsy when given for neuro-protective effect (RR 0.71 [0.55 to 0.91]) (Doyle et al, 2009a, 2009b). Optimal practice management guidelines for its use have yet to be evaluated. Current recommendation is for physicians to develop guidelines for inclusion criteria and treatment regimens in accordance with those used in one of the larger trials (Table 13-3) (American College of Obstetricians and Gynecologists Committee on Obstetric Practice, ACOG Committee Opinion No. 455, 2010).

- Calcium channel blocker (nifedipine most commonly used and studied)
  - Inhibits myosin and decreasing myometrial contractility by directly blocking influx of calcium ions through the cell membrane and increasing calcium efflux from the cell
  - No large randomized control trials assessing the effect of calcium channel blockers as compared to placebo or no drug
  - Meta-analysis of 12 trials including 1000 patients did not show any benefit for delivery less than 48 hours when compared to other tocolytics; there was improved benefit for delivery less than 7 days and less than 34 weeks (King et al, 2003).
  - Subanalysis of nine trials comparing calcium channel blockers to beta-adrenergic agonists found calcium channel blockers to significantly reduce the risk of birth prior to 48 hours
  - Calcium channel blockers were also found to confer reduced neonatal morbidity
  - Maternal side effects
    - Headache
    - Flushing
    - Palpitations
    - Nausea
    - Decreased mean arterial blood pressure
    - Use with caution in women with congestive heart failure and left ventricular dysfunction
  - Fetal side effects
    - Animal data suggest concern for decreased uterine blood flow and decreased oxygen saturation
    - Fetal Doppler studies of uteroplacental blood flow have been reassuring
  - Dosing
    - No optimal regimens have been defined

- Initially, nifedipine 20 mg orally followed by 20 mg in 90 minutes versus 10 mg every 20 minutes for up to four doses
- Maintenance dosing is commonly 10 to 20 mg every 6 hours
- Cyclooxygenase (COX) inhibitors
  - Indomethacin is most common for this class
  - Decreases prostaglandin synthesis
  - Comparison studies with placebo did not show a difference in delivery less than 48 hours or 7 days (King et al, 2005); however, the numbers enrolled were very small
  - No differences were detected in neonatal outcomes, including no increased risk of premature closure of the ductus arteriosus
  - When compared to other tocolytic agents, there was a significant benefit of decreased delivery before 48 hours when COX inhibitors were compared to beta-adrenergic agonists
  - Maternal side effects
    - Gastroesophageal reflux
    - Gastritis
    - Nausea and vomiting
    - Contraindicated in women with platelet dysfunction, bleeding disorders, gastrointestinal ulcerative disease, liver disease, renal disease, and hypersensitivity to aspirin
  - Fetal side effects
    - Concern for narrowing of ductus (appears to be safe if used prior to 32 weeks' gestation and for no more than 48 hours)
    - Oligohydramnios
    - Possible association with necrotizing enterocolitis (NEC) in preterm neonates after recent treatment (<48 hours predelivery)
  - Dosing
    - 50 to 100 mg loading (oral or rectal) followed by 25 mg orally every 4 to 6 hours up to 48 hours
    - Ultrasound for amniotic fluid index and evidence of ductal constriction should be performed if therapy is to exceed 48 hours

ANTIBIOTICS

- No trial has demonstrated reduced rates of preterm birth by administering prophylactic antibiotics including high-risk groups with abnormal vaginal flora, history of preterm delivery, or positive fetal fibronectin
- Antibiotics given to women in the acute phase of preterm labor with intact membranes fail to show a benefit in neonatal outcomes in randomized control trials and raise concerns about increased neonatal mortality (King et al, 2002)
- Oracle II randomized women with intact membranes in spontaneous preterm labor to receive amoxicillin-clavulanate, erythromycin, placebo, or both antibiotics for 10 days or until delivery and showed no benefit of any antibiotic regimen in their primary outcome of composite neonatal morbidity

UPDATE #5

Long-term follow-up data from the Oracle II trial found an unexpected increase in cerebral palsy for those exposed to either antibiotic and functional impairment in those exposed to erythromycin alone (Kenyon et al, 2008).

TABLE 13-3   **Results from Large Trials on Tocolytics for Preterm Labor**

Study	Total Number of Participants	Inclusions	Dose	Duration	Death and Cerebral Palsy	Death	Cerebral Palsy
Crowther	1255	Less than 30 weeks of gestation; likely delivery within 24 hours	4g load 1g/hr	Up to 24 hours	RR, 0.83; 95% CI, 0.66-1.03	RR, 0.83; 95% CI, 0.64-1.09	RR, 0.83; 95% CI, 0.54-1.27
Marret	688	Less than 33 weeks of gestation	4g load only	Loading dose only	OR, 0.80; 95% CI, 0.58-1.10	OR, 0.85; 95% CI, 0.55-1.32	OR, 0.70; 95% CI, 0.41-1.19
Rouse	2241	24-31 weeks of gestation; at high risk of spontaneous birth	6g load 2g/hr	Up to 12 hours; treatment resumed when delivery imminent	RR, 0.97; 95% CI, 0.77-1.23	RR, 1.12; 95% CI, 0.85-1.47	RR, 0.55; 95% CI, 0.32-0.95

CI, confidence interval; OR, odds ratio; RR, relative risk.
Data from Crowther CA, Hiller JE, Doyle LW, Haslam RR: Effect of magnesium sulfate given for neuroprotection before preterm birth: a randomized controlled trial, Australasian Collaborative Trial of Magnesium Sulfate (ACTOMg SO4) Collaborative Group, *JAMA* 290:2669-2676, 2003; Marret S, Marpeau L, Zupan-Simunek V, et al: Magnesium sulfate given before very-preterm birth to protect infant brain: the randomised controlled PREMAG trial. PREMAG trial group, *BJOG* 114:310-318, 2007; and Rouse DJ, Hirtz DG, Thom E, et al: A randomized, controlled trial of magnesium sulfate for the prevention of cerebral palsy, Eunice Kennedy Shriver NICHD Maternal-Fetal Medicine Units Network, *N Engl J Med* 359:895-905, 2008.

- Antibiotics for the treatment of group B streptococcus (GBS) should be utilized in women thought to be at risk for imminent delivery (Schrag et al, 2002)
  - GBS culture swab should be obtained upon presentation
  - Intrapartum treatment for GBS is indicated until culture results are available or threat or delivery is averted
    - If the culture returns negative, intrapartum antibiotics are no longer warranted
    - If a negative culture was obtained in the previous 4 weeks, treatment is not necessary
    - If labor is arrested and delivery does not ensue for 4 weeks, the recommendation is to repeat the culture at the 4-week mark
- The current recommendation for treatment of GBS is penicillin G 5 million units IV × 1, then 2.5 million units IV every 4 hours until delivery; if penicillin G is not available, ampicillin is an acceptable alternative (2 g IV × 1, then 1 g IV every 4 hours)
  - Women who are allergic to penicillin and who are not at high risk for anaphylaxis should be treated with cefazolin 2 g IV × 1, then 1 g every 8 hours until delivery
  - Penicillin-allergic women who are at high risk for anaphylaxis should be treated with vancomycin 1 g IV every 12 hours until delivery
  - Clindamycin (900 mg IV every 8 hours until delivery) and erythromycin (500 mg IV every 6 hours until delivery) may be used in penicillin-allergic women only if susceptibility testing has been done and if isolates are deemed sensitive to these antibiotics; if a strain is resistant to erythromycin but appears to be sensitive to clindamycin, susceptibility to clindamycin may be reduced (Figure 13-4)

Maternal Transport

- Delivery in high-volume tertiary care centers has been shown to improve neonatal outcomes among very low birth weight neonates (Phibbs et al, 2007)

- For those at significant risk of impending preterm birth, maternal transport to a regional perinatal center prior to delivery may have neonatal benefits (Hohlagschwandtner et al, 2001; Modanlou et al, 1980)

Prevention of Preterm Delivery

- Progestogens
  - There is increasing evidence that progesterone supplementation may reduce the risk of preterm birth in certain high-risk populations

UPDATE #6

It has been shown that 17-OH progesterone caproate (250 mg IM weekly) starting at 16 to 20 weeks significantly reduced the rate of preterm delivery <32 weeks (RR 0.58 [CI 0.37 to 0.91]), preterm birth <35 weeks (RR 0.67 [CI 0.48 to 0.93]), and neonatal morbidity in women with a history of prior preterm birth (Meis et al, 2003).

- Vaginal progesterone (100 mg daily) was also shown to decrease the risk of preterm birth in a population of women at high risk for preterm delivery (de Fonseca et al, 2003)
- A randomized control trial also demonstrated that asymptomatic women found to have a short cervix (less than 15 mm) between 20 and 25 weeks had a reduced rate of preterm delivery (<34 weeks) when treated with vaginal progesterone (200 mg) daily (Fonseca et al, 2007)

UPDATE #7

Randomized placebo control trials evaluating the use of 250 mg weekly administration of 17-OH progesterone caproate in twin and triplet gestations found no reduction in the rates of preterm birth (Combs et al, 2010; Rouse et al, 2007).

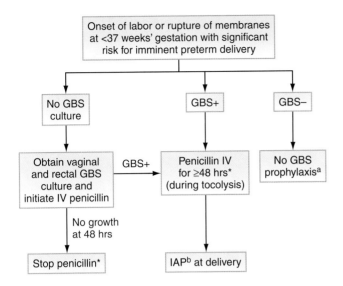

* Penicillin should be continued for a total of at least 48 hours, unless delivery occurs sooner. At the physician's discretion, antibiotic prophylaxis may be continued beyond 48 hours in a GBS culture-positive woman if delivery has not yet occurred. For women who are GBS culture positive, antibiotic prophylaxis should be reinitiated when labor likely to proceed to delivery occurs or recurs.
a If delivery has not occurred within 4 weeks, a vaginal and rectal GBS screening culture should be repeated and the patient should be managed as described, based on the result of the repeat culture.
b Intrapartum antibiotic prophylaxis.

Figure 13-4. Algorithm for group beta *streptococcus* in the setting of threatened preterm labor. (Adapted from Schrag S, Gorwitz R, Fultz-Butts K, et al: Prevention of perinatal group B streptococcal disease: revised guidelines from CDC, *MMWR Recomm Rep* 51(RR-11), Figure 3, 2002.)

• Cervical cerclage
  • Placement of cerclage remains controversial in the prevention of spontaneous preterm birth; however, it may be useful in some populations

UPDATE #8

In a prospective randomized controlled trial, women with a prior history of spontaneous preterm birth benefited from cerclage placement with reduced rates of preterm birth if the cervical length was less than 15 mm at less than 22 weeks' gestation (Owen et al, 2009).

• Observational studies suggest that smoking cessation may reduce risk of preterm birth (Kabir et al, 2009).
• The efficacy of decreased work fatigue has not been studied in randomized trials for the prevention of spontaneous preterm birth; however, high cumulative work fatigue has been identified as a risk factor for preterm delivery (Mozurkewich et al, 2000)

• Reports on the role of nutritional supplementation for the prevention of preterm birth are inconclusive
  • Some studies suggest that fish oil supplements reduce the risk of preterm birth prior to 34 weeks; however, the proportion of subjects delivering prior to 37 weeks was similar (Makrides et al, 2006)
  • Protein supplements have not demonstrated efficacy in preventing preterm birth (Kramer et al, 2003)
• There is no evidence to support or refute the use of home or hospital bed rest for the prevention of preterm delivery (Sosa et al, 2004)

SUGGESTED READINGS

Risk Factors

Michalowicz BS, Hodges JS, DiAngelis AJ, et al: Treatment of periodontal disease and the risk of preterm birth, *N Engl J Med* 355(18):1885–1894, 2006.

Late Preterm Birth

Khashu M, Narayanan M, Bhargava S, Osiovich H: Perinatal outcomes associated with preterm birth at 33-36 weeks' gestation: a population based cohort study, *Pediatrics* 123(1):109–113, 2009.

Management

Steroids

Garite TJ, Kurtzman J, Maurel K, Clark R: Impact of a rescue course of antenatal corticosteroids: a multicenter randomized placebo-controlled trial, *Am J Obstet Gynecol* 200(3): 248.e1-e9, 2009.

Tocolysis

Doyle LW, Crowther CA, Middleton P, Marret S: Antenatal magnesium sulfate and neurologic outcome in preterm infants: a systematic review, *Obstet Gynecol* 113(6):1327–1333, 2009.

Antibiotics

Kenyon S, Pike K, Jones DR, et al: Childhood outcomes after prescription of antibiotics to pregnant women with spontaneous preterm labour: 7 year follow up of the ORACLE II trial, *Lancet* 372(9646):1319–1327, 2008.

Prevention of Preterm Delivery

Combs A, Garite TJ, Maurel K, et al: Failure of 17-hydroxyprogesterone to reduce neonatal morbidity or prolong triplet pregnancy: a double-blind randomized clinical trial, *Am J Obstet Gynecol* 203(3):e1–e9, 2010.
Fonseca EB, Celik E, Parra M, et al: Progesterone and the risk of preterm birth among women with a short cervix, *N Engl J Med* 357(5):462–469, 2007.
Meis PH, Klebanoff M, Thom E, et al: Prevention of recurrent preterm delivery by 17 alpha-hydroxyprogesterone caproate, *N Eng J Med* 348(24):2379–2385, 2003.
Owen J, Hankins G, Iams JD, et al: Multicenter randomized trial of cerclage for preterm birth prevention in high-risk women with shortened midtrimester cervical length, *Am J Obstet Gynecol* 201(4): 375.e1-e8, 2009.
Rouse DJ, Caritis SN, Peaceman AM, et al: A trial of 17 alpha-hydroxyprogesterone caproate to prevent prematurity in twins, *N Engl J Med* 357(5):454–461, 2007.

References

Please go to expertconsult.com to view references.

Chapter 14

Cervical Ripening, Induction of Labor, and Prolonged Pregnancy

NICOLE M. PETROSSI • SARA ARIAN • DEBORAH A. WING*

KEY UPDATES

1 The rate of induction continues to rise in this country as a result of a variety of medical and social factors.

2 Labor induction protocols are amenable to quality assurance measures.

3 Elective inductions contribute to the overall increase in induction frequency, but they are not without risk. A growing body of evidence suggests an individualized approach to prenatal care and delivery planning known as active management of risk in pregnancy at term (AMOR-IPAT), with early pregnancy ultrasound for accurate assignment of gestational age, may hold promise.

4 Optimal management of prolonged pregnancies is controversial.

5 Methods of cervical ripening and labor induction are varied. Pharmacologic methods include vaginal administration of prostaglandin E1 (misoprostol) and prostaglandin E2 (dinoprostone), orally administered misoprostol, and transcervical Foley balloon catheter placement.

6 Extra-amniotic saline infusion with transcervical Foley balloon catheter placement does not appear to be effective.

7 Standardized protocols for oxytocin administration are gaining favor in an attempt to reduce administration errors and improve patient safety; however, none of the proposed regimens has been subjected to scientific scrutiny.

8 Development of a time-released vaginal misoprostol insert is under way.

Introduction

- Induction of labor is one of the most commonly performed obstetrical procedures in the United States.
- Induction of labor refers to the iatrogenic stimulation of uterine contractions prior to the onset of spontaneous labor to accomplish vaginal delivery.
- Augmentation of labor refers to increasing the frequency and improving the intensity of existing uterine contractions in a patient who is in labor and not progressing adequately, in order to accomplish vaginal delivery.
- Between 1990 and 2006, the frequency of labor induction approximately doubled, rising from 9.5% to 22.5% (Martin et al, 2010).
- Reasons for this increase include the availability of better cervical ripening agents, patients' and clinicians' desire to arrange a convenient time of delivery, and more relaxed attitudes toward marginal indications for induction (Rayburn et al, 2002).

- Patient or provider concerns about the risk of fetal demise with expectant management near term or postterm have also contributed to the increased rate of induction.

UPDATE #1
The rate of induction continues to rise in this country as a result of a variety of medical and social factors (Martin et al, 2007).

Indications and Contraindications

- Induction of labor is indicated when the benefits of prompt delivery to either mother or fetus outweigh the risk of continuing the pregnancy (American College of Obstetricians and Gynecologists: ACOG Committee on Practice Bulletins—Obstetrics, ACOG Practice Bulletin No. 107, 2009).
- There are many accepted medical and obstetrical indications for labor induction and several relative indications for labor induction (Table 14-1).
- Appropriately timed induction of women with these pregnancy complications can improve maternal-fetal outcomes (Nicholson et al, 2008).

---

*Dr. Wing is a principal investigator for Cytokine Pharmasciences, Inc., developer of the misoprostol time-released vaginal insert.

TABLE 14-1 Indications for Labor Induction	
Accepted Absolute Indications	**Relative Indications**
HYPERTENSIVE DISORDERS Preeclampsia/eclampsia	**HYPERTENSIVE DISORDERS** Chronic hypertension
Maternal Medical Conditions Diabetes mellitus Renal disease Chronic pulmonary disease	*Maternal Medical Conditions* Systemic lupus erythematosus Gestational diabetes
Prelabor Rupture of Membranes	
Chorioamnionitis	
Fetal Compromise Fetal growth restriction Isoimmunization Nonreassuring antepartum fetal testing	*Logistic Factors* Risk of rapid labor Distance from hospital Psychosocial indications
Fetal demise	*Previous stillbirth*
Postdates pregnancy (>42 weeks)	

TABLE 14-2 Contraindications to Labor Induction	
Accepted Absolute Contraindications	**Relative Contraindications**
Prior classical uterine incision or transfundal uterine surgery	
Active Genital Herpes Infection	**Cervical Carcinoma**
Placenta or vasa previa Umbilical cord prolapse Transverse or oblique fetal lie	Funic presentation Malpresentation (breech)
Absolute cephalopelvic disproportion (as in women with pelvic deformities)	

- However, there is only limited high-quality evidence establishing any benefits for specific medical and obstetrical indications for induction (Mozurkewich et al, 2009), with the recent exception of gestational hypertension beyond 36 weeks wherein induction was associated with improved maternal outcomes (Koopmans et al, 2009).
- Contraindications are those that preclude vaginal delivery (Table 14-2), as well as other clinical scenarios (e.g., active genital herpes infection, previous classical cesarean delivery, nonreactive nonstress testing), which may be associated with an increased risk of maternal or fetal morbidity during induction.
- Relative contraindications, such as previous low transverse cesarean delivery and multifetal pregnancy, warrant close monitoring during induction and a low threshold for intervention if labor is not progressing or there are no reassuring signs of fetal well-being.

ELECTIVE INDUCTION OF LABOR

- Elective induction of labor refers to the initiation of labor in an individual with a term pregnancy that is free of medical or obstetrical indications.
- The rate of elective induction in the United States increased dramatically from 9.5% to 19.4% from 1989 to 1998 (Moore et al, 2006; Zhang et al, 2002).
- Although elective induction is not recommended or encouraged, it may be appropriate for women with a history of very short labors, those who live a great distance from the hospital, or those who have experienced a prior stillbirth at or near term.
- In addition, certain maternal medical conditions require multispecialty participation, and the availability of experienced personnel can be a great benefit to a planned delivery.
- Examples of such cases are pregnancies with maternal cardiac disease, which may require invasive monitoring during labor, or those complicated by chronic renal disease where considerations for hemodialysis may dictate a scheduled birth.

RISKS ASSOCIATED WITH ELECTIVE INDUCTION

- The major risks of elective induction of labor at term are thought to be increased rates of cesarean delivery (especially in nulliparas), increased neonatal morbidity, and cost.
- Currently, there are insufficient high-quality data to support a policy of routine elective induction of labor at term.
- Large, randomized trials with emphasis on maternal and neonatal safety, determination of neonatal benefit as a reflection of reduced unexplained fetal death, and cost-effectiveness/cost-benefit analyses are needed.
- An overarching concern regarding higher cesarean rates following induction prevails.
- Labor induction protocols lend themselves well to quality assurance measures.
- In the future, individual provider induction rates may be monitored and evaluated using evidence-based obstetric care quality measures, especially if the induction rates and ensuing cesarean birth rates are extreme (Fisch et al, 2009).

UPDATE #2

Labor induction protocols are amenable to quality assurance measures (Fisch et al, 2009).

RISK OF CESAREAN DELIVERY FOLLOWING ELECTIVE INDUCTION AT TERM

- The risk of cesarean delivery following elective induction and associated costs, especially for the nullipara with an unfavorable cervix, has been clearly established in the literature with several cohort and case-control studies (Cammu et al, 2002; Maslow et al, 2000; Seyb et al, 1999).
- These studies revealed an increased risk of cesarean that was at least twice the risk of spontaneously laboring patients.
- Seyb and colleagues also noted in their investigation that the mean time spent on labor and delivery was almost twice as long, and postpartum stays were prolonged if labor induction was undertaken.
- The total cost associated with hospitalization for elective induction was 17.4% higher than for spontaneous labor, including costs for labor and delivery, pharmacy, and postpartum care.

TABLE 14-3   Criteria for Confirmation of Gestational Age or Fetal Pulmonary Maturity

	Parameters
Confirmation of gestational age	Fetal heart tones have been documented as present for ≥30 weeks by Doppler ultrasound.
	≥36 weeks have elapsed since a positive serum or urine human chorionic gonadotropin pregnancy test.
	Ultrasound measurement at less than 20 weeks of gestation supports gestational age of 39 weeks or greater.
Fetal pulmonary maturity	If term gestation cannot be confirmed by two or more of the preceding obstetric clinical or laboratory criteria, then amniotic fluid analyses can be used to provide evidence of fetal lung maturity. Various tests are available. The parameters for evidence of fetal pulmonary maturity are as follows:
	1. Lecithin/sphingomyelin (L/S) ratio >2.1
	2. Presence of phosphatidylglycerol (PG)
	3. TDxFLM assay ≥70 mg surfactant per 1g albumin present
	4. Presence of saturated phosphatidylcholine (SPC) ≥500 ng/mL in nondiabetic patients (≥1000 ng/mL for pregestational diabetic patients)

Modified data from Induction of Labor: American College of Obstetricians and Gynecologists: ACOG practice bulletin no 107, *Obstet Gynecol* 114:386, 2009.

- Caughey and colleagues (2009) published a meta-analysis of nine randomized controlled trials comparing expectant management (rather than spontaneous labor) to elective induction.
- The rationale for the choice of comparison group was to examine the clinical decision-making at 38 or 39 weeks' gestation between expectant management and induction of labor.
- In contrast to the previously published cohort studies, the meta-analysis of randomized controlled trials revealed a decreased risk of cesarean in the induction group compared to the expectantly managed group (relative risk [RR] 1.17, 95% confidence interval [CI] 1.05 to 1.29).
- As well, a Cochrane Library review including 19 trials involving 7984 women reported that the women induced at 37 to 40 completed weeks were more likely to have a cesarean with expectant management than those who underwent labor induction (RR 0.58, 95% CI 0.34 to 0.99) (Gulmezoglu et al, 2006).
- Caughey and colleagues (2006) also examined the risk of cesarean delivery for each week of gestational age ranging from 38 to 41 weeks and found that cesarean delivery occurred less commonly with expectant management than with induction.
- In contrast, emerging data from the Consortium of Safe Labor, which involves 115,528 deliveries from 10 U.S. institutions from 2002 to 2008 (Bailit et al, 2010), reveal that the incidence of cesarean delivery increased with elective induction compared to spontaneous labor, particularly at 37 to 38 completed weeks' gestation and at 41 weeks' gestation.
- When the outcomes were adjusted for race, maternal age, parity, preeclampsia, eclampsia, chronic hypertension, diabetes, and group B streptococcus (GBS) status, the odds ratio for electively induced patients from 37 to 42 weeks' gestation to undergo cesarean was 1.58 compared to spontaneously laboring patients (95% CI 1.48 to 1.69).

RISK OF NEONATAL MORBIDITY FOLLOWING ELECTIVE INDUCTION AT TERM

- Neonatal respiratory problems, sepsis, and asphyxia are the major pediatric concerns when mothers undergo elective delivery.

- Respiratory problems can result from inadvertent delivery of a premature infant or transient tachypnea related to cesarean delivery after failed induction.
- This is counterbalanced by observations that fewer electively induced infants have meconium passage when compared to spontaneously labored infants and therefore, likely have a reduced incidence of meconium aspiration syndrome (Caughey et al, 2009).
- Macrosomia also may be reduced, as noted in an ecologic study performed by Zhang et al (2010).
- This study revealed that the increased induction rate between 1992 and 2003 (14% to 27%) was significantly associated with reduced mean fetal birth weight (r = −0.54, 95% CI −0.71 to −0.29) and rate of macrosomia (r = −0.55, 95% CI −0.74 to −0.32).
- Guidelines to help ensure that gestational age is at least 39 weeks before elective delivery are listed in Table 14-3.
- The risk of respiratory morbidity was illustrated in a retrospective review of the infants with respiratory distress or transient tachypnea of the newborn admitted to the neonatal intensive care unit following elective delivery at term (Morrison et al, 1995).
- The data were stratified by gestational age and route of delivery:
  - Baseline incidence of respiratory distress syndrome and transient tachypnea at term were 2.2/1000 deliveries (95% CI 1.7 to 2.7/1000) and 5.7/1000 deliveries (95% confidence interval [CI] 4.9 to 6.5/1000), respectively.
- The frequencies of respiratory morbidity following vaginal delivery were as follows:
  - Week 37 + 0 to 37 + 6: 12.6 (7.6 to 19.6)/1000 deliveries with odds ratio (OR) 2.5 (95% CI 1.5 to 4.2)
  - Week 38 + 0 to 38 + 6: 7 (4.6 to 10.2)/1000 deliveries with OR 1.4 (95% CI 0.8 to 2.2)
  - Week 39 + 0 to 39 + 6: 3.2 (1.8 to 4.5)/1000 deliveries with OR 0.6 (95% CI 0.4 to 1).
- The frequencies of respiratory morbidity with cesarean delivery following labor (as would occur following an induction attempt) were as follows:
  - Week 37 + 0 to 37 + 6: 57.7 (26.7 to 107.1)/1000 deliveries with OR 11.2 (95% CI 5.4 to 13.1)

- Week 38 + 0 to 38 + 6: 9.4 (1.9 to 27.2)/1000 deliveries with OR 1.8 (95% CI 0.6 to 5.9)
- Week 39 + 0 to 39 + 6: 16.2 (5.9 to 35.5)/1000 deliveries with OR 3.2 (95% CI 1.4 to 7.4)
- Delivery by cesarean section without preceding labor increased the frequencies of respiratory morbidities even higher across all gestational ages.
- These data provide support for delaying elective delivery until 39 weeks of gestation.
- Further support can be found in a prospective observational study of 27 hospitals, including 17,794 deliveries (Clark et al, 2009).
- Of them, 44% were planned, and 73% of those deliveries were considered elective.
- The percentage of the electively induced infants admitted to the neonatal intensive care unit (NICU) at 37 weeks was 15.2% (n = 112), at 38 weeks it was 7% (n = 678), and at 39 weeks it was 6% (n = 2004).
- However, the Consortium of Safe Labor provides a conflicting result for neonatal morbidity in elective inductions, such that infants born to electively induced mothers were less likely to receive ventilatory support, become septic, or be admitted to the NICU (Bailit et al, 2010).

RISK OF INCREASED COSTS FOLLOWING ELECTIVE INDUCTION AT TERM

- Kaufman et al. studied the economic consequences of elective induction of labor at term (Kaufman et al, 2002).
- Using decision analysis, these researchers examined a hypothetical cohort of 100,000 pregnant patients for whom an initial decision was made to either induce labor at 39 weeks or to follow the patient expectantly through the remainder of pregnancy.
- All patients in this model underwent elective induction at 42 weeks.
- For women undergoing expectant management, different clinical outcomes of patients through their continuing gestations were evaluated.
- Using baseline estimates, the investigators concluded that elective induction would result in more than 12,000 excess cesarean deliveries and impose an annual cost to the medical system of nearly $100 million.
- A policy of induction at any gestational age, regardless of parity or cervical ripeness, required economic expenditures by the medical system.
- Although never cost saving, inductions were less expensive at later gestational ages, for multiparous patients, and for those women with a favorable cervix.
- The inductions most costly to the health care system were those performed in nulliparas with unfavorable cervices at 39 weeks.
- When nulliparous women with favorable cervices undergo labor induction, the estimated cost is approximately halved.

ACTIVE MANAGEMENT OF RISK IN PREGNANCY AT TERM (AMOR-IPAT): AN APPROACH TO CONTROL THE CESAREAN RATE FOLLOWING INDUCTION?

- One approach called the *active management of risk in pregnancy at term* (AMOR-IPAT) provides promise for reducing the risk of cesarean following induction of labor.

- AMOR-IPAT was first described as a retrospective cohort in which delivery outcomes of 100 women with a tailored approach to prenatal care and individualization of risk of cesarean birth were compared with 300 nonexposed women.
- Consideration was given to the most common indications for nonelective cesarean: cephalopelvic disproportion and uteroplacental insufficiency.
- A hypothetic ceiling for gestational age at delivery was set for each subject, always less than or equal to 41 weeks and more than or equal to 38 weeks.
- Cervical ripening was used for all women with Bishop scores of less than 5.
- Despite an increase in the labor induction rate in the women exposed to AMOR-IPAT (63% versus 26%, p < 0.001), there was a significant reduction in the cesarean births in this same group (4% versus 17%, p < 0.001).
- In a similar retrospective cohort study from the same authors, a protocol of risk-guided prostaglandin-assisted preventive labor induction with differing intensity was applied (Nicholson et al, 2007).
- Compared with nonexposed subjects, the exposed group (n = 794) had a significantly higher rate of labor induction (31.4% versus 20.4%) and use of prostaglandin E2 (23.3% versus 15.7%), and they had a significantly lower cesarean delivery rate (5.3% 11.8%).
- A small prospective trial of AMOR-IPAT, however, failed to confirm these promising results.
- Lack of a difference in the cesarean delivery rates (10.3% in the AMOR-IPAT group versus 14.9% in the conventional management group; P = 0.25) may have been because the sample size was too small to reveal a true difference between treatment groups (Nicholson et al, 2008).
- Larger, randomized, controlled, multicenter investigations are planned. In addition, neonatal outcomes need to be thoroughly evaluated because delivery before 39 weeks of gestation without assessment of fetal pulmonary maturity may result in higher neonatal respiratory morbidity.
- This risk may outweigh any benefit gained from the reduction of the cesarean delivery rate.

UPDATE #3

Elective inductions contribute to the overall increase in induction frequency, but they are not without risk. A growing body of evidence suggests an individualized approach to prenatal care and delivery planning known as active management of risk in pregnancy at term [AMOR-IPAT], with early pregnancy ultrasound for accurate assignment of gestational age, may hold promise (Nicholson et al, 2007).

Prolonged Pregnancy

ASSESSMENT OF GESTATIONAL AGE

- A pregnancy that has progressed to or beyond 42 weeks of gestation (294 days, or estimated date of delivery [EDD] +14 days) is considered a postterm pregnancy.
- The definition of the upper limit of a normal pregnancy is somewhat subjective and inexact.

- The definition of prolonged pregnancy is based on data derived before the common use of ultrasound for pregnancy dating.
- The incidence of prolonged pregnancy varies depending on which criteria are used to define gestational age at birth.
- It is estimated that 4% to 19% of pregnancies reach or exceed 42 weeks' gestation and 2% to 7% complete 43 weeks' gestation.
- In addition to being a common clinical occurrence, prolonged pregnancy is also associated with an increased financial burden, principally because of increased utilization of sonography, fetal testing, induction of labor, and cesarean delivery.
- Gestational age is an important determinant of the perinatal outcome.
- A high amount of attention to this issue has been focused on predicting and preventing preterm births, defined as delivery before 37 weeks of gestation.
- This is appropriate, because preterm birth accounts for the majority of perinatal morbidity, mortality, and costs (Saigal et al, 2008; Schmidt et al, 2006).
- However, postterm births are also associated with increased neonatal morbidity and mortality (Cotzias et al, 1999) and are easily preventable through induction of labor.

RISKS OF PROLONGED PREGNANCY

- Recent studies have shown that the risks to the fetus (Caughey et al, 2004, 2005; Froen et al, 2001; Heimstad et al, 2008; Kahn et al, 2003; Smith 2001; Yoder et al, 2008) and to the mother (Alexander et al, 2000; Caughey et al, 2003, 2006, 2007; Heimstad et al, 2008; Treger et al, 2002) of continuing the pregnancy beyond the estimated date of delivery have traditionally been underestimated for two reasons.
  - First, earlier studies were published before the habitual use of obstetric ultrasound and, as a result, likely included many pregnancies that were not truly postterm. Such a misclassification would falsely lower the complication rates of pregnancies designated postterm and increase the complication rates in those designated "term." This would reduce the difference between term and postterm pregnancies.
- The second issue relates to the definition of stillbirth rates. Traditionally, stillbirth rates were calculated using all pregnancies delivered at a given gestational age as the denominator. However, once a fetus is delivered, it is no longer at risk of intrauterine fetal demise, and use of this denominator has traditionally underestimated the risk of stillbirth. The proper denominator is not all deliveries at a given gestational age but ongoing (undelivered) pregnancies (Caughey et al, 2003). In one retrospective study of more than 170,000 singleton births, for example, Hilder and colleagues (Hilder et al, 1998) demonstrated that the stillbirth rate increased sixfold (from 0.35 to 2.12 per 1000 pregnancies) when the denominator was changed from all deliveries to ongoing (undelivered) pregnancies.

RISKS TO THE FETUS OF PROLONGED PREGNANCY

- Postterm pregnancy is associated with significant risks to the fetus.

- Antepartum stillbirths account for more perinatal deaths than either complications of prematurity or sudden infant death syndrome (Cotzias et al, 1999).
- According to epidemiologic studies, the perinatal mortality rate (stillbirths plus early neonatal deaths) at greater than 42 weeks of gestation is twice that at term (4 to 7 deaths versus 2 to 3 deaths per 1000 deliveries) and increases sixfold and higher at 43 weeks of gestation and beyond (Smith, 2001).
- However, several other epidemiologic studies suggested that other risk factors (such as congenital malformations and intrauterine growth restriction) outweighed prolonged pregnancy as the cause of neonatal mortality.
- Weaknesses of these studies overall included a lack of recording of the actual cause of death for many of the infants, as well as pregnancy dating by last menstrual period rather than early ultrasounds, and possible inequality or poor access to care of the populations evaluated.
- Two more recent studies consisted of prospective cohort evaluations of singleton pregnancies based on ultrasound dating (Heimstad et al, 2006; Nakling et al, 2006).
- Nakling et al. found an incidence of postterm pregnancies to be 7.6% in his cohort, with 0.3% of pregnancies progressing to 301 days (43 weeks' gestation) if inductions were not permitted prior to 43 weeks.
- A significantly increased rate of perinatal mortality after 41 weeks' gestation was also found, although causality was not ascertained in this study.
- In contrast, Heimstad et al. found an increased trend toward intrauterine fetal demise at 42 weeks' gestation compared to 38 weeks, but inductions were permitted prior to 43 weeks and there was no perinatal mortality rate calculation.
- Factors that may contribute to the increased rate of perinatal deaths are uteroplacental insufficiency, meconium aspiration, intrauterine growth restriction, and intrauterine infection (Hannah et al, 1993).
- For these reasons, the tendency has been to deliver by 41 completed weeks of gestation (42 weeks, 294 days, EDD +14 days).
- In 1954, approximately 20% of postterm fetuses were diagnosed with dysmaturity syndrome, with characteristics resembling chronic intrauterine growth restriction from uteroplacental deficiency (Clifford, 1954).
- These pregnancies were considered at increased risk of umbilical cord compression from oligohydramnios, meconium aspiration, and short-term neonatal complications (such as hypoglycemia, seizures, and respiratory insufficiency) and had an increased incidence of nonreassuring fetal testing, both antepartum and intrapartum.
- Whether such infants also are at risk of long-term neurologic sequelae was not apparent.
- In a large, prospective, follow-up study of children from 1 to 2 years of age, the general physical milestones, intelligence quotient, and frequency of intercurrent illnesses were not significantly different between normal infants born at term and those born postterm (Shime et al, 1986).

• Again, these infants might have increased neonatal complications secondary to intrauterine growth restriction and uteroplacental insufficiency, rather than from prolonged pregnancy itself.

RISKS TO THE PREGNANT WOMAN OF PROLONGED PREGNANCY

• Postterm pregnancy is also associated with significant risks to the pregnant woman, including an increase in labor dystocia (9% to 12% versus 2% to 7% at term), which is denoted by an increase in severe perineal injury related to macrosomia (3.3% versus 2.6% at term), and a doubling in the rate of cesarean delivery (Alexander et al, 2000, 2001; Caughey et al, 2004, 2006, 2007; Heimstad et al, 2006; Yoder et al, 2002).

• Cesarean delivery is associated with higher risks of complications, such as hemorrhage, endometritis, and thromboembolic disease.

• In a recent randomized, controlled trial of women at 41 weeks of gestation, those who were induced would desire the same management 74% of the time, whereas women with serial antenatal monitoring desired the same management only 38% of the time (Heimstad et al, 2007).

UPDATE #4

Optimal management of prolonged pregnancies is controversial (Gulmezoglu et al, 2006).

Clinical Considerations and Recommendations

EVIDENCE BASE FOR INDUCTION VERSUS EXPECTANT MANAGEMENT

• Management of low-risk postterm pregnancy is controversial.

• A recent meta-analysis included 19 studies that compared induction and expectant management for uncomplicated, singleton pregnancies of at least 41 weeks' gestation (Gulmezoglu et al, 2006).

• There was no difference in cesarean delivery rates (RR 0.92; 95% CI 0.76 to 1.12; RR 0.97; 95% CI 0.72 to 1.31) for women induced at 41 and 42 completed weeks, respectively.

• There was a small and statistically significant reduction in perinatal mortality rates, but none in neonatal intensive care admission rates, meconium aspiration, or abnormal Apgar scores.

• In this subset of women, elective labor induction may be justified.

• The preventive approach to postterm pregnancy management, however, revealed that women induced at 37 to 40 completed weeks were more likely to have a cesarean birth with expectant management than those in the labor induction group (RR 0.58; 95% CI 0.34 to 0.99).

PROLONGED PREGNANCY WITH A FAVORABLE CERVIX

• Many studies of postterm pregnancies comparing the outcomes of labor induction with those of expectant management excluded women with favorable cervices

(Dyson et al, 1987; Martin et al, 1989; Hannah et al, 1992; Herabutya et al, 1992; National Institute of Child Health and Human Development Network of Maternal-Fetal Medicine Units, 1994; Shaw et al, 1992).

• Also, when women allocated to expectant management experienced a change in cervical status, expectant management ceased and labor induction was initiated (Augensen et al, 1987; Dyson et al, 1987; Herabutya et al, 1992; National Institute of Child Health and Human Development Network of Maternal-Fetal Medicine Units, 1994; Witter et al, 1987).

• In studies on monitored postterm pregnancies in which women with favorable cervices were managed expectantly, there was no indication that expectant management had an injurious effect on the outcome.

• However, results were not stratified according to the condition of the cervix (Almstrom et al, 1995; Augensen et al, 1987; Bergsjo et al, 1989; Cardozo et al, 1986; Chanrachakul et al, 2003; James et al, 2001).

• In general, there is agreement that there is insufficient information to determine whether labor induction or expectant management results in the best outcome in women with a prolonged pregnancy and a favorable cervix.

• As a result, most practitioners feel that if the likelihood of a successful vaginal delivery is high enough, then there is no reason to expose the patient to the potential added risks associated with prolongation of pregnancy.

• Therefore, induction of labor in women with prolonged pregnancy and a favorable cervix is a reasonable approach in the absence of randomized controlled trials.

PROLONGED PREGNANCY WITH AN UNFAVORABLE CERVIX

• The crux of the debate regarding optimal management of prolonged pregnancies focuses on women with unfavorable cervices.

• Managing these patients could consist of either expectant management (i.e., antenatal surveillance until there are signs of fetal jeopardy, or until the patient presents in either spontaneous labor or with a favorable cervix) or induction of labor any time after 41 weeks' gestation.

• Although most authors agree that induction of labor is indicated in women with an "inducible" uterine cervix, there is lack of agreement as to the management of the patient whose cervix is considered "unfavorable."

• The introduction of preinduction cervical maturation has resulted in fewer failed and serial inductions, reduced medical cost, reduced fetal and maternal morbidity, and possibly a reduced rate of cesarean delivery in the general obstetric population (Crowley, 2004; Hannah et al, 1992; National Institute of Child Health and Human Development Network of Maternal-Fetal Medicine Units, 1994; Sanchez-Ramos et al, 2002).

OPTIMAL TIMING FOR A DELIVERY OF A PROLONGED PREGNANCY

• Delivery is typically recommended when the risks to the fetus by continuing the pregnancy outweigh those faced by the neonate after birth.

- High-risk patients (e.g., those with gestational diabetes or chronic hypertension) should not be permitted to progress beyond 41 weeks of gestation because, in these pregnancies, the balance seems to shift in favor of delivery at approximately 38 to 39 weeks of gestation (Badawi et al, 1998).
- Because delivery cannot always be brought about readily, maternal risks from cesarean delivery and the impact on future pregnancies from cesarean delivery need to be considered.
- Several recent studies have demonstrated the risks of abnormal placentation from multiple cesarean deliveries (Silver et al, 2006).
- Also, with the declining rates of vaginal birth after cesarean, once the first cesarean has occurred, there is a less than 10% chance that future pregnancies will be delivered vaginally (Martin et al, 2010).

PREVENTION OF POSTTERM PREGNANCY

- The most impactful way to prevent postterm pregnancy is to induce labor before 42 weeks' gestation.
- However, because complications rise during 40 and 41 weeks of gestation and both clinicians and patients are concerned about the risks of induction of labor, it is perceivably better for women to go into spontaneous labor at 39 weeks of gestation on their own.
- Minimally invasive interventions can be recommended to encourage the onset of labor at term and prevent postterm pregnancy, including membrane stripping.
- Although stripping of the membranes may be able to lessen the interval to spontaneous onset of labor, there is no dependable evidence of a reduction in operative vaginal delivery, cesarean delivery rates, or maternal or neonatal morbidity (Boulvain et al, 2005; de Miranda et al, 2006; Kashanian et al, 2006).

Preinduction Assessment

- Careful examination of the maternal and fetal condition is required prior to undergoing labor induction.
- Indications and contraindications for induction should be reviewed, in addition to the alternatives.
- Risks and benefits of labor induction should be discussed with the patient, including the risk of cesarean delivery as mentioned earlier.
- Confirmation of gestational age and evaluation of fetal lung maturity status should be performed (see Table 14-3).
- In preterm gestations, administration of steroids is indicated if time permits.
- Other prerequisites include an estimate of fetal weight, clinical pelvimetry, evaluation of fetal presentation, and cervical examination, which should all be documented.
- In addition, labor induction should be performed at a location where personnel are available who are familiar with the process and its potential complications.
- Uterine activity and electronic fetal monitoring (EFM) are recommended for any gravida receiving uterotonic drugs.

PREDICTING A SUCCESSFUL INDUCTION

- Because of the risk of cesarean delivery and the rising costs of health care associated with labor induction, some researchers have tried to identify, with varying success, biochemical and biophysical assays to predict the probability of vaginal delivery following labor induction (Chandra et al, 2001; Kiss et al, 2000; Ojutiku et al, 2002; Pandis et al, 2001).
- These measures include digital evaluation of the cervix (Bishop score), ultrasonographic cervical length measurements, and the use of fetal fibronectin prior to the labor induction attempt.
- Cervical status is one of the most important factors for predicting the likelihood of successfully inducing labor.
- Several cervical scoring systems are available for this purpose (e.g., Bishop system; Fields system; Burnett, Caldor, and Friedman modifications of the Bishop system) (Baacke et al, 2006).
- In observational studies, other characteristics associated with successful induction include multiparity, tall stature (over 5 feet 5 inches), increasing gestational age, nonobese maternal weight or body mass index, and infant birth weight less than 3.5 kg (Crane, 2006; Pevzner et al, 2009).
- However, these characteristics are predictive of success even in spontaneous labors, which suggests they are more predictive of the route of delivery than the likelihood the patient will reach the active phase of labor.

Bishop Score

The modified Bishop score is the system most commonly used in clinical practice in the United States (Bishop, 1964).

- This system tabulates a score based upon the station of the presenting part and four characteristics of the cervix: dilatation, effacement, consistency, and position (Table 14-4).
- If the Bishop score is high (variously defined as ≥5 or ≥8), the likelihood of vaginal delivery is similar whether labor is spontaneous or induced (Table 14-5) (Xenakis et al, 1997).

TABLE 14-4 **Modified Bishop Score**

Score	0	1	2	3
Parameter				
Dilatation (cm)	Closed	1-2	3-4	5 or more
Effacement (%)	0-30	40-50	60-70	80 or more
Length (cm)	>4	2-4	1-2	1-2
Station	−3	−2	−1 or 0	+1 or +2
Consistency	Firm	Medium	Soft	
Cervical position	Posterior	Midposition	Anterior	

*Modification by Calder AA, Brennand, JE: Labor and normal delivery: induction of labor, *Curr Opin Obstet Gynecol* 3:764-71), 1991. This modification replaces percentage of effacement as one of the parameters of the Bishop score.
From Bishop EH: Pelvic scoring for elective induction, *Obstet Gynecol* 24:266, 1964.

TABLE 14-5 Failed Induction Rate and Cesarean Delivery Rate after Induction by Bishop Score and Parity, circa 1997 (prostaglandins available)

Bishop Score	Primipara	Multipara	Overall
Failed Induction Rate, Percentage			
0-3	13.3	5.1	9.4
>3	0.7	0.8	0.7
Cesarean Delivery Rate after Induction, Percentage			
0-3	34	23	29
>3	20	13	15

Adapted from Xenakis EM, Piper JM, Conway DL, Langer O: Induction of labor in the nineties; conquering the unfavorable cervix, *Obstet Gynecol* 90:235, 1997.

- In contrast, a low Bishop score predicts that induction will fail and result in vaginal delivery.
- These relationships are particularly strong in nulliparous women who undergo induction (Johnson et al, 2003; Vrouenraets et al, 2005).
- The relationship between a low Bishop score and failed induction, prolonged labor, and a high cesarean birth rate was first described prior to widespread use of cervical ripening agents (Arulkumaran et al, 1985).

Fetal Fibronectin

The presence of an elevated fetal fibronectin (fFN) concentration in cervicovaginal secretions has also been used to predict uterine readiness for induction.

- fFN is thought to represent a disruption or inflammation of the chorionic-decidual interface.
- In several studies, women with a positive fFN result had a significantly shorter interval until delivery than those with a negative fFN result (Kiss et al, 2000) and there was reduction in the frequency of cesarean delivery (Sciscione et al, 2005).
- Positive fFN results were predictive of a shorter interval to delivery, even in nulliparas with low (<5) Bishop scores (Garite et al, 1996).
- However, there are others who have not confirmed these findings (Ojutiku et al, 2002; Reis et al, 2003).
- Bailit et al. used a decision analysis to determine if the vaginal delivery rate is increased in nulliparous women undergoing elective labor induction following fetal fibronectin testing (Bailit et al, 2002).
- In this model, three management strategies were tested presuming fetal fibronectin testing was performed in select groups at 39 weeks of pregnancy: (1) no elective induction of labor for any candidate until 41 weeks' gestation (spontaneous labor), (2) induction only of those patients with a positive fetal fibronectin result at 39 weeks, and (3) elective induction for every woman who is at least 39 weeks without performance of a fetal fibronectin test.
- They based estimates and assumptions for their statistical model on previously published clinical studies regarding rates of cesarean delivery for women in spontaneous labor, rates of cesarean delivery in postdates induction, distribution of fetal fibronectin results at 39 weeks' gestation, and percentage of pregnancies beyond 41 weeks.
- Investigators found that the spontaneous labor strategy had the highest rate of vaginal delivery (90%) and the elective induction strategy had the lowest vaginal delivery rate (79%).
- When fetal fibronectin test results were used to screen candidates for elective induction, the vaginal delivery rate was higher than the induction strategy but lower than the spontaneous labor strategy (83%).
- These investigators concluded that the best strategy to improve vaginal delivery rates was to avoid elective induction in nulliparous women.
- Fetal fibronectin may however improve chances of vaginal delivery over nonselective induction.
- Larger trials are needed to further clarify the role of fetal fibronectin in predicting the success of labor induction in the nulliparous patient as well and the cost effectiveness of this approach.

Sonographically Measured Cervical Length

In pregnant women, the risk of preterm birth increases as cervical length decreases.

- Cervical length also predicts the likelihood of spontaneous onset of labor postterm (Vankayalapati et al, 2008).
- Sonographic assessment of cervical length for predicting the outcome of labor induction has been evaluated in numerous studies.
- A systematic review of 20 prospective studies found that cervical length was predictive of successful induction (likelihood ratio of a positive test, 1.66; 95% CI 1.20 to 2.31) and failed induction (likelihood ratio of a negative test, 0.51; 95% CI, 0.39 to 0.67) (Hatfield et al, 2007).
- However, sonographic cervical length performed poorly for predicting vaginal delivery within 24 hours (sensitivity 59%, specificity 65%), vaginal delivery (sensitivity 67%, specificity 58%), achieving active labor (sensitivity 57%, specificity 60%), and delivery within 24 hours (sensitivity 56%, specificity 47%), and did not perform significantly better than the Bishop score for predicting a successful induction.
- These data are limited by substantial heterogeneity among the studies.
- As with fFN, the role of ultrasound examination as a tool for selecting women likely to have a successful induction is uncertain.
- More data, including cost-benefit analysis, are needed before this test can be recommended in choosing candidates for semielective induction.
- Despite these biochemical and radiologic advancements, the Bishop score continues to be the best available tool for predicting the likelihood that induction will result in vaginal delivery.
- This conclusion is based on systematic reviews of controlled studies that found the Bishop score was as, or more, predictive of the outcome of labor induction than fFN (Crane et al, 2006; Hatfield et al, 2007; Tanir et al, 2008) and that dilatation was the single most important element of the Bishop score (Crane et al, 2006).

Cervical Ripening

- Cervical ripening is a complex process that results in physical softening and distensibility of the cervix, ultimately leading to partial cervical effacement and dilatation (Maul et al, 2006).
- Remodeling of the cervix involves enzymatic dissolution of collagen fibrils, increase in water content, and chemical changes.
- These changes are induced by hormones (estrogen, progesterone, relaxin), as well as cytokines, prostaglandin, and nitric oxide synthesis enzymes (Maul et al, 2006).
- Cervical ripening methods fall into two main categories: pharmacologic and mechanical (Table 14-6).

UPDATE #5

Methods of cervical ripening and labor induction are varied. Pharmacologic methods include vaginal administration of prostaglandin E1 (misoprostol) and prostaglandin E2 (dinoprostone), orally administered misoprostol, and transcervical Foley balloon catheter placement (Maul et al, 2006).

TECHNIQUES FOR CERVICAL RIPENING AND LABOR INDUCTION
Mechanical Methods

- Mechanical methods are among the oldest approaches used to promote cervical ripening.
- Advantages of these techniques compared to pharmacologic methods include their low cost, low risk of tachysystole, few systemic side effects, and convenient storage requirements (no refrigeration or expiration) (Boulvain et al, 2001).
- Comparing mechanical methods with placebo/no treatment, hyperstimulation with fetal heart rate changes was not reported.

TABLE 14-6   Methods of Cervical Ripening

Pharmacologic Methods	Mechanical Methods
Oxytocin	Membrane stripping
Prostaglandins	Amniotomy
— E$_2$ (dinoprostone, Prepidil gel, and Cervidil time-released vaginal insert)	
— E$_1$ (misoprostol, Cytotec)	
Estrogen	Mechanical dilators
	— Laminaria tents
	— Dilapan
	— Lamicel
Relaxin	Transcervical balloon catheters
	— With extra-amniotic saline infusion
	— With concomitant oxytocin administration
Hyaluronic acid	
Progesterone receptor antagonists	

- The risk of cesarean birth was similar between groups (34%; RR 1.00; 95% CI: 0.76 to 1.30, n = 416, six studies).
- There were no reported cases of severe neonatal and maternal morbidity among them.
- The risk of hyperstimulation was reduced when compared with all prostaglandins (intracervical, intravaginal, or misoprostol).
- Compared with oxytocin in women with unfavorable cervix, mechanical methods reduce the risk of caesarean delivery.
- Disadvantages include a small increase in the risk of maternal and neonatal infection from introduction of a foreign body (Heinemann et al, 2008), the potential for disruption of a low-lying placenta, and some maternal discomfort upon manipulation of the cervix.
- The most common mechanical methods are stripping (or sweeping) of the fetal membranes, placement of hygroscopic dilators within the endocervical canal, and insertion of a balloon catheter above the internal cervical os (with or without infusion of extra-amniotic saline).
- All of these methods likely work, at least in part, by causing the release of prostaglandin F2-alpha from the decidua and adjacent membranes or prostaglandin E2 from the cervix.
- The latter two methods physically cause gradual cervical dilatation with minimal discomfort to the patient.

Membrane Stripping

- Stripping or sweeping of the membranes is a widely utilized technique, though it is often undocumented.
- This technique involves inserting the examiner's finger beyond the internal cervical os and then rotating the finger circumferentially along the lower uterine segment to detach the fetal membranes.
- Membrane stripping is typically performed during an office visit in pregnant women with a partially dilated cervix who wish to hasten the onset of spontaneous labor.
- Many investigations have been conducted using routine membrane stripping at 38 or 39 weeks to either prevent postterm pregnancies or decrease the frequency of more formal inductions occurring after 41 weeks (Berghella et al, 1996; Cammu et al, 1998; Crane et al, 1997).
- Two randomized trials compared outcomes of women who underwent membrane stripping or no membrane stripping at initiation of labor induction with oxytocin (Foong et al, 2000; Tan et al, 2006).
- The results of these trials suggested that membrane stripping increased the rate of spontaneous vaginal delivery and shortened the induction to delivery interval.
- However, differences in study design and management of induction preclude definitive conclusions.
- As an example, in one trial (Foong et al, 2000), these benefits were only observed in nulliparas, and, in the other trial (Tan et al, 2006), induction was performed using amniotomy or dinoprostone pessary.
- Other randomized trials have tried to assess whether membrane stripping hastens the onset of spontaneous labor.

- In one randomized trial, women assigned to membrane stripping had a significant reduction in the subsequent duration of pregnancy (2 days compared to 5 days in controls) and frequency of induction (8.1% versus 18.8% in controls) (Allott et al, 1993), whereas two other randomized trials found no beneficial effects from membrane sweeping (Hamdan et al, 2009; Hill et al, 2008).
- None of these trials reported harmful side effects that could be attributed to the procedure.
- Routine membrane stripping is not recommended given that there is no evidence this practice improves maternal or neonatal outcome.
- However, weekly membrane stripping at term shortens the interval of time to onset of spontaneous labor and reduces the need for formal induction.
- For this reason, membrane stripping after 39 weeks of gestation may be offered to patients who wish to hasten the onset of spontaneous labor.
- Although the existing meta-analysis on the use of membrane stripping (Boulvain et al, 2005) was not associated with an increase in either maternal or neonatal infection, it is unclear if the included studies involved carriers of group B streptococcus (GBS).
- There are no studies currently in the literature specifically designed to address the safety of membrane stripping in known carriers of GBS and, as a result, this is not considered a contraindication to membrane stripping (Centers for Disease Control and Prevention, 2010).
- Complications that can result from membrane stripping include rupture of membranes, hemorrhage from disruption of an occult placenta previa, and the development of chorioamnionitis.
- Most commonly, however, membrane stripping is associated with maternal discomfort and clinically insignificant vaginal bleeding.

Amniotomy

- Amniotomy, artificial rupture of membranes, is a technique involving the perforation of the chorioamniotic membranes.
- It is an effective method of labor induction performed in women with favorable cervices (Booth et al, 1970).
- Combined use of amniotomy and intravenous oxytocin is more effective than amniotomy alone with fewer women undelivered vaginally after 24 hours (Howarth et al, 2001).
- In the meta-analysis of amniotomy, 17 trials involving 2,566 women were included.
- Amniotomy and intravenous oxytocin were found to result in (1) fewer women being undelivered vaginally at 24 hours than amniotomy alone (RR 0.03, 95% CI 0.001 to 0.49, n = 100, 1 study), (2) significantly fewer instrumental vaginal deliveries than placebo (RR 0.18, CI 0.05 to 0.58), and (3) more postpartum hemorrhage than vaginal prostaglandins (RR 5.5, CI 1.26 to 24.07).
- There is also more dissatisfaction with amniotomy and intravenous oxytocin when compared with vaginal prostaglandins (RR 53, CI 3.32 to 846.51) (Howarth et al, 2001).

Hygroscopic Dilators

- Mechanical dilators placed in the lower uterine segment release endogenous prostaglandins from the fetal membranes and maternal decidua.
- In addition, the osmotic properties of hygroscopic dilators promote cervical ripening.
- There are two types of hygroscopic dilators: one is made from natural seaweed (laminaria tents) and the other is a synthetic product (e.g., Lamicel).
- Hygroscopic dilators are safe and effective for dilating the cervix, although they are used primarily during pregnancy termination rather than for preinduction cervical ripening of term pregnancies.
- Hygroscopic dilators are designed to absorb moisture and thus gradually expand within the cervical canal.
- They function by disrupting the chorioamniotic decidual interface, causing lysosomal destruction and prostaglandin release.
- These events lead to active stretching of the cervix beyond the passive mechanical stretching provided by the dilator itself.
- A meta-analysis of randomized trials comparing hygroscopic dilators to placebo/no treatment found that pregnant women in both groups had similar rates of not achieving a vaginal delivery by 24 hours (RR = 0.90, 95% CI: 0.64 to 1.26), cesarean deliveries (RR = 0.98, 95% CI: 0.74 to 1.30), and infection (Boulvain et al, 2001).
- These data suggest that although hygroscopic dilators can dilate the cervix, they are inadequate for improving the outcome of induction.
- However, no large trials have been performed, and there are no decent comparative studies evaluating the optimal use of hygroscopic dilators with other modalities, such as amniotomy, to improve the rate of successful induction.

Transcervical Balloon Catheters

- A deflated Foley catheter (usually a no. 16F 30 mL balloon) can be passed through an undilated cervix into the extra-amniotic space and then inflated.
- The catheter can be left in place until it is extruded (typically within 12 hours); most clinicians remove nonextruded catheters after 24 hours.
- This technique appears to be as effective for preinduction cervical ripening as prostaglandin E2 gel and intravaginal misoprostol in most studies (Chung et al, 2003; St Onge et al, 1995; Sciscione et al, 2001).
- The combination of a balloon catheter plus the administration of a prostaglandin does not appear to be more effective than prostaglandins alone (Chung et al, 2003).
- Although the risk of infection may theoretically be associated with the insertion of foreign object in the cervix, existing meta-analysis data did not show evidence of an increased risk of infectious morbidity (Boulvain et al, 2001).
- Transcervical Foley catheter placement is a superior method of preinduction cervical ripening when compared with intravenous oxytocin and was associated with a lower cesarean section rate in one investigation (Boulvain et al, 2001).

- Some studies show more rapid cervical ripening, shortened induction to delivery interval, and reduced frequency of patients undelivered in 24 hours when combining a transcervical balloon catheter with a pharmacologic method of cervical ripening such as a prostaglandin (Perry et al, 1998) whereas others do not (Chung et al, 2003).
- No increased risk of preterm delivery in subsequent pregnancies following the placement of balloon catheters in the lower uterine segment was found by Sciscione et al. in 126 women (Sciscione et al, 2004).
- The use of the Atad double-balloon device has also been described in a limited group of studies (Atad et al, 1991, 1996, 1997).
- One investigation included 95 women with Bishop scores no more than 4 and randomly assigned them to vaginally administered prostaglandin E2 (PGE_2), Atad balloon dilator technique, or continuous oxytocin for labor induction.
- They found a significant mean change in Bishop score after 12 hours in the PGE_2 group and Atad balloon dilator group (5) compared to the oxytocin group (2.5).
- In addition, they found a higher rate of failed induction in the oxytocin group (58%) compared to 20% in the PGE_2 and 5.7% in the Atad balloon dilator groups.
- Vaginal delivery rates in the oxytocin group were 26.7% compared to 77% and 70% in the Atad balloon dilator and PGE_2 groups, respectively.

Extra-Amniotic Saline Infusion (EASI)

- Extra-amniotic saline infusion (EASI) is a procedure in which sterile saline is infused continuously via a catheter placed in the extra-amniotic space.
- The hypothesis for this approach is that the disruption at the fetal-maternal interface will result in added release of endogenous prostaglandins and other parturition-related hormones to facilitate the onset of spontaneous uterine activity.
- Most commonly, isotonic saline is used, hence the name extra-amniotic saline infusion, or EASI, and is infused continuously at rates of 20 to 40 mL/hour.
- The use of EASI with a transcervical Foley balloon catheter appears to be effective for cervical ripening when compared with intravaginal prostaglandins (Lyndrup et al, 1994; Vengalil et al, 1998), although EASI does not appear to improve induction outcomes over those observed with the use of Foley catheter alone (Guinn et al, 2004).
- In three randomized trials, both techniques resulted in similar rates of delivery <24 hours, cesarean delivery, and complications (Guinn et al, 2004; Karjane et al, 2006; Lin et al, 2007), although one trial reported a shorter induction-to-vaginal-delivery time with the combined method (Karjane et al, 2006).
- A Cochrane review of EASI to any prostaglandin for cervical ripening showed EASI infusion was significantly less likely to result in vaginal delivery within 24 hours (42% versus 57% RR 1.33, 95% CI 1.02 to 1.75), had a higher risk of cesarean delivery (31% versus 22% RR 1.48, 95% CI 1.14 to 1.90), and did not reduce the risk of hyperstimulation (Boulvain et al, 2001).
- From these data, there is little support for the use of EASI as an adjunct to transcervical balloon catheter placement.

UPDATE #6
Extra-amniotic saline infusion with transcervical Foley balloon catheter placement does not appear to be effective (Boulvain et al, 2001).

Pharmacologic Methods

Oxytocin

- Oxytocin is a polypeptide hormone produced in the hypothalamus and secreted from the posterior lobe of the pituitary gland in a pulsatile fashion.
- It is identical to its synthetic analogue, which is among the most potent uterotonic agents known.
- Synthetic oxytocin is an effective means of labor induction (Kelly et al, 2001).
- Exogenous oxytocin administration produces periodic uterine contractions first demonstrable at approximately 20 weeks of gestation, with increasing responsiveness with advancing gestational age primarily because of an increase in myometrial oxytocin binding sites (Fuchs et al, 1984).
- There is little change in myometrial sensitivity to oxytocin from 34 weeks to term; however, once spontaneous labor begins, the uterine sensitivity to oxytocin increases rapidly (Caldeyro-Barcia et al, 1959).
- This physiologic mechanism makes oxytocin a more effective augmenter of labor as opposed to an inducer, and even less successful as a cervical ripening agent.
- Oxytocin is most often given intravenously.
- It cannot be given orally because the polypeptide is degraded to small, inactive forms by gastrointestinal enzymes.
- The plasma half-life is short, estimated at 3 to 6 minutes (Ryden et al, 1971), and steady-state concentrations are reached within 30 to 40 minutes of initiation or dose change (Seitchik et al, 1984).
- Synthetic oxytocin is generally diluted by placing 10 units in 1000 mL of an isotonic solution, such as normal saline, yielding an oxytocin concentration of 10 mU/mL.
- It is given by infusion pump to allow continuous, precise control of the dose administered.
- A common practice is to make a solution of 60 units in 1000 mL crystalloid to allow the infusion pump setting to match the dose administered (e.g., 1 mU per minute equals a pump infusion rate of 1 mL per hour).
- Several experts have suggested that implementation of a standardized protocol is desirable to minimize errors in oxytocin administration (Clark et al, 2007; Freeman et al, 2007; Hayes et al, 2008).
- However, no protocol has been subjected to the scientific scrutiny necessary to demonstrate its superiority in both efficacy and safety over another.

UPDATE #7
Standardized protocols for oxytocin administration are gaining favor in an attempt to reduce administration errors and improve patient safety; however, none of the proposed regimens has been subjected to scientific scrutiny (Clark et al, 2007; Freeman et al, 2007; Hayes et al, 2008).

- Although oxytocin is an effective means of labor induction in women with favorable cervices, it is less effective as a cervical ripening agent.
- Many randomized controlled trials comparing oxytocin to various prostaglandin (PG) formulations and other methods of cervical ripening confirm this observation.
- In a Cochrane review of 110 trials including more than 12,000 women comparing oxytocin to any vaginal prostaglandin formulation for labor induction, oxytocin alone was associated with an increase in unsuccessful vaginal delivery within 24 hours (70% versus 21%, RR 3.33, 95% CI 1.61 to 6.89).
- There was no difference in cesarean section rates between groups.
- When intracervical prostaglandins were compared to oxytocin alone for labor induction, oxytocin alone was associated with an increase in unsuccessful vaginal delivery within 24 hours (50.4% versus 34.6%, RR 1.47, 95% CI 1.10 to 1.96) and an increase in cesarean sections (19.1% versus 13.7%, RR 1.37, 95% CI 1.08 to 1.74) in the oxytocin group.
- The authors concluded that oxytocin alone may increase the likelihood of interventions in labor (Kelly et al, 2001).
- In the setting of premature rupture of membranes (PROM) at term (defined as rupture of membranes before the onset of labor), labor induction is recommended because as the time between rupture of membranes and the onset of labor increases, so may the risk of maternal and fetal infection (Hannah et al, 1996; Tan et al, 2000).
- A series of systematic reviews examined the outcomes of pregnancies with PROM at or near term (Hannah et al, 1996; Tan et al, 2000).
- One trial accounts for most of the patients included in the analysis (Hannah et al, 1996).
- Hannah et al. studied 5041 women with premature rupture of membranes at term.
- Subjects were randomly assigned to receive intravenous oxytocin, vaginal prostaglandin E$_2$ gel, or expectant management for up to four days, with labor induced through either intravenous oxytocin or vaginal prostaglandin E$_2$ gel.
- Those randomized to the expectant management group were induced if complications such as chorioamnionitis developed.
- The rates of neonatal infection and cesarean delivery were not statistically different between the groups.
- Rates of clinical chorioamnionitis were less in the group receiving intravenous oxytocin.
- When oxytocin alone was compared to vaginal prostaglandins in 14 trials for labor induction after PROM by Cochrane reviewers, both medications were found to be equally efficacious (Kelly et al, 2001).
- Both can be utilized in this clinical setting and, because the majority of women with PROM will labor spontaneously within the ensuing 12 to 96 hours (Savitz et al, 1997), a policy of expectant management for up to 96 hours is not unreasonable.
- The optimal regimen for oxytocin administration is debatable, although success rates for varying protocols are similar.

TABLE 14-7   Labor Stimulation with Oxytocin: Examples of Low- and High-Dose Oxytocin Dosing Regimens

Regimen	Starting Dose (mU/minutes)	Incremental Increase (mU/minutes)	Dosage Interval (minutes)
Low dose	0.5-2	1-2	15-40
High dose	6	3-6*	15-40

*The incremental increase is reduced to 3 mU/min in the presence of hyperstimulation and reduced to 1 mU/min with recurrent hyperstimulation.
From American College of Obstetricians and Gynecologists: Induction of Labor: ACOG practice bulletin no. 107, *Obstet Gynecol* 114:386, 2009. ©ACOG, 2009, Washington, DC.

- Protocols differ as to the initial dose (0.5 to 6 mU/min), incremental time period (10 to 60 minutes), and steady-state dose (Table 14-7) (ACOG Committee on Practice Bulletins—Obstetrics, ACOG Practice Bulletin No. 107, 2009).
- A maximum oxytocin dose has not been established, but most protocols do not exceed 42 mU/min.
- A literature review of randomized clinical trials of high- versus low-dose oxytocin regimens published from 1966 to 2003 concluded high-dose oxytocin decreased the time from admission to vaginal delivery but did not decrease the incidence of cesarean delivery compared with low-dose therapy (Patka et al, 2005).
- Only one double-blinded randomized trial has been published, and it had the same findings (Merrill et al, 1999).
- High-dose regimens are associated with a higher rate of tachysystole than low-dose regimes, and in some studies this has resulted in a higher rate of cesarean delivery for fetal distress (Satin et al, 1992) but no significant difference in neonatal outcomes (Smith et al, 2006).
- The dose is typically increased until there is normal progression of labor, or strong contractions occurring at 2-to-3-minute intervals, or uterine activity reaches 150 to 350 Montevideo units (i.e., the peak strength of contractions in mmHg measured by an internal monitor multiplied by their frequency per 10 minutes).
- There is no benefit to increasing the dose after one of these end points has been achieved.
- In addition, two randomized trials found there was no significant benefit in continuing oxytocin infusion after the onset of active labor (Daniel-Spiegel et al, 2004; Ustunyurt et al, 2007).
- Continuing oxytocin may result in a higher rate of cesarean delivery. When uterotonic drugs are administered, continuous monitoring of uterine activity and fetal heart rate are important so the dose can be adjusted if excessive or inadequate uterine activity is noted.
- Some examples of oxytocin regimens are described in Table 14-8.

Low-Dose Oxytocin Dosing

- Low-dose protocols mimic endogenous maternal physiology and are associated with lower rates of uterine tachysystole.

TABLE 14-8   Oxytocin Regimen Examples

Dilution: 10 mU oxytocin in 1000 mL normal saline for resultant concentration of 10 mU oxytocin/mL

Infusion rate: 2 mU/min or 12 mL/hour

Incremental increase: 2 mU/min or 12 mL/hour every 45 minutes until contraction frequency adequate

Maximum dose: 16 mU/min or 96 mL/hour

From Hayes EJ, Weinstein L: Improving patient safety and uniformity of care by a standardized regimen for the use of oxytocin, *Am J Obstet Gynecol* 198(6):622.e1-7, 2008. Epub March 20, 2008.

- Proponents of low-dose oxytocin administration maintain that a slow rate of oxytocin administration is as effective for inducing labor and labor augmentation as faster rates of increase, while at the same time minimizing oxytocin requirements with lower rates of uterine overactivity (Blakemore et al, 1990).
- Low-dose oxytocin is initiated at 0.5 to 1 mU and increased by 1 mU per minute at 40 to 60 minute intervals.
- Slightly higher doses beginning at 1 to 2 mU/min increased by 1 to 2 mU/min with shorter incremental time intervals of 15 to 30 minutes have also been recommended (Blakemore et al, 1990).

High-Dose Oxytocin Dosing

- High-dose oxytocin regimens are often employed in active management of labor protocols.
- These regimens are largely used for labor augmentation, rather than for labor induction.
- Examples of these protocols start with an initial oxytocin dose of 6 mU/min increased by 6 mU/min at 20-minute intervals (O'Driscoll et al, 1984) or start at 4 mU/min with 4 mU/min incremental increases (Xenakis et al, 1997).
- A prospective study was undertaken involving nearly 5000 women at Parkland Hospital in Dallas, Texas; it compared low-dose with high-dose oxytocin regimens for labor induction and augmentation (Satin et al, 1992).
- The high-dose protocol allowed for reduction of the dosage to 3 mU/min in the presence of uterine tachysystole.
- The results indicated that subjects given the high-dose regimen had a significantly shorter mean admission to delivery time, fewer failed inductions, fewer forceps deliveries, fewer cesarean sections for failure to progress, less chorioamnionitis, and less neonatal sepsis than subjects given the low-dose regimen.
- Notably, these subjects had a higher rate of cesarean section performed for "fetal distress," but no difference in neonatal outcomes was observed.
- Merrill and Zlatnik conducted a randomized, double-masked trial including 1307 patients, comparing high-dose (4.5 mU/minute initially increased by 4.5 mU/minute every 30 minutes) with low-dose (1.5 mU/minute initially, increased by 1.5 mU/minute every 30 minutes) oxytocin for augmentation and induction of labor (Merrill et al, 1999).
- Oxytocin solutions were prepared by a central pharmacy, and infusion volumes were identical to ensure double masking.

- In the group receiving high-dose oxytocin, labor was significantly shortened when used for induction (8.5 versus 10.5 hours, P < 0.001) and augmentation (4.4 versus 5.1 hours, P = 0.3).
- There was no significant difference in cesarean section rates between the two regimens (15% versus 11.3%, P = 0.17).
- There were, however, more decreases or discontinuations of oxytocin in the high-dose group, both for uterine tachysystole and fetal heart rate abnormalities.
- Discontinuation of oxytocin did not appear to have an adverse impact on cesarean section rates or lengthening of labor.
- Neonatal outcomes were observed to be similar in both groups.
- In contemporary obstetric practice, based on this evidence, oxytocin is most often used to augment labor in patients with inadequate uterine activity or to induce labor in a patient with a favorable cervical status.
- One of many dosing regimens may be used depending on the standard practice in the community or the preference of the individual practitioner.
- Satin et al. studied the differences in outcomes when oxytocin is used to augment as opposed to induce labor (Satin et al, 1992).
- These investigators prospectively studied 2788 consecutive women with singleton pregnancies.
- Indications for oxytocin stimulation were divided into augmentation (n = 1676) and induction (n = 1112).
- The low-dose regimen consisted of a starting dose of 1 mU/minute with incremental increases of 1 mU/minute at 20-minute intervals until 8 mU/minute, then 2 mU/minute increases up to a maximum of 20 mU/minute, and was used first for 5 months in 1251 pregnancies.
- The high-dose regimen consisted of a starting dose of 6 mU/minute with increases of 6 mU/minute at 20-minute intervals up to a maximum dose of 42 mU/minutes and was used for the subsequent 5 months in 1537 pregnancies.
- Labor augmentation was more than 3 hours shorter in the high-dose group compared to low-dose group.
- High-dose augmentation resulted in fewer cesarean sections for labor dystocia when compared to low-dose augmentation, although cesareans for fetal distress were performed more frequently in the high-dose group.
- Failed induction was less frequent in the high-dose induction group compared to low-dose oxytocin, although, again, the cesarean deliveries for fetal distress increased when subjects used the high-dose regimen.
- In summary, high-dose oxytocin use resulted in less labor dystocia when used as a labor augmenter and resulted in more cesarean sections for fetal distress when used for labor induction.
- It is important to note that the low-dose regimen did not clinically significantly lengthen labor (3 hours), whereas the higher-dose regimen resulted in more cesarean births for fetal distress.
- When making decisions regarding which oxytocin regimen to utilize, the risks and benefits need to be carefully considered depending on the ultimate outcome desired.

Oxytocin Dosing Intervals

- Varying dosing intervals have also been studied (Orhue, 1993a, 1993b) and, in contemporary practice, vary from 15 to 40 minutes.
- All appear to be efficacious.
- One comparison of the efficacy and outcomes with differing oxytocin-dosing intervals (Satin et al, 1994) included 1801 consecutive pregnancies receiving high-dose oxytocin (starting dose of 6 mU/minute with incremental increases of 6 mU/min) at 20- and 40-minute intervals; 949 women received oxytocin at 20-minute intervals (n = 603 labor augmentations and n = 346 labor inductions), and 852 women received oxytocin at 40-minute dosing intervals (n = 564 labor augmentations and n = 288 labor inductions).
- The rates of cesarean delivery for dystocia or fetal distress were not statistically different between groups; however, the 20-minute regimen for augmentation was associated with a significant reduction in cesareans for dystocia (8% versus 12%, P = 0.05).
- The incidence of uterine tachysystole was greater with the 20-minute regimen for induction compared to the 40-minute regimen (40% versus 31%; P = 0.02).
- Neonatal outcomes were unaffected by the dosing interval.
- The authors concluded that the 40-minute dosing interval offered no clear advantage over the 20-minute dosing interval and that both regimens were safe and efficacious.

Prostaglandins (PG)

- Administration of PG results in dissolution of collagen bundles and an increase in submucosal water content of the cervix (Rayburn et al, 1994).
- These changes in cervical connective tissue at term are similar to those observed in early labor.
- Prostaglandins are endogenous compounds found in the myometrium, decidua, and fetal membranes during pregnancy.
- Side effects include fever, chills, vomiting, and diarrhea (Brindley et al, 1988).
- The efficacy of locally applied PG (vaginal or intracervical) for cervical ripening and labor induction with comparisons to a variety of other approaches including oxytocin (alone or in combination with amniotomy) and vaginal misoprostol has been demonstrated in a Cochrane review involving more than 10,000 women.
- Vaginal PGE_2 compared with placebo or no treatment reduced the likelihood of vaginal delivery not being achieved within 24 hours, the risk of the cervix remaining unfavorable or unchanged, and the need for oxytocin augmentation when PGE_2 was compared to placebo.
- There was no difference between cesarean rates, although with PGE_2 the risk of uterine tachysystole with fetal heart rate changes increased.
- The various administration vehicles (tablet, gel, and timed-release pessary) appear to be equally efficacious (Kelly et al, 2001).
- The optimal route, frequency, and dose of prostaglandins of all types and formulations for cervical ripening and labor induction have not been determined.
- Also, prostaglandin formulations of any kind should be avoided in women with a prior uterine scar such as prior cesarean section or myomectomy because their use appears to increase the risk for uterine rupture (Lydon-Rochelle et al, 2001; Wing et al, 1998).
- Uterine activity and fetal heart rate monitoring are indicated for 0.5 to 2 hours after administration of prostaglandins for cervical ripening and should be maintained as long as regular uterine activity is present (ACOG Committee on Practice Bulletins—Obstetrics, ACOG Practice Bulletin No. 107, 2009).

PROSTAGLANDIN E2 (PGE₂)

- In a classic review, Rayburn and colleagues (Rayburn et al, 1989) summarized the experience with over 3313 pregnancies representing 59 prospective clinical trials in which either intracervical or intravaginal PGE_2 was used for cervical ripening before the induction of labor.
- They concluded that local administration of PGE_2 is effective in enhancing cervical effacement and dilatation, reducing failed induction rates, shortening induction to delivery interval, and reducing oxytocin use and cesarean section for failure to progress.
- These findings were confirmed in the recent meta-analysis of 63 controlled trials performed worldwide and involving more than 10,000 women using various PG compounds and dosing regimens (Kelly et al, 2009).
- This review includes data for the commercially available sustained release vaginal pessary for PGE_2.
- Currently, the U.S. Food and Drug Administration (FDA) has approved two PGE_2 preparations for cervical ripening.
- Various other PGE_2 compounds, such as suppositories, are available in the United States, and tablets are available in Europe, although the FDA has not approved these latter formulations for use for cervical ripening.
- Many clinicians and pharmacists may prepare their own formulations of PGE_2 gel by thawing and resuspending 20 mg PGE_2 suppositories in small amounts of methylcellulose gel.
- The resulting gel preparation is then frozen in plastic syringes in various doses ranging from 1 to 6 mg.
- Prepidil (Upjohn Pharmaceuticals, Kalamazoo, Michigan) contains 0.5 mg of dinoprostone in 2.5 mL of gel for intracervical administration.
- The dose can be repeated in 6 to 12 hours if there is inadequate cervical change and minimal uterine activity following the first dose.
- The manufacturer recommends that the maximum cumulative dose of dinoprostone not exceed 1.5 mg (three doses) within a 24-hour period.
- Oxytocin should be initiated 6 to 12 hours after the last dose because of the potential for uterine tachysystole with concurrent oxytocin and prostaglandin administration.
- Cervidil (Forest Pharmaceuticals, St. Louis, Missouri) is a vaginal insert containing 10 mg of dinoprostone in a timed-release formulation.
- The vaginal insert administers the medication at 0.3 mg/hr and may be left in place for up to 12 hours.

- An advantage of the vaginal insert over the gel formulation is that the insert may be removed with the onset of active labor, rupture of membranes, or development of uterine overactivity.
- Per the manufacturer's recommendations, oxytocin may be initiated 30 to 60 minutes after removal of the insert.
- Both Prepidil and Cervidil require refrigerated storage and become unstable at room temperature.

PROSTAGLANDIN E1

- Misoprostol (Cytotec, Searle Pharmaceuticals, Chicago, Illinois) is a synthetic prostaglandin E1 analogue available as 100-mcg and 200-mcg tablets.
- The current FDA-approved use for misoprostol is for the treatment and prevention of peptic ulcer disease related to chronic nonsteroidal anti-inflammatory use.
- The American College of Obstetricians and Gynecologists (ACOG) considers the administration of misoprostol for preinduction cervical ripening to be a safe and effective "off-label" use (American College of Obstetricians and Gynecologists, ACOG Committee Opinion No. 283, 2003).
- Misoprostol is inexpensive and stable at room temperature.
- Misoprostol can be administered both orally or placed vaginally with few systemic side effects. Although not scored, the tablets are usually divided to provide 25- or 50-mcg doses.

VAGINAL ADMINISTRATION

- The most recent meta-analysis of 70 trials revealed the following points regarding the use of misoprostol compared with other methods of cervical ripening and labor induction (Hofmeyr et al, 2003): (1) misoprostol improved cervical ripening compared to placebo and was associated with a reduced failure to achieve vaginal delivery within 24 hours (RR 0.36, 95% CI 0.19 to 0.68.); (2) compared with other vaginal prostaglandins for labor induction, vaginal misoprostol was more effective in achieving vaginal delivery within 24 hours (RR 0.80, 95% CI 0.73 to 0.87); (3) compared with vaginal or intracervical PGE$_2$, oxytocin augmentation was less common with misoprostol (RR 0.64, 95% CI 0.56 to 0.73).
- However, uterine tachysystole with fetal heart rate changes (RR = 2.32, 95% CI: 1.62 to 3.32) and meconium stained amniotic fluid (RR = 1.45, 95% CI: 1.05 to 2) were more common with misoprostol use.
- Most studies also revealed that when using misoprostol doses above 25 mcg every 4 hours, uterine tachysystole with and without fetal heart rate changes occurred more frequently as well as an increased incidence of meconium passage compared to lower doses.
- Importantly, there were no significant differences in immediate neonatal outcomes.
- Although the American College of Obstetricians and Gynecologists, based on its review of the existing evidence, recommends 25 mcg dosing every 3 to 6 hours of vaginally applied misoprostol, the optimal dose and timing interval is not known (ACOG Committee on Practice Bulletins— Obstetrics, ACOG Practice Bulletin No. 107, 2009).

- Oxytocin may be initiated, if necessary, 4 hours after the final misoprostol dose.
- A meta-analysis comparing 25-mcg to 50-mcg dosing reported that 50-mcg dosing resulted in a higher rate of vaginal delivery within 24 hours with higher rates of uterine tachysystole and meconium passage without compromise in neonatal outcomes (Sanchez-Ramos et al, 1997).
- A statistically significant difference in fetal acidosis defined as an umbilical arterial pH of <7.16 was found in infants born to mothers given 50 mcg q3h of intravaginally applied misoprostol compared to those born to mothers given 25 mcg q3h has been reported (Farah et al, 1997; Sanchez-Ramos et al, 2002).
- In their committee opinions on the use of misoprostol for labor induction, ACOG concluded that safety using the higher 50-mcg dosing could not be adequately evaluated and suggested that the higher dose could be used in select circumstances (Sanchez-Ramos et al, 2002).
- A time-released misoprostol vaginal insert (MVI) is under development.
- In a three-arm phase III investigation, an MVI dose of 100 mcg did not have appreciably better clinical outcomes than Cervidil (Wing et al, 2008).

> **UPDATE #8**
>
> Development of a time-released vaginal misoprostol insert is under way (Wing et al, 2008, 2011).

- Misoprostol is not used in term pregnancies in women with a prior cesarean birth or other prior major uterine surgeries (e.g., extensive myomectomies and hysterotomies) because of the increased risk for uterine rupture (Lydon-Rochelle et al, 2001).

ORAL ADMINISTRATION

- Oral administration of misoprostol for cervical ripening has also been studied.
- This type of administration has the promise for offering more patient comfort and satisfaction and convenience of administration by mouth.
- Most of these studies compared lower oral doses of misoprostol such as 50 mcg given every 3 to 6 hours to similar vaginal misoprostol dosing regimens such as 25 to 50 mcg given every 3 to 6 hours.
- This oral regimen of dosing appears to be no more effective than vaginal administration for achieving vaginal delivery or affecting cesarean rates, but it may be associated with less uterine tachysystole.
- A clear positive dose-response relationship is observed between the dosage of oral misoprostol and the rate of tachysystole.
- With the 25- and 50-mcg dosages, there is a lower tachysystole rate, whereas it is higher in those given 200 mcg (Alfirevic et al, 2006).
- In this meta-analysis, oral misoprostol use was clearly superior to placebo, as women administered oral misoprostol were more likely to deliver vaginally within 24 hours, needed less oxytocin, and had a lower cesarean rate.

- Some investigators have described titrating oral misoprostol to its desired effect (Dällenbach et al, 2003; Hofmeyr et al, 2001).
- This method appears to achieve vaginal delivery rates similar to vaginally administered misoprostol with less uterine hyperstimulation.
- Low doses of oral misoprostol were achieved by making a solution (e.g., dissolving a 200-mcg tablet in 200 mL of tap water), as this was believed to provide more accurate dosing than simply cutting the tablet into pieces.
- Because oral dosing has a short (2-hour) duration of action, administration was repeated at 2-hour intervals.
- The authors of this Cochrane review recommended that if clinicians choose to use oral misoprostol, a dose of 20 to 25 mcg in solution is preferred for safety considerations and addressed concerns regarding imprecision of dividing misoprostol tablets for recommended dosages.
- There are concerns, however, that the pharmacy and nursing administration needed for dose titration is complex (Alfirevic et al, 2006).
- More data are needed to shed light on the optimal dosing, safety, and cost considerations of oral misoprostol for cervical ripening and labor induction.

BUCCAL AND SUBLINGUAL ADMINISTRATION

- Other novel approaches include buccal and sublingual misoprostol administration.
- The theory is that avoiding first pass hepatic circulation from oral administration will lead to bioavailability similar to that achieved with vaginal administration.
- This hypothesis has been substantiated by pharmacokinetic studies, which have shown that the buccal and sublingual routes of administration are associated with rapid onset of action and greater bioavailability than other routes (Tang et al, 2002).
- An additional potential advantage is the avoidance of direct cervicouterine effects, including uterine tachysystole.
- In a randomized controlled trial including 250 women admitted for labor induction, 50 mcg of sublingual misoprostol was compared to 100 mg orally administered misoprostol given every 4 hours to a maximum of five doses.
- Sublingual misoprostol appeared to have the same efficacy as orally administered misoprostol to achieve vaginal delivery within 24 hours with no increase in uterine overactivity (Shetty et al, 2002).
- A randomized controlled trial including 152 women received either 200 mcg of buccal misoprostol every 6 hours or 50 mcg vaginally administered misoprostol every 6 hours (Carlan et al, 2002).
- There was no statistically significant difference in time interval to vaginal delivery, rates of vaginal delivery, or rates of uterine tachysystole between the two groups.
- The buccal route was associated with a trend toward fewer cesarean births than with the vaginal route.
- Based on only three small trials included in the Cochrane meta-analysis, sublingual misoprostol appears to be at least as effective as when the same dose is administered orally.

- There are inadequate data to comment on the relative complications and side effects.
- More data are needed to clarify the safety and efficacy of buccal and sublingual misoprostol use as well (Muzonzin et al, 2004).
- Optimal dosing regimens are yet to be defined, and concern exists because of the greater bioavailability associated with these routes of administration when compared to vaginal use.

OUTPATIENT CERVICAL RIPENING

- Outpatient or ambulatory approaches to cervical ripening and labor induction for elective or marginal indications could be useful in reducing the duration of hospitalization and the staffing requirements of labor and delivery.
- The body of evidence to support this approach, however, is limited (Chang et al, 2005; Incerpi et al, 2001; Kelly et al, 2009; McKenna et al, 2004a, 2004b; Meyer et al, 2005; O'Brien et al, 1995; Sawai et al, 1991, 1995; Sciscione et al, 2001).
- Relevant published studies reflect a variety of approaches to cervical ripening, including local applications of prostaglandin compounds and placement of Foley balloon catheters to the lower uterine segment with or without immediate hospitalization for further labor management.
- To adequately address safety of any outpatient cervical ripening and labor induction technique, large numbers of subjects will be necessary.
- For this reason, outpatient cervical ripening and labor induction is not recommended at this time, other than in a research setting.

COMPLICATIONS OF LABOR INDUCTION

- All methods of labor induction carry risks.

UTERINE OVERACTIVITY

- The most frequently encountered complication of oxytocin or prostaglandin administration is uterine overactivity.
- Historically, the most commonly used terms to describe this activity were hyperstimulation, tachysystole, and hypertonus.
- Because there were no uniform definitions for these terms, and in an attempt to reduce miscommunication among obstetrical care providers, the National Institute of Child Health and Development (NICHD) has issued standardized definitions for fetal heart rate and uterine contraction patterns (Macones et al, 2008).
- With these new guidelines, *tachysystole* is defined as more than five uterine contractions in 10 minutes averaged over a 30-minute window, and the terms *hyperstimulation* and *hypercontractility* have been abandoned.
- Importantly, tachysystole may occur with spontaneous or stimulated labor. It may also be associated with or without fetal heart rate abnormalities.
- Other authorities have used alternative terminology (Curtis et al, 1987; Hofmeyr et al, 2003), and the semantic differences can be a source of confusion if the reader is unaware of the discrepancies.

- Increased uterine activity is associated with a significantly higher incidence of an umbilical artery pH of 7.11 or less, lower fetal oxygen saturation, and more nonreassuring fetal heart rate patterns (Bakker et al, 2007; Jonsson et al, 2008; Peebles et al, 1994; Simpson et al, 2008).
- Rarely, tachysystole may cause uterine rupture; this is more common in multigravidas than primigravida (Catanzarite et al, 2006; Flannelly et al, 1993).
- The various PGE_2 preparations have up to a 5% rate of uterine tachysystole, which is usually well tolerated and not associated with an adverse outcome.
- The reported risk of tachysystole with oxytocin varies widely.
- Tachysystole occurs more frequently when higher doses of oxytocin, PGE_2, or misoprostol are used (Flannelly et al, 1993; Smith et al, 2006; Wing et al, 1997).
- Concurrent administration of oxytocin and a prostaglandin is believed to increase the risk of tachysystole, as both drugs carry a risk of this complication.
- Additionally, data from human and animal studies show that prostaglandin administration increases uterine sensitivity to oxytocin (Baguma-Nibasheka et al, 1998; Brummer, 1971; Chan et al, 1983; Gillespie, 1973; Wikland et al, 1983).
- Although some studies have not observed a statistically significant increase in excessive uterine activity with concurrent use, this is likely because of the small numbers of patients in these studies, differences in methodology (e.g., uterine activity was not continuously monitored), and the relatively low frequency of adverse events (Coleman et al, 1997; Khan et al, 2007; Tan et al, 2007, 2009).
- In one such trial, the frequency of uterine tachysystole with concurrent dinoprostone and oxytocin administration was 14% versus 5% with oxytocin alone (p = 0.20) (Tan et al, 2009).

MANAGEMENT OF FETAL HEART RATE AND UTERINE CONTRACTION ABNORMALITIES ENCOUNTERED WITH LABOR INDUCTION

- Removing the PGE_2 vaginal insert will usually reverse the effects of tachysystole.
- If prostaglandin gel was applied locally, cervical/vaginal lavage is not helpful for removing the drug or reversing adverse effects.
- One of the advantages of oxytocin administration is that if uterine overactivity is encountered, the infusion can quickly be stopped.
- This usually results in the resolution of such uterine tachysystole.
- In addition, placing the woman in the left lateral position, administering oxygen, and increasing intravenous fluids may be of benefit.
- If fetal heart rate tracing abnormalities persist and excessive uterine activity is ongoing, the use of a tocolytic such as terbutaline (0.25 mg subcutaneously) may be considered.
- Oxytocin may then be reinitiated if appropriate once uterine tone has returned to baseline and fetal status is reassuring.

WATER INTOXICATION

- Oxytocin is structurally and functionally related to vasopressin, or antidiuretic hormone.
- It binds to vasopressin and oxytocin receptors in the kidney and the brain.
- Oxytocin can have an antidiuretic effect at high doses, and in extreme situations it results in water intoxication.
- Severe symptomatic hyponatremia can result if oxytocin is administered at high concentrations (e.g., 40 mU/min) in large quantities of hypotonic solutions (over 3 liters) for prolonged periods of time (Whalley et al, 1963).
- Symptoms of severe acute hyponatremia include headache, anorexia, nausea, vomiting, abdominal pain, lethargy, drowsiness, unconsciousness, grand mal type seizures, and potentially irreversible neurologic injury.
- If water intoxication occurs, oxytocin and any hypotonic solutions should be stopped.
- Correction of hyponatremia must be performed carefully and consist of restricting water intake and careful administration of hypertonic saline.
- Correction of hyponatremia must occur slowly and cautiously because overly rapid correction can be deleterious.

HYPOTENSION

- Hypotension can result from rapid intravenous injection of oxytocin; however, studies demonstrating this effect were performed in men, nonpregnant women, and first-trimester women under general anesthesia.
- A randomized trial of oxytocin bolus versus slow infusion in women at delivery of the anterior shoulder did not find clinically significant differences in hemodynamic responses (Davies et al, 2005).
- Because bolus injections of oxytocin can cause hypotension (Weis et al, 1975), it should be administered by infusion pump or slow drip.
- Mean arterial blood pressure and peripheral vascular resistance have been noted to decrease 30% and 50%, respectively, after oxytocin bolus injection of 5 to 10 units.
- This caused a 30% increase in heart rate, a 25% increase in stroke volume, and a 50% increase in cardiac output over patients receiving slow dilute infusions.
- Fewer cardiovascular side effects are observed when it is given as a slow intravenous infusion or intramuscularly as may be needed for third-stage labor management.

UTERINE RUPTURE

- Induction of labor has been consistently found to be a risk factor for uterine rupture, although the incidence of rupture is low and most cases occur in women with a scarred uterus.
- Uterine rupture in the unscarred uterus has been reported with the use of oxytocin, misoprostol (PGE_1), and PGE_2 preparations.
- In a series of 41 true uterine ruptures occurring in a hospital system in 2006, 27 occurred in women with prior uterine surgery (cesarean delivery or other uterine surgery),

and 12 of the remaining 14 ruptures occurred in patients who received uterotonic drugs (2 of these women were nulliparous) (Porreco et al, 2009).

- Oxytocin should always be administered in the lowest dose within a low-dose or high-dose regimen that produces regular contractions and cervical change.
- Prostaglandins should be given according to the manufacturer's recommendations or established protocols.
- Misoprostol should not be used in a woman in the third trimester with scarred uterus (ACOG Committee on Practice Bulletins—Obstetrics, ACOG Practice Bulletin No. 107, 2009; Wing et al, 1998).

FAILED INDUCTION

- Induction of labor usually culminates in vaginal delivery, but, as discussed previously, this occurs less often than when women enter labor spontaneously.
- There are no standards for what constitutes a failed induction. It is important to allow adequate time for cervical ripening and development of an active labor pattern before determining that an induction has failed.
- The importance of allowing enough time to progress from the latent phase of labor to the active phase was illustrated in the following studies:
  - In one large prospective study, the mean duration of the latent phase of labor (defined as the interval from initiation of induction with either prostaglandins or oxytocin to a cervical dilatation of 4 cm) in women with a Bishop score of 0 to 3 was 12 hours in multiparas women and 16 hours in nulliparas women (Xenakis et al, 1997).
  - In another study, requiring a minimum of 12 hours of oxytocin administration after membrane rupture before diagnosing failed labor induction led to vaginal deliveries in 75% of nulliparas women and eliminated failed labor induction as an indication for cesarean birth in parous women (Rouse et al, 2000).
  - A third series found that 73% of women who ultimately delivered vaginally had a latent phase of up to 18 hours (Simon et al, 2005).
- Latent phase was defined as the interval from initiation of oxytocin/amniotomy to the beginning of the active phase (i.e., cervical dilation of 4 cm with 80% effacement or 5 cm dilation).
- The definition of failed induction should be derived from what is known about the pattern of labor progression in women undergoing induced labor who ultimately achieve vaginal delivery.
- The goal is to minimize the number of cesarean deliveries performed for failed induction in patients who are progressing slowly because they are still in the latent phase of labor (Rouse et al, 2000; Simon et al, 2005; Xenakis et al, 1997).
- Once induced women enter active labor, progression should be comparable to progression in women with spontaneous active labor, or faster (Hoffman et al, 2006).
- One group proposed that failed induction be defined as the inability to achieve cervical dilatation of 4 cm and 80% effacement or 5 cm (regardless of effacement) after a minimum of 12 to 18 hours of both oxytocin administration and membrane rupture (Lin et al, 2006).

- They also specified that uterine contractile activity should reach five contractions/10 minutes or 250 Montevideo units, which is the minimum level achieved by most women whose labor is progressing normally.
- The cervical criteria were based on the observation that most women have entered the active phase when dilatation reached 4 to 5 cm; thus intervention before this dilatation is likely to represent a latent phase delivery rather than a protracted or arrested active phase.
- The duration of oxytocin administration was based on the observational studies cited previously, which described the maximum duration of latent phase in over 70% of induced women who went on to deliver vaginally.
- The membrane rupture requirement established a clear time point for "starting the clock," removed the time required for preinduction cervical ripening from the latent phase, and acknowledged the contribution of amniotomy as a method of induction.
- An Australian researcher evaluated a group of 978 nulliparous women after either artificial or spontaneous rupture of membranes to determine factors that could predict failed induction (Beckmann, 2007).
- There was a direct correlation between increasing duration of the latent phase and the probability of cesarean birth.
- After 10 hours of oxytocin administration, the 8% of women not in the active phase of labor had an approximately 75% chance of being delivered by cesarean for failed induction; after 12 hours of oxytocin administration, the chance of cesarean was almost 90%.
- Multivariable analysis showed that short maternal stature and use of pharmacologic or mechanical methods of cervical ripening contributed to an increased probability of cesarean delivery.
- Similarly, there was a linear relationship between lack of cervical dilatation and cesarean birth.
- The authors concluded that the continuation of oxytocin after amniotomy for women who had not yet reached at least 4 cm dilatation was not unreasonable, but that beyond 12 hours the benefit was unclear.

AMNIOTIC FLUID EMBOLISM

- A population-based retrospective cohort study including 3 million deliveries reported that medical induction of labor was associated with an increased risk of amniotic fluid embolism (adjusted OR 1.8, 95% CI 1.2 to 2.7) (Kramer et al, 2006).
- However, the absolute risk was small, 10.3 per 100,000 births with medical induction versus 5.2 per 100,000 births without medical induction.
- Moreover, given that these women were induced for medical indications, not inducing labor could potentially result in greater maternal-fetal morbidity/mortality than inducing labor.
- Others should confirm these findings before changes in the management of induction are considered.

SUGGESTED READINGS

Introduction

Martin JA, Hamilton BE, Sutton PD, et al: Births: final data for 2007, *Natl Vital Stat Rep* 58(24):1–85, 2010.

Indications and Contraindications

American College of Obstetricians and Gynecologists Committee on Practice Bulletins—Obstetrics: ACOG practice bulletin no. 107: induction of labor, *Obstet Gynecol* 114(2 Pt 1):386–397, 2009.

Elective Induction of Labor

Moore LE, Rayburn WF: Elective induction of labor, *Clin Obstet Gynecol* 49(3):698–704, 2006.

Risks Associated with Elective Induction

Fisch JM, English D, Pedaline S, Brooks K, Simhan HN: Labor induction process improvement: a patient quality-of-care initiative, *Obstet Gynecol* 113(4):797–803, 2009.

Risk of Cesarean Delivery Following Elective Induction at Term

Bailit JL, Gregory KD, Reddy UM, et al: Maternal and neonatal outcomes by labor onset type and gestational age, *Am J Obstet Gynecol* 202(3): 245e1–245e12, 2010.

Cammu H, Haitsma V: Sweeping of the membranes at 39 weeks in nulliparous women: a randomised controlled trial, *BJOG* 105(1):41–44, 1998.

Gülmezoglu AM, Crowther CA, Middleton P: Induction of labour for improving birth outcomes for women at or beyond term, *Cochrane Database Syst Rev*(4)CD004945, 2006.

Risk of Neonatal Morbidity Following Elective Induction at Term

Caughey AB, Sundaram V, Kaimal AJ, et al: Systematic review: elective induction of labor versus expectant management of pregnancy, *Ann Intern Med* 151(4):252–263, 2009.

Clark SL, Miller DD, Belfort MA, et al: Neonatal and maternal outcomes associated with elective term delivery, *Am J Obstet Gynecol* 200(2): 156.e1–156.e4, 2009.

Risk of Increased Costs Following Elective Induction at Term

Kaufman KE, Bailit JL, Grobman W: Elective induction: an analysis of economic and health consequences, *Am J Obstet Gynecol* 187(4):858–863, 2002.

Active Management of Risk in Pregnancy at Term (AMOR-IPAT): An Approach to Control the Cesarean Rate Following Induction?

Nicholson JM, Parry S, Caughey AB, et al: The impact of the active management of risk in pregnancy at term on birth outcomes: a randomized clinical trial, *Am J Obstet Gynecol* 198(5):511e1–511e15, 2008.

Prolonged Pregnancy

Risks of Prolonged Pregnancy

Alexander JM, McIntire DD, Leveno KJ: Forty weeks and beyond: pregnancy outcomes by week of gestation, *Obstet Gynecol* 96(2):291–294, 2000.

Smith GC: Life-table analysis of the risk of perinatal death at term and post term in singleton pregnancies, *Am J Obstet Gynecol* 184(3):489–496, 2001.

Clinical Considerations and Recommendations

Prolonged Patient with a Favorable Cervix

Hannah ME, Hannah WJ, Hellman J, et al: Induction of labor as compared with serial antenatal monitoring in post-term pregnancy: a randomized controlled trial. The Canadian Multicenter Post-term Pregnancy Trial Group, *N Engl J Med* 326(24):1587–1592, 1992.

Prolonged Patient with an Unfavorable Cervix

Interventions for preventing or improving the outcome of delivery at or beyond term. *The Cochrane library, issue 2*, Chicester, UK, 2004, John Wiley & Sons.

Optimal Timing for a Delivery of a Prolonged Pregnancy

Silver RM, Landon MB, Rouse DJ, et al: Maternal morbidity associated with multiple repeat cesarean deliveries, *Obstet Gynecol* 107(6):1226–1232, 2006.

Prevention of Postterm Pregnancy

Boulvain M, Stan C, Irion O: Membrane sweeping for induction of labour, *Cochrane Database Syst Rev* (1):CD000451, 2005.

Preinduction Assessment

Predicting a Successful Induction

Bailit JL, Downs SM, Thorp JM: Reducing the caesarean delivery risk in elective inductions of labour: a decision analysis, *Paediatr Perinat Epidemiol* 16(1):90–96, 2002.

Bishop EH: Pelvic scoring for elective induction, *Obstet Gynecol* 24:266–268, 1964.

Xenakis EM, Piper JM, Conway DL, Langer O: Induction of labor in the nineties: conquering the unfavorable cervix, *Obstet Gynecol* 90(2):235–239, 1997.

Membrane Stripping

Centers for Disease Control and Prevention: Provisional recommendations for the prevention of perinatal Group B Streptococcal disease (website). www.cdc.gov/groupbstrep/guidelines/downloads/provisional-recommendations-508.pdf. Accessed July 10, 2011.

Amniotomy

Howarth G, Botha DJ: Amniotomy plus intravenous oxytocin for induction of labour, *Cochrane Database Syst Rev* (3):CD003250, 2001.

Transcervical Balloon Catheters

Boulvain M, Kelly A, Lohse C, et al: Mechanical methods for induction of labour, *Cochrane Database Syst Rev* (4):CD001233, 2001.

Pharmacologic Methods

Oxytocin

Clark S, Belfort M, Saade G, et al: Implementation of a conservative checklist-based protocol for oxytocin administration: maternal and newborn outcomes, *Am J Obstet Gynecol* 197(5):480.e1–480.e5, 2007.

Hannah ME, Ohlsson A, Farine D, et al: Induction of labor compared with expectant management for prelabor rupture of the membranes at term. TERMPROM Study Group, *N Engl J Med* 334(16):1005–1010, 1996.

Seitchik J, Amico J, Robinson AG, Castillo M: Oxytocin augmentation of dysfunctional labor. IV. Oxytocin pharmacokinetics, *Am J Obstet Gynecol* 150(3):225–228, 1984.

Tan BP, Hannah ME: Prostaglandins for prelabour rupture of membranes at or near term, *Cochrane Database Syst Rev* (2):CD000178, 2000.

High-Dose Oxytocin Dosing

Merrill DC, Zlatnik FJ: Randomized, double-masked comparison of oxytocin dosage in induction and augmentation of labor, *Obstet Gynecol* 94(3): 455–463, 1999.

Prostaglandins (PG)

Kelly AJ, Kavanagh J, Thomas J: Vaginal prostaglandin (PGE2 and PGF2a) for induction of labour at term, *Cochrane Database Syst Rev* (2):CD003101, 2001.

Prostaglandin E1

American College of Obstetricians and Gynecologists: ACOG committee opinion no. 283, May 2003: new U.S. Food and Drug Administration labeling on Cytotec (misoprostol) use and pregnancy, *Obstet Gynecol* 101(5 Pt 1):1049–1050, 2003.

Vaginal Administration

Hofmeyr GJ, Gulmezoglu AM: Vaginal misoprostol for cervical ripening and induction of labour, *Cochrane Database Syst Rev* (1):CD000941, 2003.

Lydon-Rochelle M, Holt VL, Easterling TR, Martin DP: Risk of uterine rupture during labor among women with a prior cesarean delivery, *N Engl J Med* 345(1):3–8, 2001.

Wing DA: Misoprostol Vaginal Insert Consortium: Misoprostol vaginal insert compared with dinoprostone vaginal insert: a randomized controlled trial, *Obstet Gynecol* 112(4):801–812, 2008.

Oral Administration

Alfirevic Z, Weeks A: Oral misoprostol for induction of labour, *Cochrane Database Syst Rev* (2):CD001338, 2006.

Hofmeyr GJ, Alfirevic Z, Matonhodze B, et al: Titrated oral misoprostol solution for induction of labour: a multi-centre, randomised trial, *BJOG* 108(9):952–959, 2001.

Outpatient Cervical Ripening

Kelly AJ, Alfirevic Z, Dowswell T: Outpatient versus inpatient induction of labour for improving birth outcomes, *Cochrane Database Syst Rev* (2):CD007372, 2009.

Complications of Labor Induction

Uterine Overactivity

Macones GA, Hankins GD, Spong CY, et al: The 2008 National Institute of Child Health and Human Development Research Workshop Report on electronic fetal heart rate monitoring, *Obstet Gynecol* 112(3):661–666, 2008.

Uterine Rupture

Porreco RP, Clark SL, Belfort MA, et al: The changing specter of uterine rupture, *Am J Obstet Gynecol* 200(3):269.e1–269.e4, 2009.

Failed Induction

Lin MG, Rouse DJ: What is a failed labor induction? *Clin Obstet Gynecol* 49(3):585–593, 2006.

Rouse DJ, Owen J, Hauth JC: Criteria for failed labor induction: prospective evaluation of a standardized protocol, *Obstet Gynecol* 96(5 Pt 1):671-617, 2000.

References

Please go to expertconsult.com to view references.

Chapter 15

Perinatal Infections

CHRISTINE K. FARINELLI • AFSHAN B. HAMEED

KEY UPDATES

1 In a prospective cohort study, 261 women underwent polymerase chain reaction (PCR) analysis of their amniotic fluid for the detection of *Toxoplasma gondii*. Sensitivity of the test was found to be 92.2%; specificity, 100%; negative predictive value, 98.1%; and positive predictive value, 100%. Four negative results occurred in children who were infected.

2 In patients exposed to cytomegalovirus (CMV), ultrasound abnormalities predict symptomatic congenital infection in only a third of cases in which the fetal infection status is unknown. However, ultrasound is a useful adjunct in predicting symptomatic postnatal disease.

3 Vaccines consisting of recombinant CMV envelope glycoprotein B have been produced and are undergoing trials. In a recent placebo-controlled, randomized, double-blind trial, 234 subjects received the vaccine and 230 received placebo. The vaccine group was more likely to remain uninfected at 42 months postvaccination with an efficacy of 50%.

4 Some specialists recommend cesarean delivery for women with newly acquired herpes simplex virus (HSV) in the third trimester regardless of symptoms or signs at the time of labor because (a) 6 to 12 weeks are required for the mother to produce type-specific antibodies that can transverse the placenta and protect their neonate; (b) the risk of neonatal herpes is 30% to 50% in women subclinically shedding virus at the time of labor as a result of acquiring genital herpes in the third trimester; (c) high titers of the virus persist in genital secretions for many months after the initial infection.

5 Screening for human immunodeficiency virus (HIV) is recommended for all pregnant women after they have been notified that they will be tested for HIV infection as part of the routine panel of prenatal blood tests unless they decline the test. This is called "opt-out" screening. The American College of Obstetricians and Gynecologists (ACOG) also currently recommends repeat HIV testing in the third trimester in areas with high HIV prevalence, for women at high risk for acquiring the infection, and for women who declined testing earlier in the pregnancy; rapid HIV testing should be used in labor for women with undocumented status.

6 During the H1N1 influenza pandemic in 2009, significant morbidity (22% admission to intensive care) and mortality (8%) occurred in pregnant and postpartum women. Regardless of the results of rapid antigen testing, prompt evaluation and antiviral treatment of influenza-like illness should be considered for these women. As well, all pregnant women should be encouraged to receive annual influenza vaccinations.

Toxoplasmosis

BACKGROUND

- Infection by protozoan *Toxoplasma gondii*
- Transmission occurs by eating cysts in undercooked meat of infected animals or from oocysts from the feces of an infected cat

CLINICAL

- Primary infection is usually asymptomatic during pregnancy but may cause congenital infection in the fetus
  - Risk of fetal infection is highest if maternal infection occurs in third trimester (60%), but risk of severe fetal injury is highest if maternal infection occurs in first trimester (transmission 10% to 15%)

- Fetal infection occurs in one third of cases
- Complications of fetal infection include fetal demise, impaired vision resulting from chorioretinitis in 4% to 27%, uveitis, seizures, mental retardation, enlarged spleen and liver, disseminated purpuric rash, and significant learning disabilities
- The classic triad consists of chorioretinitis, hydrocephalus, and intracranial calcifications

DIAGNOSIS

- Routine screening is not recommended
- Serologic testing in the mother, fetus, or neonate
- PCR testing can be performed on amniotic fluid samples
- Ultrasound findings: ventriculomegaly, intracranial calcifications, microcephaly, ascites, hepatosplenomegaly, intrauterine growth restriction

UPDATE #1

In a prospective cohort study, 261 women underwent PCR analysis of their amniotic fluid for the detection of *Toxoplasma gondii*. Sensitivity of the test was found to be 92.2%; specificity, 100%; negative predictive value, 98.1%; and positive predictive value, 100%. Four negative results occurred in children who were infected (Wallon et al, 2010).

TREATMENT

- Acutely in pregnancy: spiramycin may reduce the risk of congenital infection by 50% (only available through the Food and Drug Administration [FDA] after serologic confirmation)
- Additional therapy with pyrimethamine and sulfadiazine is indicated if the diagnosis is confirmed in the fetus
- Folinic acid must be administered with pyrimethamine to rescue human cells

PROGNOSIS

- In untreated neonates with congenital infection: poor prognosis with high rates of chorioretinitis, seizures, and severe psychomotor retardation

Syphilis

BACKGROUND

- Infection by spirochete *Treponema pallidum*
- Transmission by direct sexual contact with ulcerative lesions on skin or mucous membranes
- Congenital infection results from transplacental passage of spirochetes, which has the highest risk in the second half of pregnancy and in mothers with primary or secondary syphilis

CLINICAL

- Congenital infection may result in stillbirth (25%), fetal hydrops, preterm labor
- In the neonate, early (onset <2 years of age) syphilis results in cutaneous lesions on palms and soles, hepatosplenomegaly, jaundice, anemia, snuffles, and periostitis
- Late neonatal manifestations include frontal bossing, short maxilla, high palatal arch, mulberry molars, Hutchinson

teeth, interstitial keratitis, eighth nerve deafness, saddle nose, saber shins, and perioral fissures—these stigmata are due to scarring from early lesions or reactions to persistent inflammation
- These complications can be prevented by treatment within the first 3 months of birth

DIAGNOSIS

- ACOG recommends routine screening for syphilis as part of the first prenatal visit
- Direct visualization of the spirochetes under darkfield microscopy or direct fluorescent antibody tests from the lesion
- Serologic tests include nontreponemal tests such as Venereal Disease Research Laboratory (VDRL) or Rapid Plasma Reagin (RPR), which are primarily used for screening
- Once screening tests are positive, specific treponemal tests (microhemagglutination and fluorescent treponemal antibody absorption) are used for confirmation
- Treponemal tests remain positive for life with or without treatment
- Ultrasound findings: fetal hepatomegaly, ascites, hydrops, thickened placenta

TREATMENT

- Parenteral penicillin remains the drug of choice for all stages of syphilis
- Jarisch-Herxheimer reaction:
  - Occurs within several hours of treatment of primary or secondary syphilis and resolves by 24 to 36 hours
  - Fever, chills, malaise, headache, hypotension, transient worsening of cutaneous lesions
  - Increases risk of preterm labor or fetal distress if treatment given in second half of pregnancy with this reaction

Rubella (German Measles)

BACKGROUND

- Single-strand RNA virus
- Transmission via respiratory droplets
- Fetal transmission via hematogenous dissemination across the placenta and frequency of infection is dependent on time of exposure to virus:
  - 50% to 80% of infants exposed to virus within 12 weeks after conception will manifest signs of congenital infection
  - Rate declines with advancing gestational age (few fetuses are affected if infection occurs after 18 weeks' gestation)

CLINICAL

- Causes mild, self-limited (3 to 5 days) illness in adults; characteristic widely disseminated, nonpruritic, erythematous, maculopapular rash
- Congenital infection may lead to neurosensory deafness, cataracts, cardiac malformations (especially patent ductus arteriosus; supravalvular pulmonic stenosis pathognomonic), meningoencephalitis, behavioral disorders, and mental retardation

- Newborn may have hepatosplenomegaly, thrombocytopenia, purpuric skin lesions (blueberry muffin lesions) because of extramedullary hematopoiesis and hyperbilirubinemia
- Approximately 60% of infected fetuses will have intrauterine growth restriction

DIAGNOSIS

- ACOG recommends routine screening for rubella as part of the first prenatal visit (10% to 20% of women in the United States remain susceptible)
- Isolation of the virus from nasal secretions, throat swab, blood, urine, or cerebrospinal fluid (CSF)
- Serologic testing with fourfold increase in the antibody titer indicates infection
- Rubella specific IgM antibody represents acute infection, and rising titers of IgG are suggestive of congenital infection
- Ultrasound findings: growth restriction, microcephaly, central nervous system abnormalities, cardiac abnormalities

TREATMENT

- None

Cytomegalovirus (CMV)

BACKGROUND

- Double-stranded DNA herpesvirus transmitted by close personal contact
- CMV remains latent in host cells after initial infection but can undergo reactivation and recurrent infection
- Even though ~ 50% to 80% of women have serologic evidence of CMV infection, presence of antibodies is not entirely protective
- Congenital infection may result from transplacental passage of virus to the fetus
- Risk of fetal infection is highest if the mother has a primary CMV infection in the third trimester
- Risk of severe fetal sequelae is highest if infection occurs in the first trimester
- Neonates are at risk of infection from direct exposure to genital secretions at the time of delivery or through breast-feeding
- Most common congenital infection, affecting 0.2% to 2.2% of all neonates; leading cause of congenital hearing loss
- Risk of transmission with primary maternal CMV infection is 30% to 40%; the risk with recurrent maternal infection is 0.15% to 2%

CLINICAL

- Asymptomatic in adults; occasionally mild flulike illness
- 85% to 90% of infants with congenital CMV are asymptomatic; of these, 10% to 15% develop hearing loss, chorioretinitis, dental defects by age 2 years
- Severe, symptomatic disease in the neonate: hepatosplenomegaly, jaundice, thrombocytopenia with petechiae, hyperbilirubinemia, hepatitis, intracranial calcifications, microcephaly, chorioretinitis, hearing loss, growth restriction, and nonimmune hydrops

- Approximately 30% of severely infected infants die, and 80% of survivors have major morbidity

DIAGNOSIS

- Routine screening is not recommended
- Maternal diagnosis: seroconversion from negative to positive or greater than fourfold increase in anti-CMV IgG titers is evidence of infection
- Presence of CMV in the amniotic fluid either by culture or PCR
- Fetal ultrasonographic findings consistent with severe injury: intracerebral calcifications, ventriculomegaly, microcephaly, oligohydramnios, growth restriction, and hydrops (less common: heart block, echogenic bowel, meconium peritonitis, renal dysplasia, ascites, pleural effusions)

> **UPDATE #2**
>
> In patients exposed to CMV, ultrasound abnormalities predict symptomatic congenital infection in only a third of cases in which the fetal infection status is unknown. However, ultrasound is a useful adjunct in predicting symptomatic postnatal disease (Guerra et al, 2008).

TREATMENT

- Intravenous CMV-specific hyperimmune globulin every month throughout the pregnancy

> **UPDATE #3**
>
> Vaccines consisting of recombinant CMV envelope glycoprotein B have been produced and are undergoing trials. In a recent placebo-controlled, randomized, double-blind trial, 234 subjects received the vaccine and 230 received placebo. The vaccine group was more likely to remain uninfected at 42 months post-vaccination with an efficacy of 50% (Pass et al, 2009).

Herpes Simplex Virus (HSV)

BACKGROUND

- Oropharyngeal or genital infection by double-stranded DNA herpesvirus
- Transmission via sexual contact
- First episode of primary genital herpes infection refers to an infection by HSV-1 or HSV-2 without antibodies to either one
- First episode nonprimary genital herpes is an infection by HSV-1 or HSV-2 with antibodies to the other viral serotype
- Recurrent genital herpes infection is mild and the episodes brief (3 to 10 days) due to preexisting antibodies
- Fetal infection primarily occurs via transplacental passage of the virus in the presence of maternal viremia; higher risk of this occurring late in pregnancy with primary infection
- Neonatal infection is more common than fetal infection because of direct contact with genital secretions at the time of birth
  - Risk is very high (30% to 60%) if mother has recent infection (i.e., presence of virus in genital tract but without development of type-specific antibodies)

- If recurrent, clinically evident infection, transmission risk is 1% to 2%
- Transmission can occur in asymptomatic infected mothers as well

CLINICAL

- In the adult, primary infection manifests as painful crops of vesicles and ulcers at various stages of evolution, tender inguinal adenopathy, fever, and constitutional symptoms that resolve in 3 to 6 weeks; rarely, meningitis
- Recurrent infection is encountered in ~50% of individuals within 6 months
- Neonatal disease presents at the end of the first week of life with skin lesions, cough, cyanosis, tachypnea, dyspnea, jaundice, seizures, disseminated intravascular coagulopathy (DIC)
  - Can be classified as disseminated (25%), central nervous system disease (30%), disease limited to the skin, eyes, or mouth (45%)
- Infants with disseminated herpes have risk of mortality or serious morbidity of ~30% to 40%, even with antiviral therapy; ~20% of survivors of neonatal herpes have long-term neurologic sequelae

DIAGNOSIS

- Routine screening is not recommended
- Viral culture of the vesicle fluid; results are usually available in 48 to 72 hours
- PCR for the viral DNA is a relatively quick test that may detect viral shedding in an asymptomatic carrier

TREATMENT

- For adults: supportive measures including oral analgesics, topical anesthetics, frequent bathing followed by drying affected area with hair dryer; oral acyclovir therapy; other options include valacyclovir and famciclovir
- Neonatal infection can be prevented by elective cesarean delivery in the presence of typical herpes lesions
- Of note, women with nongenital herpes should utilize barriers and avoid contact of the newborn with the infected maternal skin until the lesions have encrusted

PREVENTION

- In women with active recurrent genital herpes who are pregnant, suppressive viral therapy should be encouraged at or beyond 36 weeks' gestation

---

UPDATE #4

Some specialists recommend cesarean delivery for women with newly acquired HSV in the third trimester regardless of symptoms or signs at the time of labor because (1) 6 to 12 weeks are required for the mother to produce type-specific antibodies, which can transverse the placenta and protect their neonate; (2) the risk of neonatal herpes is 30% to 50% in women subclinically shedding virus at the time of labor as a result of acquiring genital herpes in the third trimester; (3) high titers of the virus persist in genital secretions for many months after the initial infection (Brown et al, 2005).

Gonorrhea

BACKGROUND

- Gram-negative diplococcus *Neisseria gonorrhoeae*
- Sexually transmitted; second most commonly reported communicable disease in United States
- Risk of transmission from infected male to female partner is ~50% to 90% with single exposure
- Prevalence of infection in pregnancy ranges from 0 to 10%
- Newborns acquire infection via infected birth canal

CLINICAL

- Most women are asymptomatic but may report vaginal discharge or dysuria
- Women in second and third trimesters are at increased risk of disseminated disease:
  - First stage: chills, fevers, vesicles that become pustules with hemorrhagic base; rarely, perihepatitis, endocarditis, meningitis
  - Second stage: septic arthritis
- Increased risks of premature rupture of membranes (PROM), chorioamnionitis, preterm delivery, intrauterine growth restriction, neonatal sepsis, postpartum endometritis
- Neonatal sequelae include ophthalmia neonatorum (frank purulent bilateral conjunctivitis, which can lead to corneal ulceration and blindness if untreated) and disseminated gonococcal infection

DIAGNOSIS

- The Centers for Disease Control and Prevention (CDC) recommends screening during pregnancy if prevalence is >1%
- The CDC and the ACOG recommend a third-trimester rescreen for at-risk women
- Tests include culture, nucleic acid hybridization, and nucleic acid amplification

TREATMENT

- For women with uncomplicated gonorrhea: ceftriaxone 125 mg IM × 1 dose
- For women with complicated gonorrhea (i.e., disseminated): ceftriaxone 1 gm IM or IV q24 hr
- Because there is a high frequency (20% to 50%) of coinfection with chlamydia, the CDC recommends treating for chlamydia if the patient tests positive for gonorrhea (amoxicillin or azithromycin)
- For neonates, prevention of ophthalmia neonatorum with erythromycin (0.5%) ophthalmic ointment, tetracycline (1%) ophthalmic ointment, and silver nitrate (1%) aqueous solution

Group B Streptococcal (GBS) Infection

BACKGROUND

- Caused by *Streptococcus agalactiae* (Gram-positive bacteria)
- In 1995, rate of perinatal sepsis was 1.3 per 1000 liveborn infants; in 2008, ~ 0.4 per 1000 liveborn infants
- Overall case fatality rate of 4% to 6%: 2% to 3% in term, 16% to 30% in preterm infants

- Risk factors for neonatal GBS sepsis: prematurity, maternal intrapartum fever, membrane rupture >18 hours, a previous infant with GBS disease, GBS bacteriuria in current pregnancy

CLINICAL

- Asymptomatic rectovaginal colonization occurs in ~20% of pregnant women (this colonization may be transient, intermittent, or persistent)
- Without intervention, ~1% to 2% of infants born to colonized mothers will develop early onset infection
- Early onset neonatal infection (within first week of life, usually in first 48 hours): rapid clinical deterioration and high mortality rate; may lead to death within hours from septic shock and respiratory distress despite appropriate antibiotic coverage; meningitis occurs in 10% to 30%
- Late-onset neonatal infection (usually after first week of life): usually presents as meningitis; 50% have neurologic sequelae; can be transmitted nosocomially

DIAGNOSIS

- Culture is the gold standard; some PCR-based tests

TREATMENT

- Penicillin G (5 million units initially, then 2.5 million units every 4 hours IV) or, if patient is allergic, check susceptibilities (Figure 15-1)
- Beta-lactam antibiotics administered ≥4 hours before delivery are highly effective at preventing vertical transmission (exact duration of antibiotics needed remains unknown)
- High rate of resistance to erythromycin

PREVENTION

- Has dramatically decreased incidence of early-onset GBS sepsis
- Screen all pregnant women at 35 to 37 weeks' gestation for vaginorectal colonization using a culture; if colonized, patient should receive intrapartum antibiotic prophylaxis (IAP) at labor or rupture of membranes
- Negative predictive value of GBS cultures performed ≤5 weeks' gestation before delivery is 95% to 98% (clinical utility decreases at >5 weeks before delivery)
- Give IAP to women with GBS in urine (prenatal screening at 35 to 37 weeks' gestation is not indicated)
  - Treat bacteriuria as usual at the time of culture positivity
  - This will not eradicate recolonization from genitourinary and gastrointestinal tracts; therefore, IAP still indicated
- Women with previous birth of infant with GBS disease should receive IAP (do not require prenatal screening)
- Give IAP if GBS culture is unknown and patient is <37 weeks' gestation, rupture of membranes >18 hours, or temperature ≥100.4° F (Table 15-1)
- Collection of samples should be from distal vagina and anorectum (through the anal sphincter); do not use speculum

Human Immunodeficiency Virus (HIV)

BACKGROUND

- Caused by an RNA retrovirus
- Mechanism of transmission: heterosexual contact, IV drug use; rarely, organ donation, artificial insemination, blood transfusion
- Risk of perinatal transmission is 25% in the absence of any intervention; decreases to 2% with intervention (most cases

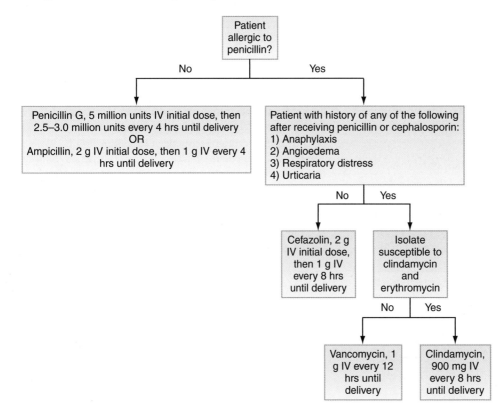

Figure 15-1. Recommended regimens for intrapartum antimicrobial prophylaxis for perinatal GBS disease prevention. (Adapted from Centers for Disease Control and Prevention: Revised guidelines for prevention of perinatal group B streptococcal disease, *MMWR* 9(RR-10):1-32, 2010.)

TABLE 15-1 **Indications for Intrapartum Antibiotic Prophylaxis to Prevent Early Onset GBS Disease**

Intrapartum Prophylaxis Indicated	Intrapartum Prophylaxis Not Indicated
Previous infant with invasive GBS disease	Colonization with GBS during previous pregnancy
GBS bacteriuria at any time during current pregnancy	GBS bacteriuria during previous pregnancy
Positive GBS vaginal-rectal screening culture in late gestation during current pregnancy	Negative vaginal-rectal GBS screening culture in late gestation during current pregnancy
Unknown GBS status at onset of labor and — Delivery <37 weeks — Amniotic membranes rupture >18 hours — Intrapartum temperature ≥100.4°F — Intrapartum nucleic acid amplification test positive for GBS (rapid test)	Cesarean performed before onset of labor on woman with intact membranes (regardless of gestational age, colonization status)

Adapted from Centers for Disease Control and Prevention: revised guidelines for prevention of perinatal group B streptococcal disease, *MMWR* 59(RR-10):1-32, 2010.

occur at delivery, but some occur antenatally from invasive procedures, postnatal from breast-feeding)
- Risk factors for perinatal transmission: history of previously infected infant, severe maternal disease, preterm delivery, intrapartum blood exposure (vaginal lacerations, episiotomy, instrumental delivery), time since rupture of membranes >4 hours, invasive antepartum procedures, chorioamnionitis, concurrent sexually transmitted diseases (STDs), vaginal delivery in the presence of an elevated viral load

CLINICAL
- Four stages in adults:
  1. Acute retroviral illness: severe flulike illness, malaise, poor appetite, weight loss, low-grade fever, generalized lymphadenopathy
  2. Latent phase: viral load is low, virus concentrates in lymphatic tissue and replicates slowly
  3. Symptomatic phase: viral load increases
  4. Acquired immunodeficiency syndrome
- Hallmark of disease: opportunistic infections such as *Pneumocystis pneumonia* and *Mycobacterium avium-intracellulare*; also tuberculosis, toxoplasmosis, CMV, candidiasis, non-Hodgkin lymphoma

DIAGNOSIS
- Screening test is enzyme immunoassay (EIA) for HIV-1, HIV-2
- Confirmatory tests are Western blot or immunofluorescent assay (IFA)
- The CDC and the ACOG currently recommend universal prenatal screening, with "opt-out" strategy to ensure compliance

UPDATE #5
HIV screening is recommended for all pregnant women after they have been notified that they will be tested for HIV infection as part of the routine panel of prenatal blood tests unless they decline the test. This is called "opt-out" screening. ACOG also currently recommends repeat HIV testing in the third trimester in areas with high HIV prevalence, women at high risk for acquiring the infection, and women who declined testing earlier in the pregnancy; rapid HIV testing should be used in labor for women with undocumented status (American College of Obstetrics and Gynecology Committee on Obstetric Practice, Committee Opinion No. 418, 2008).

TREATMENT
- Highly active antiretroviral therapy (HAART)
- First prenatal appointment: measure CD4 count and viral load; screen for gonorrhea, chlamydia, syphilis, hepatitis B and C; test for tuberculosis, toxoplasmosis, CMV
- Vaccinate HIV-positive pregnant women with pneumococcal, influenza, hepatitis A and B, meningococcal vaccines
- If CD4 <200 cells/mm^3, start trimethoprim-sulfamethoxazole-double strength prophylaxis (for *Pneumocystis pneumonia*)
- If protein purified derivative test (ppd) is positive and chest x-ray negative, treat with isoniazid and pyridoxine
- If CD4 <50 to 75 cells/mm^3, then start azithromycin prophylaxis (for *Mycobacterium avium-intracellulare*)
- If recurrent candidiasis, can give daily fluconazole; should also be given if CD4 <50 cells/mm^3 to prevent cryptococcal infection
- If recurrent herpes infection, give acyclovir 400 mg po bid
- Vaginal delivery is acceptable if viral load is <1000 copies/mL; avoid amniotomy, scalp monitoring, scalp pH assessment, episiotomy, instrumental delivery
- If viral load >1000 copies/mL, deliver at 38 weeks' gestation (prior to labor and rupture of membranes)
- Patient should receive intravenous zidovudine during delivery: 2 mg/kg for 1 hour, then 1 mg/kg/hr until delivery or at least 4 hours prior to scheduled cesarean
- Infants of infected mothers are treated for 6 weeks

Listeriosis

BACKGROUND
- Caused by *Listeria monocytogenes*: a motile, non-spore-forming, Gram-positive bacillus
- Most common transmission to fetus is via hematogenous dissemination through the placenta, forming placental abscesses and fetal septicemia
- Associated with food contamination: fresh, unpasteurized cheeses (Mexican "queso fresco") and processed meats (hot dogs)

CLINICAL

- Stillbirth, preterm labor, fetal infection with high perinatal morbidity and mortality rates
- Early-onset (manifests in first few hours to days of life): diffuse sepsis with involvement of multiple organs; high rate of stillbirth and neonatal mortality rate; more frequent in low birth weight infants
- Late-onset (manifests several days to weeks of life): usually meningitis in term infants born to mothers with uneventful prenatal course; common to have neurologic sequelae including hydrocephalus and mental retardation; mortality rate approaching 40%
- Most women are asymptomatic; some with flulike symptoms of fever, malaise, chills, back pain, upper respiratory discomfort

DIAGNOSIS

- Culture from cervix and blood

TREATMENT

- Penicillin G and ampicillin (plus aminoglycoside for mother)
- Case studies suggest that early diagnosis and aggressive antibiotic management may significantly improve perinatal mortality

Parvovirus

BACKGROUND

- Caused by a single-stranded DNA virus
- Transmission via respiratory droplets, hand-to-mouth, and infected blood products
- Approximately 50% to 60% of reproductive-age women show prior infection, with long-term immunity
- Fetal transmission is via transplacental passage of virus, which then infects fetal red cell progenitors and suppresses erythropoiesis

CLINICAL

- Erythema infectiosum (fifth disease): low-grade fever, malaise, myalgias, arthralgias, "slapped cheek" facial rash; erythematous lacelike rash on torso and upper extremities
- Transient aplastic crisis in children and adults with hemoglobinopathy
- Fetal manifestations: severe anemia resulting in high output congestive heart failure, some fetuses with confounding cardiomyopathy; spontaneous abortion; stillbirth
- Ultrasound: fetal hydrops (hematocrit <20%)
  - Risk is directly related to gestational age: if infection before 12 weeks, risk of hydrops is 5% to 10%; if infection between 13 and 20 weeks, risk is 5% or less; if infection beyond 20 weeks, risk is <1%

DIAGNOSIS

- Serologic testing of mother: IgM persists for one to several months and indicates recent infection; IgG persists indefinitely and alone indicates prior infection and immunity

- If confirmed infection, surveillance of fetus for anemia including middle cerebral artery (MCA) Doppler for peak systolic velocity (PSV) for at least 8 weeks after maternal seroconversion

TREATMENT

- If MCA PSV indicates anemia, recommend cordocentesis to evaluate hematocrit and be prepared to proceed with intrauterine blood transfusion if severe anemia is confirmed
- If infant survives intrauterine infection, the prognosis is excellent but there have been case reports of neurologic sequelae

Varicella-Zoster Virus (VZV)

BACKGROUND

- DNA virus, which causes varicella (chickenpox) and herpes zoster infections (shingles)
- Herpes zoster poses essentially no risk to fetus or neonate because patient already has antibody to VZV (however, someone who has not been exposed previously should avoid the lesions for risk of new infection)
- However, varicella poses significant risk to mother, fetus, and neonate
- Transmission via respiratory droplets and direct contact with vesicular lesions

CLINICAL

- Typical rash: disseminated, pruritic, vesicular rash in multiple stages of evolution
- Mild, self-limited in children
- 20% of adults develop pneumonia, 1% encephalitis
- Fetal complications include spontaneous abortion, fetal death, congenital anomalies (risk is <1% at less than 12 weeks' gestation and ~2% weeks 13 to 20)
  - Anomalies include skin scarring, limb hypoplasia, chorioretinitis, microcephaly
- Approximately 40% of infected fetuses will have intrauterine growth restriction
- Neonatal varicella occurs when mother develops acute varicella between 5 days prior to delivery to 2 days after delivery
  - Manifestations: disseminated mucocutaneous lesions, visceral infection, pneumonia, encephalitis; 30% will die without immediate treatment

DIAGNOSIS

- Identification of anti-VZV IgM antibody
- Ultrasound findings: intrauterine growth restriction, microcephaly, ventriculomegaly, echogenic foci in the liver and bowel, limb anomalies, hydrops

TREATMENT

- If susceptible pregnant patient is exposed to varicella, she should receive IM varicella zoster immune globulin (VZIG) or oral acyclovir within 72 to 96 hours

PREVENTION

- Varicella vaccine is a live virus vaccine
- Contraindicated in pregnancy, immunodeficiencies, high dose corticosteroid therapy, untreated tuberculosis, severe systemic illness, allergy to neomycin
- If rash develops after vaccine, small risk of transmission to susceptible patients

Viral Influenza

BACKGROUND

- RNA virus of the myxovirus family
- Antigenic drift allows virus to change enough to evade immune system response and leads to yearly epidemics; profound mutations occur approximately every 20 to 40 years
- Transmitted via respiratory droplets and direct contact (limited extent)
- Most commonly occurs in late fall and winter

CLINICAL

- Ranges in severity from mild illness to life-threatening pneumonia
- Malaise, myalgia, headache, fever, cough, coryza, mild dyspnea, sore throat
- Not associated with spontaneous abortion, stillbirth, congenital anomalies
- Neonates are susceptible if delivered to an acutely ill patient

DIAGNOSIS

- Mainly by clinical picture; also culture the virus from respiratory secretions
- Document serum antibody to influenza A and B

TREATMENT

- Symptomatic relief (bed rest, analgesia, fluids, fever control with acetaminophen)
- Zanamivir or oseltamivir
- If pneumonia, prompt hospitalization with broad spectrum antibiotic coverage for superinfecting bacteria (i.e., *Streptococcus aureus*, *Streptococcus pneumonia*, *Haemophilus influenza*); consider respiratory support

PREVENTION

- Annual vaccination with killed, inactivated virus

UPDATE #6

In the most recent pandemic with H1N1 influenza in 2009, significant morbidity (22% admission to intensive care) and mortality (8%) occurred in pregnant and postpartum women. Regardless of results of rapid antigen testing, prompt evaluation and antiviral treatment of influenza-like illness should be considered in these women. As well, all pregnant women should be encouraged to receive annual influenza vaccinations (Louie et al, 2010).

TABLE 15-2 Serologic Markers of HBV Infection

Clinical Condition	HBsAg	HBsAb	HBcAb Total	HBcAb IgM	HBeAg
Acute infection	Pos	Neg	Pos	Strong Pos	Pos to Neg
Resolving infection	Pos	Neg	Pos	Pos	Neg
Immune status (exposure)	Neg	Pos	Pos	Neg	Neg
Immune status (vaccination)	Neg	Pos	Neg	Neg	Neg
Chronic infection or carrier	Pos	Neg	Pos	Pos or Neg	Pos or Neg

Viral Hepatitis

HEPATITIS A

- Second most common form of viral hepatitis in the United States
- RNA virus transmitted via fecal-oral route
- Clinical: low-grade fever, malaise, poor appetite, right upper quadrant pain and tenderness, jaundice, acholic stools
- Diagnosis: detection of IgM antibody for hepatitis A virus
- Virtually no perinatal transmission
- Prevention: inactivated vaccine

HEPATITIS E

- RNA virus, endemic in developing countries where mortality rate ranges from 10% to 20% (especially maternal mortality rates)
- Hepatitis E infection in women co-infected with HIV has mortality of 100%
- Very similar to hepatitis A in clinical picture; diagnosed via electron microscopy of stool
- Perinatal transmission is rare

HEPATITIS B

- DNA virus transmitted parenterally, via sexual contact, and can be transmitted perinatally
- Approximately 90% of patients who acquire hepatitis B completely clear their infection, <1% die from fulminate hepatitis, ~10% acquire chronic carrier state (Table 15-2, Figure 15-2)
- Chronic carriers may ultimately develop severe chronic liver disease including active hepatitis, cirrhosis, hepatocellular carcinoma; more likely if co-infected with hepatitis D or C
- Without intervention, ~20% of mothers who are seropositive for hepatitis B surface antigen will transmit infection to neonates; ~90% of mothers who are positive for surface antigen and e antigen will transmit infection
- Perinatal infection carries an 85% to 90% risk of persistence or chronic infection, with a 25% to 30% lifetime risk of serious or fatal liver disease
- Immunoprophylaxis for neonates: hepatitis B immune globulin (HBIG) within 12 hours after birth plus vaccination series to begin prior to discharge from hospital

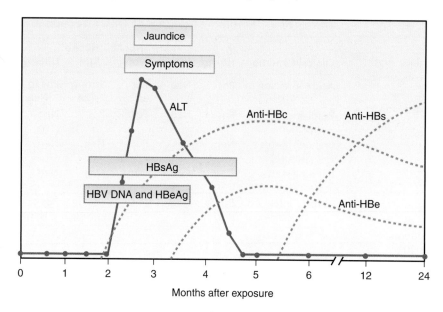

Figure 15-2. Serologic events in acute hepatitis B infection. (Adapted from White DO, Fenner F: *Hepadnaviridae and Deltavirus.* In *Medical Virology*, ed. 4, San Diego, 1994, Academic Press.)

- CDC recommends universal vaccination for all infants as well as offers of the vaccine for all women of reproductive age
- Breast-feeding is encouraged if mother is HbsAg positive and infant receiving HBIG and vaccines; no data regarding breast-feeding if patient is HBeAg positive

HEPATITIS D

- RNA virus that is dependent on co-infection with B for replication
- Chronic hepatitis D produces severe disease with 70% to 80% of patients developing cirrhosis and portal hypertension with a more rapid progression; mortality approaches 25%
- Perinatal transmission can occur, but immunoprophylaxis for B is highly effective against D as well

HEPATITIS C

- RNA virus that is transmitted parenterally, via sexual contact, and perinatally
- Often asymptomatic initially
- Diagnosis by serology: screen with EIA, confirm with recombinant immunoblot assay (RIBA)
- If RNA load is low and patient not co-infected with HIV, perinatal transmission is <5%
- If RNA load is high or co-infected with HIV, perinatal transmission is 25%
- May consider elective cesarean section if viral load is high, but no definitive recommendations at this time
- Breast-feeding is not contraindicated

HEPATITIS G

- RNA virus related to C (more prevalent, less virulent)
- Usually asymptomatic but can cause chronic carrier state; perinatal transmission can occur, but no significant infections in mother or baby have been seen

SUGGESTED READINGS

General Review

American College of Obstetricians and Gynecologists: ACOG practice bulletin no. 20: perinatal viral and parasitic infections, *Obstet Gynecol* 96(3), Sep 2000.

American College of Obstetricians and Gynecologists: ACOG practice bulletin no. 12: intrauterine growth restriction, *Obstet Gynecol* 95(1), Jan 2000.

Duff P, Sweet R, Edwards R: Maternal and fetal infections. In Creasy R, Resnik R, Iams J, editors: *Creasy & Resnick's maternal-fetal medicine: principles and practice*, ed 6, Philadelphia, 2009, Saunders/Elsevier, pp 739–795.

Toxoplasmosis

Wallon M, Franck J, Thulliez P, et al: Accuracy of real-time polymerase chain reaction for Toxoplasma gondii in amniotic fluid, *Obstet Gynecol* 115(4):727–733, 2010.

Cytomegalovirus

Duff P: Immunotherapy for congenital cytomegalovirus infection, *N Engl J Med* 353(13):1402–1404, 2005.

Duff P, Barth WH Jr, Post MD: Case records of the Massachusetts General Hospital: case 4-2009: a 39-year-old pregnant woman with fever after a trip to Africa, *N Engl J Med* 360(5):508–516, 2009.

Guerra B, Simonazzi G, Puccetti C, et al: Ultrasound prediction of symptomatic congenital cytomegalovirus infection, *Am J Obstet Gynecol* 198(4):380.e1–e7, 2008.

Nigro G, Adler SP, La Torre R, Best AM: Congenital Cytomegalovirus Collaborating Group: Passive immunization during pregnancy for congenital cytomegalovirus infection, *N Engl J Med* 353(13):1350–1362, 2005.

Pass RF, Zhang C, Evans A, et al: Vaccine prevention of maternal cytomegalovirus infection, *N Engl J Med* 360(12):1191–1199, 2009.

Herpes Simplex Virus

American College of Obstetricians and Gynecologists Committee on Practice Bulletins: ACOG practice bulletin no 82: clinical management guidelines for obstetrician-gynecologists: management of herpes in pregnancy, *Obstet Gynecol* 109:1489–1498, 2007.

Brown ZA, Gardella C, Wald A, et al: Genital herpes complicating pregnancy, *Obstet Gynecol* 106(5):845–856, 2005.

Group B Streptococcus

Edwards RK, Novak-Weekley SM, Koty PP, et al: Rapid group B streptococci screening using a real-time polymerase chain reaction assay, *Obstet Gynecol* 111(6):1335–1341, 2008.

Gibbs RS, Schrag S, Schuchat A: Perinatal infections due to group B streptococci, *Obstet Gynecol* 104(5 Pt 1):1062–1076, 2004.

Jamie WE, Edwards RK, Duff P: Vaginal-perianal compared with vaginal-rectal cultures for identification of group B streptococci, *Obstet Gynecol* 104(5 Pt 1):1058–1061, 2004.

Verani JR, McGee L, Schraq SJ, et al: Prevention of perinatal group B streptococcal disease—revised guidelines from CDC, 2010, *MMWR Recomm Rep* 59(RR-10):1–36, 2010.

Human Immunodeficiency Virus

American College of Obstetrics and Gynecology Committee on Obstetric Practice: ACOG committee opinion no. 418: prenatal and perinatal human immunodeficiency virus testing: expanded recommendations, *Obstet Gynecol* 112(3):739–742, 2008.

Chou R, Smits AK, Huffman LH, et al: Prenatal screening for HIV: a review of the evidence for the U.S. Preventive Services Task Force, *Ann Intern Med* 143(1):38–54, 2005.

Louis J, Landon MB, Gersnoviez RJ, et al: Perioperative morbidity and mortality among human immunodeficiency virus infected women undergoing cesarean delivery, *Obstet Gynecol* 110(2 Pt 1):385–390, 2007.

Parvovirus

Nagel HT, de Haan TR, Vandenbussche FP, et al: Long-term outcome after fetal transfusion for hydrops associated with parvovirus B19 infection, *Obstet Gynecol* 109(1):42–47, 2007.

Influenza

Louie J, Acosta M, Jamieson DJ, et al: Severe 2009 H1N1 influenza in pregnant and postpartum women in California, *N Engl J Med* 362(1):27–35, 2010.

Hepatitis

American College of Obstetricians and Gynecologists: ACOG practice bulletin no. 86: viral hepatitis in pregnancy, *Obstet Gynecol* 110(4):941–956, 2007.

White DO, Fenner F, Hepadnaviridae, Deltavirus. In: *Medical virology*, ed 4, San Diego, 1994, Academic Press, pp 359-379.

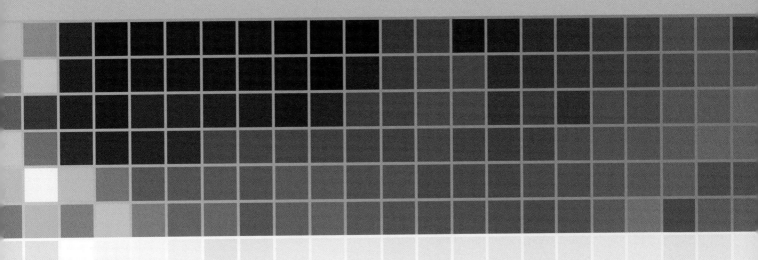

Childbirth: Intrapartum Care and Puerperium

Chapter 16

Intrapartum Fetal Monitoring

ANDREW D. HULL • KRISTEN H. QUINN

KEY UPDATES

1 The recommendations of the 2008 National Institute of Child Health and Human Development (NICHD), American College of Obstetricians and Gynecologists (ACOG), and Society for Maternal-Fetal Medicine (SMFM) workshop on electronic fetal monitoring (EFM) form the basis of ACOG Practice Bulletin 106 and together constitute the contemporary interpretation and management of fetal heart rate monitoring in the United States.

2 EFM has poor inter- and intra-observer reliability and a high false positive rate for the detection of fetal compromise.

3 A full description of an EFM tracing requires both qualitative and quantitative assessment of:

 i Uterine contractions

 ii Baseline fetal heart rate (FHR)

 iii Baseline FHR variability

 iv Presence of accelerations

 v Periodic or episodic decelerations

 vi Changes or trends of FHR over time

4 FHR tracings should be categorized as category I, II, or III according to the new Three-Tier FHR Interpretation System.

5 Category I FHR tracings are normal; category II tracings are indeterminate and require reevaluation, surveillance, and reevaluation; and category III tracings are abnormal, require prompt evaluation and treatment, and mandate delivery if they do not resolve.

6 Both regional and parenteral obstetric anesthesia may lead to transient changes in FHR tracings.

7 A fetal scalp blood sample for measuring pH or lactate may be helpful in the management of a labor with a category III fetal heart tracing.

8 A fetal heart rate acceleration in response to fetal scalp stimulation in the presence of a nonreassuring fetal heart tracing suggests that the fetus may not be acidotic, but close surveillance should be continued.

9 There is no evidence to support the safety and efficacy of vibroacoustic stimulation used to assess fetal well-being in labor in the presence of a nonreassuring fetal heart tracing.

10 The use of fetal pulse oximetry does not improve neonatal outcomes or reduce the cesarean section rate.

11 The use of ST segment analysis (STAN) as an adjunct to conventional cardiotocography appears to reduce the rate of neonatal encephalopathy and may reduce acidosis at birth.

12 Computer-assisted interpretation of fetal heart tracing is an area of promising research.

13 The use of fetal Doppler velocimetry in labor does not improve neonatal outcomes or reduce the cesarean section rate.

Electronic Fetal Monitoring

GUIDELINES

> **UPDATE #1**
>
> The recommendations of the 2008 NICHD, ACOG, and SMFM workshop on electronic fetal monitoring (EFM) form the basis of ACOG Practice Bulletin 106 and together constitute the contemporary interpretation and management of fetal heart rate monitoring in the United States (ACOG Practice Bulletin No. 106, 2009).

- Since the late 1990s or so, the National Institute of Child Health and Human Development (NICHD) has organized a series of workshops intended to develop standardized definitions for fetal heart rate (FHR) tracings and to generate recommendations for their interpretation.
- Guidelines for FHR interpretation have been published by national bodies in the UK, Royal College of Obstetricians and Gynaecologists (RCOG) (National Collaborating Centre for Women's and Children's Health, 2011) and Canada, Society of Obstetricians and Gynaecologists of Canada (SOGC) (Liston et al, 2007). These include classification of FHR tracings as normal; suspicious, pathologic, and normal; and atypical and abnormal, respectively.
- Individual authors have studied more complex FHR grading systems, but they have not been widely adopted (Parer et al, 2007).
- In 2008 the NICHD, the American College of Obstetricians and Gynecologists (ACOG), and the Society for Maternal-Fetal Medicine (SMFM) convened a joint workshop on electronic fetal monitoring. The workshop had three distinct aims:
  - To review and update the FHR pattern categories from the previous workshops
  - To assess all existing FHR classification and interpretation systems and recommend a system for general usage in the United States
  - To make recommendations for research priorities in EFM
- The published findings of the 2008 workshop (Macones et al, 2008) form the basis of the 2009 ACOG Practice Bulletin on Intrapartum Fetal Heart Rate Monitoring (ACOG Practice Bulletin No. 106, 2009).

BACKGROUND AND BASIC PRINCIPLES

> **UPDATE #2**
>
> EFM has poor inter- and intraobserver reliability and a high false positive rate for the detection of fetal compromise (ACOG Practice Bulletin No. 106, 2009).

- More than 85% of laboring women undergo EFM
- External monitoring is performed using a Doppler ultrasound device
- Internal monitoring uses a fetal spiral electrode attached directly to the fetus
- FHR monitoring is used to indirectly assess fetal oxygenation
- Despite its widespread use, FHR monitoring is of uncertain efficacy
- EFM has poor inter- and intraobserver reliability and a high false-positive rate for the detection of fetal compromise

- A meta-analysis of EFM versus intermittent auscultation of FHR showed the following results:
  - EFM increased the overall cesarean section rate and the rate for delivery for abnormal FHR
  - EFM increased the operative vaginal delivery rate
  - EFM did not reduce perinatal mortality
  - EFM did reduce the risk of neonatal seizures
  - EFM did not reduce cerebral palsy rates
- Given this information, either EFM or intermittent auscultation is acceptable for low-risk patients
- High-risk patients have not been studied with intermittent auscultation and should receive EFM
- Intermittent auscultation requires effectively one-to-one care to ensure adequate observations
- The optimal strategy for intermittent auscultation is unknown, but a frequency of every 15 minutes in the first stage of labor and every 5 minutes in the second stage seems reasonable

NEW DEFINITIONS FOR EFM

> **UPDATE #3**
>
> A full description of an EFM tracing requires both qualitative and quantitative assessment of the following:
> - Uterine contractions
> - Baseline FHR
> - Baseline FHR variability
> - Presence of accelerations
> - Periodic or episodic decelerations
> - Changes or trends of FHR over time (ACOG Practice Bulletin No. 106, 2009)

- Uterine activity is a key component in the interpretation of EFM; key definitions are given in Table 16-1
- The terms *hyperstimulation* and *hypercontractility* should be abandoned
- The new EFM definitions are listed in Table 16-2
- Baseline must be for a minimum of 2 minutes in any 10-minute segment; if the baseline for a segment cannot be determined, the prior 10-minute segment should be used
  - Normal 110 to 160 beats per minute (bpm)
  - Tachycardia >160 bpm
  - Bradycardia <110 bpm
- Baseline variability
  - Absent: amplitude range undetectable
  - Minimal: amplitude range detectable but ≤5 bpm
  - Moderate: (normal) amplitude range 6 to 25 bpm
  - Marked: amplitude range >25 bpm

TABLE 16-1   **Terminology Used to Describe Normal and Abnormal Uterine Activity**

Term	
Normal activity	≤5 contractions every 10 minutes averaged over 30 minutes
Tachysystole	≥5 contractions every 10 minutes averaged over 30 minutes
	Tachysystole applies to both spontaneous and induced labor
	Tachysystole should always be defined by the presence or absence of FHR decelerations

TABLE 16-2 EFM Definitions and Descriptions Based on 2008 NICHD Working Group Findings

Pattern	Definition
Baseline	Mean FHR to nearest 5 bpm over a 10-minute segment *excluding* periodic or episodic changes, periods of marked FHR variability, and segments of baseline that differ by >25 bpm
Baseline variability	Fluctuations in the baseline FHR that are irregular in amplitude and frequency, quantitated as the amplitude of the peak to trough in bpm
Acceleration	A visually apparent abrupt increase in FHR—must reach peak in <30 seconds For GA ≥32 weeks accelerations must be ≥15 bpm above baseline for ≥15 seconds and <2 minutes from onset to return to baseline For GA <32 weeks accelerations must be ≥10 bpm above baseline for ≥10 seconds and <2 minutes from onset to return to baseline
Deceleration	Late, early, or variable (see Table 16-3)
Sinusoidal pattern	A specific visually apparent smooth sine wave–like undulating pattern in FHR baseline with a cycle frequency of 3 to 5/min that persists for ≥20 mins

GA, Gestational age.

TABLE 16-3 Characteristics of Decelerations Based on 2008 NICHD Working Group Findings

Deceleration	Characteristics
Late *utroplacenta insuff.*	Visually apparent usually symmetrical gradual decrease and return of the FHR associated with a uterine contraction A gradual FHR decrease is defined as from the onset to the FHR nadir of ≥30 secs The decrease in FHR is calculated from the onset to the nadir of the deceleration The deceleration is delayed in timing, with the nadir of the deceleration occurring after the peak of the contraction In most cases, the onset, nadir, and recovery of the deceleration occur after the beginning, peak, and ending of the contraction, respectively
Early *Head*	Visually apparent usually symmetrical gradual decrease and return of the FHR associated with a uterine contraction A gradual FHR decrease is defined as from the onset to the FHR nadir of ≥30 secs The decrease in FHR is calculated from the onset to the nadir of the deceleration The nadir of the deceleration occurs at the same time as the peak of the contraction In most cases, the onset, nadir, and recovery of the deceleration are coincident with the beginning, peak, and ending of the contraction, respectively
Variable *Cord*	Visually apparent abrupt decrease in FHR An abrupt FHR decrease is defined as from the onset of the deceleration to the beginning of the FHR nadir of <30 secs The decrease in FHR is calculated from the onset to the nadir of the deceleration The decrease in FHR is ≥15 bpm, lasting ≥15 secs and < 2 mins in duration When variable decelerations are associated with uterine contractions, their onset, depth, and duration commonly vary with successive contractions
Prolonged	Visually apparent decrease in the FHR below baseline Decrease in FHR from the baseline that is ≥15 bpm or lasting ≥2 mins but <10 mins in duration If a deceleration lasts >10 mins it is a baseline change

- Acceleration
  - A prolonged acceleration lasts ≥2 minutes and <10 minutes
  - An acceleration lasting ≥10 minutes is a baseline change
- Decelerations (see Table 16-3).
- Decelerations are recurrent if they occur with ≥50% of uterine contractions in any 20-minute window
- Decelerations are intermittent if they occur with <50% of uterine contractions in any 20-minute window

INTERPRETATION AND CLASSIFICATION OF FHR PATTERNS

UPDATE #4

FHR tracings should be categorized as category I, II or III according to the new Three-Tier FHR Interpretation System (ACOG Practice Bulletin No. 106, 2009).

- Any system of FHR interpretation should be simple to use and apply to clinical practice
- FHR responses are dynamic and change over time; FHR tracings may move from one category to another and require constant review
- FHR tracings should be interpreted in the context of clinical events
- FHR accelerations reliably predict the absence of fetal metabolic acidemia
- The absence of accelerations does *not* reliably predict fetal acidemia
- Moderate FHR variability reliably predicts the absence of fetal metabolic acidemia at the time it is observed
- Minimal or absent FHR variability *alone* does *not* reliably predict fetal metabolic acidemia or hypoxemia

TABLE 16-4 Three-Tiered Fetal Heart Rate Interpretation System Based on 2008 NICHD Working Group Findings

Category I
Include *all* of the following:
Baseline rate 110 to 160 bpm
Baseline FHR variability: moderate
Late or variable decelerations: absent
Early decelerations: present or absent
Accelerations: present or absent

Category II
Includes all FHR tracings not categorized as category I or III. They may make up a substantial proportion of clinical cases. Examples of category II FHR tracings include any of the following:

Baseline Rate
Bradycardia not accompanied by absent baseline variability
Tachycardia

Baseline FHR Variability
Minimal baseline variability
Absent baseline variability with no recurrent decelerations
Marked baseline variability

Accelerations
Absence of induced accelerations after fetal stimulation

Periodic or Episodic Decelerations
Recurrent variable decelerations accompanied by minimal or moderate baseline variability
Prolonged deceleration >2 mins but <10 mins
Recurrent late decelerations with moderate baseline variability
Variable decelerations with other characteristics such as slow return to baseline, overshoots, or "shoulders"

Category III
Either of the following:
Absent baseline FHR variability and any of the following:
 — Recurrent late decelerations
 — Recurrent variable decelerations
 — Bradycardia
OR
Sinusoidal FHR pattern

- FHR tracings should be reviewed every 30 minutes in the first stage of labor and every 15 minutes in the second stage of labor in uncomplicated pregnancies
- FHR tracings should be reviewed every 15 minutes in the first stage of labor and every 5 minutes in the second stage of labor in pregnancies complicated by intrauterine growth restriction (IUGR), preeclampsia, or other significant fetal or maternal disorders
- The new Three-Tier FHR Interpretation System should be used to categorize all FHR tracings (Table 16-4)

RESPONSE TO FHR CATEGORIES

UPDATE #5
Category I FHR tracings are normal; category II tracings are indeterminate and require surveillance, and reevaluation; and category III tracings are abnormal, require prompt evaluation and treatment, and mandate delivery if they do not resolve (ACOG Practice Bulletin No. 106, 2009).

- Category I FHR tracings (Figures 16-1 and 16-2) are reassuring, are predictive of normal fetal acid-base balance, and do not require any further action other than continued surveillance
- Category II FHR tracings (Figures 16-3 and 16-4) are indeterminate, and they do not predict abnormal fetal acid-base balance reliably; further tests to evaluate fetal well-being (such as scalp stimulation) may be indicated, or resuscitative measures may be employed
- Category III FHR tracings (Figures 16-5, 16-6, and 16-7) are abnormal; they are associated with abnormal fetal acid-base balance; they require prompt evaluation
- Maneuvers that may help resolve category III FHR tracings are shown in Table 16-5
- Category III FHR tracings that do not respond to such measures mandate delivery

MEDICATIONS AND FHR TRACING

UPDATE #6
Both regional and parenteral obstetric anesthesia may lead to transient changes in FHR tracings (ACOG Practice Bulletin No. 106, 2009).

- Epidural anesthesia may lead to postural hypotension, producing FHR tracing abnormalities that can be corrected by administering a maternal fluid bolus, ephedrine, or both
- Independent of this effect, the local anesthetics and narcotics used in epidurals may produce other transient FHR tracing abnormalities
- Parenteral analgesics may produce similar effects at a similar rate
- Combined spinal-epidural anesthesia is more likely to cause FHR abnormalities than epidural anesthesia
- Other medications produce a variety of effects on FHR tracings (Table 16-6)

Fetal Scalp Blood Sampling

UPDATE #7
A fetal scalp blood sample for measuring pH or lactate may be helpful in the management of a labor with a category III fetal heart tracing (Young et al, 1980).

A sample of fetal scalp blood can be obtained by scalp puncture and be analyzed for pH or lactate:
- A scalp pH of ≤7.21 or less predicts a cord pH of ≤7 with a sensitivity of 36% and a positive predictive value of 9%
- A scalp pH of ≤7.21 or less predicts hypoxic-ischemic encephalopathy with a sensitivity of 50% and a positive predictive value of 3%
- A scalp pH ≥7.21 has a negative predictive value for hypoxic-ischemic encephalopathy of 97% to 99% (Kruger et al, 1999)
- Scalp blood lactate levels provide similar predictive value to pH measurements
- Scalp blood pH measurement may reduce the number of cesarean sections performed for "fetal distress"

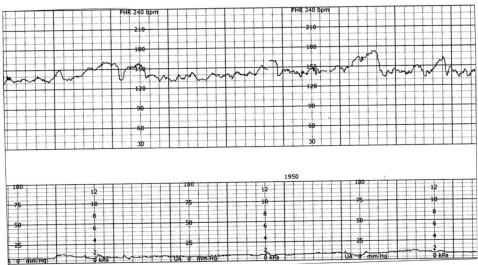

Figure 16-1. Category I FHR tracing with baseline rate 125 bpm, moderate variability, accelerations and no decelerations.

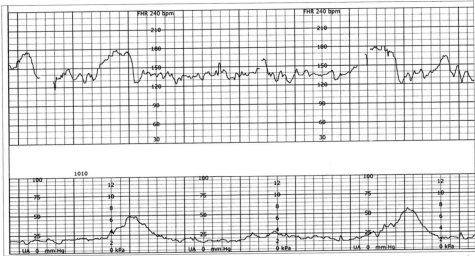

Figure 16-2. Category I FHR tracing with baseline rate 140 bpm, moderate variability, accelerations and no decelerations.

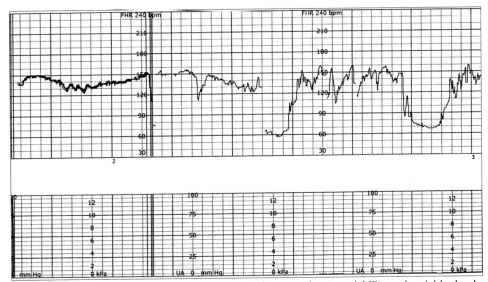

Figure 16-3. Category II FHR tracing with baseline rate 140 bpm, moderate variability and variable decelerations.

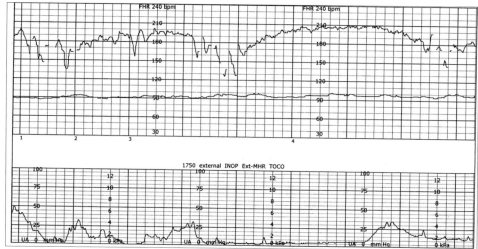

Figure 16-4. Category II FHR tracing with baseline tachycardia 190 bpm, moderate variability and variable decelerations.

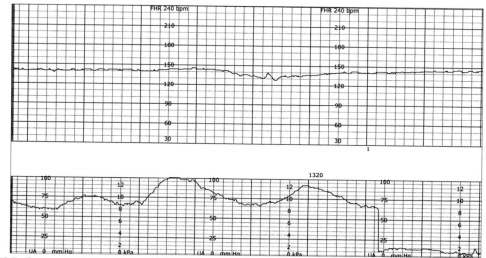

Figure 16-5. Category III FHR tracing with baseline rate 140 bpm, absent to minimal variability and late decelerations.

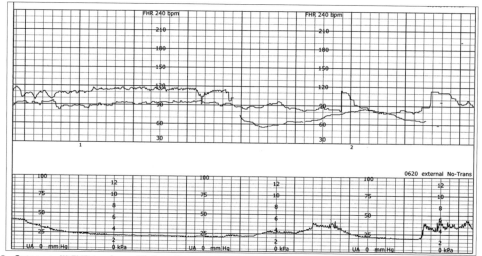

Figure 16-6. Category III FHR tracing with baseline rate 110 bpm, absent to minimal variability and terminal bradycardia.

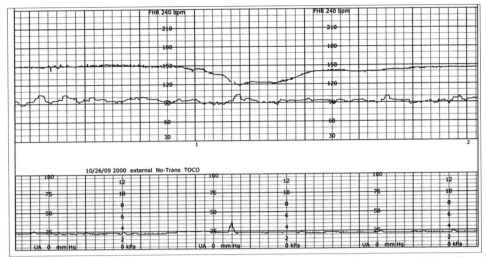

Figure 16-7. Category III FHR tracing with baseline 150 bpm, absent variability and variable deceleration.

TABLE 16-5 Management of Category III and II Tracings

Action

Cervical examination to check for cord prolapsed or rapid cervical dilation or descent of the fetal head

Discontinue any oxytocics

Change maternal position to obviate postural hypotension

Treat hypotension with fluid bolus, ephedrine, or both, especially if regional anesthesia is in use

Evaluate and treat tachysystole with terbutaline

Consider amnioinfusion for recurrent variable decelerations

- Scalp blood sampling has almost disappeared in U.S. practice, is not even available in many tertiary centers, and has largely been replaced by scalp stimulation tests (Goodwin et al, 1994)

Scalp Stimulation

> **UPDATE #8**
>
> A fetal heart rate acceleration in response to fetal scalp stimulation in the presence of a nonreassuring fetal heart tracing suggests that the fetus may not be acidotic, but close surveillance should be continued (Clark et al, 1984).

- Several authors noted that fetuses undergoing scalp pH measurement who had a fetal heart rate acceleration in response to scalp puncture were likely to have a normal pH
- Conversely, those not showing a fetal heart rate acceleration in response to scalp puncture were more likely to be acidotic (pH <7.2) (Spencer, 1991)
- A later study showed that 15 seconds of firm digital scalp stimulation produced fetal heart accelerations only in fetuses subsequently shown to have scalp pH >7.2; fetuses with scalp pH <7.2 did not show fetal heart rate accelerations (Elimian et al, 1997)
- A meta-analysis of published studies of scalp stimulation concluded that scalp puncture, scalp stimulation with

TABLE 16-6 Effects of Drugs on FHR Tracing

Medication	Effect on FHR Tracing
Narcotics	Decrease in variability Decrease in accelerations
Butorphanol	Transient sinusoidal FHR pattern
Cocaine	Decreased long-term variability
Betamethasone	Decrease in FHR variability with beta-methasone
Magnesium sulfate	Decrease in short-term variability, decreased accelerations
Terbutaline	Increase in baseline FHR Increase in tachycardia
Zidovudine	No effect

From American College of Obstetricians and Gynecologists: ACOG practice bulletin no. 106: intrapartum fetal heart rate monitoring: nomenclature. Interpretation, and general management principles, *Obstet Gynecol* 114:192-202, 2009.

an Allis clamp, and digital scalp stimulation had similar predictive values for both the presence and absence of acidemia (Table 16-7); the authors further stated that "The very low negative likelihood ratios warrant the use of these tests when a non-reassuring intrapartum FHR pattern appears. Because these tests are less than perfect, caution is advised; careful continued monitoring with repeat testing during the course of labor should be performed as long as suspicious FHR patterns persist. Fetal scalp pH should be determined whenever possible after a positive stimulation test (lack of acceleration)" (Skupski et al, 2002)

Vibroacoustic Stimulation

> **UPDATE #9**
>
> There is no evidence to support the safety and efficacy of vibroacoustic stimulation used to assess fetal well-being in labor in the presence of a nonreassuring fetal heart tracing (Lin et al, 2001).

- In nonlaboring patients, fetal vibroacoustic stimulation using an electrical artificial larynx buzzer has been used to

TABLE 16-7 Positive and Negative Likelihood Ratios (LR) and Confidence Intervals (CI) for Different Techniques of Scalp Stimulation in Predicting Presence of Fetal Academia (Positive Test) or Absence of Academia (Negative Test)

Type of scalp stimulation	Positive Test (no acceleration in FHR after stimulation)		Negative Test (acceleration in FHR after stimulation)	
	LR	CI	LR	CI
Scalp puncture	8.54	1.28-56.96	0.12	0.02-0.78
Allis clamp	10.4	1.47-73.61	0.1	0.01-0.68
Digital stimulation	15.68	3.22-76.24	0.06	0.01-0.31

elicit a fetal heart acceleration as part of an antenatal fetal health assessment

- There are no randomized studies of the use of vibroacoustic stimulation to assess fetal well being in labor (East et al, 2005)
- Fetal heart rate responses to vibroacoustic stimulation do not provide reliable evidence of fetal well-being in the presence of a non-reassuring fetal heart tracing
- Fetal heart rate accelerations in response to vibroacoustic stimulation in the second stage of labor do not reliably predict a lack of acidosis at delivery (Anyaegbunam et al, 1994)

Fetal Pulse Oximetry

UPDATE #10

The use of fetal pulse oximetry does not improve neonatal outcomes or reduce the cesarean section rate (East et al, 2007).

- Fetal pulse oximetry allows continuous measurement of the oxygen saturation of fetal hemoglobin using an optical sensor placed on the fetus
- Reliable measurements may be obtained in 70% to 90% of laboring women for 50% to 88% of their labors
- The lower limit for fetal oxygen saturation is generally accepted to be 30%, although the normal range of oxygen saturation of the cord blood of healthy infants at delivery ranges from 5% to 75%
- Saturation levels below 30% lasting >2 minutes are said to be associated with an increased risk of poor fetal outcome
- A Cochrane review has compared the effectiveness and safety of fetal pulse oximetry plus cardiotocography to cardiotocography; five trials with a total of 7424 pregnancies were studied; there were no significant differences in the overall cesarean section rate between the two groups; additionally, neonatal outcomes were not improved by the use of fetal pulse oximetry
- Some authorities have expressed concern over the safety of fetal pulse oximetry; there have been several reports in the literature of acidotic neonates who did not have a documented fetal pulse oximetry of less than 30% (East et al, 2007)
- Sales of fetal pulse oximetry equipment in the United States were discontinued in 2005

Fetal Electrocardiogram (EKG) and ST Segment Analysis (STAN)

UPDATE #11

The use of ST segment analysis (STAN) as an adjunct to conventional cardiotocography appears to reduce the rate of neonatal encephalopathy and may reduce acidosis at birth (Neilson, 2006).

- The fetal EKG has been evaluated for the prediction of intrapartum fetal acidemia; studies have focused on the PR/RR ratio, T/QRS ratio, and, most successfully, the ST waveform
- ST waveform changes can indicate that the fetal heart is utilizing anaerobic metabolism (increased T wave amplitude) or when the heart is not fully capable of responding to stress (ST segment depression)
- A Cochrane review gave some support for the use of fetal ST waveform analysis together with cardiotocography during labor; compared to conventional monitoring, STAN was associated with fewer cases of neonatal encephalopathy (RR 0.37, 95% CI 0.14, 1.00) and fewer operative deliveries (RR 0.89, 95% CI 0.81, 0.98). There were no significant differences in neonates with metabolic acidosis at birth, cesarean section rates, Apgar scores less than 7 at 5 minutes, or admission to the special care unit (Neilson, 2006)
- There are strict guidelines for the use of the commercially available monitoring device, STAN (S31 Fetal Heart Monitor; Neoventa Medical AB, Mölndal, Sweden), which must be followed closely to avoid false reassurance from the ST segment analysis
- The device has been tested in the United States with similar results to those obtained overseas
- A recent Swedish prospective study of STAN usage in Sweden showed a reduction in the cord metabolic acidosis rate from 0.72% to 0.06%. (Norén et al, 2010)

Computer-Aided Analysis of Fetal Heart Tracing

UPDATE #12

Computer-assisted interpretation of fetal heart tracing is an area of promising research (Costa et al, 2010).

- Interpretation of intrapartum fetal heart rate tracings is subject to high rates of inter- and intraobserver variability

- Normal reassuring tracings are more likely to be similarly graded
- Retrospective analysis of fetal heart tracings is often confounded by knowledge of outcome
- There have been numerous attempts to develop computer-aided analysis of fetal heart tracing; there is some evidence that such systems will reduce inter and intraobserver variation (Costa et al, 2010)
- Newer techniques offer promising hints of things to come, but as yet no systems are ready for use outside of a research and development setting

Fetal Doppler Velocimetry

UPDATE #13
The use of fetal Doppler velocimetry in labor does not improve neonatal outcomes or reduce the cesarean section rate (Farrell et al, 1999).

- A meta-analysis of eight studies involving 2700 pregnancies in which fetal umbilical artery Doppler was used intrapartum showed poor predictive value for low Apgar scores, fetal heart rate abnormality in labor, acidotic cord pH at delivery, and risk of cesarean section (Farrell et al, 1999)

SUGGESTED READINGS

Electronic Fetal Monitoring

Guidelines

American College of Obstetricians and Gynecologists: ACOG practice bulletin no. 106: intrapartum fetal heart rate monitoring: nomenclature, interpretation, and general management principles, *Obstet Gynecol* 114:192–202, 2009.

American College of Obstetricians and Gynecologists: ACOG practice bulletin no. 116: management of intrapartum fetal heart rate tracings, *Obstet Gynecol* 116(5):1232–1240, 2010.

Liston RL, Sawchuck D, Young D: Society of Obstetricians and Gynaecologists of Canada: Fetal health surveillance: antepartum and intrapartum consensus guideline, *J Obstet Gynaecol Can* 29(9 Suppl 4):S3–S56, 2007.

Macones GA, Hankins GD, Spong CY, et al: The 2008 National Institute of Child Health and Human Development workshop report on electronic fetal monitoring: update on definitions, interpretation, and research guidelines, *Obstet Gynecol* 112(3):661–666, 2008.

National Collaborating Centre for Women's and Children's Health: *Intrapartum care: care of healthy women and their babies during childbirth* (website). www.nice.org.uk/nicemedia/live/11837/36275/36275.pdf Accessed July 10, 2011.

Parer JT, Ikeda T: A framework for standardized management of intrapartum fetal heart rate patterns, *Am J Obstet Gynecol* 197(1):26.e1-e6, 2007.

Background and Basic Principles

Cunningham F, Leveno K, Bloom S, et al, editors: Intrapartum assessment. In *Williams obstetrics*, ed 23, New York, 2009, McGraw-Hill Professional, pp 410-443.

Fetal Scalp Blood Sampling

Goodwin TM, Milner-Masterson L, Paul RH: Elimination of fetal scalp blood sampling on a large clinical service, *Obstet Gynecol* 83(6):971–974, 1994.

Kruger K, Hallberg B, Blennow M, et al: Predictive value of fetal scalp blood lactate concentration and pH as markers of neurologic disability, *Am J Obstet Gynecol* 181(5 Pt 1):1072–1078, 1999.

Wiberg-Itzel E, Lipponer C, Norman M, et al: Determination of pH or lactate in fetal scalp blood in management of intrapartum fetal distress: randomised controlled multicentre trial, *BMJ* 336(7656):1284–1287, 2008.

Young DC, Gray JH, Luther ER, et al: Fetal scalp blood pH sampling: its value in an active obstetric unit, *Am J Obstet Gynecol* 136(3):276–281, 1980.

Scalp Stimulation

Clark SL, Gimovsky ML, Miller FC: The scalp stimulation test: a clinical alternative to fetal scalp blood sampling, *Am J Obstet Gynecol* 148(3):274–277, 1984.

Elimian A, Figueroa R, Tejani N: Intrapartum assessment of fetal well-being: a comparison of scalp stimulation with scalp blood pH sampling, *Obstet Gynecol* 89(3):373–376, 1997.

Skupski DW, Rosenberg CR, Eglinton GS: Intrapartum fetal stimulation tests: a meta-analysis, *Obstet Gynecol* 99(1):129–134, 2002.

Spencer JA: Predictive value of a fetal heart rate acceleration at the time of fetal blood sampling in labour, *J Perinat Med* 19(3):207–215, 1991.

Vibroacoustic Stimulation

Anyaegbunam AM, Ditchik A, Stoessel R, et al: Vibroacoustic stimulation of the fetus entering the second stage of labor, *Obstet Gynecol* 83(6):963–966, 1994.

East CE, Smyth R, Leader LR, et al: Vibroacoustic stimulation for fetal assessment in labour in the presence of a nonreassuring fetal heart rate trace, *Cochrane Database Syst Rev*(2):CD004664, 2005.

Lin CC, Vassallo B, Mittendorf R: Is intrapartum vibroacoustic stimulation an effective predictor of fetal acidosis? *J Perinat Med* 29(6):506–512, 2001.

Fetal Pulse Oximetry

Arikan GM, Scholz HS, Petru E, et al: Cord blood oxygen saturation in vigorous infants at birth: what is normal? *BJOG* 107(8):987–994, 2000.

Bloom SL, Spong CY, Thorn E, et al: Fetal pulse oximetry and cesarean delivery, *N Engl J Med* 355(21):2195–2202, 2006.

East CE, Chan FY, Colditz PB, et al: Fetal pulse oximetry for fetal assessment in labour, *Cochrane Database Syst Rev*(2):CD004075, 2007.

Tekin A, Ozkan S, Caliskan E, et al: Fetal pulse oximetry: correlation with intrapartum fetal heart rate patterns and neonatal outcome, *J Obstet Gynaecol Res* 34(5):824–831, 2008.

Fetal EKG and ST Segment Analysis (STAN)

Amer-Wahlin I, Arulkumaran S, Hagberg H, et al: Fetal electrocardiogram: ST waveform analysis in intrapartum surveillance, *BJOG* 114(10): 1191–1193, 2007.

Devoe ID, Ross M, Wilde C, et al: United States multicenter clinical usage study of the STAN 21 electronic fetal monitoring system, *Am J Obstet Gynecol* 195(3):729–734, 2006.

Luttkus AK, Noren H, Stupin JH, et al: Fetal scalp pH and ST analysis of the fetal ECG as an adjunct to CTG. A multi-center, observational study, *J Perinat Med* 32(6):486–494, 2004.

Neilson JP: Fetal electrocardiogram (ECG) for fetal monitoring during labour, *Cochrane Database Syst Rev*(3):CD000116, 2006.

Norén H, Carlsson A: Reduced prevalence of metabolic acidosis at birth: an analysis of established STAN usage in the total population of deliveries in a Swedish district hospital, *Am J Obstet Gynecol* 202(6):546.e1-e7, 2010.

Westerhuis ME, Kwee A, van Ginkel AA, et al: Limitations of ST analysis in clinical practice: three cases of intrapartum metabolic acidosis, *BJOG* 114(10):1194–1201, 2007.

Computer-Aided Analysis of Fetal Heart Tracing

Costa MA, Ayres-de-Campos D, Machado AP, et al: Comparison of a computer system evaluation of intrapartum cardiotocographic events and a consensus of clinicians, *J Perinat Med* 38(2):191–195, 2010.

Devoe L, Golde S, Kilman Y, et al: A comparison of visual analyses of intrapartum fetal heart rate tracings according to the new national institute of child health and human development guidelines with computer analyses by an automated fetal heart rate monitoring system, *Am J Obstet Gynecol* 183(2):361–366, 2000.

Salamalekis E, Hintipas E, Salloum I, et al: Computerized analysis of fetal heart rate variability using the matching pursuit technique as an indicator of fetal hypoxia during labor, *J Matern Fetal Neonatal Med* 19(3):165–169, 2006.

Taylor GM, Mires GJ, Abel EW, et al: The development and validation of an algorithm for real-time computerised fetal heart rate monitoring in labour, *BJOG* 107(9):1130–1137, 2000.

Fetal Doppler Velocimetry

Farrell T, Chien PF, Gordon A: Intrapartum umbilical artery Doppler velocimetry as a predictor of adverse perinatal outcome: a systematic review, *BJOG* 106(8):783–792, 1999.

Chapter 17

Management of Labor

STEPHEN HEBERT

KEY UPDATES

1 Classical labor curves of Friedman may underestimate the times of normal labor in current practice.

2 Evidence does not support routine artificial rupture of membranes (AROM) in normal spontaneous labor.

3 Neuraxial anesthesia may be given early without increasing the cesarean delivery rate or increasing the duration of labor.

4 The traditional "2-hour rule" for active phase arrest is probably too stringent a criterion in deciding to proceed with cesarean section.

5 Passive descent for 1 to 2 hours may be appropriate in the second stage of labor in selected patients with reassuring maternal and fetal status.

6 The evidence does not support the routine practice of suctioning of meconium at delivery to reduce meconium aspiration syndrome in vigorous neonates.

7 Active management of the third stage of labor is associated with reduced postpartum blood loss.

8 Double layer closure of the uterine incision decreases rupture rate in vaginal birth after cesarean (VBAC).

9 Expectant management of premature rupture of membranes (PROM) near term does not reduce cesarean delivery rates and is associated with increased rates of maternal infection.

Definitions: Labor Is the Process of Uterine Activity Leading to Delivery of the Fetus

A. First stage: generally defined as the period from the onset of painful contractions with cervical change until reaching complete dilation
   • Reported mean duration varies because of various definitions of onset
   • Composed of two phases:
      • Latent phase: begins with the onset of cervical change and ends with the acceleration of the rate of dilation:
         • Usually 3 to 4 cm in nullipara
         • Occasionally up to 5 to 6 cm, especially in multipara (Greulich et al, 2007)
      • Active phase: onset with the acceleration of dilation (coinciding with the end of the latent phase) until complete dilation
         • Originally further subdivided into three phases by Friedman (Friedman, 1995)
         • Acceleration phase, phase of maximum slope, and deceleration phase
         • Existence of a deceleration phase has been disputed (Cesario, 2004; Zhang et al, 2002)

B. Second stage: time from complete dilation to expulsion of the fetus; characterized by the following:
   • Descent
   • Delivery
C. Third stage: time from delivery of the fetus until delivery of the placenta and membranes

UPDATE #1

The original labor curves were first described in a classical observational paper published in 1955, in which 500 primiparous patients were followed in spontaneous labor at term (Friedman, 1955). Subsequent authors have reevaluated the rates of cervical change and duration of labor in modern patient populations with more current management practices (Cesario, 2004; Zhang et al, 2002). They have found that although the average length of labor is similar, there is likely a wider range of "normal" and the typical rates of cervical change are slower (often less than 1 cm per hour). The *deceleration phase* originally described was also not observed in the majority of patients in the newer studies. Further, the length of the second stage was also increased compared to Friedman's early description (Figure 17-1)

General Management Considerations (Berghella et al, 2008)

A. Evidence suggesting improved outcome or reduced complications (should probably be incorporated into practice):
- Hospital birth settings
- Delayed admission to labor and delivery (L&D)
- Doula support
- Upright positions in the second stage

B. Evidence suggesting increased complications or poorer outcome without sufficient benefit (should probably be avoided):
- Homelike births
- Enemas
- Pubic hair shaving
- Vaginal irrigation
- Early amniotomy
- "Hands-on" delivery technique (i.e., Ritgen maneuver)
- Fundal pressure
- Episiotomy
- Radiographic pelvimetry

C. Insufficient evidence to recommend (studies of poor quality, underpowered or conflicting results):
- Fetal admission tests (electronic monitoring, amniotic fluid assessment, biometry)
- Fluid intake, (intravenous [IV] or oral [PO])
- Ambulation
- Massage, water birth, aromatherapy
- Active management of labor
- Intrauterine pressure catheter (IUPC)
- Delayed pushing, closed glottis pushing
- Perineal massage

D. Routine care for uncomplicated labor
- Initial evaluation/history and physical
  - Estimated gestational age
  - Review of prenatal care and pregnancy complications including group B streptococcal (GBS) status, HIV status, and blood type
  - Review of past obstetric history and pertinent medical history
  - Thorough physical examination including vital signs, cardiovascular system, abdominal and pelvic exam
  - Baseline assessment of amniotic membrane status, uterine activity, and fetal heart rate
  - Assessment of fetal position, estimated size, and clinical pelvimetry
- Laboratory tests: complete blood count (CBC), urinalysis for protein, and specimen for blood bank (clot to hold or type and screen)
- Monitoring: external electronic or intermittent auscultation
- Repeat cervical examinations
  - Intervals of 1 to 4 hours in the first stage, hourly in the second stage
  - Prior to interventions such as epidural, amniotomy, or placement of internal fetal or uterine monitors
  - With recognition of fetal heart rate abnormalities
  - With the urge to push

E. Initiate GBS antibiotic prophylaxis if indicated per Centers for Disease Control and Prevention (CDC) guidelines (see Table 17-1 and Figures 17-2 and 17-3)
- Term infant, group B streptococcus (GBS) negative: no prophylaxis
- Term infant, GBS positive, prior infant with invasive GBS disease or GBS bacteruria in current pregnancy: start penicillin (PCN) if nonallergic, Ancef if low-risk allergy (i.e., no anaphylaxis) or third-line therapy based on sensitivities
- Preterm infant or GBS unknown: treat for risk factors in labor (i.e., estimated gestational age (EGA) <37 weeks, fever in labor, PROM ≥18 hours
- Despite the recommendations to screen and treat positives, compliance is still suboptimal

F. If HIV status unknown, offer rapid HIV screening and treat if positive per CDC guidelines (see Table 17-2 and Figure 17-4))
- Rapid HIV screening should be available at all labor and delivery units and offered to all pregnant patients
- Intrapartum treatment with zidovudine (ZDV) dramatically reduces the risk of vertical transmission of HIV

Latent Phase

A. Normal: difficult to define, as the exact onset and end are poorly defined and often hard to pinpoint

B. According to Friedman (1950s' data), mean duration is 6.4 and 4.8 hours for nulliparas and multiparas respectively (Friedman, 1995)

C. Prolonged: >20 hours for nullipara and >14 hours for multipara (> 2SD's, 95% tile above the mean)
- Prolonged latent phase associated with increased cesarean delivery
- Largest risk factors are PROM and entering labor with a low Bishop's score

D. More recent data suggest the normal labor curves are longer with current labor management practices of today's patients (Kilpatrick et al, 1989; Zhang et al, 2002)
- Possible contributing factors are numerous
- More inductions, epidurals, increased maternal body mass index (BMI), larger fetuses

E. Distinction between "false" and "latent" labor
- False or "prelabor" is characterized by lack of cervical change
- May simply reflect inadequate period of observation to detect cervical change
- May actually be more painful than "true" labor

F. Therapeutic options
- Delayed admission: reduces need for cesarean birth, oxytocin use, epidural anesthesia, and obstetric interventions (Greulich et al, 2007)
- Membrane sweeping: controversial (Boulvain et al, 2010)
  - No change in need for cesarean
  - Decreases need for induction after 41 weeks
  - Increases maternal discomfort
  - Not routinely recommended
- Therapeutic rest: allows for labor progress while patient sleeps with the aid of parenteral narcotics or sedatives
  - Morphine sulfate 15 mg intramuscular (IM) (or 5 mg IV + 5 mg IM) ± Phenergan 25 mg IV
  - Nubain 10 mg IV + Phenergan 25 mg IV

TABLE 17-1 **Compliance with GBS Prophylaxis**

Type of Population Sampled (reference number)	Deliveries Receiving Intrapartum Antibiotics, %*	Delivers with Prolonged ROM* Receiving Intrapartum Antibiotics, %*	Preterm Deliveries Receiving Intrapartum Antibiotics, %*	Women Screened Overall, %	GBS Culture-Positive Women Receiving Intrapartum Antibiotics, %*
Risk-Based Strategy Evaluated					
Two HMO* hospitals, California (49)	—†	88	81	N/A†	N/A
University hospital, Florida (50)	—	20 in 1992 / 72 in 1995	13 in 1992 / 42 in 1995	N/A	N/A
Single hospital, Vienna, Austria (51)	11.9	—	—	N/A	N/A
Single hospital, Massachusetts (52)	—	81	—	N/A	N/A
Connecticut (statewide), 1996 (53)	15.2	45	53	N/A	N/A
Screening-Based Strategy Evaluated					
Community hospital, New York (54)	—	N/A	76	91	86
University hospital, North Carolina (55)	12.9 for GBS prophylaxis	N/A	—	98	92
Single hospital, Sydney, Australia (42)	—	N/A	—	90	—
Single hospital, Vienna, Austria (51)	14.5	N/A	96	98.6	91
University hospital, New Mexico (56)	—	N/A	—	81	72
Single hospital, California (59)	26.3	N/A	91	89.8	94.4
Single hospital, Pennsylvania (57)	—	N/A	—	92	86
Two HMO hospitals, Washington State (58)	—	N/A	53	91	74 (automated data) / 87 (chart review)
Single hospital, Massachusetts (52)	—	N/A	—	N/A	100
Connecticut (statewide), 1996 (53)	15.2	N/A	——	(36% of births in Connecticut)	78

*Given for any reason.
†ROM, rupture of membranes; HMO, health maintenance organization; —, data not available; N/A, not applicable.
From Schrag S, Gorwitz R, Fultz-Butts K, Schuchat A: Prevention of perinatal group B streptococcal disease, *CDC MMWR* 51(RR11):1-22, 2002.

- Zolpidem 5 mg PO, diphenhydramine 50 mg PO, hydroxyzine 50 to 100 mg PO/IM, or secobarbital 100 mg PO
- Ambulation: may potentiate cervical change in the latent phase via Ferguson's reflex
- Amniotomy: controversial (see the discussion presented later)

UPDATE #2

The evidence does not support routine use of amniotomy in normally progressing spontaneous labor. In a recent meta-analysis (Smyth et al, 2007), 14 studies involving 4893 women were assessed regarding the effects of amniotomy on spontaneous labor. No shortening of the first stage of labor was identified with a possible increase in the cesarean section rate. Increased maternal pain was not addressed. Although amniotomy is commonly practiced around the world, this Cochrane review suggested little evidence to support this practice to shorten labor in view of the potential risks of cord accidents and increased infection.

- Uterotonics: oxytocin augmentation is indicated, especially if therapeutic rest has failed, cervix is favorable at ≥39 weeks, postterm gestation ≥41 weeks, or oligohydramnios
- Cesarean delivery is generally not advised for "failed induction" unless maternal or fetal factors dictate or after a minimum of 12 hours of oxytocin following amniotomy (Rouse et al, 2000)
- Neuraxial anesthesia may be used to provide adequate analgesia (Wong et al, 2005)

UPDATE #3

Neuraxial anesthesia may be administered early in labor without untoward effect. In the past, it was commonly assumed that initiation of an epidural too early in labor could prolong labor, increase the need for cesarean, and relax the pelvic floor, thus increasing difficulties with abnormal fetal positions in the second stage. However, a randomized trial of 750 nulliparous women in spontaneous labor or with spontaneous rupture of membranes

(SROM) and dilation less than 4 cm failed to show an increased cesarean rate (Wong et al, 2005). Patients in the study group were given intrathecal fentanyl at the first request for analgesia and epidural at the second request. Neuraxial anesthesia provided better analgesia and shorter duration of labor (by approximately 80 to 90 minutes).

Active Phase

A. Normal: rapid rate of cervical change (usually >1 cm/hour) (Friedman, 1978)
- Mean for nullipara = 4.6 hours (1.2 cm/hour lower limit of normal)
- Mean for multipara = 2.4 hours (1.5 cm/hour lower limit of normal)

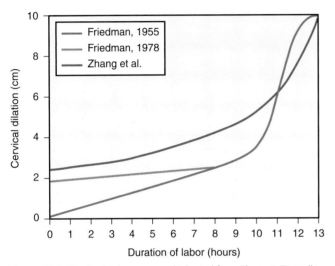

Figure 17-1. **Revised labor curves.** (Adapted from Zhang J, Troendle J, Yancey M: Transactions of the twenty-second annual meeting of the Society for Maternal-Fetal Medicine: reassessing the labor curve in nulliparous women, *Am J Obstet Gynecol* 187[4]:824-828, 2001.)

B. Longer active phase has been described in more recent data sets (Zhang et al, 2002)
- Duration of 5.5 hours from 4 to 10 cm for nullipara
- Fifth percentile rates all <1 cm/hour: 0.5 to 0.7 cm/hour for both nullipara and multipara

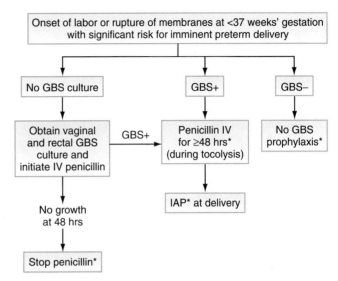

*Penicillin should be continued for a total of at least 48 hours, unless delivery occurs sooner. At the physician's discretion, antibiotic prophylaxis may be continued beyond 48 hours in a GBS culture-positive woman if delivery has not yet occurred. For women who are GBS culture positive, antibiotic prophylaxis should be reinitiated when labor likely to proceed to delivery occurs or recurs.
*If delivery has not occurred within 4 weeks, a vaginal and rectal GBS screening culture should be repeated and the patient should be managed as described, based on the result of the repeat culture.
*Intrapartum antibiotic prophylaxis.

Figure 17-3. **Management of GBS with threatened preterm delivery.** (From Schrag S, Gorwitz R, Fultz- Butts K, Schuchat A: Prevention of perinatal group B streptococcal disease, *MMWR* 51[RR11]:1-22, 2002.)

Vaginal and rectal GBS screening cultures at 35–37 weeks' gestation for **ALL** pregnant women (unless patient had GBS bacteriuria during the current pregnancy or a previous infant with invasive GBS disease)

Intrapartum prophylaxis indicated
- Previous infant with invasive GBS disease
- GBS bacteriuria during current pregnancy
- Positive GBS screening culture during current pregnancy (unless a planned cesarean delivery, in the absence of labor or amniotic membrane rupture, is performed)
- Unknown GBS status (culture not done, incomplete, or results unknown) and any of the following:
  - Delivery at <37 weeks' gestation*
  - Amniotic membrane rupture ≥18 hours
  - Intrapartum temperature 100.4°F (≥38.0°C)†

Intrapartum prophylaxis not indicated
- Previous pregnancy with a positive GBS screening culture (unless a culture was also positive during the current pregnancy)
- Planned cesarean delivery performed in the absence of labor or membrane rupture (regardless of maternal GBS culture status)
- Negative vaginal and rectal GBS screening culture in late gestation during the current pregnancy, regardless of intrapartum risk factors

*If onset of labor or rupture of amniotic membranes occurs at <37 weeks' gestation and there is a significant risk for preterm delivery (as assessed by the clinician), a suggested algorithm for GBS prophylaxis management is provided (Figure 3).
†If amnionitis is suspected, broad-spectrum antibiotic therapy that includes an agent known to be active against GBS should replace GBS prophylaxis.

Figure 17-2. **Algorithm for GBS prophylaxis.** (From Schrag S, Gorwitz R, Fultz-Butts K, Schuchat A: Prevention of perinatal group B streptococcal disease, *MMWR* 51[RR11]:1-22, 2002.)

- No deceleration phase
- Before 7 cm, no change over 2 hours is common

C. Dysfunctional patterns/dystocia
  - Defined as abnormal labor because of abnormalities of the power (uterine contractions or pushing), passenger (presentation, position, or size), or passage (pelvis or soft tissue) (American College of Obstetricians and Gynecologists, 2003)
  - Protraction disorders: abnormally slow rate of cervical dilation
  - Arrest disorders: lack of dilation for ≥2 to 4 hours
  - Most common causes are hypotonic uterine dysfunction and relative fetopelvic disproportion
  - Lack of progress accounts for ~2/3 of unplanned cesarean sections in patients with vertex presentation (Gifford et al, 2002)

D. Dystocia in the first stage of labor: risk factors
  - Advanced maternal age, poor obstetric history
  - History of hypertension, diabetes, infertility
  - Preterm premature rupture of membranes (PPROM)
  - Abnormal amniotic fluid volume
  - Chorioamnionitis
  - Epidural: conflicting data
    - Not shown to increase cesarean rates
    - Prolongs labor by 40 to 90 minutes and increases the need for oxytocin
    - Increased need for operative vaginal delivery

E. Diagnosis/prediction
  - Predictive models have low sensitivity, specificity, and positive predictive values
  - Magnetic resonance imaging (MRI) or x-ray pelvimetry in conjunction with sonographic biometry remains investigational

F. Complications
  - Maternal or fetal infectious morbidity
  - Pelvic floor injury in prolonged obstructed labor
  - Asphyxial risk unrelated to duration of labor in the absence of fetal heart rate abnormalities

G. Therapeutic options
  - Mainstay of therapy is oxytocin augmentation to achieve "adequate" labor (the only drug approved for this purpose by the Food and Drug Administration)
    - Minimally effective labor: 3 contractions in 10 minutes, 25 mm Hg above baseline (75 Montevideo units [mvu])
    - Adequate: ≥ 200 mvu
    - Expected range: 95 to 395

- Goal is to achieve labor adequacy (>200 mvu) without evidence of fetal heart rate (FHR) abnormalities and ≤5 contractions in 10 minutes (attainable in 54% of patients) (Hauth et al, 1991; Rouse et al, 2001)
- Many protocols exist for oxytocin administration: all via IV infusion and titrated to effect
  - "Low" dose: for example, 1 mU start, increase by 1 mU Q 30 to 45 minutes
  - "High" dose: for example, 2 to 6 mU increase Q 20 minutes
    - Usually associated with shorter labor and reduced cesarean rates
    - Less maternal and neonatal infection
    - More tachysystole
    - Inappropriate for VBAC
- Use of IUPC
  - Evidence does not support routine use
  - May be beneficial when clinical assessment of contraction strength is suboptimal in the face of poor progress in labor
- Use of electronic fetal monitoring (EFM) during augmentation
  - Has not been shown superior to intermittent auscultation
  - Associated with decrease in neonatal seizures
  - No difference in low Apgar, cerebral palsy, neonatal intensive care unit (NICU) admission, or perinatal mortality
  - Increased rates of cesarean birth
- Early amniotomy and oxytocin ("active management of labor" [AML]) (Brown et al, 2009; Hinshaw et al, 2008; Rouse et al, 1994; Wei et al, 2009)
  - Risks include tachysystole and FHR abnormalities
  - Decreased duration of labor by 1.1 hours
  - Slight reduction in cesarean rates
  - Unclear effects on maternal satisfaction
- Lack of progress as a diagnostic criteria for active phase arrest
  - Current recommendations suggest that maintaining augmentation of beyond 2 hours of no progress can lead to vaginal delivery without undo risk (Rouse et al, 1999, 2001)

UPDATE #4

The traditional "2-hour rule" is overly restrictive in managing the active phase of labor. So-called lack of progress is one of the most common reasons for performing cesarean, accounting for 68% of

---

TABLE 17-2   Protocol for Prevention of Vertical HIV Transmission with ZDV

Time of ZDV Administration	Regimen
Antepartum	Oral administration of 100 mg ZDV five times daily,* initiated at 14-34 weeks' gestation and continued throughout the pregnancy.
Intrapartum	During labor, intravenous administration of ZDV in a 1-hour initial dose of 2 mg/kg body weight, followed by a continuous infusion of 1mg/kg body weight per hour until delivery.
Postpartum	Oral administration of ADV to the newborn (ZDV syrup at 2 mg/kg body weight/dose every 6 hours) for the first 6 weeks of life, beginning at 8-12 hours after birth.†

*Oral ZDV, administered as 200 mg three times daily or 300 mg twice daily, is used in general clinical practice and is an acceptable alternative regimen to 100 mg orally five times daily.
†Intravenous dosage for infants who cannot tolerate oral intake is 1.5 mg/kg body weight intravenously every 6 hours.
From Mofenson L: U.S. Public Health Service Task Force recommendations for use of antiretroviral drugs in pregnant HIV-1 infected women for maternal health and interventions to reduce perinatal HIV-1 transmission in the United States, *CDC MMWR* 51(RR18):1-38, 2002.

1. HIV-1-infected pregnant women who have not received prior antiretroviral therapy

- Pregnant women with HIV-1 infection must receive standard clinical immunologic, and virologic evaluation. Recommendations for initiation and choice of antiretroviral therapy should be based on the same parameters used for persons who are not pregnant, although the known and unknown risks and benefits of such therapy during pregnancy must be considered and discussed.
- The three-part zidovudine (ZDV) chemoprophylaxis regimen, initiated after the first trimester, should be recommended for all pregnant women with HIV-1 infection regardless of antenatal HIV-1 RNA copy number to reduce the risk for perinatal transmission.
- The combination of ZDV chemoprophylaxis with additional antiretroviral drugs for treatment of HIV-1 infection is recommended for infected women whose clinical, immunologic, or virologic status requires treatment or whose HIV-1 RNA is >1,000 copies/mL regardless of clinical or immunologic status.
- Women who are in the first trimester of pregnancy may consider delaying initiation of therapy until after 10–12 weeks' gestation.

2. HIV-1 infected women receiving antiretroviral therapy during the current pregnancy

- HIV-1 infected women receiving antiretroviral therapy whose pregnancy is identified after the first trimester should continue therapy. ZDV should be a component of the antenatal antiretroviral treatment regimen after the first trimester whenever possible, although this may not always be feasible.
- Women receiving antiretroviral therapy whose pregnancy is recognized during the first trimester should be counselled regarding the benefits and potential risks of antiretroviral administration during this period, and continuation of therapy should be considered. If therapy is discontinued during the first trimester, all drugs should be stopped and reintroduced simultaneously to avoid the development of drug resistance.
- Regardless of the antepartum antiretroviral regimen, ZDV administration is recommended during the intrapartum period and for the newborn.

3. HIV-1 infected women in labor who have had no prior therapy

- Several effective regimens are also available for women who have had no prior therapy:
  - a single dose nevirapine at the the onset of labor followed by a single does of nevirapine for the newborn at age 48 hours,
  - oral ZDV and lamivudine (3TC) during labor, followed by 1 week of oral ZDV-3TC for the newborn,
  - intrapartum intravenous ZDV followed by 6 weeks of ZDV for for the newborn, or
  - the 2-dose nevirapine regimen combined with the intrapartum intravenous ZDV and 6 weeks of ZDV for the newborn.
- In the immediate postpartum period, the woman should have appropriate assessments (e.g., CD4 T-lymphocyte count and HIV-1 RNA copy number) to determine whether antiretroviral therapy is recommended for her own health.

4. Infants born to mother who have received no antiretroviral therapy during pregnancy or intrapartum

- The 6-week neonatal component of the ZDV chemoprophylactic regimen should be discussed with the mother and offered for the newborn.
- ZDV should be initiated as soon as possible after delivery, preferably within 6–12 hours of birth.
- Some clinicians might use ZDV in combination with other antiretroviral drugs, particularly if the mother is known or suspected to have ZDV-resistant virus. However, the efficacy of this approach for prevention of transmission is unknown, and appropriate dosing regimens for neonates are incompletely defined.
- In the immediate postpartum period, the woman should undergo appropriate assessments (e.g., CD4 count and HIV-1 RNA copy number) to determine if antiretroviral therapy is required for her own health. The infant should undergo early diagnostic testing, so that if he or she is HIV infected, treatment can be initiated as soon as possible.

Figure 17-4. Clinical recommendations for prevention of vertical transmission of HIV. (From Mofenson L: U.S. Public Health Service Task Force recommendations for use of antiretroviral drugs in pregnant HIV-1 infected women for maternal health and interventions to reduce perinatal HIV-1 transmission in the United States, *MMWR* 51[RR18]:1-38, 2002.)

unplanned, vertex cesareans (Gifford et al, 2000). Waiting longer than the typical 2-hour rule to declare active phase arrest often leads to successful vaginal delivery without significant complication (Rouse et al, 2001). Five hundred and one consecutive spontaneously laboring women with abnormal progress were managed by protocol to achieve adequate contractions (≥200 mu) for 4 or more hours before cesarean. The fifth percentile rate of dilation was 0.5 cm per hour, and 38 patients were arrested for >2 hours despite adequate labor. Vaginal delivery was achieved in 61%. Although rates of maternal infection and mild shoulder dystocia increased, there was no increased rate of postpartum hemorrhage or serious fetal complication.

- Alternative measures (Berghella et al, 2008)
  - Support persons/Doulas
    - Reduced cesarean, operative vaginal delivery, need for pain medication, and patient dissatisfaction
  - Ambulation: is not harmful, may improve comfort in some patients, but has no significant impact on the course of labor or its complications
  - Hydration
    - Solid food intake should be avoided for 6 to 8 hours before elective cesarean and in laboring patients
    - In general, oral intake of clear liquids in uncomplicated labor poses little risk
    - IV hydration is beneficial with epidural anesthesia and may improve uterine function

Second Stage

NORMAL COURSE AND MANAGEMENT

- Friedman reported means of 0.29 hours (17 minutes) and 0.95 hours (57 minutes) for multipara and nullipara respectively (Friedman, 1978, 1995)
  - Differs from today's data because of different rates of epidural use and high incidence of operative delivery
  - Second stage was generally arbitrarily ended after 2 hours
- More recent mean durations (Kilpatrick et al, 1989):
  - Nullipara/no epidural: 54 minutes
  - Multipara/no epidural: 19 minutes
  - Nullipara/with epidural: 79 minutes
  - Multipara/with epidural: 45 minutes
- Conduction anesthesia prolongs the second stage approximately 20 to 30 minutes
- Pushing techniques (Berghella et al, 2008)
  - Closed glottis techniques associated with shorter (13 to 18 minutes) second stage and similar neonatal outcome compared to open glottis (women's own urge)
  - Closed glottis method may result in poorer urodynamics at 3 months postpartum
  - Method should be the woman's choice, although most choose Valsalva (closed glottis)
- Maternal position (Berghella et al, 2008)
  - Upright position (without epidural) associated with 4 minute shorter second stage, less pain, fewer FHR abnormalities, and higher rates of estimated blood loss (EBL) >500 cc
  - Kneeling associated with less pain than sitting

- Perineal massage
  - Increases incidence of intact perineum in nullipara (but not multipara) when performed after 34 weeks before labor
  - In labor, may reduce the incidence of third and fourth degree tears

PROLONGED

- The 2-hour rule: based on Friedman's pioneering work
  - Not evidence based
  - Greatly different study population and labor practices compared to today
- Redefined by the American College of Obstetricians and Gynecologists (ACOG) in 2000 (American College of Obstetricians and Gynecologists, 2000)
  - "Lack of continuing progress"
  - After 2 hours in nullipara (or 3 hours with an epidural)
  - After 1 hour in multipara (or 2 hours with an epidural)

ARRESTED DESCENT

- Classification of station
  - Revised by ACOG in 1988
  - Recommendation to abandon definition of descent by one third of the pelvis above and below the ischial spines
  - More precise and reproducible method based on centimeters above and below the ischial spines (−5 cm to +5 cm)
- Failure to gain station over ≥1 hour is arrested descent

DYSTOCIA IN THE SECOND STAGE

- Risk factors (American College of Obstetricians and Gynecologists, 2003)
  - Epidural
  - EGA >41 weeks
  - Persistent occiput posterior
  - Protraction of first stage
  - Nulliparity
  - Short stature (<150 cm)
  - Macrosomia
    - High station entering the second stage (above +2)
- Management—three basic options: expectant management while optimizing labor efforts, operative vaginal delivery, or cesarean
  - Expectant management
    - Provide emotional support
    - Treat uterine hypotonic dysfunction if present
    - Consider modification of neuraxial analgesia if indicated
    - Change maternal position
    - The 2-hour rule for second stage arrest is arbitrary, and passive descent or continued pushing may be appropriate for selected patients

UPDATE #5

The PEOPLE (pushing early or pushing late with epidural) study was a multicenter randomized controlled trial that looked at waiting up to 2 hours before pushing unless the woman had an irresistible urge to push, the fetal head was visible, or there were medical indications for delivery (Fraser et al, 2000). The study found a reduced incidence of difficult deliveries and midpelvic operations (relative risk [RR] approximately 0.79 and 0.72, respectively). There was an increase in abnormal cord pH but no increase in neonatal morbidity index. Maternal morbidity was similar. Women entering the second stage with transverse or posterior positions or station above +2 are most likely to benefit. Because of the increased risk of abnormal cord pH, the authors recommend close fetal surveillance if a policy of delayed pushing is adopted. Another randomized controlled trial (Hansen et al, 2002) found that delayed pushing was (not surprisingly) associated with longer second stages (up to 4.9 hours) but also observed no adverse outcomes. There were decreased pushing times, decreased maternal fatigue in primips, and fewer fetal heart rate decelerations.

- Prolonged second stage in nullipara (>4 hour) is associated with increased maternal morbidity (cesarean, operative delivery, chorioamnionitis, uterine atony, and perineal trauma) but no increased poor neonatal outcome with close fetal surveillance (Cheng et al, 2004; Rouse et al, 2009)
- In multipara, a second stage of ≥3 hours has been associated with both increased maternal morbidity (operative vaginal delivery, chorioamnionitis, and perineal trauma) and neonatal morbidity (low Apgar, low pH, and NICU admission) despite relatively high vaginal delivery rates (Cheng et al, 2007)
  - A prolonged second stage is much less common in multiparas but may signify true cephalopelvic disproportion (CPD) and portend poorer outcomes
- Operative vaginal delivery (American College of Obstetricians and Gynecologists, 2000)
  - Indications: per ACOG
    - Prolonged second stage as defined previously (>1 or 2 hours of pushing in multipara or >2 or 3 hours of pushing in nullipara)
    - Suspicion of immediate or potential fetal compromise
    - Shortening of second stage for maternal benefit
  - Criteria and classification
    - Outlet: scalp visible or fetal head on the perineum, occiput anterior (OA) or occiput posterior (OP) ± 45 degrees
    - Low: leading point of the fetal skull is at station +2 or below; rotation <45 degrees; rotation >45 degrees
    - Mid: above station +2 but head engaged
    - High: not defined, presumably unengaged
  - Midpelvic delivery: still appropriate albeit only for adequately trained providers
  - Sequential use of vacuum and forceps is associated with increased neonatal head trauma
- Cesarean delivery: best option if operative vaginal delivery is not deemed likely to succeed
  - When performed in the second stage, associated with longer operative times, epidural anesthesia, chorioamnionitis and higher birthweights
  - Composite maternal morbidity is increased and neonatal morbidity unchanged with cesarean in the second stage of labor (Alexander et al, 2007)

VI. Delivery Techniques

A. "Hands on" method of Ritgen versus "hands poised"
- "Hands on" involves pressure on the fetal head upon crowning and upward pressure on the perineal or perianal area
- May increase third-degree tears

B. Fundal pressure
- Inadequately studied in trials
- Unknown benefit in assisting vaginal birth
- Is contraindicated in managing shoulder dystocia

C. Episiotomy: should not be performed routinely (Berghella et al, 2008)
- Use is associated with increased perineal trauma, poor healing, later dyspareunia, and subsequent incontinence
- If required, the best technique (i.e., mediolateral versus midline) is controversial
- May be indicated to facilitate delivery of the posterior arm in difficult shoulder dystocia when there is inadequate room posteriorly

D. Meconium stained fluid: recommendations for amnioinfusion and suctioning have changed (Ahanya et al, 2005; American College of Obstetricians and Gynecologists, 2007; Cuttini, 2004; Fraser et al, 2005; Ross, 2005; Vain et al, 2004)

UPDATE #6

Amnioinfusion, although it may ameliorate variable decelerations, has also been associated with adverse events such as uterine hypertonus, uterine rupture, fetal heart rate abnormalities, chorioamnionitis, and abruption. In a large multicenter trial of 1998 patients, it was not shown to prevent meconium aspiration syndrome (Fraser et al, 2005).

The routine suctioning of meconium at delivery is no longer considered necessary or beneficial to the neonate. Meconium passage usually occurs within 24 to 48 hours after birth. Fetal passage of meconium and meconium stained amniotic fluid occurs in approximately 12% of all pregnancies (Ahanya et al, 2005; Ross, 2005). Up to 4% of these infants develop meconium aspiration syndrome (MAS) and account for 2% of perinatal mortality (Ross, 2005). Intrapartum oropharyngeal or nasopharyngeal suctioning and immediate postpartum endotracheal suctioning were considered to be standard of care in the past. A randomized multicenter trial of 2514 patients did not support the practice of suctioning before the delivery of the shoulders, as it did not prevent MAS, need for mechanical ventilation, or mortality (Cuttini, 2004; Vain et al, 2004). Thus, ACOG no longer recommends intrapartum suctioning. If meconium is present and the newborn is depressed, intubation and suction are still recommended but are not necessary if the infant is vigorous and the heart rate is >100.

E. Shoulder dystocia (American College of Obstetricians and Gynecologists, 2002)
- Generally unpredictable
- Risk factors:
  - Macrosomia
  - Diabetes
  - Protracted active phase
  - Prolonged second stage
  - Need for midpelvic delivery
- Complications:
  - Maternal soft tissue injuries and perineal trauma

- Neonatal asphyxia and birth trauma (especially brachial plexus injury)
- Elective cesarean section or early induction of labor is generally not indicated for prophylaxis except in special cases after informed consent:
  - Estimated fetal weight (EFW) >5000 grams in women without diabetes, >4500 grams in women with diabetes
  - Prior history of severe shoulder dystocia
- Management
  - Call for help
  - Initial maneuvers (recommended with scant evidence): McRobert's and suprapubic pressure
  - Secondary maneuvers: delivery of the posterior arm, rotational maneuvers (i.e., Rubin's, Wood's corkscrew or combination), Gaskin all-fours position
  - Tertiary maneuvers: Zavanelli maneuver (replacement of the fetal head followed by cesarean) or abdominal surgical rescue; these procedures are methods of last resort

Third Stage

NORMAL

- Generally averages 5 to 6 minutes
- Prolonged third stage exceeds 30 minutes

PROLONGED THIRD STAGE: RISK FACTORS

- Preterm delivery
- Abnormal placentation

COMPLICATIONS

- Postpartum hemorrhage (discussed later)
- Retained placental tissue
- Uterine inversion

MANAGEMENT OPTIONS

- Expectant
- Cord traction, cord drainage (Giacolone et al, 2000; Soltani et al, 2009)
- Uterotonics
  - Oxytocin: 10 to 40 units/1000 cc IV or 10 units IV bolus or 10 units IM
  - Ergot alkaloids (e.g., methylergonovine) 0.2 mg IM or PO (not IV): contraindicated with hypertension
  - Prostaglandins: for example, prostaglandin F2α (Hemabate 250 micrograms IM, contraindicated in asthma) or prostaglandin E1 analog (misoprostol 800 micrograms per rectum)
    - Less effective than oxytocin or oxytocin-Methergine for active management (Villar et al, 2002)
    - Advantages: cheaper, can be given PO, do not require refrigeration
    - Long-acting oxytocin agonists (carbetocin): not available in the United States
- Active management (i.e., early oxytocin, early cord clamping ± drainage, cord traction, and fundal massage) has been shown to be superior to expectant management (Jackson et al, 2001; Leduc et al, 2009; Prendaville et al, 2009)

Postpartum Hemorrhage (American College of Obstetricians and Gynecologists, 1998)

DEFINITION

- >500 cc (approximately 4% of vaginal deliveries) or >1000 cc (approximately 6% to 7% of cesarean sections)

MATERNAL MORTALITY

- Third leading cause of maternal mortality in developed countries (after venous thromboembolism [VTE] and hypertensive disorders)
- Leading cause of preventable deaths
- Even more prevalent in developing countries

RISK FACTORS

- Rapid or prolonged labor, dystocia
- High parity
- Use of magnesium sulfate or general anesthesia
- History of retained placenta or prior history of postpartum hemorrhage (PPH)
- Chorioamnionitis
- Obesity
- Preeclampsia

CAUSES

- Atony: most common
- Obstetric trauma, lacerations, or uterine rupture or inversion
- Retained placental tissue
- Coagulopathy: rare in the absence of disseminated intravascular coagulation (DIC)

MANAGEMENT OPTIONS: BASED ON THE UNDERLYING CAUSE

- Call for help (nursing, anesthesia, hemorrhage protocols)
- Obtain good IV access
- Treat for atony aggressively with bimanual massage and uterotonics
- Assess for lacerations, uterine rupture or inversion
- Dilation and curettage (D&C) with sonographic guidance if suspected retained tissue
- *Avoid delay and denial*
- Prompt use of blood products and fluid resuscitation in cases >1000 cc; consider moving to an operating room (OR) if >1500 cc and ongoing bleeding

- In stable patient, consider interventional radiology for embolization or Bakri balloon for tamponade of lower segment bleeding if there is good uterine tone
- Move to surgical options in cases >2000 cc with ongoing blood loss
  - Laparotomy
  - B-Lynch sutures
  - Bakri balloon
  - Uterine artery or hypogastric artery ligation
  - Hysterectomy
- Recombinant activated factor VII: may show promise for intractable obstetric hemorrhage (Franchini, 2007)
  - Off-label use
  - Expensive
  - Useful for select patients with inherited bleeding disorders
  - Major risk is thrombosis
  - Controlled trials are needed

Special Considerations

VBAC (American College of Obstetricians and Gynecologists, 2004)

- Appropriate to offer in selected patients after informed consent
- Uterine scar rupture rate of 0.7% with one prior lower segment scar and similar rates with unknown scar
- Inappropriate for patients with classical incisions or uterine surgery with deep myometrial incision (i.e., certain myomectomies)
- Induction of labor increases risk of uterine scar rupture
- Cervical ripening with prostaglandins generally contraindicated because of high scar rupture rate (Lydon-Rochelle, et al, 2001)
- Oxytocin augmentation for active phase dystocia should be used with extreme caution
- Signs of uterine scar rupture
  - New onset of significant variable FHR decelerations or bradycardia
  - Sudden loss of station
  - New-onset of vaginal bleeding
  - New-onset of lower abdominal pain
- Prompt recognition and treatment of dystocia (with repeat cesarean) can prevent up to 42% of uterine ruptures (Hamilton et al, 2001)
- Should be undertaken only at hospitals where an obstetrical provider able to perform cesarean section is immediately available

UPDATE #8

An observational cohort study examined risk factors for uterine rupture (Bugold et al, 2002). This large study of 2142 women found a fourfold risk of uterine rupture associated with single-layer closure of the uterus. Double-layer closure of the uterine incision is probably most appropriate for patients who may be candidates for VBAC in the future. Whether it may also decrease the rate of placenta accreta remains to be studied.

MANAGEMENT OF PROM AT TERM

- Rupture of membranes before the onset of labor occurs in approximately 8% of term pregnancies
- Treatment can be expectant or active (i.e., induction of labor)
- Patient preference often drives the choice of management
- The primary concern for expectant management is infectious morbidity (both maternal and neonatal), and the primary concern for active management is failed induction and cesarean

UPDATE #9

Expectant management of PROM at term remains controversial. The largest published randomized study to address this issue involved 5041 women with PROM at term (Hannah et al, 1996). Patients were randomized to undergo induction of labor with oxytocin or prostaglandin or expectant management of up to 4 days. The neonatal infection rates and cesarean rates were similar between all groups. However, the maternal infectious morbidity was increased in the expectant management group, and the women who were induced viewed their experience more positively.

SUGGESTED READINGS

Labor Management: General

Berghella V, Baxter J, Chauhan SP: Evidence-based labor and delivery management, *Am J Obstet Gynecol* 199(5):445–454, 2008.
Cesario S: Reevaluation of Friedman's labor curve: a pilot study, *JOGNN Clinical Research* 33(6):713–722, 2004.
Friedman EA: Primigravid labor: a graphicostatistical analysis, *Obstet Gynecol* 6(6):567–589, 1955.
Mofenson L: U.S. Public Health Service Task Force recommendations for use of antiretroviral drugs in pregnant HIV-1 infected women for maternal health and interventions to reduce perinatal HIV-1 transmission in the United States, *MMWR* 51(RR18):1–38, 2002.
Schrag S, Gorwitz R, Fultz-Butts K, Schuchat A: Prevention of perinatal group B streptococcal disease, *MMWR* 51(RR11):1–22, 2002.
Zhang J, Troendle J, Yancey M: Transactions of the twenty-second annual meeting of the Society for Maternal-Fetal Medicine: reassessing the labor curve in nulliparous women, *Am J Obstet Gynecol* 187(4):824–828, 2002.

Latent Phase

Rouse DJ, Owen J, Hauth J: Criteria for failed labor induction: prospective evaluation of a standardized protocol, *Obstet Gynecol* 96(5):671–677, 2000.
Smyth RMD, Alldred SK, Markham C: Amniotomy for shortening spontaneous labour (Review), *The Cochrane Collaboration* 2:1–15, 2010.
Wong CA, Scavone BM, Peaceman AM, et al: The risk of cesarean delivery with neuraxial analgesia given early versus late in labor, *N Engl J Med* 352(7):655–720, 2005.

Active Phase

American College of Gynecologists and Obstetricians: *ACOG practice bulletin no. 49: dystocia and augmentation of labor* 102(6):1445–1454, 2003.
Brown HC, Paranjothy S, Dowswell T, Thomas J: Package of care for active management in labour for reducing caesarean section rates in low-risk women, *Obstet Gynecol* 113(1):218–220, 2009.
Gifford DS, Morton SC, Fiske M, et al: Lack of Progress in labor as a reason for cesarean, *Obstet Gynecol* 95(4):589–595, 2000.
Hinshaw K, Simpson S, Cummings S, et al: A randomized controlled trial of early versus delayed oxytocin augmentation to treat primary dysfunctional labour in nulliparous women, *BJOG* 115:1289–1296, 2008.
Rouse DJ, Owen J, Savage KG, Hauth JC: Active phase labor arrest: revisiting the 2-hour minimum, *Obstet Gynecol* 98(4):550–554, 2001.
Wei S, Wo BL, Xu H, et al: Early amniotomy and early oxytocin for prevention of, or therapy for; delay in first stage spontaneous labour compared with routine care (Review), *The Cochrane Collaboration* 4:1–29, 2009.

Second Stage

Alexander JM, Leveno KJ, Rouse DJ, et al: Comparison of maternal and infant outcomes from primary cesarean delivery during the second compared with first stage of labor, *Obstet Gynecol* 109(4):917–921, 2007.

American College of Obstetricians and Gynecologists: ACOG practice bulletin no. 17; June 2000, Operative vaginal delivery, *Obstet Gynecol* 95:998–1005. www.acog.org/publication/educational_bulletin/pb017.cfm.

Cheng YW, Hopkins LM, Caughey AB: How long is too long: does a prolonged second stage of labor in nulliparous women affect maternal and neonatal outcomes? *Am J Obstet Gynecol* 191:933–938, 2004.

Cheng YW, Hopkins LM, Laros RK Jr, Caughey AB: Duration of the second stage of labor in multiparous women: maternal and neonatal outcomes, *Am J Obstet Gynecol* 196:585.e1-585.e6, 2007.

Fraser WD, Marcoux S, Krauss I, et al: Multicenter, randomized, controlled trial of delayed pushing for nulliparous women in the second stage of labor with continuous epidural analgesia, *Am J Obstet Gynecol* 182(5): 1165–1172, 2000.

Hansen SL, Clark SL, Foster JC: Active pushing versus passive fetal descent in the second stage of labor: a randomized controlled trial, *Obstet Gynecol* 99(1):29–34, 2002.

Rouse DJ, Weiner SJ, Bloom SL, et al: Second-stage labor duration in nulliparous women: relationship to maternal and perinatal outcomes, *Am J Obstet Gynecol* 201:357.e1-e7, 2009.

Delivery

Ahanya A, Lakshmanan J, Morgan B, Ross M: Meconium passage in utero: mechanisms, consequences, and manuscripts, *Obstet Gynecol* 60(1): 45–56, 2005.

American College of Obstetricians and Gynecologists: ACOG opinion no. 379: management of delivery of a newborn with meconium-stained amniotic fluid, *Obstet Gynecol* 110(3):739, 2007.

American College of Obstetricians and Gynecologists: ACOG practice bulletin 40: shoulder dystocia, *Obstet Gynecol* 100(5):1045–1049, 2002.

Fraser WK, Hofmeyr J, Lede R, et al: Amnioinfusion for the prevention of the meconium aspiration syndrome, *N Engl J Med* 353(9):909–917, 2005.

Vain NE, Szyld EG, Prudent LM, et al: Oropharyngeal and nasopharyngeal suctioning of meconium-stained neonates before delivery of their shoulders: multicentre, randomized controlled trial, *Lancet* 364:597–602, 2004.

Third Stage

American College of Obstetricians and Gynecologists: ACOG educational bulletin no. 243; January 1998, Postpartum hemorrhage, *Obstet Gynecol* 1–6.

Jackson KW Jr, Allbert JR, Schemmer GK, et al: A randomized controlled trial comparing oxytocin administration before and after placental delivery in the prevention of postpartum hemorrhage, *Am J Obstet Gynecol* 185(4):873–877, 2001.

Leduc D, Senikas V, Lalonde AB: active management of the third stage of labour: prevention and treatment of postpartum hemorrhage (SOGC Clinical Practice Guideline), *JOGC* 235:980–993, 2009.

Prendville WJP, Elbourne D, McDonald SJ: Active versus expectant management in the third stage of labour (Review), *The Cochrane Collaboration* 3:1–2, 2009.

Special Topics

American College of Obstetricians and Gynecologists: ACOG practice bulletin no. 54: vaginal birth after previous cesarean delivery, *Obstet Gynecol* 104(1):203–211, 2004.

Bugold E, Bujold C, Hamilton EF, et al: The impact of a single-layer or double-layer closure on uterine rupture, *Am J Obstet Gynecol* 186(6): 1326–1330, 2002.

Hamilton EF, Bujold E, McNamara H, et al: Dystocia among women with symptomatic uterine rupture, *Am J Obstet Gynecol* 184(4):620–624, 2001.

Hannah ME, Ohlsson A, Farine D, et al: Induction of labor compared with expectant management for prelabor rupture of the membranes at term, *N Engl J Med* 334(16):1005–1011, 1996.

Lydon-Rochelle M, Holt VL, Easterling TR, Martin DP: Risk of uterine rupture during labor among women with a prior cesarean delivery, *N Engl J Med* 345(1):3–7, 54–55, 2001.

References

Please go to expertconsult.com to view references.

Chapter 18

Emergent Management of the Newborn

JAE H. KIM

KEY UPDATES

1 Continuous positive assisted pressure (CPAP) support is a viable initial alternative to intubation for the very low birth weight infant in the delivery room.

2 Suctioning at the perineum for thick meconium has not been shown to be beneficial.

3 Use of video laryngoscopy may improve chances of successful intubation as well as provide recordable visualization of the airway anatomy.

4 Fetal surgery remains an option for a limited number of infants and centers.

5 Early pulse oximetry screening may increase detection of cyanotic heart disease.

6 Early antenatal diagnosis of hypoplastic left heart disease results in better preoperative clinical status.

7 Use of corticosteroids may sensitize the infant to epinephrine and potentiate the response to other inotropic drugs.

8 Successful attempts have been made to treat homozygous alpha-thalassemia with in utero transfusions and postnatal bone marrow transplant.

9 Antenatal bowel dilatation is more specific than bowel echogenicity for postnatal bowel pathology.

10 The incidence of gastroschisis continues to rise worldwide.

11 Maternal use of beta-blockers puts infants at greater risk for hypoglycemia.

12 Increasing involvement of the hospital ethics committee for difficult end-of-life or poor-quality-of-life discussions helps the health care team.

13 In moderate to severe encephalopathy, the use of whole body cooling or selective head cooling can reduce overall combined death and neurodevelopmental morbidity at 18 months.

14 Infants with congenital myotonic dystrophy may require prolonged ventilation but may also improve over time, even greater than 30 days.

15 The molecular basis of the congenital skin disorders is increasingly detailed, but we still await specific therapies.

Respiratory Distress

CLINICAL PROFILE

- Nasal flaring, tachypnea, grunting, subcostal/intercostal retractions, cyanosis, thoracic breathing
- Cyanosis not easily detected clinically, influenced by skin color, lighting, hemoglobin level
- Oxygen saturation monitoring essential but hyperoxia not sensitive (i.e., paO_2 highly variable at 100% saturation because of sigmoidal hemoglobin-oxygen saturation curve)

UPDATE #1

Intubation is a potentially dangerous procedure with accompanying adverse effects such as bradycardia, laryngospasm, apnea, and desaturations, besides being a noxious stimulus. Ventilator-induced lung injury is inevitable the longer the duration of intubation. Increasing use of continuous positive assisted pressure (CPAP) support can normalize lung volumes with spontaneous breathing (Finer, 2010). Nasal intermittent mechanical ventilation (NIMV) is also being used to circumvent intubation in infants with poor spontaneous breathing, although additional clinical studies are still warranted.

DIFFERENTIAL DIAGNOSIS

- Transient tachypnea of the newborn
- Respiratory distress syndrome
- Pneumonia
- Pneumothorax
- Airway obstruction (see the Airway Obstruction section)
- Aspiration syndrome (blood, amniotic fluid, meconium) (see the Meconium Aspiration Syndrome section)
- Pulmonary hemorrhage
- Sepsis/metabolic acidosis
- Congenital diaphragmatic hernia (see the Congenital Diaphragmatic Hernia section)
- Pulmonary hypoplasia

MANAGEMENT

- Provide oxygen to maintain oxygen saturations in the 95% to 99% range
- Term infants often do not tolerate continuous positive airway pressure (CPAP) very well
- Intubation may be necessary if oxygenation or ventilation is inadequate
- In nonemergent circumstances, intubation using premedication (e.g., analgesic, anticholinergic, muscle relaxant) is recommended (Kumar et al, 2010)

Meconium Aspiration Syndrome (MAS)

CLINICAL PROFILE

- One in every seven pregnancies is associated with meconium-stained amniotic fluid, and about 5% of these infants develop MAS
- MAS is a life-threatening condition at birth
- Meconium is detectable in the gastrointestinal tract of the fetus by 20 weeks
- The healthy fetus normally does not pass stool in utero, but a stressed fetus may pass meconium
- Meconium is composed of a mixture of water, desquamated cells, carbohydrates, protein, fat, bilirubin, and digestive enzymes that can incite an inflammatory reaction in the airways and alveolar space when inhaled
- In severe cases, persistent pulmonary hypertension (PPHN) becomes the major management problem, often greater than the aspiration

UPDATE #2

Suctioning at the perineum has not been shown to be beneficial. Nonsuctioning is as safe as routine suctioning at the perineum for infants born with meconium-stained amniotic fluid (Velaphi et al, 2006).

MANAGEMENT

- No suctioning at the perineum is required (Velaphi et al, 2006)
- Oropharyngeal suctioning with a bulb suction or suction catheter may cause apnea, bradycardia, or poor respiratory recovery
- Endotracheal intubation and suctioning are currently recommended only for nonvigorous infants

- Amnioinfusion to dilute the meconium in the amniotic fluid has not been proven to be effective in reducing the morbidity of MAS (Xu et al, 2008)
- Postpartum management of the vigorous newborn with thick meconium does not require immediate intubation and endotracheal suctioning
- Surfactant treatment or lavage has a beneficial effect on the clearance of meconium through detergent action, as well as a reduction in pulmonary hypertension in addition to the replacement of inactivated surfactant
- Inhaled nitric oxide relaxes the pulmonary vascular tone and has been shown to reduce morbidity and mortality in infants with PPHN

Airway Obstruction

CLINICAL PROFILE

- Symptoms include stridor, abnormal cry, cough, paradoxical breathing, feeding abnormalities, and positional effect on symptoms
- May be present anywhere, from the nose to lung alveoli

UPDATE #3

Use of video laryngoscopy may improve chances of successful intubation, as well as provide recordable visualization of the airway anatomy (Hackell et al, 2009).

CAUSE OF OBSTRUCTION

- Nasal
  - Nasal congestion
  - Choanal atresia
- Oropharynx
  - Macroglossia
  - Pierre Robin sequence
  - Cystic hygroma
  - Microstomia
- Trachea
  - Congenital tracheal stenosis
  - Tracheomalacia
  - Cyst
  - Tumor
  - Vascular ring
  - Vernix aspiration
  - Meconium aspiration
- Larynx
  - Laryngomalacia
  - Congenital/acquired vocal cord paralysis
  - Congenital/acquired subglottic stenosis
  - Acute laryngospasm
  - Laryngeal atresia
  - Laryngeal web/cysts
- Hemangiomata

MANAGEMENT

- Good head and neck positioning is crucial to maintaining a patent airway
- A nasal or oral airway device using endotracheal tube, nasal trumpet, or other fixed airway device is very effective in establishing a patent airway

- Ex utero intrapartum therapy (EXIT) procedure: this specialized surgical technique for babies born with difficult airways is a limited procedure for use in specialized hospitals that have an organized team assembled

Congenital Diaphragmatic Hernia

CLINICAL PROFILE

- Failure of the diaphragm to close during fetal development
- Association with genetic syndromes, particularly with cardiac anomalies
- Left-sided lesion much more common than right (~85%)
- Associated with pulmonary hypoplasia and pulmonary hypertension
- Bowel sounds present in the chest
- High mortality rate of 40% to 62%

UPDATE #4

Fetal surgery has been an option for a limited number of infants and centers. Tracheal occlusion did not improve survival or morbidity outcomes. Conclusive evidence for the efficacy of fetal diaphragmatic repair is not available, limiting the availability of this option (Mitanchez, 2008).

MANAGEMENT

- Request antenatal chromosomes and fetal echocardiogram
- Discuss the use of early antenatal steroids to accelerate lung maturation
- Request latest gestation as possible for elective C-section
- Resuscitate with 100% and limit peak pressures to 24 cm H_2O (Finer et al, 1998)
- Avoid bag and mask ventilation, and immediately place endotracheal tube, nasogastric tube, and vascular access with umbilical venous catheter (UVC)
- Accept lower oxygen saturation targets (i.e., >70%)
- Limit spontaneous breathing with heavy sedation or paralysis (morphine/fentanyl +/− vecuronium)
- If severe hypoxia, trial-test a dose of surfactant (0.5 to 1.0 mL intratracheal)

The Cyanotic Newborn

CLINICAL PROFILE

- Central cyanosis without respiratory distress = cyanotic heart disease
- Need 5 g/dL hemoglobin in blood to make blue color readily visible
- Most common cause of early cyanosis is transposition of the great arteries (TGA) with an intact ventricular septum (poor mixing)
- Defects without murmur more difficult to detect, picked up 26% by clinical exam (e.g., total anomalous pulmonary venous drainage, atrial septal defect, coarctation)

UPDATE #5

The antenatal diagnosis of congenital heart disease has better prepared the pediatric team at delivery. Early pulse oximetry screening may be able to increase detection of cyanotic heart disease, reducing the risk of discharge with undiagnosed congenital heart disease by at least 75% (Valmari, 2007).

MANAGEMENT

- If clinical suspicion, best to place a postductal pulse oximetry probe
- Assess relationship of degree of respiratory distress to oxygen saturation
- If available, determine early the anatomic diagnosis by two-dimensional echocardiography

Suspected Congenital Heart Disease (CHD)

CLINICAL PROFILE

- Fetal ultrasound diagnosis of congenital CHD has improved the readiness of the neonatal team in managing the cyanotic newborn
- Lesions divided into ductus-dependent lesions and ductus-independent lesions
- Lesions with significant mixing of left and right circulations will lead to lower baseline oxygen saturations

UPDATE #6

Early antenatal diagnosis of hypoplastic left heart disease results in better preoperative clinical status, including earlier start of prostaglandin, better arterial gases, lower oxygen requirements, and reduced need for mechanical ventilation (Sivarajan et al, 2009).

DIFFERENTIAL DIAGNOSIS

- Ductus-dependent lesions
- Transposition of the great arteries
- Right-sided obstructive lesions
  - Pulmonary atresia/stenosis
  - Tetralogy of Fallot
  - Total anomalous pulmonary venous return
  - Tricuspid atresia
  - Truncus arteriosus
- Ebstein's anomaly (not duct dependent)
- Left-sided obstruction
  - Interrupted aortic arch
- Coarctation of the aorta

MANAGEMENT

- Infants with known duct-dependent lesions are resuscitated in the standard manner
- Keep oxygen low to prevent premature or accelerated closure of the oxygen sensitive patent ductus arteriosus
- Initiate prostaglandin E1 (PGE1) as infusion at 0.01 to 0.05 mcg/kg/min to maintain duct patency
- At lower rates of PGE1 infusion, less likely to encounter apnea
- More favorable to secure airway with intubation in infants who require long transportation to another facility

Shock

CLINICAL PROFILE

- Sign of inadequate delivery of substrates and oxygen to meet the metabolic needs of the tissues (Jones et al, 2009)
- Sudden and unexpected blood loss may lead to significant cardiovascular destabilization
- Hypovolemic versus cardiogenic

UPDATE #7

Defining what is considered hypotension for any given infant of a gestational age is still debated. There is no absolutely accepted standard or test to confirm adequate tissue perfusion. Controversies are still present with determining best inotropic drug for hypotension (Dempsey et al, 2009). Numeric blood pressure is approximately the same as gestational age on day 1 but rises over the first week of life. Use of corticosteroids may sensitize the infant to epinephrine and potentiate the response to other inotropic drugs.

DIFFERENTIAL DIAGNOSIS

- Hypovolemia
  - Fetomaternal hemorrhage
  - Placental abruption
- Cardiogenic
  - Uterine rupture
  - Sepsis
- Hypoxic ischemic damage

MANAGEMENT

- Match resuscitation therapy to type of shock
- In acute hypovolemia, administer crystalloid such as normal saline or Ringer's lactate, stat order unmatched O-neg blood (Dempsey et al, 2009)
- In asphyxial shock, extra caution should be taken for administration of volume expansion and not cause undue cardiac stress
- Dopamine is effective in raising numeric systemic blood pressure but can also restrict blood flow to end organs at high doses

Congenital Hydrops

CLINICAL PROFILE

- Abnormal accumulation of fluid in at least two fetal body compartments such as peritoneal, pleural, or pericardial space
- Accompanied by significant peripheral edema
- Immune hydrops mostly the result of severe anemia caused by isoimmunization with red cell antigens such as Rh
- Nonimmune hydrops may be caused by cardiogenic causes or anemia (Sosa, 1999)
- An imbalance of interstitial fluid production and the lymphatic return
- Causes of non-immune hydrops (NIH) include cardiovascular diseases, chromosomal disorders, infections, lung, stomach, intestinal, kidneys, urinary tract and blood diseases, metabolic disorders, and tumors

UPDATE #8

Successful attempts have been made to treat homozygous alpha-thalassemia (hemoglobin H) with in utero transfusions and postnatal bone marrow transplant (Vichinsky, 2009).

DIFFERENTIAL DIAGNOSIS

- Cardiovascular (21.7%)
- Hematologic (10.4%)
- Chromosomal (13.4%)
- Syndromic (4.4%)
- Lymphatic dysplasia (5.7%)
- Inborn errors of metabolism (1.1%)
- Infections (6.7%)
- Thoracic (6%)
- Urinary tract malformations (2.3%)
- Extrathoracic tumors (0.7%)
- Placental (5.6%)
- Gastrointestinal (GI) (0.5%)
- Miscellaneous (3.7%)
- Idiopathic (17.8%)

MANAGEMENT

- Large pleural effusions may need to be needled (thoracentesis) emergently during the newborn resuscitation to permit adequate gas exchange
- Care with excessive volume resuscitation in chronic anemia because of compensated normal intravascular volume

Gastrointestinal Obstruction

CLINICAL PROFILE

- Proximal GI obstructions (i.e., esophageal, gastric, or duodenal) present earliest
- Tracheoesophageal fistula (TEF)/esophageal atresia (EA)
  - Most common form is EA with distal TEF (trachea communicates with lower esophagus)
  - Sometimes detected inadvertently in the delivery room with passage of naso/orogastric catheter
  - Presents often with vomiting or regurgitation with feeding and associated respiratory distress
- Duodenal atresia
  - Obstruction leads to dilated duodenal bulb and stomach ("double bubble" on radiograph)
- Meconium ileus
  - Meconium ileus is caused by the inspissation of meconium in the small or large bowel leading to obstruction in utero
  - This obstruction may result in dilatation of a segment of bowel, perforation, peritonitis, bowel volvulus, bowel atresias, or formation of a pseudocyst (walled-off perforation)
  - Clinically may appear normal or have marked abdominal distension
  - Echogenic bowel by ultrasound (US) or multiple calcifications on plain abdominal radiographs
  - Associated with pancreatic insufficient cystic fibrosis (CF), presenting manifestation in 10% to 15% of CF (Chaudry et al, 2006)

- Meconium plug syndrome
  - Obstructive firm meconium plugs in the colon
  - Often associated with infant of a diabetic mother (i.e., small left colon syndrome)
  - Also seen in extremely low-birth-weight infants
- Imperforate anus
  - May be associated with rectovaginal or rectovesicular fistula, with appearance of passage of stool

UPDATE #9

Antenatal bowel dilatation is more specific than bowel echogenicity for postnatal bowel pathology (Jackson et al, 2010).

MANAGEMENT

- To prevent aspiration, place large suction catheter/Replogle under continuous or intermittent suction
- Care must be taken with mask or endotracheal ventilation in TEF because of the potential for gas trapping in the stomach; sometimes, elective right mainstem intubation is required to establish adequate ventilation
- Rarely the stomach is needled or gastrostomy tube placed to decompress it temporarily if unable to ventilate properly
- With meconium ileus or plug syndrome, abdominal ultrasound and contrast enema are performed to evaluate anatomy and offer possible therapeutic benefit, especially for meconium plug syndrome
- In imperforate anus, may be missed if low-lying defect; important to spread anus during exam

Abdominal Wall Defects

CLINICAL PROFILE

- Gastroschisis
  - Condition in which abdominal contents, typically the intestine and sometimes the bladder, are extruded through a small abdominal wall defect lateral (mostly right side) to the umbilical cord (Banyard et al, 2010)
  - Occurs before the 12th week of gestation
  - Detected by the first trimester antenatal ultrasound
  - Associated with significant bowel dysmotility resulting from the damage from the serosal side of the bowel
- Omphalocele
  - Central herniation of abdominal contents encased within the umbilical cord
  - High association with other congenital and chromosomal abnormalities (~50%)
  - Large omphaloceles are associated with pulmonary hypoplasia

UPDATE #10

The incidence of gastroschisis continues to rise worldwide. There is an association of change in paternity in multigravida mothers (Chambers et al, 2007). Delayed reduction of moderate to large gastroschisis avoids abdominal compartment syndrome. Sutureless closure that incorporates the use of the umbilical stump may be an alternative method that does not significantly increase the time to reach full enteral feeding or hospital discharge. Environmental exposure to herbicides such as atrazine has been linked with increased gastroschisis rates (Mattix et al, 2007).

MANAGEMENT

- Delay of immediate primary closure may be accomplished with the use of preformed silos (synthetic translucent bags) that protect the exposed bowel (Allotey et al, 2007)
- Silos are not associated with worse outcomes and may provide time for bowel edema to settle, reducing the risk for abdominal compartment syndrome
- The bowel should be immediately wrapped in plastic and supported to prevent any abrupt changes of the blood supply
- In some cases, bowel obstruction may occur with occult bowel atresias
- A Replogle suction catheter under intermittent suction helps to prevent further bowel distension
- Initiation of feeding should take place as soon as signs of bowel motility are present (i.e., bowel sounds, stooling)

Hypoglycemia
CLINICAL PROFILE

- Glucose is primary energy source for organs
- Cerebral glucose use accounts for almost 90% of total glucose consumption
- The newborn brain has higher metabolic demands than the adult brain
- Glucose utilization rates are 5 to 8 mg/kg/minute
- Gluconeogenic enzymes induced slower in preterm infants
- The duration of hypoglycemia correlates with poor long-term neurodevelopmental outcomes
- Most metabolically active parts of the brain are at greatest risk for injury (basal ganglia, parieto-occipital cortex)
- Signs: apnea, jitteriness, irritability, grunting, seizures, or asymptomatic behaviors

UPDATE #11

The maternal use of beta-blockers puts infants at greater risk for hypoglycemia (Davis et al, 2010). Asymmetric large for gestational age (LGA) infants are at higher risk for morbidity than symmetric LGA and non-LGA infants (Bollepalli et al, 2010).

MANAGEMENT

- Aim for early correction and stabilization of serum glucose levels
- Treatment should escalate in proportion to the duration of hypoglycemia (i.e., increasing glucose administration the longer the hypoglycemic episode)
- Second-line therapies include glucagon, diazoxide, and octreotide

Dysmorphic Newborn
CLINICAL PROFILE

- Trisomy 21, 18, and 13 are the most common trisomies, in order of decreasing frequency
- Turner's syndrome (46,XO) is often associated with cystic hygroma involving the neck or the chest

- The common trisomies frequently have associated cardiac anomalies in addition to numerous GI emergencies such as bowel obstruction because of duodenal atresia, esophageal atresia, or imperforate anus

UPDATE #12

The increasing involvement of hospital ethics committees for cases that present issues surrounding corrective surgery for cardiac and GI anomalies helps improve the health care team's and parental discussion of difficult ethical challenges (Mercurio, 2010).

MANAGEMENT

- Good parental communication is essential
- Immediate assessment of general clinical features should alert you to possible syndromic diagnosis
- Look for abnormalities of the face, head, skin, extremities, chest, abdomen, and genitalia
- Low oxygen saturation, a heart murmur, or any abnormalities on cardiac exam should trigger a full cardiac evaluation
- Ultrasounds for renal anomalies of the abdomen and for dysgenesis of the brain are important for early evaluations

Hypoxic Ischemic Encephalopathy (HIE)

CLINICAL PROFILE

- Acute perinatal event versus intermittent subacute events
- Presence of severe metabolic acidosis at birth with a cord gas of pH <7 and a base deficit less than 15 mmol/L
- Presence of altered level of consciousness and seizures, as well as evidence of other end organ injury besides the brain such as oliguria, liver enzyme elevation, and poor cardiac output

UPDATE #13

In moderate to severe encephalopathy, the use of whole body cooling or selective head cooling can reduce overall combined death and neurodevelopmental morbidity at 18 months (Edwards et al, 2010).

DIFFERENTIAL DIAGNOSIS

- Idiopathic
- Cord prolapse
- Cord compression
- Uterine rupture

MANAGEMENT

- In delivery room, if HIE is suspected, passive cooling should be initiated by not warming with radiant warmer
- Cooling to 33.5° C started for 72 hours if infant meets criteria according to published protocols (National Institute of Child Health and Development [NICHD], Cool Cap, or total body cooling [TOBY] trials) (Edwards et al, 2010)

Hypotonia

CLINICAL PROFILE

- Flaccid limbs, poor truncal tone, weak cry, poor respiratory effort (Bodamer et al, 2009; Bodensteiner 2008)
- Most have central causes
- In severe neuromuscular disorders, infants are described as "rag doll," and family history may be helpful (e.g., myotonic dystrophy dominantly inherited)
- In congenital conditions, associated oligohydramnios resulting from poor swallowing may be present
- The infant with a spinal cord injury will display active facial muscles but be flaccid below the neck

UPDATE #14

Infants with congenital myotonic dystrophy may require prolonged ventilation but may also improve over time, even greater than 30 days (Campbell et al, 2004).

DIFFERENTIAL DIAGNOSIS

- Central causes
  - Hypoxic ischemic encephalopathy
  - Intracranial hemorrhage
  - Cerebral malformations
  - Chromosomal abnormalities (e.g., trisomy 21, Prader-Willi syndrome)
  - Congenital infections such as toxoplasmosis, rubella, cytomegalovirus, herpes simplex (TORCH)
  - Acquired infections
  - Peroxisomal disorders
  - Drug effects (e.g., hypermagnesemia, narcotics, benzodiazepines)
  - Others
- Includes spinal cord injury, spinal muscular atrophy, myasthenia gravis, congenital myasthenia gravis, central core disease, metabolic inborn errors of metabolism

MANAGEMENT

- Important to ensure a secure airway is present
- Generally easy to bag and mask ventilate
- Assess degree of hypotonia (central and peripheral tone, head lag) and level of alertness
- Elicit deep tendon reflexes to help differentiate upper from lower motor neuron disease
- Obtain a good family history of weakness or neuromuscular disorders and maternal drug use prior to and at delivery

Congenital Skin Disorders

CLINICAL PROFILE

- Diffuse skin lesions with breakdown of normal skin barrier raising risk for infection
- Severe lesions can be vesicular, bullous, or ichthyotic skin
- Vesicular lesions most suspicious for herpes infection (herpes simplex or zoster)
- Bullous lesions lead to rapid skin breakdown and greater risk for infection

- Difficult to discern lethal versus nonlethal
- Heat intolerance in infants with thickened skin caused by inadequate sweating

UPDATE #15

The molecular basis of the congenital skin disorders is increasingly detailed, but we are still awaiting specific therapies (Langan et al, 2009).

DIFFERENTIAL DIAGNOSIS

- Infectious: herpes simplex, varicella zoster
- Epidermolysis bullosa (EB)
- Ichthyoses: harlequin ichthyosis, lamellar ichthyosis, and nonbullous congenital ichthyosiform erythroderma

MANAGEMENT

- Start protection of skin with barrier ointment
- No effective treatment known for EB (Langan et al, 2009)
- Instigate early consultation of dermatologist and clinical genetics
- Avoid prognosticating until full consultations occur

SUGGESTED READINGS

Respiratory Distress

Finer NN, Carlo WA, Walsh MC, et al: Early CPAP versus surfactant in extremely preterm infants, *N Engl J Med* 362(21):1970–1979, 2010.

Kumar P, Denson SE, Mancuso TJ: Premedication for nonemergency endotracheal intubation in the neonate, *Pediatrics* 125(3):608–615, 2010.

Meconium Aspiration

Velaphi S, Vidyasagar D: Intrapartum and postdelivery management of infants born to mothers with meconium-stained amniotic fluid: evidence-based recommendations, *Clin Perinatol* 33(1):29–42, 2006. v-vi.

Xu H, Wei S, Fraser WD: Obstetric approaches to the prevention of meconium aspiration syndrome, *J Perinatol* 28(Suppl 3):S14–S18, 2008.

Airway Obstruction

Hackell RS, Held LD, Stricker PA, et al: Management of the difficult infant airway with the Storz Video Laryngoscope: a case series, *Anesth Analg* 109(3):763–766, 2009.

Congenital Diaphragmatic Hernia

Finer NN, Tierney A, Etches PC, et al: Congenital diaphragmatic hernia: developing a protocolized approach, *J Pediatr Surg* 33(9):1331–1337, 1998.

Mitanchez D: Antenatal treatment of congenital diaphragmatic hernia: an update, *Arch Pediatr* 15(8):1320–1325, 2008.

Cyanotic Newborn

Valmari P: Should pulse oximetry be used to screen for congenital heart disease? *Arch Dis Child Fetal Neonatal Ed* 92(3):F219–F224, 2007.

Suspected Congenital Heart Disease

Sivarajan V, Penny DJ, Filan P, et al: Impact of antenatal diagnosis of hypoplastic left heart syndrome on the clinical presentation and surgical outcomes: the Australian experience, *J Paediatr Child Health* 45(3):112–117, 2009.

Shock

Dempsey EM, Barrington KJ: Evaluation and treatment of hypotension in the preterm infant, *Clin Perinatol* 36(1):75–85, 2009.

Jones JG, Smith SL: Shock in the critically ill neonate, *J Perinat Neonatal Nurs* 23(4):346–354, 2009.

Congenital Hydrops

Sosa ME: Nonimmune hydrops fetalis, *J Perinat Neonatal Nurs* 13(3):33–44, 1999.

Vichinsky EP: Alpha thalassemia major: new mutations, intrauterine management, and outcomes, *Hematology Am Soc Hematol Educ Program* 1:35–41, 2009.

Gastrointestinal Obstruction

Chaudry G, Navarro OM, Levine DS, et al: Abdominal manifestations of cystic fibrosis in children, *Pediatr Radiol* 36(3):233–240, 2006.

Jackson CR, Orford J, Minutillo C, et al: Dilated and echogenic fetal bowel and postnatal outcomes: a surgical perspective: case series and literature review, *Eur J Pediatr Surg* 20(3):191–193, 2010.

Abdominal Wall Defects

Banyard D, Ramones T, Phillips SE, et al: Method to our madness: an 18-year retrospective analysis on gastroschisis closure, *J Pediatr Surg* 45(3):579–584, 2010.

Chambers CD, Chen BH, Kalla K, et al: Novel risk factor in gastroschisis: change of paternity, *Am J Med Genet A* 143(7):653–659, 2007.

Mattix KD, Winchester PD, Scherer LR: Incidence of abdominal wall defects is related to surface water atrazine and nitrate levels, *J Pediatr Surg* 42(6):947–949, 2007.

Hypoglycemia

Allotey J, Davenport M, Njere I, et al: Benefit of preformed silos in the management of gastroschisis, *Pediatr Surg Int* 23(11):1065–1069, 2007.

Bollepalli S, Dolan LM, Miodovnik M, et al: Asymmetric large-for-gestational-age infants of type 1 diabetic women: morbidity and abdominal growth, *Am J Perinatol* 27(8):603–610, 2010.

Davis R, Andrade S, Rubanowice D, et al: C-a4-03: risks to the newborn associated with in-utero exposure to beta-blockers and calcium-channel blockers, *Clin Med Res* 8(1):57, 2010.

Dysmorphic Newborn

Mercurio MR: The role of a pediatric ethics committee in the newborn intensive care unit, *J Perinatol* 31(1):1–9, 2010.

Hypoxic Ischemic Encephalopathy

Edwards AD, Brocklehurst P, Gunn AJ, et al: Neurological outcomes at 18 months of age after moderate hypothermia for perinatal hypoxic ischaemic encephalopathy: synthesis and meta-analysis of trial data, *BMJ* 340:c363, 2010.

Hypotonia

Bodamer OA, Miller G: Approach to the infant with hypotonia and weakness, *UpToDate Version* 17, ed 3, 2009.

Bodensteiner JB: The evaluation of the hypotonic infant, *Semin Pediatr Neurol* 15(1):10–20, 2008.

Campbell C, Sherlock R, Jacob P, et al: Congenital myotonic dystrophy: assisted ventilation duration and outcome, *Pediatrics* 113(4):811–816, 2004.

Congenital Skin Disorders

Langan SM, Williams HC: A systematic review of randomized controlled trials of treatments for inherited forms of epidermolysis bullosa, *Clin Exp Dermatol* 34(1):20–25, 2009.

References

Please go to expertconsult.com to view references.

Chapter 19

Puerperium

ANDREW H. SPENCER • MARYAM TARSA

KEY UPDATES

1 At the time of diagnosis for postpartum cardiomyopathy, an ejection fraction of less than 25% is associated with poor outcomes.

2 Breast-feeding has protective cardiovascular role.

3 Domperidone increases breast milk volume in mothers with preterm delivery.

4 Recombinant activated factor VIIa can be used for postpartum hemorrhage when standard treatments have failed.

5 Emergent postpartum hysterectomy is associated with significant maternal morbidity.

6 Postpartum incontinence is more common in women with incontinence during pregnancy.

7 Personalized clinical care may decrease postpartum cesarean wound complication.

8 Risk of postpartum depression is higher in mothers with premature infants.

9 Selective serotonin reuptake inhibitor (SSRI) use in late pregnancy has been associated with the development of pulmonary hypertension of the newborn.

Definition

Puerperium refers to the time period from the delivery of the placenta through the first 6 weeks after delivery. This is considered the time during which the female body returns to the nonpregnant state.

Normal Puerperium

SYSTEMIC PUERPERAL CHANGES

- Abdominal wall: remains soft for many weeks depending on level of maternal exercise
- Separation of rectus muscles may result in diastasis recti
- Cardiovascular system: though most cardiac indices return to baseline by 6 to 8 weeks postpartum, the rate of return to basal remains unknown
  - Cardiac output increases significantly immediately postpartum due to autotransfusion
  - Cardiac output, stroke volume, end-diastolic volume, and systemic vascular resistance remain elevated for about 12 weeks postpartum (Capeless et al, 1991)

UPDATE #1

One of the rare complications of this period is peripartal cardiomyopathy. The prognosis is related to the recovery of left ventricular function. Counseling for the outcome of subsequent pregnancy is based on limited current information. Recent data suggest that a left ventricular ejection fraction of 25% or less at the time of diagnosis is associated with poor long-term outcome and a higher rate of cardiac transplantation. This is regardless of subsequent recovery of left ventricular function in the follow-up period (Habli et al, 2008).

- Renal: glomerular filtration rate returns to nongravid state by 6 weeks postpartum
  - Dilation of renal calyces, pelvis, and ureters may persist for several months postpartum
- Urinary tract: Bladder function is altered in postpartum
  - Mucosal injury to bladder is related to length of labor
  - Bladder distension immediately postpartum is due to increased capacity and insensitivity to excess fluid volume
  - Traumatized bladder, poor bladder emptying, residual hydronephrosis, and hydroureter increase the risk of urinary tract infection in this period
  - Liver: estrogen-induced increases in clotting factors and binding globulins of hepatic origin return to nonpregnant state within 3 weeks postpartum

PELVIC ORGAN CHANGES

- Return of ovulation and menstruation: chorionic gonadotropin is eliminated from circulation within the first 2 weeks
  - Return of ovulation and menstruation depends on the duration of lactation and maternal adiposity
- Uterus: reduction in size and weight within the first 2 weeks
  - Lochia: vaginal discharge lasting approximately 5 weeks and changing from red (rubra) to brown (serosa) and finally to yellow (alba)
  - Involution of the uterus begins by day 2 postpartum; individual muscle fibers decrease in size rather than numbers

176

- Subinvolution may cause erratic and at times heavy bleeding; short course of Methergine has been suggested with unproven benefit
- Cervix: external os accommodates only two fingers by the end of first week
  - Parous cervix remains wider with bilateral outward depression
  - Epithelium undergoes remodeling with a chance of regression of cervical dysplasia
- Vagina: Does not fully return to prepregnant state
  - Vaginal epithelium is atrophic for up to 10 weeks
  - Breast-feeding delays restoration of normal epithelium

PUERPERAL BREAST CHANGES

- Physiologic breast changes
  - Enlargement of the breasts occurs in the postpartum period as a result of edema and milk production
  - Lactation suppression can be achieved in 70% of women by binding the breasts
  - Acetaminophen, ibuprofen, and cold compresses may be used for symptomatic relief
- Lactation: Lactogenesis begins in pregnancy (stage I)
  - Stage II begins after delivery with copious milk secretion resulting from the decreased progesterone level
    - The components of human milk play a role in neonatal immune system modulation, digestion, and promotion of growth
    - Milk composition changes in the first 4 days
    - Immediately postpartum, concentration of sodium, chloride, and immunoglobulin is high (colostrum)
    - Colostrum stimulates maturation of neonatal B lymphocytes and increases the activity of macrophages
    - Progressively, concentration of lactose, protein, and lipid and the overall volume of milk increase (Neville et al, 2001)
- Breast-feeding: the let-down (ejection) reflex is the most important factor in the initiation of lactation
  - Oxytocin promotes milk ejection
    - Exclusive breast-feeding is recommended for the first 6 months after birth and should be continued, with the addition of solid foods, for at least 12 months (Gartner et al, 2005)
    - Benefits to the neonate of human milk include improvement in gastrointestinal function and immune response, and reduction of acute illnesses during the time of breast-feeding (American College of Obstetricians and Gynecologists, ACOG Education Bulletin 258, 2000)
  - Contraindications to breast-feeding: these include women with herpetic breast lesions (American Academy of Pediatrics, 2009), women who are susceptible to varicella infection, and those who came into contact with contagious individuals (also see Table 19-1)

UPDATE #2

Recent data suggest that breast-feeding has a protective role in maternal cardiovascular health. Breast-feeding for at least 3 months decreases the chances of aortic and coronary artery calcification (Schwarz et al, 2010).

TABLE 19-1   Conditions in Which Breast-Feeding Should Be Avoided

Breast-feeding is not advisable if one of the following conditions exists:
1. Infant has galactosemia
2. Mother is infected with human immunodeficiency virus
3. Mother is taking antiretroviral
4. Mother has active tuberculosis
5. Mother is infected with human T-cell lymphotropic virus
6. Mother is dependent or actively using illicit drug
7. Mother is taking chemotherapeutic agents
8. Mother is undergoing radiation therapy

Modified and adapted from Center Disease Control and Prevention. cdcinfo@cdc.gov.

UPDATE #3

Domperidone is sometimes prescribed to increase breast milk volume. Recent data suggests that it increases the breast milk volume in preterm mothers with lactation failure without significantly altering breast milk composition (Campbell et al, 2010).

Abnormal Puerperium

HEMORRHAGE

- Accounts for 30% of direct maternal death worldwide (Khan et al, 2006); defined by the World Health Organization as blood loss greater than 500 mL
- Early postpartum hemorrhage (PPH): 4% to 6% of all deliveries within the first 24 hours; Figure 19-1 shows summary of approach
  - Causes: atony, lacerations, retained products of conception, and abnormal coagulation
  - Disorders of coagulation should be suspected in patients with a family history and in the absence of any other causes; the workup is summarized in Figure 19-2 (Silver et al, 2010)

UPDATE #4

Multiple case reports document the use of activated recombinant factor VIIa in addressing postpartum hemorrhage when the usual treatments have failed. The suggested dose is 40 to 60 micrograms/kg. This can be repeated in 15 to 30 minutes if there is no clinical improvement (Franchini et al, 2007).

- Late PPH: 1% to 3% of all deliveries between 24 hours and 6 weeks
- Mostly because of retained placenta
- Emergent postpartum hysterectomy: in the United States, incidence is 0.8 to 2.3 per 1000 deliveries (Whiteman et al, 2006)
  - Risks include placenta previa, placenta accreta, placenta increta, placenta percreta, uterine rupture, and number of previous cesarean sections

UPDATE #5

A recent meta-analysis has suggested maternal morbidity in 55.8% of cases of emergent postpartum hysterectomy. Morbidities include fever (26%), disseminated intravascular coagulation (22%), infection (16%), genitourinary and pulmonary injury (24%) (Rossi et al, 2010). Risk of blood transfusion was 43.6%, and postoperative maternal death complicated 2.6% of cases.

LOWER GENITAL TRACT LACERATIONS

- Risk factors: large baby, nulliparity, episiotomy, operative delivery, and precipitous birth
  - Higher-degree laceration and mediolateral episiotomy have an increased incidence of wound disruption

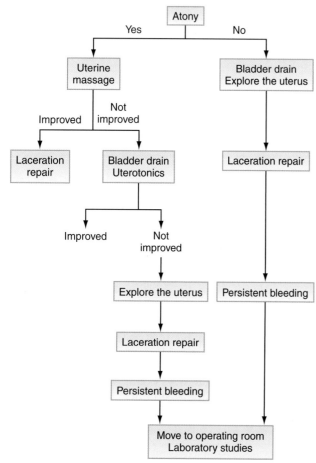

POSTPARTUM HEMORRHAGE

Figure 19-1. Management of postpartum hemorrhage. (Modified and adapted from Quiñones JN, Uxer JB, Gogle J, et al: Clinical evaluation during postpartum hemorrhage, *Clin Obstet Gynecol* 53(1):157-164, 2010.)

- Routine episiotomy should be avoided
- Mediolateral episiotomy results in fewer third- and fourth-degree lacerations
- Incontinence: vaginal birth is a major determinant of anal and urinary incontinence
  - Instrumental deliveries and episiotomy compound the risk

INFECTION

- Puerperal fever is defined as an "oral temperature of 38.0° C or more on any 2 of the first 10 days postpartum" by United States Joint Commission on Maternal Welfare
- Most organizations extend this period to 42 days postpartum
- Endometritis: most severe cases are caused by group A streptococci
  - More common after cesarean delivery
  - Infection is polymicrobial aerobic and anaerobic
  - A combination of clindamycin and aminoglycoside is an appropriate regimen
- Urinary tract infection: frequency, urgency, and a urine specimen containing $\geq 10^5$ colony-forming U/ml
  - *Escherichia coli* followed by *Proteus mirabilis* and *Klebsiella pneumoniae* are the most common organisms
  - A 3-day course of antibiotic is usually sufficient
  - Systemic symptoms such as fever, flank pain, nausea, and vomiting should raise the suspicion for pyelonephritis
  - Early and aggressive treatment of pyelonephritis with antibiotics is recommended to prevent sepsis
- Mastitis: painful, localized breast inflammation associated with fever that occurs in breast-feeding women
  - Occurs in up to 10% of breast-feeding women (American College of Obstetricians and Gynecologists, Opinion No. 361, 2007) and can result in poor breast-feeding

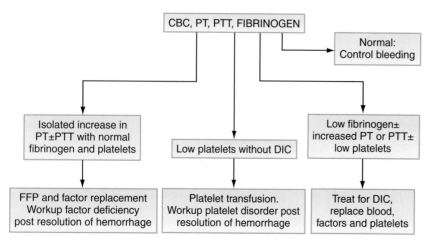

Figure 19-2. Workup for coagulation disorders. (Modified and adapted from Silver RM, Major H: Maternal coagulation disorders and postpartum hemorrhage, *Clin Obstet Gynecol* 53(1):252-264, 2010)

- Risk factors include a previous history of mastitis, prolonged unilateral breast engorgement, poor milk drainage, and nipple cracking
- Diagnosis is suspected if a fever of >38° C, erythema, induration and painful swelling of one breast, associated myalgias, chills, or flulike symptoms exist
- Staphylococcus aureus is the usual organism
- If mastitis is refractory to antibiotics, ultrasound may reveal an underlying abscess (Dener et al, 2003)
- Cold-compresses, anti-inflammatory medications, emptying of the breast by pumping, or breast-feeding can aid in treatment (Thomsen et al, 1984)
- Antibiotics should be prescribed if symptoms do not resolve by 72 hours
- Wound infection: complicates up to 16% of cesarean sections
  - The rate of infection is related to length of labor, internal monitoring, number of vaginal examinations, maternal weight, and significant blood loss during surgery
  - Clostridial infection can cause cellulites, tissue necrosis, and significant maternal systemic compromise including hemolysis, renal failure, and cardiovascular collapse
  - Necrotizing fasciitis can be caused commonly by group A beta-hemolytic streptococci or *Staphylococcus aureus* and will require surgical excision

UPDATE #7

To reduce wound complications post cesarean section, the following has been suggested (Sarsam et al, 2005):
1. Placement of sutures in the subcutaneous layer during abdominal closure in obese patients
2. Stringent glucose control in diabetic patients
3. Prophylactic antibiotics at or prior to umbilical cord clamping
4. Blood transfusion in patients with significant anemia
5. Placement of a closed drain system in patients receiving anticoagulation medications or with a coagulation disorder
6. Avoidance of perioperative hypothermia

- Perineal infection: pain, swelling, erythema are characteristic
  - Treatment should start with sitz baths unless abscess is present
  - Infection beyond Camper's fascia may result in necrotizing fasciitis
  - Retroperitoneal, gluteal muscle, levator ani, retropsoas abscess should be considered if not responding to treatment; exploration, debridement, and drainage may be necessary
- Septic pelvic thrombophlebitis: risk is higher in patients post cesarean section
  - Diagnosis suspected with failed antibiotic treatment for suspected endometritis
  - Computed tomography for magnetic resonance imaging is used to make a diagnosis
  - Treatment includes anticoagulation and broad-spectrum antibiotics
  - Length of treatment is a matter of debate
  - Patients are at increased risk for pulmonary embolus

- Pelvic abscess: despite extensive, broad-spectrum antibiotic treatment, patients with pelvic abscess continue to have persistent spiking fever
  - Ultrasound or computed tomography can be used to diagnose abscess
  - Treatment of choice is drainage

ENDOCRINE DISORDERS

- Postpartum thyroiditis: thyroiditis that occurs within 1 year of delivery; mean prevalence is 7% to 11% (Abalovich et al, 2007; Golden et al, 2009)
  - Diagnosis: can be hyperthyroidism, hypothyroidism, or transient hyperthyroidism followed by hypothyroidism
  - Usually mild disease, with minimal thyroid enlargement
  - Usually resolves within 4 weeks of parturition, which can also be used to distinguish it from Graves disease (Abalovich et al, 2007)
  - There has been no proven association between postpartum thyroiditis and postpartum depression (Kent et al, 1999)
  - Laboratory findings can include abnormal thyroid stimulating hormone (TSH), T4, and T3, along with elevated thyroglobulin, and peroxidase antibodies
  - Treatment: symptoms of postpartum thyroiditis usually resolve with no treatment; patients with moderate symptoms may be treated with a beta-blocker until thyroid levels return to normal
  - Patients with symptomatic hypothyroidism are usually treated with thyroxine for 4 to 6 weeks followed by reevaluation
- Postpartum Graves disease
  - Usually more severe than postpartum thyroiditis and does not resolve within 4 weeks of parturition
  - Caused by long-acting autoantibodies that are directed against the TSH receptor causing follicular hypertrophy and hyperplasia
  - Results in classic symptoms of hyperthyroidism such as tremor, anxiety, weakness, palpitations, tachycardia, sweating, and exophthalmos
  - If untreated, can cause severe thyrotoxicosis, which results in catabolism of bone and muscle, as well as deterioration of skin, eye, brain, and heart function
  - Therapy for Graves disease in the postpartum period is usually radioactive iodine; the use of radioactive iodine is a contraindication to breast-feeding
- Pituitary infarction: infarction of the pituitary gland caused by severe hypotension as a result of postpartum hemorrhage
  - Pituitary infarction remains a common cause of hypopituitarism in underdeveloped countries, where severe hemorrhage is more common (Zargar et al, 2005)
  - Symptoms include inability to lactate, weight loss, lethargy, anorexia, and failure to resume menstruation (Dokmetas et al, 2006)
  - Diagnosis can be made by finding abnormalities in levels of growth hormone, prolactin, gonadotropins, TSH, and adrenocorticotropic hormone (ACTH)
  - Treatment includes replacement with hydrocortisone, L-thyroxine, growth hormone, and estrogen and progesterone

- Pulsatile gonadotropin releasing hormone (GnRH) can be used to induce ovulation if pregnancy is desired
- Lymphocytic hypophysitis
  - Rare condition caused by enlargement and lymphocytic infiltration of the pituitary gland followed by destruction of pituitary cells
  - This condition is thought to be autoimmune in origin
  - Symptoms include headache, thyroid abnormalities, diabetes insipidus, elevated prolactin and growth hormone, and adrenal insufficiency (Sato et al, 1998)
  - Magnetic resonance imaging (MRI) or computed tomography (CT) evaluation of the pituitary can often show enhancement of the anterior pituitary and occasionally what appears to be a pituitary adenoma or mass (Powrie et al, 1995)
  - Lymphocytic hypophysitis results in progressive pituitary atrophy
  - Recovery of pituitary function can occur with high-dose glucocorticoid therapy (Kristof et al, 1999)

PSYCHIATRIC DISORDERS

- Postpartum blues: a temporary condition characterized by mild and sudden mood swings ranging from euphoria to grief, crying spells, irritability, nervousness, decreased concentration, and insomnia (O'Hara et al, 1991)
  - From 40% to 80% of postpartum women develop mood changes, generally within 2 to 3 days of delivery (Steiner, 1990)
  - Symptoms of postpartum blues generally peak at the end of the first week and taper off around 2 weeks after delivery

- Postpartum blues generally resolve over time with conservative management
- Occasionally, patients will require low-dose benzodiazepines to control insomnia
- Postpartum depression is defined as depression with an onset within 12 months of delivery
  - Postpartum depression affects approximately 5% to 10% of women (American Psychiatric Association, 1994)
  - Largest risk factor is a personal history of depression (Lee et al, 2001)
  - Diagnosis: symptoms of depression are present every day for at least 2 weeks
  - Screening for depression during the postpartum period should be considered using tools such as the Edinburgh Postnatal Depression Scale
  - Treatment: ensure the patient is not a threat to herself or anyone else
  - Psychotherapy is recommended as the initial therapy for mild to moderate postpartum depression (Rojas et al, 2007)
  - Pharmacotherapy is an acceptable treatment when psychotherapy is ineffective
  - In nonlactating mothers, the drug of choice is the same as that used for nonpuerperal depression
  - Most medications are transferred through breast milk
  - Selective serotonin reuptake inhibitor (SSRI) levels detected in breast milk are very low
  - For breast-feeding women, measuring the psychotropic drug level in the infant is not recommended
  - Benefits of breast-feeding should be weighed against the potential risk of the medication (Table 19-2)

TABLE 19-2   **Selected Psychiatric Medications in Lactation**

Generic Name	Trade Name	American Academy of Pediatrics Rating	Lactation Risk Category*
Anxiolytic Medications			
Benzodiazepines			
Diazepam	Valium	Unknown, of concern	L3, L4 if chronic use
Lorazepam	Ativan	Unknown, of concern	L3
Alprazolam	Xanax	Unknown, of concern	L3
Nonbenzodiazepine Anxiolytic			
Zolpidem	Ambien	N/A	L3
Antiepileptic and Mood Stabilizing			
Lithium carbonate	Lithonate	Contraindicated	L4
Valproic acid	Depakote	Compatible	L2
Antidepressants			
Fluoxetine	Prozac	Unknown, of concern	L2 in older infants, L3 in neonates
Paroxetine	Paxil	Unknown, of concern	L2
Sertraline	Zoloft	Unknown, of concern	L2
Antipsychotic Medications			
Haloperidol	Haldol	Unknown, of concern	L2
Risperidone	Risperidal	N/A	L3

*Lactation risk categories are as follows: L1, safest; L2, safer; L3, moderately safe; L4, possibly hazardous; L5, contraindicated.
Modified from The American College of Obstetrician and Gynecologists Compendium, American College of Obstetricians and Gynecologists (ACOG). Use of psychiatric medications during pregnancy and lactation. Washington (DC); American College of Obstetricians and Gynecologists (ACOG); 2008 Apr 20 p. (ACOG practice bulletin; no. 92).

UPDATE #8

The risk for postpartum depression is as high as 40% among women with premature infants (Vigod et al, 2010).

UPDATE #9

There appears to be an association between exposure of a mother to an SSRI during late pregnancy and the occurrence of persistent pulmonary hypertension of the newborn in her infant (Chambers et al, 2006).

- Postpartum psychosis is defined as the onset of psychotic symptoms following childbirth, usually within the first 6 weeks of delivery
  - Women are more likely to develop a psychotic illness in the postpartum period than at any other time in their lives (Videbech et al, 1995), with primiparous mothers at the greatest risk (Munk-Olsen et al, 2006)
  - Risk factors include a history of postpartum psychosis in a previous delivery (relapse rate up to 70%), a history of bipolar disorder (relapse rate up to 50%), and a family history of puerperal psychosis
  - Diagnosis of postpartum psychosis is based on DSM-IV criteria
  - Postpartum psychosis is considered a medical emergency, and the mother should be hospitalized under the care of a psychiatrist until stable
  - Electroconvulsive therapy can be used in patients who are at high risk for suicide or infanticide, for those who are acutely agitated, or for patients who refuse medication

SUGGESTED READINGS

Normal Puerperium

Breast

Campbell ML, Allen AC, Joseph KS, et al: Effect of domperidone on the composition of preterm human breast milk, *Pediatrics* 125(1):e107–e114, 2010.

Schwarz EB, McClure CK, Tepper PG, et al: Lactation and maternal measures of subclinical cardiovascular disease, *Obstet Gynecol* 115(1):41–48, 2010.

Cardiovascular System

Habli M, O'Brien T, Nowack E, et al: Peripartum cardiomyopathy: prognostic factors for long-term maternal outcome, *Am J Obstet Gynecol* 199(4):415.e1–e5, 2008.

Hemorrhage

Franchini M, Lippi G, Franchi M: The use of recombinant activated factor VII in obstetric and gynaecological haemorrhage, *BJOG* 114(1):8–15, 2007.

Rossi CA, Lee RH, Chamit RH: Emergency postpartum hysterectomy for uncontrolled postpartum bleeding, *Obstet Gynecol* 115(3):637–644, 2010.

Lower Genital Tract

Solans-Domenech M, Sanchez E, Espuna-Pons M (Pelvic Floor Research Group): Urinary and anal incontinence during pregnancy and postpartum, *Obstet Gynecol* 115(3):618–628, 2010.

Infection

Sarsam SE, Elliott JP, Lam GK: Management of wound complications from cesarean delivery, *Obstet Gynecol Surv* 60(5):462–473, 2005.

Psychiatric Disorders

Chambers CD, Hernandez-Diaz S, Van Marter LJ, et al: Selective serotonin-reuptake inhibitors and risk of persistent pulmonary hypertension of the newborn, *N Engl J Med* 354(6):579–587, 2006.

Vigod SN, Villegas N, Dennis CL, Ross LE: Prevalence and risk factor for postpartum depression among women with preterm and low birth weight infants: a systemic review, *BJOG* 117(5):540–550, 2010.

References

Please go to expertconsult.com to view references.

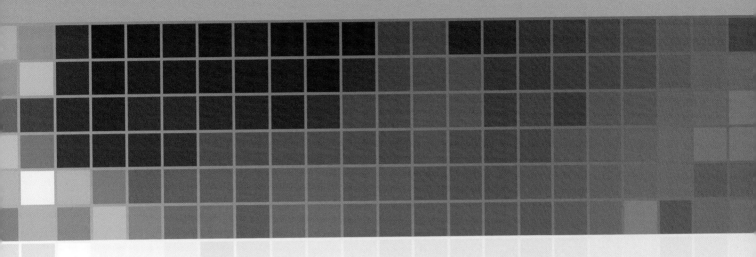

SECTION 6

Maternal Diseases Complicating Pregnancy

Chapter 20

Cardiac and Pulmonary Disorders in Pregnancy

DOUGLAS A. WOELKERS

KEY UPDATES

Cardiovascular Diseases

1 Prospective studies do not show an increased risk of preeclampsia in women with inherited thrombophilias.

2 Anti-angiogenic factors secreted by the placenta are elevated in women who have, or who are destined to develop, preeclampsia.

3 Severe systolic hypertension (>160 mmHg) is more strongly related to the risk of stroke than is severe diastolic hypertension.

4 Women with a history of preeclampsia are at increased future risk of cardiovascular and renal disease.

5 Iatrogenic preterm delivery for preeclampsia may prevent stillbirth, but these infants are at higher risk for diseases of prematurity than age-matched controls.

6 Magnesium sulfate is the agent of choice for seizure prophylaxis in preeclampsia. Selective use of prophylaxis will increase the rate of eclampsia.

7 Exposure to angiotensin-converting enzyme (ACE) inhibitors in pregnancy is associated with congenital anomalies.

8 Antioxidants do not reduce the risk of preeclampsia in high- or low-risk women.

9 Women with a history of peripartum cardiomyopathy are at high risk for recurrent heart failure in subsequent pregnancies.

Pulmonary Diseases

10 Pregnant women with asthma and depressed FEV_1 <80% are at risk for adverse pregnancy outcomes.

11 Appropriate intensive care unit (ICU) management of the pregnant woman requires input from the obstetrician and a collaborative approach to decision making.

12 Pregnancy alters the pharmacokinetics of low-molecular-weight heparin. Therapeutic dosing should be adjusted based on monitoring of anti-Factor Xa levels.

13 A history of thrombosis with thrombophilia or a prior idiopathic thrombosis is a risk factor for recurrent antepartum thrombosis during pregnancy.

Cardiovascular Disorders

HYPERTENSIVE DISORDERS OF PREGNANCY

- Classification of hypertension in pregnancy
  - Four recognized hypertensive disorders of pregnancy
    - Chronic hypertension
    - Preeclampsia-eclampsia
    - Superimposed preeclampsia with chronic hypertension
    - Gestational hypertension
  - Gestational hypertension is a temporary diagnosis, used to identify women with a new diagnosis of hypertension in pregnancy but without evidence of

the preeclampsia syndrome; if the hypertension does not resolve postpartum, then the patient has chronic hypertension; if the hypertension does resolve, then she had transient hypertension of pregnancy
- Pregnancy-induced hypertension (or PIH) is not a specific condition, and its use is discouraged
- Additional preeclampsia-like syndromes and atypical presentations include the following (Sibai et al, 2009):
  - Syndrome of hemolysis, elevated liver enzymes, and low platelets (HELLP)
  - Severe gestational hypertension
  - Gestational proteinuria

- Late postpartum preeclampsia-eclampsia
- Early (≤ 20 weeks') preeclampsia
- Etiology: most theories invoke a two-stage model of preeclampsia
  - Stage I
    - Shallow placentation with failed trophoblast invasion of maternal spiral arterioles, followed by placental ischemia/injury related to underperfusion, infarction, or thrombosis
    - The cause of the primary placental events in preeclampsia is not known; evidence suggests defects in trophoblast expression of surface adhesion molecules (integrins) and vascular growth factors, leading to failed acquisition of an invasive endothelial phenotype (Ilekis et al, 2007)

UPDATE #1

Contrary to initial evidence, large, prospective trials have *not* found that common inherited thrombophilias contribute significantly to the risk of preeclampsia (Kahn et al, 2009; Said et al, 2010; Silver et al, 2010).

  - Stage II
    - Factors released by the placenta into the maternal circulation lead to endothelial dysfunction and the clinical end points of preeclampsia (such as hypertension, proteinuria, and end-organ injury)
    - Many vasoactive factors are implicated in the pathology of preeclampsia, including cytokines, prostaglandins, lipid peroxides, trophoblast debris, and angiogenic growth factors

UPDATE #2

Increased placental secretion of soluble anti-angiogenic factors precedes the clinical onset of preeclampsia and is associated with the timing and severity of hypertensive disorders in pregnancy (Levine et al, 2006).

    - Anti-angiogenic factors, including the soluble receptor for vascular endothelial growth factor (VEGF) (sVEGF R1, or sFlt-1) and soluble endoglin (sEnd) may disrupt the balance of pro-angiogenic growth factors (such as placental growth factor, PlGF), which are secreted in high concentrations during normal pregnancy (Levine et al, 2004); women with elevations of sFlt-1 and sEndoglin, above the fourth quartile have a 30-fold increased risk of developing preeclampsia compared to those in the first quartile (Levine et al, 2006)
- Diagnosis and definitions
  - Preeclampsia is a *de novo* disorder of pregnancy; its diagnosis depends on establishing the baseline blood pressure and degree of proteinuria before 20 weeks of gestation
  - Women with hypertension or proteinuria prior to 20 weeks should be investigated further to determine the cause and duration of their condition (e.g., molar pregnancy or aneuploidy)
  - Diagnosis of hypertension

  - Blood pressure is a finding that shows great variability; correct measurement technique must be followed to minimize errors (Pickering et al, 2005)
  - Definition of hypertension: systolic blood pressure ≥140 mmHg or diastolic blood pressure ≥90 mmHg
    - Severe hypertension: systolic blood pressure ≥160 mmHg or diastolic blood pressure ≥110 mmHg on two occasions at least 6 hours apart at rest
- Diagnosis of proteinuria
  - Proteinuria is determined qualitatively by urine dipstick or quantitatively by a timed protein excretion (i.e., 24-hour collection) or a random urine protein-to-creatinine ratio (P/C ratio).
  - Dipstick is an unreliable measure of proteinuria. A reading of ≥1+ will usually correlate to 30 mg/dL, or approximately 300 mg per 24-hour collection. A reading of ≥3+ is considered a criterion for severe proteinuria. Nonetheless, urine dipstick fails to detect proteinuria in 33% of cases (Meyer et al, 1994) and shows great interobserver variability.
  - The 24-hour protein excretion is considered the gold standard of urine protein assessment. Proteinuria is defined as excretion of ≥300 mg per 24 hours. Severe proteinuria is defined as ≥5000 mg per 24 hours (ACOG, 2002). Errors in collection can lead to excessive variability in up to 20% of repeat collections (Cote et al, 2008).
  - A protein-to-creatinine ratio (P/C ratio) provides a quantitative assessment of random proteinuria that correlates closely to the 24-hour collection. It is calculated as the ratio of the urine protein concentration (mg/dL) divided by the urine creatinine concentration (mg/dL). A value of 0.30 is usually accepted as a surrogate for 300 mg of protein per day, although other cutoffs have been proposed. A meta-analysis of seven studies in pregnancy evaluating the P/C ratio versus the 24-hour threshold of 300 mg suggested an acceptable negative cutoff of 0.15 and a positive cutoff of 0.60, with only 2% to 5% discrepancy beyond these criteria (Papanna et al, 2008).
- Chronic hypertension is hypertension that is present or observable before 20 weeks, or hypertension that is first diagnosed in pregnancy and does not resolve postpartum
- Preeclampsia is the development of new onset hypertension and proteinuria after 20 weeks of pregnancy
  - In the absence of proteinuria the disease is highly suspect when increased blood pressure appears accompanied by the symptoms of headache, blurred vision, and abdominal pain, or with abnormal laboratory tests, specifically, low platelet counts, and abnormal liver enzymes
- Severe preeclampsia is preeclampsia accompanied by one or more severe criteria as follows (ACOG, 2002):
  - Severe hypertension
  - Severe proteinuria
  - Oliguria <500 ml in 24 hours
  - Cerebral or visual disturbances
  - Pulmonary edema or cyanosis
  - Epigastric or right upper-quadrant pain

- Impaired liver function
- Thrombocytopenia
- Fetal growth restriction
- Eclampsia is the presence of seizures in a woman with preeclampsia that cannot be attributed to another cause
- HELLP syndrome and other atypical variants of preeclampsia require a high index of suspicion and often present as a spectrum of clinical and laboratory findings that may evolve over time
  - In general, the diagnosis of HELLP syndrome or preeclampsia should not be given to women with isolated laboratory abnormalities in the absence of other symptomatic or physical markers of the syndrome
- Superimposed preeclampsia is chronic hypertension with suspected preeclampsia; this diagnosis is likely in cases of chronic hypertension with the following:
  - New onset proteinuria
  - Sudden increase in proteinuria
  - Sudden increase in blood pressure in previously well controlled chronic hypertension
  - Hypertension and proteinuria before 20 weeks
  - Thrombocytopenia
  - Abnormal liver function tests
- Gestational hypertension is new-onset hypertension in pregnancy without proteinuria or other criteria for severe preeclampsia.
- Outcomes
  - Hypertensive disorders complicate 5% to 10% of pregnancies
    - Preeclampsia affects 3.9% of pregnancies, or about half of the cases of hypertension in pregnancy
    - Severe preeclampsia is reported to affect 0.90% of pregnancies

UPDATE #3

A report by Martin and colleagues has focused attention on the neurovascular risks of severe systolic hypertension (Martin et al, 2005). They reported that of 25 patients who sustained a witnessed stroke in association with severe preeclampsia or eclampsia, 24 had immediate prestroke systolic blood pressures ≥160 mmHg. In contrast, only 3 of these patients had diastolic pressures exceeding 110 mmHg, and only 5 had diastolic pressures exceeding 105 mmHg. They concluded that aggressive antihypertensive therapy is indicated in women with severe preeclampsia or eclampsia whose systolic blood pressure (BP) exceeds 160 mmHg.

- Women with mild gestational hypertension at term have a favorable prognosis with fetal outcomes that are comparable to nonhypertensive women
- Women with severe gestational hypertension (BP ≥160/110), experience high rates of abruptio placenta, preterm delivery, and fetal growth restriction that are similar to cases with severe preeclampsia (Barton et al, 2001; Buchbinder et al, 2002; Sibai 2003)
- Nearly half of women with preterm gestational hypertension (≤37 weeks) will ultimately develop preeclampsia (Barton et al, 2001)

- In the United States, complications of hypertension and preeclampsia are the third most common cause of maternal mortality, responsible for 16% of maternal deaths (Berg et al, 2003); more than half of these deaths are considered preventable

UPDATE #4

Women with a history of preeclampsia are at increased risk of future cardiovascular, metabolic, and renal disease (Thadhani et al, 2008). Vikse and colleagues reported that women with preeclampsia in their first pregnancy had a 4.7-fold increased risk of subsequent end-stage renal disease (ESRD) (Vikse et al, 2008). The risks for ESRD increased with the number of pregnancies complicated by preeclampsia and with the concomitant delivery of a low-birth-weight infant. The mechanism of this increased risk is thought to be secondary to the same underlying cardiac, renal, and metabolic risk factors that predispose to preeclampsia in the first place and not the result of any long-lasting harm induced by the woman's episode of preeclampsia. Common risk factors include latent or essential hypertension, dyslipidemia, insulin resistance, diabetes, and endothelial dysfunction. It is important to recognize that an obstetrical history of early onset preeclampsia connotes the same degree of future cardiovascular risk as does a 20-pack year history of smoking.

- Fetal risks of preeclampsia are primarily related to placental insufficiency, intrauterine growth restriction (IUGR), or iatrogenic prematurity

UPDATE #5

Preeclampsia is the number one indication for iatrogenic preterm delivery. In her analysis of the Norwegian Medical Birth Registry, Basso and colleagues demonstrated that the rate of preterm induction of labor and cesarean section for preeclampsia increased 2.6-fold between 1967 to 2001, whereas the risk of stillbirth decreased 7.6-fold in this same cohort of women (Basso et al, 2006). The rates of neonatal and childhood mortality among these offspring were virtually unchanged over time, suggesting that substantial additional risk was not shifted to the newborns. Nonetheless, infants of women whose labor was induced because of preterm hypertension or preeclampsia have higher rates of admission to the neonatal intensive care unit (NICU), RDS, and ventilatory support than gestational age-matched controls (Habli et al, 2007).

- Management
  - Preeclampsia
    - There is no cure for preeclampsia or its variants other than delivery of the fetus and placenta
    - Management should be planned to appropriately balance the mother's and the baby's risks of preeclampsia, mode of delivery, and prematurity
    - At term (≥37 weeks), immediate induction of labor yields better maternal outcomes and a lower cesarean section rate than expectant management, with no change in neonatal outcomes (Koopmans et al, 2009)
    - Preterm preeclampsia (<37 weeks) is more likely to include maternal end-organ injury or fetal growth restriction than term preeclampsia

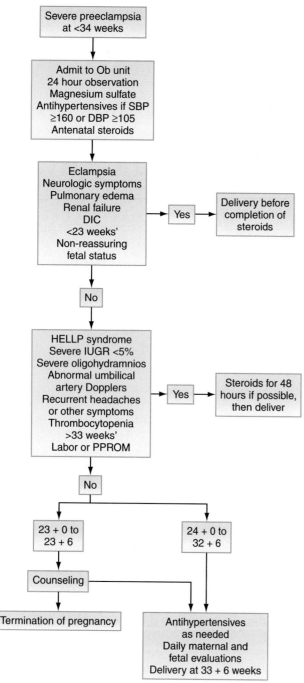

Figure 20-1. Suggested treatment for patients with severe preeclampsia at <34 weeks of gestation. (Adapted from Sibai BM, Barton JR: Expectant management of severe preeclampsia remote from term: patient selection, treatment, and delivery indications, *Am J Obstet Gynecol* 196(6):514 e1-e9, 2007.)

- Expectant management of mild preterm preeclampsia is associated with improved neonatal outcomes and low risk to the mother if properly monitored
- Expectant management of severe preterm preeclampsia (between 24 and 34 weeks) in selected patients is associated with a pregnancy prolongation of about 1 to 2 weeks and improved neonatal outcomes (Figure 20-1) (Sibai et al, 2007)
  - The risk of abruption, fetal distress, and IUGR remains elevated in these patients, however

TABLE 20-1   Suggested Regimens for Treatment and Prevention of Eclamptic Seizures

Indication	Dose Type	Dose
Prophylaxis	Loading dose	4 gm IV bolus in 100 cc saline over 15-20 minutes
	Maintenance dose*	1-2 gm/hr IV
Treatment	Loading dose	6 gm IV bolus in 100 cc saline over 15-20 minutes
	Maintenance dose*	1-2 gm/hr IV
	Repeat dose	2 gm IV bolus for recurrent seizure

*Follow respirations and reflexes closely for signs of magnesium toxicity. Target serum concentration is 4.8 to 8.4 mg/dL. Half-life is 4 hours with normal renal function.

- Maternal risks of expectant management include pulmonary edema, renal failure, eclampsia, and HELLP syndrome, and this practice of expectant management is only recommended at experienced referral centers
- There is little benefit of expectant management beyond the steroid exposure window (48 hours) for women who are <25 weeks, who have HELLP syndrome, or whose infants demonstrate IUGR
- Magnesium sulfate is the optimum medication for the prevention and treatment of eclamptic seizures (Table 20-1)
  - Seizure prophylaxis is usually administered for 24 hours after delivery, although seizures may rarely occur up to 1 week postpartum

UPDATE #6

Ehrenberg and Mercer studied an abbreviated 12-hour postpartum magnesium sulfate regimen in women with mild preeclampsia (Ehrenberg et al, 2006). They reported that only 7% of subjects progressed to severe preeclampsia or required prolongation of the regimen to 24 hours. The women who progressed to severe preeclampsia had higher blood pressures at admission and were more likely to have diabetes. In a separate publication, Alexander and colleagues studied a protocol of withholding magnesium sulfate seizure prophylaxis from women with mild gestational hypertension who had <2+ proteinuria (Alexander et al, 2006). Over 4.5 years, they treated 40% fewer women with magnesium prophylaxis but noted 27 excess cases of eclampsia (a rate of 1/92) in the untreated group.

- Antihypertensive therapy is indicated to treat severe range hypertension (systolic [SBP] ≥160 mmHg; diastolic blood pressure [DBP] ≥105 mmHg)
  - The goal of acute antihypertensive therapy is to lower the blood pressure to a range that reduces the risk of stroke (135 to 145/95 to 105) (Table 20-2); overly aggressive therapy may lead to placental underperfusion and fetal compromise
  - Chronic antihypertensive therapy has not been shown to prolong pregnancies with mild or moderate preeclampsia or improve maternal or fetal outcome

TABLE 20-2   **Acute Antihypertensive Therapy in Pregnancy**

Generic Name	Labetalol	Hydralazine	Nifedipine
Trade Name	Normodyne, Trandate	Apresoline	Procardia, Adalat
Mechanism	Selective α1- & nonselective β- antagonist	Selective arteriolar vasodilator	Calcium channel blocker
Initial Dose	10-20 mg IV	5 mg IV	10 mg po
Repeat Dose and Maximum	20-80 mg IV Q 10' up to 220 mg	5-10 mg IV Q 20' up to 30 mg	10 mg po Q 30' up to 40 mg
Comments	Wide therapeutic window; oral form for maintenance if needed	Brisk hypotensive response, more maternal tachycardia	Do not administer sublingual dose; concerns about concurrent use with magnesium sulfate

- Chronic hypertension
  - Antihypertensive therapy is indicated for women with severe range (≥160/105) chronic hypertension
  - Therapy is probably beneficial at a lower threshold (DBP ≥90 mmHg) for women with evidence of renovascular disease such as left ventricular hypertrophy, chronic renal insufficiency, pregestational diabetes, or previous stroke or myocardial infarction
  - The ideal treatment threshold and target range of therapy for the uncomplicated patient with essential hypertension has not been defined; "tight" control may reduce episodes of unanticipated severe hypertension but is associated with greater reductions in fetal growth (Magee et al, 2007)
  - Antihypertensive therapy has not been shown to decrease the risk of superimposed preeclampsia, and a high index of suspicion must be maintained for this condition throughout pregnancy
  - Several commonly used first-line oral agents for blood pressure control in pregnancy are α-methyldopa (Aldomet), labetalol (Normodyne, Trandate), and nifedipine (Adalat, Procardia)
  - Atenolol is not recommended by the American College of Obstetricians and Gynecologists (ACOG) because of its association with fetal growth restriction
  - Inhibitors of the angiotensin system (ACE inhibitors and angiotensin receptor blockers) are associated with severe fetal malformation syndromes and are contraindicated in pregnancy

UPDATE #7

In a cohort study of 29,507 infants, Cooper and colleagues reported that first-trimester use of ACE inhibitors was associated with a 3.72-fold increased risk of cardiovascular malformations and a 4.39-fold increased risk of central nervous system malformations (Cooper et al, 2006).

- Gestational hypertension
  - In the absence of proteinuria or other evidence of preeclampsia, women with mild gestational hypertension and their infants experience good outcomes and can be followed expectantly
  - Because 30% to 50% of women with gestational hypertension develop preeclampsia, they should be monitored regularly for evidence of clinical deterioration

TABLE 20-3   **Risk of Preeclampsia with Abnormal Serum Analytes**

Analyte	Odds Ratio (95% CI)
PAPP-A <5th centile*	2.10 (1.57, 2.81)
AFP >2.0 MoM*	2.36 (1.46, 3.83)
HCG >2.0 MoM*	2.45 (1.57, 3.84)
INH >2.0 MoM*	6.00 (5.12, 7.03)
AFP + INH #	4.26 (1.91, 9.51)
AFP + INH + HCG†	7.04 (3.90, 12.73)

Adapted from *Morris RK, Cnossen JS, Langejans M et al: Serum screening with Down's syndrome markers to predict pre-eclampsia and small for gestational age: systematic review and meta-analysis, *BMC Pregnancy and Childbirth* 8:33, 2008; and †Dugoff L, Hobbins JC, Malone FD, et al: Quad screen as a predictor of adverse pregnancy outcome, *Obstet Gynecol* 106:260-267, 2005.

- Severe gestational hypertension (BP ≥160/110) poses maternal and fetal risks equivalent to severe preeclampsia, and these patients should be managed accordingly with prompt delivery at term and with intensive monitoring or delivery when preterm
- Prediction and prevention of preeclampsia
  - Recognized clinical and demographic risk factors for preeclampsia include extremes of age, obesity, insulin resistance, nulliparity, malnutrition, multiple gestations, diabetes, hypertension, history of preeclampsia, and molar or aneuploid pregnancy
  - Abnormalities of first and second trimester serum analytes are associated with preeclampsia (and other adverse outcomes); the risk of preeclampsia rises with the degree of the abnormality and with the number of abnormal analytes (Table 20-3) (Dugoff and Society for Maternal-Fetal, 2010)
  - Doppler ultrasound of the uterine artery assesses vascular development of the midtrimester placenta and has a modest ability to predict preeclampsia (Cnossen et al, 2008; Conde-Agudelo et al, 2004)
  - Nutritional strategies to prevent preeclampsia in high- or low-risk women have not been successful
    - Calcium supplementation is not effective in preventing preeclampsia, although it may reduce the incidence of severe disease or adverse outcomes among patients with dietary calcium deficiency

- Fish oil supplementation does not reduce the risk of preeclampsia

UPDATE #8

Compelling evidence demonstrates an association between pre-eclampsia and oxidative stress in both the maternal circulation and in the placenta. Nonetheless, the genesis of this pro-oxidant environment is not fully understood, and whether it is the cause or a consequence of preeclampsia has been debated (Jeyabalen et al, 2006). Several recent high-quality randomized trials of supplemental vitamin C and E started as early as 15 weeks have failed to demonstrate a reduction in the risk of preeclampsia or other adverse pregnancy outcomes (Poston et al, 2006; Roberts et al, 2010; Rumbold et al, 2006; Spinnato et al, 2007; Villar et al, 2009; Xu et al, 2010).

- Pharmacologic strategies to prevent preeclampsia have shown only a modest benefit.
  - Low-dose aspirin (60 to 80 mg) or anti-platelet therapy may reduce the risk of preeclampsia by approximately 10% in both low and high-risk women; the number needed to treat (NNT) in order to prevent one additional case of preeclampsia ranges from 56 in high-risk women (e.g., history of preeclampsia), to more than 500 in low-risk women (Askie et al, 2007)
  - Heparin anticoagulation, with or without low-dose aspirin therapy, has not been convincingly shown to prevent preeclampsia—even among women with various genetic or acquired thrombophilias

HEART DISEASE IN PREGNANCY

- Heart disease complicates less than 1% of pregnancies but accounts for up to 20% of direct maternal deaths
- The physiologic changes of pregnancy that may complicate heart disease include the following:
  - 45% increase in blood volume
  - 43% increase in cardiac output
  - 17% increase in heart rate
  - 17% increase in left ventricular stroke work index
  - 21% decrease in systemic vascular resistance
  - 14% decrease in colloid oncotic pressure
- Certain cardiac conditions, such as mitral valve regurgitation, are well tolerated in pregnancy, whereas other conditions, such as Marfan's syndrome or Eisenmenger's syndrome, can carry a maternal mortality risk up to 50%
- Predictors of cardiac complications in pregnancy include the following (Siu et al, 1997):
  - Baseline New York Heart Association (NYHA) class III or IV
  - Prior heart failure, transient ischemic attack (TIA), arrhythmia, or stroke
  - Left-sided valvular obstruction
  - Ejection fraction <40%

UPDATE #9

Up to one half of women with peripartum cardiomyopathy become pregnant again despite counseling and contraception (Habli et al, 2008). Of those who choose to carry their pregnancies,

29% demonstrate worsening symptoms of heart failure, despite interval recovery (>40%) of their ejection fraction. Of those with an ejection fraction <25% at initial diagnosis, more than half (57%) progress to transplant status within 4 years of the index pregnancy.

- The key to pregnancy management in women with heart disease is close cooperation with a multidisciplinary team to address patient needs

Pulmonary Disorders

NORMAL PHYSIOLOGIC ADAPTATION

- Physiologic adaptations of the pulmonary system can mimic or aggravate concurrent pulmonary disease; these adaptations include the following:
  - 40% increase in tidal volume
  - No change in respiratory rate
  - 30% increase in minute ventilation
  - 20% decrease in functional residual capacity
  - A small increase in paO_2 and a significant decrease in pCO_2 from 40 to 32 mmHg

ASTHMA

- Approximately 4% to 8% of pregnancies are complicated by asthma
- Pathologic components of asthma that interfere with maternal ventilation include the following:
  - Reversible bronchoconstriction
  - Vascular congestion/shunting
  - Mucosal edema
  - Mucous obstruction
- The effect of pregnancy upon asthma is best predicted by the baseline severity of disease
  - A review of prospective studies of asthmatics in pregnancy concluded that one third improved, one third remained stable, and one third worsened (Gluck et al, 2006)
  - With severe baseline disease, up to 50% of patients will report exacerbations in pregnancy, and approximately half will require admission
- In general, the effect of well-managed asthma upon pregnancy and perinatal outcomes is minimal
  - Women with moderate to severe asthma may have increased rates of preterm delivery, gestational hypertension, cesarean delivery, and fetal growth restriction

UPDATE #10

Adverse perinatal outcomes have not been identified in all studies of asthmatic women. In a recent observational cohort, Schatz and associates found that only a depressed FEV_1 <80% (moderate to severe asthma) was independently associated with gestational hypertension, preterm delivery, or low birth weight. Reported symptoms and medication use did not predict adverse outcomes, suggesting that objective disease monitoring is essential for optimal management (Schatz et al, 2006).

- Concerns about fetal effects lead some women to decrease or discontinue asthma medications in pregnancy

- Commonly used anti-asthma drugs are considered safe to prescribe during pregnancy (Kallen, 2007)
  - Inhaled drugs reduce medication exposure; avoid systemic use of corticosteroids in the first trimester if possible because of a possible association with midline facial clefts
- Management
  - Patient education is critical to optimal management; patients should be proficient at the following:
    - Recognizing early symptoms
    - Avoiding and removing environmental triggers
    - Performing objective testing by use of a peak flow meter
  - Formal pulmonary function testing should employed to establish baseline spirometry and provide correlation to daily self-testing
  - Chronic asthma is treated in a stepwise manner (see Table 20-4)
  - Acute asthma exacerbations are a medical emergency for the mother and fetus; treatment includes the following:
    - Low threshold for hospitalization and observation
    - Intravenous (IV) hydration
    - Oxygen supplementation to maintain O_2 sat ≥95% and PaO_2 ≥60 mmHg
    - Serial pulmonary function testing by peak flow or FEV_1
    - Fetal monitoring
    - Intensive inhaled β-agonist therapy with concomitant inhaled steroids
    - IV or PO corticosteroids if suboptimal response to inhaled agents (FEV_1 <70%).
  - Avoid use of prostaglandin $F_2\alpha$ or ergotamine derivatives in pregnant women with asthma because of the risk of bronchospasm

TUBERCULOSIS

- The incidence of tuberculosis (TB) in pregnancy is increasing, and most gravidas with the disease are asymptomatic
- Indications for purified protein deriviative (PPD) screening in pregnancy include the following:
  - Birth in country with endemic TB
  - Medically underserved population
  - Low income
  - Clinical risk factors related to exposure and immunosuppression
- Antepartum prophylaxis is prescribed (Figure 20-2) after the first trimester in patients with a negative chest x-ray and
  - A newly positive PPD (conversion within 2 years), or
  - Unknown duration of positive PPD with risk factors

TABLE 20-4   **Stepwise Therapy of Chronic Asthma in Pregnancy**

Asthma Classification	Stepwise Therapy
Intermittent	Inhaled short-acting β-agonist (e.g., albuterol) as needed
Mild	1°—low-dose inhaled steroid (e.g., budesonide)
	2°—cromolyn, leukotriene antagonists, or theophylline (serum level 5-12 ug/ml)
Moderate	1°—low-dose inhaled steroid *plus* long-acting β-agonist (salmeterol), or medium-dose inhaled steroid, or medium dose inhaled steroid plus salmeterol
	2°—low-dose or medium-dose inhaled steroid *and* either theophylline or leukotriene antagonists
Severe	1°—high-dose inhaled steroid *plus* salmeterol *plus* (if needed) oral steroids
	2°—high dose inhaled steroid *plus* theophylline *plus* (if needed) oral steroids

Adapted from American College of Obstetricians and Gynecologists: ACOG practice bulletin no. 90: asthma in pregnancy, *Obstet Gynecol* 111:457-464, 2008.

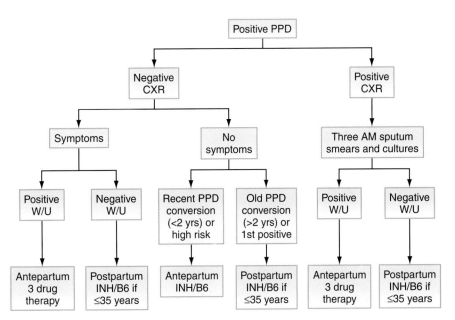

Figure 20-2. Treatment algorithm for tuberculosis in pregnancy. INH, isoniazid 300 mg/day for 6 to 9 months; B_6, pyridoxine 50 mg/day.

- Postpartum prophylaxis is recommended for women ≤ age 35 with a negative chest x-ray and
  - Long-standing (>2 years) positive PPD, or
  - Positive PPD of unknown duration

PNEUMONIA

- Physiologic changes of pregnancy place women at higher risk of complications from pneumonia in pregnancy.
  - Decreased functional residual capacity accelerates risk of hypoxia
  - Decreased colloid oncotic pressure increases risk of pulmonary edema
  - Altered immunity affects risk of acquisition and progression of certain pathogens
- Viral pneumonia is especially morbid in pregnant women
  - Pneumonitis develops in up to 5% of pregnant women with acute varicella or influenza A infection
  - Early therapy (<48 hours) with antivirals reduces morbidity and mortality (Siston et al, 2010)
- Evaluation of suspected pneumonia should include careful physical exam, chest x-ray, and blood gases
- Inpatient management is generally recommended
- Supplemental oxygen to keep the paO_2 >70 mmHg
- Sputum and blood cultures and Gram stain may be helpful to guide antibiotic therapy
- Empiric therapy begins with third-generation cephalosporin and macrolide (e.g., azithromycin)
- Preterm labor is a common complication

PULMONARY EDEMA

- Two general causes of pulmonary edema
  - Cardiogenic
    - Heart failure
  - Noncardiogenic
    - Capillary and alveolar injury
    - Sepsis, preeclampsia, etc.
- Management
  - Investigate and treat underlying causes
  - Fluid restriction
  - Diuresis
  - Oxygen
  - Mechanical ventilation if needed

ACUTE RESPIRATORY DISTRESS SYNDROME

- A syndrome of acute lung inflammation and injury followed by a delayed subacute reparative process
- Common initiators include the following:
  - Aspiration
  - Pneumonia
  - Sepsis
  - Hemorrhage
  - Embolism (amniotic fluid or air)
- Management
  - High-intensity, multidisciplinary ICU care

UPDATE #11

The key components of successful ICU care in pregnancy include (ACOG Practice Bulletin No. 100, 2009):
- Immediate, pathogen-directed antimicrobial treatment before ICU admission

---

- Collaborative decision-making between intensivists, obstetricians, nurses, and neonatologists
- Relatively unrestricted pharmacologic treatment and imaging based on maternal needs

AMNIOTIC FLUID EMBOLISM

- A heterogeneous disorder recognized by the acute onset of some or all of the following: hypotension, hypoxia, and consumptive coagulopathy
- Incidence of 7 to 8 per 100,000 births, but case-fatality rate of 22% (Abenhaim et al, 2008)
- Management is supportive, and includes mechanical ventilation, blood product replacement, delivery of fetus; no single, optimal therapy has emerged

PULMONARY EMBOLISM (PE)

- Incidence and presentation
  - PE complicates about 1 in 7000 pregnancies; about 50% of women with DVT have silent PE, and more than two thirds of women with PE have concurrent deep vein thrombosis (DVT)
  - PE causes about 10% of direct maternal deaths
  - Risk factors include cesarean section, infection, obesity, bed rest, maternal age >35, smoking, and thrombophilia
  - There is equal frequency of antepartum and postpartum events
  - Symptoms and findings are nonspecific and include the following:
    - Dyspnea
    - Pleuritic chest pain
    - Cough
    - Syncope
    - Hemostasis
    - Tachypnea
    - Tachycardia
- Diagnosis
  - Diagnosis depends on maintaining high clinical suspicion
  - There are no reliable criteria from arterial blood gas testing, although hypoxia and a large a-A gradient are suggestive
  - Serum D-Dimers are elevated in normal pregnancy, so a positive assay does not facilitate the diagnosis of DVT/PE
  - Algorithms for diagnosing PE rely on compression ultrasound of the lower extremities, computed tomography (CT) pulmonary angiography, and ventilation-perfusion imaging (Figure 20-3) (Marik et al, 2008)
  - Fetal radiation exposure from pulmonary diagnostic imaging is minimal and should not deter prompt evaluation
  - Testing for common thrombophilias is helpful to determine risk for recurrent thromboembolism and the duration and intensity of treatment (Table 20-5).
- Treatment and prevention
  - Treat PE in pregnancy or postpartum with therapeutic anticoagulation for at least 4 months, followed by prophylactic anticoagulation until at least 6 weeks postpartum

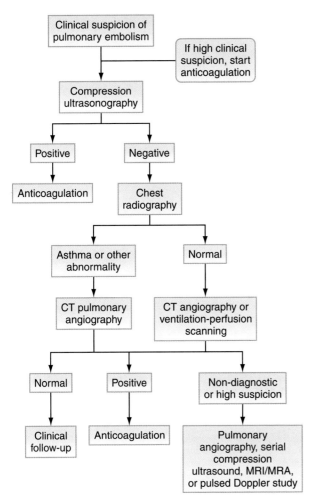

Figure 20-3. Diagnostic algorithm for suspected pulmonary embolism during pregnancy. CT, computed tomography; MRI/MRA, magnetic resonance imaging/angiography. (Adapted from Marik PE, Plante LA: Venous thromboembolic disease and pregnancy, *N Engl J Med* 359(19):2025-2033, 2008.)

TABLE 20-5 **List of Recommended Testing for Thrombophilia in Acute Pulmonary Embolism**

Factor V Leiden mutation
 (or activated protein C resistance assay)
Factor II G20110A mutation
Protein C deficiency
Antithrombin III deficiency
Lupus anticoagulant
Anticardiolipin antibody

(Protein S concentration and activity falls with normal pregnancy and hence should be tested postpartum.)

- Initial treatment with intravenous unfractionated heparin allows one to maintain a partial thromboplastin time (PTT) 2 × control until symptoms are resolved
  - In acute cases, administer IV heparin immediately, pending outcomes of diagnostic studies
- Low-molecular-weight heparins (LMWHs) are given Q12 hours for therapeutic anticoagulation,

TABLE 20-6 **Recommended Laboratory Targets for Therapeutic and Prophylactic Anticoagulation**

	Agent	aPTT	Anti-Factor Xa Assay
Prophylaxis	Unfractionated heparin	Prolonged 2-10 seconds at midinterval	0.1-0.3 U/ml
	Low-molecular weight heparin (enoxaparin)	Not reliable	0.2-0.4 U/ml
Therapeutic	Unfractionated heparin	1.6-2.3 × control at midinterval	0.3-0.6 U/ml
	Low-molecular weight heparin (enoxaparin)	Not reliable	0.5-1.0 U/ml

aPTT, Activated partial thromboplastin time.

but dosing should be adjusted by intermittent assessment of serum anti-Factor Xa activity (Table 20-6) to achieve the desired level of anticoagulation

UPDATE #12

Physiologic changes of pregnancy can alter the bioavailability of heparins, leading to unpredictable therapeutic response. Fox et al. reported that pregnant women on prophylactic doses of LMWH were within the desired heparin concentration range only 59% of the time (Duhl et al, 2007; Fox et al, 2008).

- Anticoagulation is temporarily halted for delivery
- The anticoagulant effects of LMWH must be allowed to resolve before placement of neuraxial anesthesia
  - Patients at high risk of PE and DVT may receive a low or intermediate dose of prophylactic heparin through pregnancy and postpartum

UPDATE #13

The risk of recurrent PE or DVT is highest in women whose primary event occurred in the absence of an identifiable transient risk factor (such as surgery or immobilization) and in those with thrombophilia. Of 51 such patients, the risk of a recurrent antepartum event without thromboprophylaxis was nearly 6% (Brill-Edwards et al, 2000). Most experts recommend antepartum and postpartum prophylactic anticoagulation for women with a history of DVT/PE that was idiopathic or associated with thrombophilia (Duhl et al, 2007; Marik et al, 2008).

- Routine thromboprophylaxis with pneumatic compression stockings is recommended for all patients following cesarean section (Quinones et al, 2005)

SUGGESTED READINGS

Hypertension

Cooper WO, Hernandez-Diaz S, et al: Major congenital malformations after first-trimester exposure to ACE inhibitors, *N Engl J Med* 354(23):2443–2451, 2006.

Heart Disease

Habli M, O'Brien T, et al: Peripartum cardiomyopathy: prognostic factors for long-term maternal outcome, *Am J Obstet Gynecol* 199(4):415e1–e5, 2008.

Preeclampsia

Alexander JM, McIntire DD, et al: Selective magnesium sulfate prophylaxis for the prevention of eclampsia in women with gestational hypertension, *Obstet Gynecol* 108(4):826–832, 2006.

Basso O, Rasmussen S, et al: Trends in fetal and infant survival following preeclampsia, *JAMA* 296(11):1357–1362, 2006.

Ehrenberg HM, Mercer BM: Abbreviated postpartum magnesium sulfate therapy for women with mild preeclampsia: a randomized controlled trial, *Obstet Gynecol* 108(4):833–838, 2006.

Habli M, Levine RJ, et al: Neonatal outcomes in pregnancies with preeclampsia or gestational hypertension and in normotensive pregnancies that delivered at 35, 36, or 37 weeks of gestation, *Obstet Gynecol* 197(4):406e1–e7, 2007.

Ilekis JV, Reddy UM, et al: Preeclampsia—a pressing problem: an executive summary of a National Institute of Child Health and Human Development workshop, *Reprod Sci* 14(6):508–523, 2007.

Jeyabalan A, Caritis SN: Antioxidants and the prevention of preeclampsia: unresolved issues, *N Engl J Med* 354(17):1841–1843, 2006.

Kahn SR, Platt R, et al: Inherited thrombophilia and preeclampsia within a multicenter cohort: the Montreal Preeclampsia Study, *Obstet Gynecol* 200(2):151e1–e9; discussion e1-5, 2009.

Levine RJ, Lam C, et al: Soluble endoglin and other circulating antiangiogenic factors in preeclampsia, *N Engl J Med* 355(10):992–1005, 2006.

Levine RJ, Maynard SE, et al: Circulating angiogenic factors and the risk of preeclampsia, *N Engl J Med* 350(7):672–683, 2004.

Martin JN Jr, Thigpen BD, et al: Stroke and severe preeclampsia and eclampsia: a paradigm shift focusing on systolic blood pressure, *Obstet Gynecol* 105(2):246–254, 2005.

Poston L, Briley AL, et al: Vitamin C and vitamin E in pregnant women at risk for pre-eclampsia (VIP trial): randomised placebo-controlled trial, *Lancet* 367(9517):1145–1154, 2006.

Roberts JM, Myatt L, et al: Vitamins C and E to prevent complications of pregnancy-associated hypertension, *N Engl J Med* 362(14):1282–1291, 2010.

Rumbold AR, Crowther CA, et al: Vitamins C and E and the risks of preeclampsia and perinatal complications, *N Engl J Med* 354(17):1796–1806, 2006.

Said JM, Higgins JR, et al: Inherited thrombophilia polymorphisms and pregnancy outcomes in nulliparous women, *Obstet Gynecol* 115(1):5–13, 2010.

Silver RM, Zhao Y, et al: Prothrombin gene G20210A mutation and obstetric complications, *Obstet Gynecol* 115(1):14–20, 2010.

Spinnato JA 2nd, Freire S, et al: Antioxidant therapy to prevent preeclampsia: a randomized controlled trial, *Obstet Gynecol* 110(6):1311–1318, 2007.

Thadhani R, Solomon CG: Preeclampsia: a glimpse into the future? *N Engl J Med* 359(8):858–860, 2008.

Vikse BE, Irgens LM, et al: Preeclampsia and the risk of end-stage renal disease, *N Engl J Med* 359(8):800–809, 2008.

Villar J, Purwar M, et al: World Health Organisation multicentre randomised trial of supplementation with vitamins C and E among pregnant women at high risk for pre-eclampsia in populations of low nutritional status from developing countries, *BJOG* 116(6):780–788, 2009.

Xu H, Perez-Cuevas R, et al: An international trial of antioxidants in the prevention of preeclampsia (INTAPP), *Am J Obstet Gynecol* 202(3):239e1–239e10, 2010.

Asthma

American College of Obstetricians and Gynecologists: ACOG practice bulletin no. 60: asthma in pregnancy, *Obstet Gynecol* 111:457–464, 2008.

Schatz M, Dombrowski MP, et al: Spirometry is related to perinatal outcomes in pregnant women with asthma, *Obstet Gynecol* 194(1):120–126, 2006.

Pulmonary Embolism

Brill-Edwards P, Ginsberg JS, et al: Safety of withholding heparin in pregnant women with a history of venous thromboembolism: recurrence of clot in this pregnancy study group, *N Engl J Med* 343(20):1439–1444, 2000.

Duhl AJ, Paidas MJ, et al: Antithrombotic therapy and pregnancy: consensus report and recommendations for prevention and treatment of venous thromboembolism and adverse pregnancy outcomes, *Obstet Gynecol* 197(5):457e1–21, 2007.

Fox NS, Laughon SK, et al: Anti-factor Xa plasma levels in pregnant women receiving low molecular weight heparin thromboprophylaxis, *Obstet Gynecol* 112(4):884–889, 2008.

Marik PE, Plante LA: Venous thromboembolic disease and pregnancy, *N Engl J Med* 359(19):2025–2033, 2008.

Critical Care

American College of Obstetricians and Gynecologists: ACOG practice bulletin no. 100: critical care in pregnancy, *Obstet Gynecol* 113(2 Pt 1):443–450, 2009.

Siston AM, Rasmussen SA, et al: Pandemic 2009 influenza A (H1N1) virus illness among pregnant women in the United States, *JAMA* 303(15):1517–1525, 2010.

References

Please go to expertconsult.com to view references.

Chapter 21

Renal Disease in Pregnancy

RICHARD B. WOLF

KEY UPDATES

1 Preeclampsia increases the risk of developing future end-stage renal disease (ESRD).

2 In addition to ESRD, preeclampsia predisposes women for chronic medical conditions such as hypertension, stroke, ischemic heart disease, and type 2 diabetes.

3 Potential complications of pregnancy in renal transplant patients include hypertension, preeclampsia, allograft dysfunction, and effects of immunosuppressive medications on the fetus.

4 Pregnancy in renal transplant patients should be planned and monitored closely using a multidisciplinary approach for optimum maternal and neonatal outcomes.

5 Given the potential for maternal and fetal complications in renal transplant patients, physicians should be proactive in discussing timing, risks, and alternatives of pregnancy.

Physiologic Renal Changes in Pregnancy

KIDNEY SIZE AND DILATION

- Relaxed smooth muscle resulting from progesterone and relaxin causes increased renal vascular volume
- Kidney size increases by approximately 30% and length increases by 1 cm
- Physiologic *hydronephrosis of pregnancy* (right greater than left) is seen in 90% of pregnant women, as early as the first trimester
  - Renal pelves, calyces, and ureters markedly dilated as early as first trimester
  - Dextrorotation of gravid uterus compresses the right ureter
  - Urinary stasis and vesicoureteral reflux are increased
  - Increased risk of urinary tract infection (UTI) and pyelonephritis

ALTERED FUNCTION (Table 21-1)

- Glomerular filtration rate (GFR) increases up to 50% over prepregnancy rate due to increased renal plasma flow
  - Renal plasma flow (RPF) increases up to 80% above prepregnant levels
  - Altered function resulting from progesterone-mediated decreased renal vascular resistance and increased plasma volume (1.2 L above prepregnancy volume)
  - Begins in first trimester, plateaus at 16 weeks, and is sustained through remainder of pregnancy

- Creatinine clearance increases to 110 to 150 mL/min
- Urine concentration of sodium and potassium are unchanged
- Increased clearance of creatinine, urea, and uric acid, along with total volume increase produces lowered concentrations in serum
  - Creatinine: 0.5 mg/dL
  - Blood urea nitrogen (BUN): 10 mg/dL
  - Uric acid: 4.0 mg/dL
  - Sodium: 136 mM/L
- Glucose reabsorption is decreased in the loop of Henle, produces glucosuria
- Fractional excretions of amino acids variously increase, decrease, or remain unchanged, but *proteinuria should not exceed 300 mg/24 hours*

Urinary Tract Infection

ASYMPTOMATIC BACTERIURIA

- Bacteria present in the urine without associated inflammatory response or symptoms
- Incidence in pregnancy is 2% to 7%
- Urine culture contains $\geq 10^5$ bacteria/mL
- Untreated can lead to pyelonephritis in 25% of patients
- Most frequent bacterial cause is *Escherichia coli*, which accounts for 80% to 90% of community-acquired UTIs and 50% of hospital-acquired UTIs
- Antibiotic treatment typically consists of a minimum 3-day course of ampicillin or nitrofurantoin (Table 21-2)

TABLE 21-1   **Physiologic Renal Changes in Pregnancy**

Plasma volume	1.2 L increase
Glomerular filtration rate	50% increase
Renal vascular resistance	Decreased
Creatinine clearance	Increased
Systemic blood pressure	Decreased
Urine concentration	Unchanged
Proteinuria	Up to 300 mg/24 hrs
Glucosuria	Increased
Acid-base balance	Compensated respiratory alkalosis
Serum creatinine, BUN, uric acid, sodium	Decreased

TABLE 21-2   **Antibiotic Treatment for Lower Urinary Tract Infection and Asymptomatic Bacteriuria in Pregnancy**

Single-Dose Treatment

Ampicillin	2 g
Amoxicillin	3 g
Cephalexin	2 g
Nitrofurantoin	200 mg
Trimethoprim-sulfamethoxazole	320/1600 mg

3-Day Course

Ampicillin	250 mg 4 times per day
Amoxicillin	500 mg 3 times per day
Cephalexin	250 mg 4 times per day
Nitrofurantoin	100 mg twice per day
Trimethoprim-sulfamethoxazole	160/800 mg twice per day

7- to 14-Day Course

Nitrofurantoin	100 mg at bedtime
Nitrofurantoin	100 mg 4 times per day
Prophylactic suppression for remainder of pregnancy	
Nitrofurantoin	100 mg at bedtime
Cephalexin	250 mg at bedtime

Modified from Sheffield JS, Cunningham FG: Urinary tract infection in women, *Obstet Gynecol* 106:1085-1092, 2005.

- Trimethoprim-sulfisoxazole can be used, but should be avoided late in pregnancy because of competitive albumin binding of bilirubin, which can lead to neonatal kernicterus
- Fluoroquinolone derivatives are not generally used as first-line treatment in pregnancy because of the potential teratogenicity to the fetal cartilage; however, they can be used for resistant infection
- Recurrence rate is approximately 30%

TABLE 21-3   **Antibiotic Treatment for Pyelonephritis in Pregnancy**

Intravenous Therapy

Cefepime	2 g every 8 hours
Cefotetan	2 g every 12 hours
Ticarcillin-sulfamethoxazole	3.1 g every 6 hours
Trimethoprim-sulfamethoxazole	2 mg/kg every 6 hours
Ceftriaxone	1-2 g every 12-24 hours
Gentamycin	3-5 mg/kg/day
Ampicillin (if suspected enterococcus)	2 g every 6 hours
Aztreonam	2 g every 8 hours
Cefotaxime	1-2 g every 8 hours
Outpatient oral regimen (10- 14-day treatment) in	Select cases
Amoxicillin-clavulanate	875/125 mg twice per day
Trimethoprim-sulfamethoxazole	160/800 mg twice per day

Modified from Sheffield JS, Cunningham FG: Urinary tract infection in women, *Obstet Gynecol* 106:1085-1092, 2005.

LOWER URINARY TRACT INFECTION

- Cystitis and urethritis are inflammatory processes caused by bacterial infection, producing symptoms of urgency, frequency, and dysuria
- Occurs less frequently than asymptomatic bacteriuria, with approximately 1% to 2% incidence in pregnancy
- Treatment is similar to that used for asymptomatic bacteriuria

UPPER URINARY TRACT INFECTION

- Pyelonephritis is an infection of the kidney and may be acute or chronic
- Symptoms include upper back pain, fever, and chills, and approximately 25% will have associated nausea and vomiting
- Incidence in pregnancy is 1% to 2%
- Most often occurs in the second or third trimester
- Vesicoureteral reflux is a risk factor, particularly in recurrent pyelonephritis
- Has a strong association with preterm labor and birth
- Treatment is generally with intravenous antibiotics (Table 21-3) continued until clinical improvement, with subsequent conversion to oral anabolic therapy to complete a 10- to 14-day course
- Intravenous cefazolin, ampicillin plus gentamycin, and intramuscular ceftriaxone have equivalent efficacy and recurrence risks
- Outpatient antibiotic therapy used only if no signs of sepsis, respiratory insufficiency, underlying medical conditions including renal disease, or preterm labor
- Inadequate treatment can progress to urosepsis, acute renal failure, multiorgan system failure, and death
- Acute respiratory distress syndrome (ARDS) may occur in up to 10% with urosepsis because of endotoxin-mediated alveolar capillary endothelial damage
- Ultrasound or intravenous urogram should be used if the patient fails to improve to rule out urolithiasis or renal abscess

- Chronic antibiotic suppression using nitrofurantoin or cephalexin following initial treatment reduces the risk of recurrence from 30% to 40% to 3%

Urolithiasis

DEFINITION

- Urinary calculi that can obstruct the intrarenal structures and ureter(s)
- Complicates approximately 1:1500 pregnancies
- Occurs primarily in second and third trimester
- Most common subjective symptom is flank pain (84%)

ASSESSMENT

- Gross or microscopic hematuria is present in 75%
- Renal ultrasound visualizes 60% of calculi in nephrolithiasis
- Limited single-shot intravenous pyelogram is considered the gold standard and should be performed if ultrasound is negative with continued clinical suspicion for calculi

CAUSES

- Most stones are composed of calcium oxalate, resulting from hypercalciuria caused by the following:
  - Suppressed parathyroid hormone, which reduces tubular resorption of calcium
  - Increased placental formation of 1,25-dihydroxychole-calciferol

TREATMENT

- With conservative treatment (fluid hydration, antibiotics, and analgesia) 70% to 80% will spontaneously pass their stones
- Ureteroscopy with holmium:YAG laser lithotripsy or basket extraction can be performed in pregnancy
- Percutaneous extracorporeal lithotripsy is contraindicated in pregnancy because of the need for fluoroscopy and potential adverse fetal effects with its use
- Ureteral stents or percutaneous nephrostomy may be required for relieving obstruction during pregnancy with definitive ureteroscopic laser treatment or extracorporeal shock wave lithotripsy delayed until postpartum

Acute Renal Failure

DEFINITION

- Glomerular filtration rate (GFR) deteriorates abruptly:
  - Oliguria with urine output <400 mL/24 hours
  - Acute rise in serum creatinine, BUN
  - Often reversible

ASSESSMENT (Figure 21-1)

- Complete history and physical examination
- Renal ultrasound
- Laboratory studies
  - Electrolyte panel, creatinine, uric acid, calcium, albumin, phosphorus
  - Complete blood cell count
  - Liver function studies

- Urinalysis with microscopic assessment
- Urine protein:creatinine ratio to estimate proteinuria, with 24-hour urine collection to follow for total protein and creatinine clearance
- Fractional excretion of sodium (FE_{Na}) in oliguric renal failure:

$$FE_{Na} = \frac{Urine[Na]\,/\,Serum[Na]}{Urine[Cr]\,/\,Serum[Cr]} \times 100$$

CAUSES

- Prerenal disease
  - Because of *hypoperfusion* states:
    - Volume depletion from dehydration (e.g., hyperemesis gravidarum)
    - Acute hemorrhage (e.g., postpartum hemorrhage or abruption)
    - Marked peripheral edema (e.g., third space losses from hypoalbuminemia in nephrotic syndrome)
    - Decreased peripheral vascular tone (e.g., sepsis)
    - Decreased cardiac output (e.g., congestive heart failure)
    - Increased renal vascular resistance (e.g., prostaglandin inhibitors, including nonsteroidal anti-inflammatory drugs [NSAIDs])
  - Low fractional excretion of sodium (FE_{Na}), <1%
  - Postural hypotension common
- Intrinsic renal disease
  - Tubular disease
    - *Acute tubular necrosis* (ATN) from renal ischemia (e.g., hypotension or sepsis) (Table 21-4)
      - Historically, septic abortion was most common cause, but diminished incidence with legalized sterile termination procedures available in the United States (still common in developing nations); today in the United States, preeclampsia is the most common cause
      - Inadequate treatment can lead to acute *cortical* necrosis with irreversible renal impairment
    - Acute damage from toxins
      - Nephrotoxic exposures (e.g., aminoglycosides, radiocontrast media, ethylene glycol)
      - Endogenous toxins (e.g., incompatible blood transfusion, myoglobinuria from rhabdomyolysis)
  - Acute glomerulonephritis
    - Immune complex deposition (e.g., lupus nephritis, membranoproliferative nephropathy)
    - Without immune deposits (e.g., Wegener's granulomatosis)
  - Interstitial nephritis
    - Pyelonephritis
    - Drug toxicity or allergies (e.g., antibiotics)
  - Vascular disease
    - Acute renal artery stenosis (e.g., thromboembolic disease)
    - Small vessel disease (e.g., microangiopathy caused by hemolytic uremic syndrome, thrombocytopenic purpura [HELLP])
- Postrenal disease
  - Caused by ureteral *obstruction*:
    - Urolithiasis

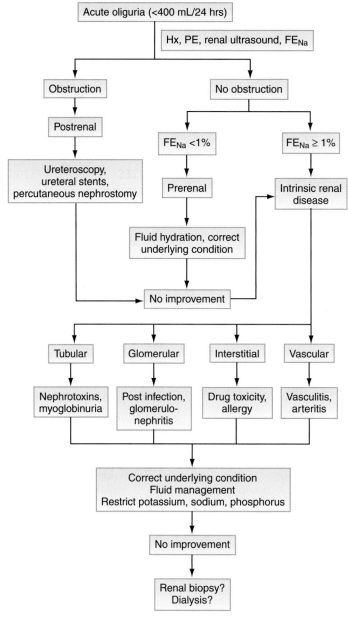

Figure 21-1. Diagnosis and treatment of acute renal failure. *FE*$_{Na}$, Fractional excretion of sodium.

**TABLE 21-4   Causes of Acute Tubular Necrosis
in Pregnancy**

Septic abortion

Hemorrhage

Hyperemesis gravidarum (with prolonged volume depletion)

Preeclampsia/HELLP syndrome

Placental abruption

Acute fatty liver

- Compression of the ureters by overdistended uterus (e.g., multifetal gestation, polyhydramnios)
- Preexisting ureteropelvic junction obstruction
- Normal fractional excretion of sodium (FE_{Na}), ≥ 1%
- Pregnancy-related acute renal disease
  - Preeclampsia/HELLP: can produce ATN; renal function generally improves following delivery

- Hemolytic uremic syndrome/thrombotic thrombocytopenic purpura:
  - Typically develops postpartum with *acute cortical necrosis* causing oliguria and associated microangiopathic hemolytic anemia, thrombocytopenia, coagulopathy, and neurologic impairment
  - May require plasmapheresis to correct
- Acute fatty liver: can produce acute renal failure in up to 60%
- Amniotic fluid embolism: can produce *acute cortical necrosis* with hematuria and oliguria that persists >1 week

TREATMENT

- Correct underlying cause, if possible
  - In prerenal disease, intravenous fluid volume expansion to correct perfusion deficits

- In postrenal disease, eliminate obstruction via ureteroscopy, ureteral stents, or percutaneous nephrostomy
- Conservative treatment
  - Careful fluid management
  - Dietary restriction of potassium, sodium, and phosphorus; low-protein diet
  - Discontinue any nephrotoxic medications; avoid NSAIDs, which reduce renal blood flow
  - Adjust medication dosing based on GFR
  - Monitor electrolytes and renal function
- Indications for peritoneal or hemodialysis:
  - Volume overload with pulmonary edema or CHF
  - Hyperkalemia (K+ >5.5 mEq/L produces electrocardiogram [EKG] changes, including reduced p-waves, widened QRS, and peaked t-waves)
  - Metabolic acidosis
  - Uremic encephalopathy (serum urea nitrogen >60 to 80 mg/dL)

UPDATE #1

The overall rate of developing end-stage renal disease (ESRD), defined as the need for long-term dialysis treatment or renal transplantation, following acute renal failure in pregnancy is 3.7 per 100,000 women per year. Most of these (35%) are due to glomerulonephritis, hereditary, or congenital causes (21%) and diabetic nephropathy (14%). Those who have preeclampsia in pregnancy are at higher risk for developing ESRD. The relative risk (RR) of ESRD following one pregnancy complicated by preeclampsia is 4.7 (95% confidence interval [CI], 3.7 to 6.1); for two pregnancies with preeclampsia, the RR is 6.4 (95% CI, 3.0 to 13.5); and for three pregnancies with preeclampsia, the RR is 15.5 (95% CI, 7.8 to 30.8) (Vikse et al, 2008).

UPDATE #2

In addition to ESRD, women with a history of preeclampsia have an increased risk of hypertension, stroke, ischemic heart disease, and type 2 diabetes later in life. Some eventual ESRD may be due to renal derangements that existed prior to the pregnancy. However, histologic changes such as swelling of glomerular endothelial cells (endotheliosis) and proteinuria indicate acute glomerular damage with preeclampsia. The cellular injury may not heal completely or even progress in a small percentage of patients to eventual chronic kidney disease. Long-term control of hypertension and diabetes mellitus reduces the risk of the progression of renal disease (Thadhani et al, 2008).

Nephrotic Syndrome

DEFINITION

- Proteinuria in excess of 3 to 3.5 g/day
- Often associated with the following:
  - Hypoalbuminemia caused by urinary protein loss
  - Peripheral edema caused by low plasma oncotic pressure
  - Hyperlipidemia with elevated total and low-density lipoprotein (LDL) cholesterol, but low to normal high-density lipoprotein (HDL)
- High risk of miscarriage or perinatal mortality, growth restriction, and preterm delivery
  - With superimposed preeclampsia, there is 29% fetal loss rate
  - Inverse relationship between 24-hour urine protein and birth weight

CAUSES

- Most common cause of nephrotic range proteinuria in pregnancy is *preeclampsia*
- Renal biopsy for definitive diagnosis generally delayed until postpartum
- *Primary glomerular disease*: in reproductive age, caused by the following:
  - Proliferative glomerulonephritis (20% to 25%)
  - Membranous nephropathy (15% to 30%)
  - Focal segmental glomerulosclerosis (20%)
  - Minimal change disease (5% to 15%)
  - Other primary renal disease (15% to 20%)
- *Secondary renal disease:* that is, associated with other diseases:
  - Systemic disease (e.g., diabetes, lupus, amyloidosis)
  - Infections (e.g., chronic pyelonephritis, poststreptococcal infection, hepatitis, malaria)
  - Neoplasia (e.g., Hodgkin's lymphoma)
  - Hereditary disease (e.g., Finnish nephrosis)
  - Medication exposures (e.g., NSAIDs, lithium, heavy metals)
  - Serum sickness (e.g., blood transfusion reaction)

TREATMENT

- Corticosteroids
  - Prednisone at 1 mg/kg/day, not to exceed 80 mg/day
  - Continued for 6 weeks beyond clinical improvement and then slowly tapered
  - May take longer than 15 weeks for clinical response before being considered steroid resistant
- Cyclophosphamide is used for steroid-resistant cases and for chronic treatment to prevent recurrence
- Twenty percent of patients with nephrotic syndrome progress to ESRD within 4 years

Chronic Renal Failure

DEFINITION

- Progressive and generally irreversible deterioration of glomerular filtration rate because of chronic underlying renal disease with associated increased creatinine
  - BUN >14 mg/dL or creatinine >0.9 mg/dL may indicate preexisting renal insufficiency
- Disease severity is classified according to serum creatinine
  - <1.4 mg/dL = Mild
  - 1.4 – 2.4 mg/dL = Moderate
  - >2.4 mg/dL = Severe
- Population risk of renal disease in reproductive age women is approximately 1:1000
- Typically associated with infertility, particularly in advanced renal disease
- *Increased risk of maternal and perinatal complications*:
  - Regardless of underlying renal parenchymal lesion, but particularly if there is associated hypertension and significant renal insufficiency (Table 21-5)
  - Adverse effects on pregnancy
    - Increased fetal growth restriction

TABLE 21-5   Pregnancy Outcomes in Chronic Renal Disease

Creatinine, mg/dL	IUGR, %	PTD, %	Perinatal mortality, %	ESRD,%
<1.4	25	30	1	0
1.4-2.0	40	60	5	2
>2.0	65	>95	10	35

ESRD, End-stage renal disease; *IUGR*, intrauterine growth restriction; *PTD*, preterm delivery.
Modified from Williams D, Davison J: Chronic kidney disease in pregnancy, *BMJ* 336:211-215, 2008.

- Preterm delivery
- Higher perinatal morbidity and mortality
  - Hypertension at conception or not well controlled during pregnancy increases fetal loss rate by two to three times
  - BUN >80 mg/dL imparts a high risk of intrauterine fetal demise (IUFD)
- Adverse effects on maternal health
  - Worsening chronic hypertension; 25% will develop new onset hypertension
  - Superimposed preeclampsia can exceed 50%
  - Worsening anemia from decreased erythropoietin production
  - Worsened renal function with decreased GFR
    - Normal gestational increases in GFR typically *absent* if only mild preconception renal dysfunction (creatinine <2.0 mg/dL)
    - Accelerated *decrease* in GFR if moderate or severe preconception renal compromise (creatinine >2.0 mg/dL)
  - Approximately 23% will develop ESRD within six months postpartum
  - Approximately 45% will develop ESRD within the next few years following pregnancy
  - Worsening proteinuria in 30% to 50%
- Worse prognosis if secondarily associated with active systemic disease (e.g., periarteritis nodosa, scleroderma, active lupus nephritis)

CAUSES

- Primary glomerulopathies
  - Generally good outcomes as long as renal dysfunction is mild (creatinine <1.4 mg/dL), no hypertension, and proteinuria <3 g/day (i.e., not nephrotic range)
  - The most common form of glomerulonephritis is IgA nephropathy (Berger's disease)
  - Worst fetal loss rate is found with focal glomerulosclerosis (23% to 45%) with preterm delivery of approximately 32%; this is compared with IgA nephropathy with a loss rate of approximately 13%
  - Progressive disease is worst with membranoproliferative glomerulonephritis, IgA nephropathy, and focal and segmental glomerulosclerosis
- Diabetic nephropathy
  - Diabetes is the most frequent cause of ESRD in the United States
  - Five percent to 10% of diabetic women have nephropathy (Priscilla White class "F")

- Complications include hypertension (>60%), preeclampsia (41%), preterm delivery (22% to 30%), IUGR (16%), and increased bacteriuria
- Hypertension accelerates glomerular disease in diabetic nephropathy
- During pregnancy, 32% will have worsening renal function; 15% will have accelerated ESRD
- Associated with early death, with approximately one third dying within 10 years of diagnosis
- Lupus nephritis
  - Affects approximately 50% of systemic lupus erythematosus (SLE) patients
  - If a patient develops new onset nephrotic range proteinuria, hypertension, and renal insufficiency in pregnancy, evaluate for SLE
  - Best outcomes are achieved if in remission for *6 months* prior to conception
  - Approximately 9% will have a flare in pregnancy; lupus flares are seven times *more frequent immediately following completion* of the pregnancy compared to nonpregnant state
  - Live birthrate is 58% to 84%
  - Complications include intrauterine growth restriction (IUGR) (10% to 30%), preterm delivery (13% to 53%), and preeclampsia (15%)
  - If antiphospholipid antibodies are present (lupus anticoagulant or anticardiolipin antibodies):
    - Increased risk of IUFD and maternal thromboembolic disease
    - Adverse fetal outcomes in 76%, compared to 13% if antiphospholipid antibodies are absent
  - Renal function deteriorates in 33%
  - Lupus flare can be confused with preeclampsia
    - Both will have hypertension and increased proteinuria
    - With lupus, complement levels are decreased and anti-DNA antibodies are increased; with preeclampsia, CH_{50} levels are normal
- Polycystic kidney disease
  - Adult polycystic kidney disease represents approximately 10% of ESRD during childbearing years in the United States, but increases in frequency thereafter
  - Increased incidence of developing hypertension in late pregnancy, which often persists as chronic hypertension postpartum
  - *Genetic counseling important for this autosomal dominant disease (50% of offspring will have same disease)*

TREATMENT

- Low-protein diet
- Avoid overuse of diuretics (reduced plasma volume can produce decreased uteroplacental perfusion)
- Monitor for urinary tract infection and proteinuria
  - Start prophylactic suppression with nitrofurantoin following any UTI
  - Start thromboprophylaxis if proteinuria >1000 mg/24 hours
- Control hypertension
  - Avoid use of angiotensin converting enzyme (ACE) inhibitor and angiotensin receptor blocker (ARB) drugs, as both are category D

- Goal of therapy is to keep blood pressure below 140/90; however, overly reduced blood pressure may cause uteroplacental insufficiency and IUGR
- Tight glycemic control in diabetic nephropathy
- Monitor blood count, treat significant anemia in ESRD with recombinant EPO and iron supplementation; transfusion(s) may be required to keep hemoglobin >8 g/dL
- Adjust dosing of renally cleared medications as needed
- Avoid indomethacin or betamimetics as these can worsen real function; use nifedipine for tocolysis if needed
  - Dialysis as needed (see indications under acute renal failure)

Dialysis in Pregnancy

- Pregnancy is relatively uncommon in patients on chronic dialysis because of infertility secondary to hypothalamic-gonadal dysfunction
  - Conception rate is 1% to 7%, but spontaneous and therapeutic abortions in first trimester are common
  - Most case series are of patients who conceived with moderate renal insufficiency but progressed to dialysis-requiring ESRD during the pregnancy
  - Lower success if conceived while in dialysis
- Current limited successful pregnancy outcome, but at a cost to perinatal morbidity and worsening maternal health
  - Up to approximately 50% live-birth rate
    - Live-birth rate is higher (75%) if the patient began dialysis after becoming pregnant
    - Approximately 85% prematurity
    - Approximately 90% IUGR
  - A 70% incidence of preeclampsia
  - About 75% worsening hypertension, including hypertensive crisis
  - Approximately 50% cesarean rate
- Dialysis sessions have to be increased in frequency and duration to achieve successful pregnancy outcome, perhaps to five or more times per week
  - Avoid maternal volume depletion and hypotension
  - Consider continuous ambulatory peritoneal dialysis
    - Advantages of peritoneal dialysis
      - Fluid and electrolyte concentrations are more stable
      - Less hypotension
      - No need for anticoagulation
      - Better glucose control in diabetic nephropathy
      - Less preeclampsia
      - Higher birth weights
    - Disadvantages of peritoneal dialysis
      - Higher risk of peritonitis
      - Dialysis can induce uterine contractions and preterm delivery
- High-risk pregnancy demands close monitoring and multidisciplinary treatment by a team made up of the obstetrician, perinatologist, nephrologist, and neonatologist to optimize outcome

Renal Transplant in Pregnancy

- Following transplantation, normal renal function is returned and with it fertility resumes; therefore, pregnancy success is more common
  - Low perinatal mortality (approximately 3%)

- Pregnancy complications include miscarriage (22%), preterm delivery (55%), and growth restriction (20% to 40%)
- Renal function in the allograft kidney increases similar to normal kidneys in pregnancy
- Prognosis for pregnancy with renal transplant depends on the following:
  - Time since transplant (>1 year is optimum)
  - Origin of transplant (better if from a living donor)
  - Blood pressure control (better if ≤ single agent antihypertensive treatment)
  - Immunosuppressive drugs and dosages—best if:
    - Prednisone <15 mg/day
    - Azathioprine <2 mg/kg/day
    - Cyclosporine <4 mg/kg/day
  - Allograft function
    - Creatinine <1.4 mg/dL = 95% survival
    - Creatinine ≥1.4 mg/dL = 75% survival
- Pregnancy contraindicated if creatinine >2.3 mg/dL, creatinine clearance <70 ml/min, or proteinuria >1000 mg/day, because of diminished renal function and increased need for renal transplant replacement within 2 years
- Approximately one third will develop worsening hypertension, perhaps as superimposed preeclampsia
- Immunosuppressive effects
  - About 40% will develop urinary tract infections
  - Increased CMV risk
- Allograft rejection during pregnancy (occurrence 2% to 11%) and long-term outcomes following pregnancy in renal transplant patients are similar to that for nonpregnant transplant patients
  - Ten-year graft survival (66% versus 75%)
  - Ten-year patient survival (94% versus 92%)

UPDATE #3

With transplantation, gonadal dysfunction associated with end-stage kidney disease (and other organs) is reversed. As such, patients should be counseled on effective contraception to avoid unexpected pregnancy. Although pregnancies are reported in recipients of other solid organ transplants, the numbers of pregnancies in kidney transplant recipients far outnumber recipients of other organs. If pregnancy is desired, the optimal timing is after the second posttransplant year with normal functioning allograft tissues. These include a stable creatinine of <1.5 mg/dL, proteinuria of less than 500 mg/day, and low dosing of immunosuppressive medications. The risks of pregnancy complications include hypertension and preeclampsia (47% to 73%) and risk of allograft rejection (2% to 12%). Medications used in transplant patients including immunosuppressive drugs pass into the fetal circulation with uncertain effects. Although animal models may show some teratogenic effects, there is not a unifying pattern of malformation in the children of recipients of transplanted organs. Long-term effects of in utero exposure are not well known. Immunosuppressive drugs are passed through the breast milk, and the risk-benefit ratio of breast-feeding remains unknown (McKay et al, 2006).

UPDATE #4

Pregnancies in solid organ transplant patients are increasing, though data from the National Transplantation Pregnancy Registry show that most are renal transplant cases (1208 out of 1595 from 1991 to 2007). Complications in pregnancy include hypertension (57% to 69%), preeclampsia (29%), diabetes (5% to 12%), and rejection (2% to 4%). However, the live-birth rate is 74% to 79% with a mean gestational age at birth of 35 to 36 weeks. Cesarean delivery occurs in 49% to 59%. Immunosuppressive medications in pregnancy include corticosteroids, antimetabolites (azathioprine), calcineurin inhibitors (cyclosporine and tacrolimus), and perhaps newer immunosuppressants, which may be teratogenic. During pregnancy, transplant recipients should be assessed for infection, hypertension, preeclampsia, diabetes, anemia, and graft function. Serial ultrasound examinations should be performed for following growth, with nonstress tests initiated at 32 weeks, and ultimately delivery at term unless complications occur earlier. Cesarean is reserved for usual obstetric indications (Mastrobattista et al, 2008).

UPDATE #5

In counseling a transplant patient on whether to pursue pregnancy, the physician should inform that patient that there are potential risks to (1) the allograft (rejection or dysfunction), (2) her general health (ectopic, hypertension, infection, potential need for cesarean delivery), and (3) the fetus (exposure to immunosuppressive drugs, prematurity, low birth weight, possible neurodevelopmental disabilities). Fertility issues should be addressed, preferably prior to transplantation, to include alternatives such as adoption and surrogacy. Issues of decreased maternal life expectancy and care for the child in the event of her death should be openly discussed. The pros and cons of immunosuppressive medications should also be discussed. Ultimately, however, physicians should respect the decision the transplant recipient makes about the risks and benefits of childbearing (Ross, 2006).

SUGGESTED READINGS

Physiologic Renal Changes in Pregnancy

FitzGerald MP, Graziano S: Anatomic and functional changes of the lower urinary tract during pregnancy, *Urol Clin North Am* 34(1):7–12, 2007.

Jeyabalan A, Lain KY: Anatomic and functional changes of the upper urinary tract during pregnancy, *Urol Clin North Am* 34(1):1–6, 2007.

Urinary Tract Infection

American College of Obstetricians and Gynecologists: ACOG practice bulletin no. 91: treatment of urinary tract infections in nonpregnant women, *Obstet Gynecol* 111(3):785–794, 2008.

Macejko AM, Schaeffer AJ: Asymptomatic bacteriuria and symptomatic urinary tract infections during pregnancy, *Urol Clin North Am* 34(1): 35–42, 2007.

Sheffield JS, Cunningham FG: Urinary tract infection in women, *Obstet Gynecol* 106(5 Pt 1):1085–1092, 2005.

Urolithiasis

Biyani CS, Joyce AD: Urolithiasis in pregnancy. I: Pathophysiology, fetal considerations and diagnosis, *BJU Int* 89(8):811–818, 2002.

Cormier CM, Canzoneri BJ, Lewis DF, et al: Urolithiasis in pregnancy: current diagnosis, treatment, and pregnancy complications, *Obstet Gynecol Surv* 61(11):733–741, 2006.

McAleer SJ, Loughlin KR: Nephrolithiasis and pregnancy, *Curr Opin Urol* 14(2):123–127, 2004.

Acute Renal Failure

Gammill HS, Jeyabalan A: Acute renal failure in pregnancy, *Crit Care Med* 33(Suppl 10):S372–S384, 2005.

Khanna N, Nguyen H: Reversible acute renal failure in association with bilateral ureteral obstruction and hydronephrosis in pregnancy, *Am J Obstet Gynecol* 184(2):239–240, 2001.

Larsen CP, Ejiofor MC, Walker PD: Acute kidney failure in the third trimester of pregnancy, *Am J Kidney Dis* 53(1):175–179, 2009.

Thadhani R, Solomon CG: Preeclampsia: a glimpse into the future? *N Engl J Med* 359(8):858–860, 2008.

Vikse BE, Irgens LM, Leivestad T, et al: Preeclampsia and the risk of end-stage renal disease, *N Engl J Med* 359(8):800–809, 2008.

Nephrotic Syndrome

Hull RP, Goldsmith DJ: Nephrotic syndrome in adults, *BMJ* 336(7654): 1185–1189, 2008.

Nachman PH, Jennette JC, Falk RJ: Primary glomerular disease: glomerular diseases that cause nephrotic syndrome. In Brenner BM, editor: *Brenner and Rector's the kidney*, ed 8, Philadelphia, 2008, Saunders.

Pandya BK, Gibson SP, Robertson IG: Nephrotic syndrome in early pregnancy: is renal biopsy always necessary? *Nephrol Dial Transplant* 17(4):672–674, 2002.

Chronic Renal Failure

Davison JM: Renal disorders in pregnancy, *Curr Opin Obstet Gynecol* 13(2):109–114, 2001.

Imbasciati E, Gregorini G, Cabiddu G, et al: Pregnancy in CKD stages 3 to 5: fetal and maternal outcomes, *Am J Kidney Dis* 49(6):753–762, 2007.

Jones DC, Hayslett JP: Outcome of pregnancy in women with moderate or severe renal insufficiency, *N Engl J Med* 335(4):226–232, 1996.

Ramin SM, Vidaeff AC, Yeomans ER, Gilstrap LC: Chronic renal disease in pregnancy, *Obstet Gynecol* 108(6):1531–1539, 2006.

Williams D, Davison J: Chronic kidney disease in pregnancy, *BMJ* 336(7637):211–215, 2008.

Dialysis in Pregnancy

Chao AS, Huang JY, Lien R, et al: Pregnancy in women who undergo long-term hemodialysis, *Am J Obstet Gynecol* 187(1):152–156, 2002.

Haase M, Morgera S, Bamberg C, et al: A systematic approach to managing pregnant dialysis patients: the importance of an intensified haemodiafiltration protocol, *Nephrol Dial Transplant* 20(11):2537–2542, 2005.

Holley JL, Reddy SS: Pregnancy in dialysis patients: a review of outcomes, complications, and management, *Semin Dial* 16(5):384–388, 2003.

Renal Transplant in Pregnancy

Gill JS, Zalunardo N, Rose C, Tonelli M: The pregnancy rate and live birth rate in kidney transplant recipients, *Am J Transplant* 9(7):1541–1549, 2009.

Levidiotis V, Chang S, McDonald S: Pregnancy and maternal outcomes among kidney transplant recipients, *J Am Soc Nephrol* 20(11):2433–2440, 2009.

Mastrobattista JM, Gomez-Lobo V: Pregnancy after solid organ transplantation, *Obstet Gynecol* 112(4):919–932, 2008.

McKay DB, Josephson MA: Pregnancy in recipients of solid organs: effects on mother and child, *N Engl J Med* 354(12):1281–1293, 2006.

Ross LF: Ethical considerations related to pregnancy in transplant recipients, *N Engl J Med* 354(12):1313–1316, 2006.

References

Please go to expertconsult.com to view references.

Chapter 22

Autoimmune Diseases in Pregnancy

DOUGLAS A. WOELKERS

KEY UPDATES

1 The risk of maternal mortality is increased up to 20-fold in women with systemic lupus erythematosus (SLE) compared to those without SLE. Risk factors for adverse outcomes in pregnancy complicated by SLE include advanced age, black race, multiple gestation, and lupus comorbidities involving the kidney, heart, or lung.

2 Pregnancy outcomes are generally favorable for women with well-managed systemic lupus erythematosus who have been free of flares or active nephritis for greater than 6 months before conception.

3 Diagnosis of the antiphospholipid antibody syndrome requires *both* the presence of persistent moderate to high titers of antiphospholipid antibodies *and* a history of a prior thrombosis or adverse pregnancy event.

4 Persistence of fetal cells in maternal tissues (microchimerism) has been postulated to contribute to the genesis of systemic sclerosis and several other autoimmune diseases in women.

5 Sjögren's antibodies (SS-A or SS-B) can cross the placenta and cause congenital heart block during pregnancy.

Immunity in Pregnancy

- Normal pregnancy is characterized by the following:
  - Modest, transient suppression of pro-inflammatory T-helper and T-cytotoxic cell-mediated immunity (Th1 function)
  - Predominance of humoral immunity (Th2 function)
  - Increased hepatic production of acute phase reactants
- Clinical consequences of altered immunity in pregnancy include the following:
  - Tolerance of fetal and placental antigens
  - Modest remission of some Th1-mediated autoimmune disorders (e.g., rheumatoid arthritis, multiple sclerosis, autoimmune thyroiditis)
  - No consistent effect on activity of other autoimmune diseases or on risks of infection
  - Erythrocyte sedimentation rate (ESR) and C-reactive protein (CRP) increase in normal pregnancy, and they are not reliable markers of disease activity
  - Autoantibody titers and serum complement levels are generally unchanged
- Drugs that should be avoided before or during pregnancy include methotrexate, leflunomide (Arava), and mycophenolate (CellCept) (Table 22-1)

Systemic Lupus Erythematosus

- Systemic lupus erythematosus (SLE) is a multisystem autoimmune disease caused by antigen-antibody deposition in various tissues

DIAGNOSIS AND PRESENTATION

- SLE is characterized by a 9:1 female preponderance; incidence of 1 in 500 reproductive-aged women; fourfold increase in African-American women
- Symptoms may include malaise, arthritis, serositis, rash, fever, alopecia, oral ulcers, Reynaud's phenomenon, or seizures
- Laboratory findings may include anemia, thrombocytopenia, neutropenia, proteinuria, elevated creatinine
- Antinuclear antibodies (ANAs) are virtually always present at high titer in lupus; other autoantibodies that are relatively specific for lupus include the following:
  - Anti-double-stranded DNA (dsDNA) antibody
  - Anti-Sm antigen antibody
- The American Rheumatological Association has established 11 candidate criteria for the diagnosis of SLE; they include malar rash, discoid rash, photosensitivity, oral ulcers, arthritis, serositis, renal disorder (persistent proteinuria or cellular casts), neurologic disorder (seizures or psychosis), hematologic disorder (hemolytic anemia, leukopenia, lymphopenia, thrombocytopenia), and positive ANA
- The diagnosis is established by the presence of ≥3 clinical or laboratory findings and a positive ANA (Liang et al, 1980)

MANAGEMENT

- Preconceptional counseling is strongly recommended to optimize maternal health and provide education before contemplating pregnancy

TABLE 22-1   **Antirheumatic Drugs in Pregnancy**

Drug Classification	Drugs	Safety Category	Lactation Category	Notes
Anti-inflammatory	Corticosteroids (prednisone, prednisolone)	B	Compatible	Small risk cleft lip and palate with first trimester exposure. Avoid fluorinated steroids (dexamethasone or betamethasone), which have greater transplacental passage. Monitor hyperglycemia, hypertension, and adrenal suppression.
	NSAIDs (ibuprofen, naproxen, and similar)	B in first trimester; D in third trimester	Mostly compatible	No identified pattern of anomalies with first-trimester use. In the second and third trimesters there are risks of ductal closure and oligohydramnios.
DMARD				
Antimalarial	Hydroxychloroquine (Plaquenil)	C	Compatible	None to date.
Immunosuppressive	Methotrexate	X	Not recommended	Abortion. CNS, craniofacial, and skeletal defects. Discontinue 3 months prior to conception.
	Azathioprine	D	Caution—limited data	No identified pattern of anomalies. Possible growth restriction, preterm delivery.
	Cyclophosphamide	D	Not recommended	First-trimester teratogen. Possible fetal death. Third-trimester exposure risks are unknown.
	Leflunomide (Arava)	X	Not recommended	Major anomalies in animal studies. Lipid soluble, prolonged half-life. Check serum levels if any exposure within 2 years of planning or experiencing pregnancy. Cholestyramine tid if >0.03 mg/L.
Anti-inflammatory	Sulfasalazine	B in first trimester and second trimester; D at term	Compatible caution with prematurity or hyperbilirubinemia	No identified pattern of anomalies. Possible displacement of bilirubin in newborn blood.
TNF-α antagonists	Etanercept (Enbrel), adalimumab (Humira), and infliximab (Remicade)	B	Caution—limited data	No identified pattern of anomalies in animals. Multiple anomalies reported in humans, but no proven association with drug. Possible neonatal immunosuppression with near-term use and lactation.
BRM				
Immunosuppressive	Mycophenolate (CellCept)	D	Not recommended	Abortion, preterm delivery, congenital anomalies.
Immunoglobulin	IVIG	C	Compatible	No known adverse effect on fetal development or growth

BRM, Biologic response modifiers; CNS, central nervous system; DMARD, disease modifying antirheumatic drug.
Adapted from Elliott AB, Chakravarty EF: Immunosuppressive medications during pregnancy and lactation in women with autoimmune diseases, *Womens Health (Lond Engl)* 6(3):431-440, 2010; and Mitchell K, Kaul M, Clowse, ME: The management of rheumatic diseases in pregnancy, *Scand J Rheumatol* 39(2):99-108, 2010.

- The need for acute or maintenance pharmacotherapy is dictated primarily by maternal disease severity, with consideration of fetal consequences
  - First-line therapy includes oral prednisone or hydroxychloroquine
  - Low-dose aspirin and heparin are recommended to prevent fetal loss and maternal thrombosis in patients with antiphospholipid antibody syndrome (discussed later)
  - Intravenous immunoglobulins (IVIG), azathioprine, or nonsteroidal anti-inflammatory drugs (NSAIDs) may be occasionally necessary
- Surveillance of maternal symptoms, blood pressure, renal function, platelets, and hematocrit is warranted
  - Serologic studies for antiphospholipid antibodies (APA) and SS-A (anti-Ro) or SS-B (anti-La) antibodies (associated with congenital heart block) and baseline urine protein excretion and creatinine clearance should be obtained
- Distinguishing superimposed preeclampsia from an exacerbation of lupus nephritis is difficult
  - Extracranial symptoms (e.g. rash, arthalgia), rising anti-dsDNA antibody titers, falling complement levels, and urinary erythrocytes favor the diagnosis of lupus flare over preeclampsia
- Regular monitoring of fetal growth and antenatal testing are recommended because of risks of growth restriction and stillbirth
- Cooperative care should involve the obstetrician, neonatologist, and internist or rheumatologist

PROGNOSIS AND OUTCOME

Pregnancy probably does not alter the course of lupus—approximately one third of patients improve, one third deteriorate, and the remaining patients experience no change

UPDATE #1

Disease activity prior to conception is the best predictor of prognosis during pregnancy (Imbasciati et al, 2009).
- The likelihood of a severe lupus flare is increased (60% to 70%) in women with active disease in the 6 months prior to conception, in those with poorly controlled lupus in the year prior to conception, and in those who discontinue medications because of pregnancy.
- For women with quiescent disease in the 6 months prior to conception, less than 10% will have moderate to severe SLE during pregnancy.

- Advanced age, African-American race, and the presence of comorbidities (especially nephritis or antiphospholipid antibody syndrome) are other predictors of adverse outcome
  - Subjects with active nephritis experience high rates of preeclampsia (50% to 60%), preterm delivery (30% to 50%), and perinatal mortality (6% to 35%) (Imbasciati et al, 2009; Wagner et al, 2009)

UPDATE #2

Clowse and colleagues compared U.S. outcomes for 13,555 pregnancies with lupus to 16.7 million without lupus over a 4-year period from 2000 to 2003 (Clowse et al, 2008). Patients with lupus were 3.0-fold more likely to have preeclampsia, 2.6-fold more likely to have a growth restricted infant, and

2.4-fold more likely to have preterm labor. The risks for severe morbidity such as stroke, deep vein thrombosis (DVT), and pneumonia increased 6.5-, 7.9-, and 4.3-fold, respectively. The risk of maternal death was nearly 20-fold higher than in controls, and it was concentrated among women with prior arterial thrombosis, myocarditis, prior myocardial infarction or valve disease, uncontrolled hypertension, pulmonary hypertension, or a prior severe SLE flare during pregnancy.

- Four percent to 8% of newborns will exhibit signs of neonatal lupus, which may include thrombocytopenia, anemia, neutropenia, heart block, or cutaneous lesions

Antiphospholipid Antibody Syndrome (APAS)

- APAS is an immune-mediated vasculopathy characterized by autoantibodies to complexes of anionic phospholipids and serum or membrane-bound proteins

UPDATE #3

The APAS syndrome is defined (Miyakis et al, 2006) as a combination of the following:
1. One or more persistent, high-titer antiphospholipid antibodies (aPL)
   - Anticardiolipin antibody (IgG or IgM >40 units), or
   - Lupus anticoagulant, or
   - Anti-β2-glycoprotein-I (IgG or IgM >99th percentile)
2. One or more attributable clinical events
   - Prior arterial or venous thrombosis, or
   - Prior adverse pregnancy outcomes
     - ≥3 unexplained embryonic losses (<10 weeks)
     - ≥1 unexplained fetal death (>10 weeks)
     - Early (<34 weeks) preeclampsia, eclampsia, or intrauterine growth restriction (IUGR)

- Isolated, low-titer antiphospholipid antibodies are found incidentally in 1% to 5% of apparently healthy adults and pregnant women; but less than 1% have persistent high titers upon repeat testing (Levine et al, 2002)
  - The term *lupus anticoagulant* is a historic misnomer, because the antibodies detected by this assay are neither specific to lupus nor do they act *in vivo* as anticoagulants
    - Antibodies to other phospholipids (such as phosphatidylserine) and proteins (such as prothrombin or annexin V) may be detected, but their clinical significance is not well defined
- Additional clinical manifestations of APAS may include thrombocytopenia, hemolytic anemia, livido reticularis, or a false-positive rapid plasma reagin (RPR) test for syphilis
- Management in pregnancy
  - Therapy is directed to reduce the risk of primary or recurrent thrombosis and pregnancy loss (Table 22-2)
    - In women without a history of thrombosis:
      - Heparin (7500 to 10,000 U sq bid) and low-dose aspirin (80 mg/day) have been shown to improve the live birth rate in women with aPL and a history of recurrent pregnancy loss
      - To date, studies have not shown that anticoagulation reduces the risk of preeclampsia, IUGR, or preterm delivery

TABLE 22-2   **Management of Antiphospholipid Antibody Syndrome in Pregnancy**

Clinical History	Suggested Therapy	Timing and duration
History of prior thrombotic event	Therapeutic anticoagulation with UFH or LMWH during pregnancy; with or without LDA	From onset of pregnancy at least until 6 weeks postpartum with appropriate pause for delivery. Most subjects will be on lifelong anticoagulation. Consider warfarin for postpartum anticoagulation.
History of fetal death (≥10 weeks) or recurrent (≥3) early pregnancy losses	LDA (81 mg/day) and low dose UFH or LMWH	Starting LDA during conception and adding heparin at confirmation of fetal cardiac activity; cessation of therapy for delivery. Consideration of postpartum thromboprophylaxis with heparin or warfarin for 6 weeks.
History of prior adverse pregnancy outcome including preterm pre-eclampsia, eclampsia, or IUGR; no prior thrombosis	Insufficient data. Consider LDA and low-dose UFH or LMWH, versus LDA alone.	Starting therapy at confirmation of fetal cardiac activity. Consideration of postpartum thromboprophylaxis for 6 weeks.
Persistent high titer aPL without qualifying clinical event	Insufficient data. Consider no therapy, LDA, or various regimens of heparin	If treatment is elected, it should begin at confirmation of cardiac activity, and should continue postpartum.

aPL, Antiphospholipid antibodies; LDA, low-dose aspirin; LMWH, low-molecular-weight heparin; UFH, unfractionated heparin.
Adapted from American College of Obstetricians and Gynecologists: ACOG Practice Bulletin no. 68 (2005): Antiphospholipid Syndrome, *Obstet Gynecol* 106:1113-1121, 2005; and Bates SM, Greer IA, Pabinger I: Venous thromboembolism, thrombophilia, antithrombotic therapy, and pregnancy: American College of Chest Physicians Evidence-Based Clinical Practice Guidelines, ed 8, *Chest* 133(6 Suppl):844S-886S, 2008.

- Postpartum anticoagulation is suggested by many experts given the high risk of thrombosis in the puerperium (see Table 22-2)
- Women with a history of APAS and thrombosis require high-level prophylactic anticoagulation through pregnancy and the puerperium
  - Suggested regimens include the following (Bates et al, 2008):
    - Adjusted dose of unfractionated heparin to prolong midinterval partial thromboplastin time (PTT) greater than 1.5 × control (7500 to 20,000 U bid to tid), or
    - Twice daily low-molecular-weight heparin (e.g., enoxaparin 40 mg bid)
- Close fetal and maternal monitoring is indicated to detect early adverse events and allow appropriate ancillary management and preparation for delivery

OUTCOMES

- Obstetrical complications are frequent in women with APAS (2005); up to 80% of women with APAS have experienced at least one fetal death; the risk of preeclampsia is as high as 50%, whereas the risk of IUGR is between 15% and 30%; preterm birth because of placental insufficiency occurs in up to 33% of women with APAS
- Patients with APAS and a prior thrombosis will require lifelong anticoagulation
  - The risk of recurrent thrombosis (3.3% per year) or death (1% per year) is still elevated despite treatment (Cervera et al, 2009)

Rheumatoid Arthritis (RA)

- RA is correctly known as one of the few maternal diseases that may actually improve during pregnancy, and outcomes are generally good
  - The prevalence is approximately 4 to 8/1000

- About 75% of pregnant RA patients experience remission in pregnancy
  - Postpartum flares, however, are common (up to 90%)
- Rates of preeclampsia and preterm delivery appear to be slightly elevated
- Treatment options for women with RA in pregnancy are limited, because many disease-modifying antirheumatic drugs (DMARDs) are contraindicated in pregnant or nursing women (e.g., methotrexate, leflunomide, tumor necrosis factor [TNF] antagonists; see Table 22-1)
- Active disease is usually treated with as low a dose as possible of prednisone, sulfasalazine, or hydroxychloroquine

Scleroderma

- Also known as progressive systemic sclerosis
  - Rare disorder with a 13:1 female preponderance in the reproductive years
- Unknown etiology
  - Characterized by chronic fibrosis of skin or internal organs (lungs, GI, kidneys, etc.)

UPDATE #4

Persistent fetal cells in maternal tissues have been postulated to contribute to the genesis of systemic sclerosis, lupus, and other autoimmune disorders in women (Adams Waldorf et al, 2008).

- May present as part of a mixed connective tissue disease with lupus, rheumatoid arthritis, Sjögren's syndrome, and polymyositis
- Pregnancy outcomes depend on degree of organ involvement prior to conception
  - Favorable outcomes for women with limited cutaneous sclerosis

- No increase in pregnancy loss or disease progression in these cases
- Alarmingly high maternal and fetal mortality rates are reported in women with preexistent renal or pulmonary fibrosis

Sjögren's Syndrome

- Characterized by autoimmune destruction of exocrine glands of the
  - Eye: keratoconjunctivitis
  - Mouth: xerostomia, or
  - Mucosa: vaginal or gastrointestinal
- Frequently arises in setting of mixed connective tissue disorders including lupus and rheumatoid arthritis
  - High prevalence of autoantibodies, including the following:
    - Antinuclear antibodies
    - Antismooth muscle antibody
    - Rheumatoid factor
    - Anti-Ro (SS-A) and anti-La (SS-B) nuclear antigens

UPDATE #5

SS-A and SS-B antibodies may cross the placenta and induce fetal cardiac injury leading to congenital heart block (CHB). The risk of CHB is approximately 2% in women with no previously affected infant, but it is as high as 20% in those with such a history. Fetal echocardiography and frequent fetal heart rate monitoring are recommended between 16 and 26 weeks (Friedman et al, 2008).

  - The use of maternally administered corticosteroids to prevent the advancement of second-degree to CHB, or to ameliorate or regress established CHB, is controversial

Autoimmune Thyroid Disease

- Autoimmune activity in the thyroid may be characterized by gland stimulation, destruction, or a mixture of the two processes
  - Thyroid stimulating immunoglobulins (TSIg) activate the thyroid-stimulating hormone receptor (TSH-R), leading to hyperthyroidism (Graves' disease)
  - Hypothyroidism is related to antibody or cell-mediated glandular dysfunction
    - Anti-thyroid peroxidase (anti-TPO) antibodies are characteristic of Hashimoto's thyroiditis
    - Other antibodies may block the TSH receptor (thyroid binding inhibitory immunoglobulins, TBIIg) or bind thyroglobulin (anti-thyroglobulin immunoglobulins, anti-TG)
- Autoimmune hyperthyroidism (Graves' disease) often improves during late gestation but commonly flares postpartum
  - Graves' disease affects 1 to 2 per 1000 pregnancies
  - Pregnancy complications of Graves' disease include thyroid storm, miscarriage, preeclampsia, heart failure, preterm birth, and growth restriction
    - Neonatal hyperthyroidism resulting from transplacental passage of maternal TSIg may affect up to 1% of newborns
- Treatment with thionamides is recommended at the lowest dose necessary to keep free T4 concentration in the high-normal range (see Chapter 25 on thyroid disease in pregnancy)
- Autoimmune hypothyroidism (Hashimoto's disease) affects approximately 0.2% to 0.3% of pregnancies
  - Characterized by the presence of anti-thyroid peroxidase (TPO) or anti-thyroglobulin (TG) antibodies, an elevated thyroid stimulating hormone (TSH), and low thyroglobulin hormone (free T4)
    - Up to 4% of euthyroid women have anti-TPO antibodies
    - Several reports suggest that women with anti-TPO or anti-TG antibodies have higher rates of miscarriage, preterm delivery, or placental abruption—independent of thyroid function (Abbassi-Ghanavati et al, 2010; Männistö et al, 2009; Prummel et al, 2004)
  - Treatment of hypothyroidism should begin prior to conception, or at least by the fifth week of pregnancy (see Chapter 25 on the treatment of thyroid disease in pregnancy)
  - Hashimoto's thyroiditis is not typically associated with fetal thyroid dysfunction; only 1:180,000 offspring of affected pregnancies are estimated to have hypothyroidism
- Postpartum thyroiditis is a manifestation of altered autoimmunity following pregnancy
  - Risk is as high as 5% to 10% in first year after delivery
    - Risk is related to the presence of antithyroid antibodies in the first trimester
    - Twenty percent to 50% of apparently euthyroid women with anti-TPO antibodies in the first trimester experience postpartum thyroiditis (Pearce et al, 2003; Sakaihara et al, 2000)
  - Postpartum thyroiditis is characterized by an initial hyperthyroid phase (1 to 4 months postpartum) followed by a hypothyroid phase (4 to 12 months postpartum)
    - Approximately 40% of cases are the hyperthyroid type, 40% are the hypothyroid type, and 20% are the sequential type
    - Symptoms are nonspecific, transient, and may be attributed to the postpartum state
      - Hyperthyroid: fatigue, palpitations, heat intolerance, anxiety, irritability
      - Hypothyroid: fatigue, hair loss, depression, dry skin, inability to concentrate
    - Treatment is generally supportive given the transient nature of symptoms and the potential conflicts with breast-feeding
    - Antithyroid medications (thionamides, iodine) are not indicated in the hyperthyroid phase
      - Low-dose B-blockade may ameliorate bothersome symptoms
    - Short-term thyroid hormone replacement may be considered when indicated for 8 to 12 weeks in symptomatic hypothyroid women
    - Repeat thyroid function testing (off medication) is indicated after 12 weeks because of the high risk of subsequent hypothyroidism

SUGGESTED READINGS

Systemic Lupus Erythematosus

Clowse ME, Jamison M, Myers E, et al: A national study of the complications of lupus in pregnancy, *Am J Obstet Gynecol* 199(2):127e1–127e6, 2008.

Imbasciati E, Tincani A, Gregorini G, et al: Pregnancy in women with pre-existing lupus nephritis: predictors of fetal and maternal outcome, *Nephrol Dial Transplant* 24(2):519–525, 2009.

Liang MH, Meenan RF, Cathcart ES, et al: A screening strategy for population studies in systemic lupus erythematosus. Series design, *Arthritis Rheum* 23(2):153–157, 1980.

Wagner SJ, Craici I, Reed D, et al: Maternal and foetal outcomes in pregnant patients with active lupus nephritis, *Lupus* 18(4):342–347, 2009.

Antiphospholipid Antibody Syndrome

American College of Obstetricians and Gynecologists: ACOG practice bulletin no. 68: antiphospholipid syndrome, *Obstet Gynecol* 106(5 Pt 1):1113–1121, 2005.

Bates SM, Greer IA, Pabinger I, et al: Venous thromboembolism, thrombophilia, antithrombotic therapy, and pregnancy: American College of Chest Physicians evidence-based clinical practice guidelines, ed 8, *Chest* 133(Suppl 6):844S–886S, 2008.

Cervera R, Khamashta MA, Shoenfeld Y, et al: Morbidity and mortality in the antiphospholipid syndrome during a 5-year period: a multicentre prospective study of 1000 patients, *Ann Rheum Dis* 68(9):1428–1432, 2009.

Levine JS, Branch DW, Rauch J: The antiphospholipid syndrome, *N Engl J Med* 346(10):752–763, 2002.

Miyakis S, Lockshin MD, Atsumi T, et al: International consensus statement on an update of the classification criteria for definite antiphospholipid syndrome (APS), *J Thromb Haemost* 4(2):295–306, 2006.

Antirheumatic Agents

Elliott AB, Chakravarty EF: Immunosuppressive medications during pregnancy and lactation in women with autoimmune diseases, *Womens Health (Lond Engl)* 6(3):431–440, 2010. quiz 441-442.

Mitchell K, Kaul M, Clowse ME, et al: The management of rheumatic diseases in pregnancy, *Scand J Rheumatol* 39(2):99–108, 2010.

Systemic Sclerosis

Adams Waldorf KM, Nelson JL: Autoimmune disease during pregnancy and the microchimerism legacy of pregnancy, *Immunol Invest* 37(5):631–644, 2008.

Sjögrens Syndrome

Friedman DM, Kim MY, Copel JA, et al: Utility of cardiac monitoring in fetuses at risk for congenital heart block: the PR Interval and Dexamethasone Evaluation (PRIDE) prospective study, *Circulation* 117(4):485–493, 2008.

Autoimmune Thyroiditis

Abbassi-Ghanavati M, Casey BM, Spong CY, et al: Pregnancy outcomes in women with thyroid peroxidase antibodies, *Obstet Gynecol* 116(2 Pt 1):381–386, 2010.

Männistö T, Vääräsmäki M, Pouto A, et al: Perinatal outcome of children born to mothers with thyroid dysfunction or antibodies: a prospective population-based cohort study, *J Clin Endocrinol Metab* 94(3):772–779, 2009.

Pearce EN, Farwell AP, Braverman LE, et al: Thyroiditis, *N Engl J Med* 348(26):2646–2655, 2003.

Prummel MF, Wiersinga WM: Thyroid autoimmunity and miscarriage, *Eur J Endocrinol* 150(6):751–755, 2004.

Sakaihara M, Yamada H, Kato EH, et al: Postpartum thyroid dysfunction in women with normal thyroid function during pregnancy, *Clin Endocrinol (Oxf)* 53(4):487–492, 2000.

References

Please go to expertconsult.com to view references.

Chapter 23

Gastroenterologic Disorders in Pregnancy

THOMAS F. KELLY

KEY UPDATES

1. Pharmacologic treatment of nausea and vomiting of pregnancy should utilize a stepwise strategy that incurs the least amount of fetal and maternal risk.

2. Magnetic resonance imaging should be considered in the workup of acute appendicitis, especially if the workup is inconclusive.

3. Bariatric surgical patients have increased nutritional deficiency risks as well as surgical complications.

4. All pregnant women should be screened for hepatitis B.

5. Intrahepatic cholestasis of pregnancy appears to have an increased risk of poor fetal outcomes.

6. Acute fatty liver may be associated with a genetic mutation of the fetus involving fatty acid oxidation.

7. Patients with liver transplants can achieve successful pregnancies, but they are at higher risk of prematurity, growth restriction, and hypertensive disease.

Nausea and Vomiting of Pregnancy

CLINICAL PROFILE

- Seventy percent to 85% of pregnant women are affected
- Hyperemesis gravidarum incidence is approximately 0.5% to 2% of pregnancies, and it is the most common indication for hospitalization in the first trimester
- Etiology is unknown; theories include psychological predisposition, evolutionary adaptation, and hormonal stimulus
- Human chorionic gonadotropin and estrogen have been found to have an association
- Risk factors include increased placental mass, family history, and a prior history of hyperemesis; other risk factors include a history of migraines and motion sickness

DIAGNOSIS

- Timing is important; virtually all women present with symptoms prior to 9 weeks' gestation; if a patient experiences symptoms for the first time after 9 weeks, other conditions should be considered
- Differential diagnosis includes other gastrointestinal conditions, genitourinary tract pathology, metabolic disease, neurologic disorders, drug toxicity, and pregnancy-related conditions such as preeclampsia
  - Laboratory assessment should be used not only to assess the patient's metabolic status but to target other potential etiologies including hepatitis and pancreatitis

MANAGEMENT

- Prevention: women who take multivitamins prior to conception are less likely to need medical attention for vomiting

- Nonpharmacologic therapies include rest, avoidance of provocative sensory stimuli, and frequent small meals; ginger may improve clinical symptoms

UPDATE #1

First-line treatment of nausea and vomiting during pregnancy preferably should be vitamin B_6 with or without doxylamine. Refractory cases may require other medications of which the following have been shown to be relatively safe in pregnancy: antihistamine (H1) receptor blockers, phenothiazines, and benzamides. Severe cases may require the consideration of methylprednisolone, but given the risks associated with its use, such therapy should be considered as a last resort (American College of Obstetrics and Gynecology, 2004).

- Pharmacologic therapy (Figure 23-1)
  - Intravenous hydration should be used in women who cannot tolerate oral liquids; dextrose and vitamins, especially thiamine, should be included when prolonged vomiting is present
  - Enteral and parenteral nutrition can be considered in extreme cases. The latter is associated with increased morbidity, including line infections and thromboembolism, and should be considered only as a last resort

Gastrointestinal Reflux Disease (GERD)

CLINICAL PROFILE

- Heartburn is the most common gastrointestinal complaint in Western populations. 80% of pregnant

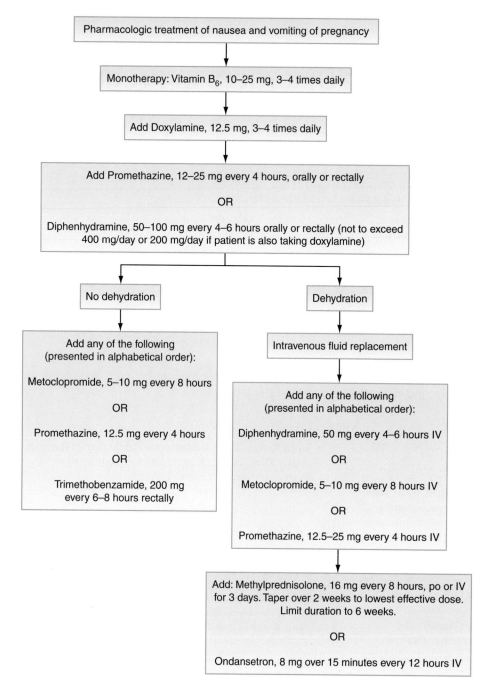

Figure 23-1. **Pharmacologic therapy for the treatment of nausea and vomiting of pregnancy.** (Adapted from American College of Obstetricians and Gynecologists: ACOG practice bulletin no. 52: nausea and vomiting of pregnancy, *Obstet Gynecol* 103:803-815, 2004).

women are symptomatic at some point, and 25% experience it daily

- Factors associated with GERD include prepregnancy symptoms, advancing gestational age, and parity
- Exact etiology is unknown; however, the lower esophageal sphincter tone is decreased during pregnancy, and there is presumed increased intra-abdominal pressure and delayed gastric emptying, all of which may contribute to the increased incidence

DIAGNOSIS

- Symptoms include substernal burning, dyspepsia, and regurgitation; extraesophageal symptoms may also be present, such as hoarseness, chronic cough, laryngitis, and asthma

- There is rarely a need for invasive testing; upper gastrointestinal endoscopy should be reserved for the exceptional cases refractory to medical management

MANAGEMENT (Figure 23-2)

- Lifestyle and dietary changes are helpful for patients with mild symptoms; these include avoidance of meals prior to bedtime and avoidance of alcohol, smoking, caffeine, chocolate, and peppermint
- Medications used in nonpregnant patients for GERD are not routinely tested in pregnant women; most recommendations rely on data from small case series
- Commonly used histamine (H2) receptor antagonists are listed as category B; proton pump inhibitors (PPIs) are in category B with the exception of omeprazole (C); misoprostol should not be used during pregnancy

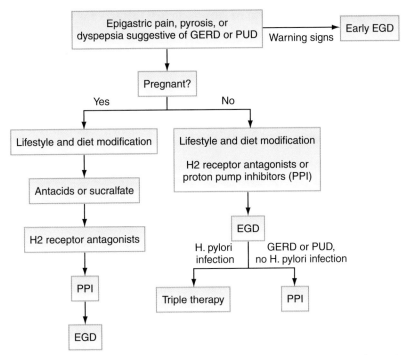

Figure 23-2. **Stepwise management of GERD or peptic ulcer disease (PUD).** (Adapted from Kelly TF, Savides TJ: Gastrointestinal disease in pregnancy. In Creasy RK, Resnik R, Iams JD, et al, editors: *Creasy & Resnik's maternal fetal medicine: principles and practice,* ed 6, Philadelphia, 2009, Saunders Elsevier, pp 1041-1057.)

Appendicitis

CLINICAL PROFILE

- Acute appendicitis is one of the most common causes of an acute abdomen in pregnancy, occurring in approximately 1 in 1500 gestations
- Fetal loss rates for appendectomy are higher than for other surgical procedures during pregnancy approximating 2.6%; loss rates may increase to 10% if peritonitis is present
- The advancing gestational age increases the rate of delayed diagnosis and appendiceal perforation

DIAGNOSIS

- Right lower quadrant pain appears to be the most common complaint; symptoms felt to be suspicious for appendicitis in the nonpregnant patient may not be reliable
- It is important to rule out urinary tract infection and pulmonary pathology, as their symptoms may mimic that of appendicitis

UPDATE #2

Computed tomography and magnetic resonance imaging are potentially useful adjuncts in the evaluation of acute appendicitis. The latter has the advantage of no fetal exposure to radiation. Pedrosa et al. (2006) suggested a high positive and negative predictive value for magnetic resonance imaging (MRI). Pooled data suggest a specificity of 99% in patients with a prior normal or inconclusive abdominal ultrasound (Basaran et al, 2009).

- Imaging options include ultrasound, computed tomography (CT), and magnetic resonance imaging (MRI); given ultrasound's poor sensitivity, inconclusive

or normal results should prompt the use of CT or MRI; Table 23-1 represents the performance of these two modalities in patients with a prior normal or inconclusive ultrasound

MANAGEMENT

- Prompt surgical intervention
- If laparotomy is performed, either a muscle splitting incision over the point of maximal tenderness or a midline approach if generalized peritonitis is present
- Laparoscopy has been used for appendectomies during pregnancy; data on outcomes and safety are based on case series, but they appear to be similar to those done via an open approach; theoretic concerns over uterine injury may preclude the laparoscopic approach in the latter part of pregnancy; however, local expertise will likely guide management
- Perioperative antibiotics should be used

Irritable Bowel Syndrome (IBS)

CLINICAL PROFILE

- Characterized by chronic recurring abdominal pain and altered bowel habits
- Very common, with a prevalence of about 15%

DIAGNOSIS

- Can be diagnosed with history, physical examination, and routine laboratory studies providing there are no warning signs (rectal bleeding, anemia, weight loss, fever, family history of colon cancer, onset at >50 years of age, or major change in symptoms)
- Rome diagnostic criteria for IBS: recurrent abdominal pain or discomfort at least 3 days per month for the

TABLE 23-1 Imaging Modalities for Evaluation of Appendicitis: Criteria for Diagnosis and Reported Detection Rates

Modality	Diagnostic Criteria	Sensitivity	Specificity	Positive Likelihood Ratio	Negative Likelihood Ratio
			(95% Confidence Intervals)		
CT	Abnormal appendix identified or calcified fecalith seen in association with periappendiceal inflammation or a diameter of >6 mm	85.7% (63.7%-97%)	97.4% (86.2%-99.9%)	10.1 (3.4-30.1)	0.21 (0.05-0.88)
MRI	Appendix diameter of >7 mm or 6-7 mm with periappendiceal inflammation	80% (44%-98%)	99% (94%-100%)	22.7 (6.0-87.5)	0.29 (0.13-0.68)

Data from Basaran A, Basaran M: Diagnosis of acute appendicitis during pregnancy: a systematic review, *Obstet Gynecol Surv* 64:481-468, 2009.

TABLE 23-2 Comparison of Ulcerative Colitis and Crohn's Disease

Feature	Ulcerative Colitis	Crohn's Disease
Extent of inflammation	Limited to mucosa	Transmural
Intestine involved	Colon only	Throughout the gastrointestinal system, especially the terminal ileum
Rectal involvement	Always	Sometimes
Pattern of spread	Contiguous	Skip lesions
Granulomas	No	Yes
Fistula	No	Yes
Strictures	No	Yes
Abscess	No	Yes
Perianal disease	No	Yes
Bloody diarrhea	Yes	Maybe
Ileal disease on computed tomography	No	Yes
Increased colon cancer risk	Yes	Maybe if colonic involvement
Cure with surgery	Yes	No
Percent of patients who will require surgery	20%	70%

Adapted from Kelly TF, Savides TJ: Gastrointestinal disease in pregnancy. In Creasy RK, Resnik R, Iams JD, et al, editors: *Creasy & Resnik's maternal fetal medicine, principles and practice,* ed 6, Philadelphia, 2009, Saunders Elsevier, pp 1041-1057.

past 3 months, associated with two or more of the following:
- Improvement with defecation
- Onset associated with a change in frequency of stool
- Onset associated with a change in form (appearance) of stool
- Differential diagnosis includes celiac disease, atypical Crohn's disease, and chronic constipation

MANAGEMENT
- Symptomatic treatment mainly targeting normalizing bowel habits

- Identify and eliminate foods that worsen symptoms
- A minority of patients will need medications; only a small number of pharmacologic treatments are supported by well-designed trials for the use in IBS
- Fiber and bulking agents used for the treatment of constipation may be associated with increased side effects of bloating in patients with IBS
- Low-dose antidepressants (paroxetine and citalopram) may be considered for the treatment or modification of the abdominal pain
- Antispasmodic medications such as hyoscyamine may be helpful

Inflammatory Bowel Disease (IBD)

CLINICAL PROFILE (Table 23-2)
- IBD refers to Crohn's disease and ulcerative colitis
- Etiology is unknown
- Women with IBD may be at increased risk for adverse pregnancy outcomes; however, most studies suggest that if the disease is quiescent, pregnancy outcomes are usually acceptable; poorly controlled disease at the time of conception does appear to increase the risk of poor obstetrical outcome

DIAGNOSIS
- Because most patients are likely diagnosed prior to pregnancy, clinical symptoms are important to assess for exacerbation of the disease
- Flexible sigmoidoscopy appears to be safe in pregnancy
- Stool cultures may be necessary to rule out intestinal infection, particularly clostridium difficile especially when considering any new immunosuppressive therapy
- Magnetic resonance imaging or computed tomography may be considered, particularly in Crohn's disease flares; these modalities should be used in carefully selected cases when the benefits outweigh the potential risks

MANAGEMENT (Table 23-3)
- 5-aminosalicylic acid (5-ASA) preparations (sulfasalazine, mesalamine, balsalazide, olsalazine) are usually the first-line drugs in the treatment of IBD; they are poorly absorbed from the intestinal tract and act locally

TABLE 23-3 Drugs Usually Used in IBD: Safety in Pregnancy

Safe to Use	Probably Safe but Limited Data	Contraindicated
Sulfasalazine	Azathioprine	Methotrexate
5-Amniosalicylates	6-Mercaptopurine	Diphenoxylate
Corticosteroids	Cyclosporine	
	Metronidazole	
	Ciprofloxacin	
	Infliximab	
	Loperamide	

Adapted from Kelly TF, Savides TJ: Gastrointestinal disease in pregnancy. In Creasy RK, Resnik R, Iams JD, et al, editors: *Creasy & Resnik's maternal fetal medicine, principles and practice,* ed 6, Philadelphia, 2009, Saunders Elsevier, pp 1041-1057.

- Corticosteroids can be used, mainly to induce remission; they are not usually used for long-term maintenance therapy
- Antibiotics, primarily metronidazole and ciprofloxacin, are occasionally used in patients with Crohn's; although the short-term use of the former is likely safe, ciprofloxacin's use during pregnancy should be reserved when the benefit clearly outweighs the theoretic risks
- Immunomodulators such as azathioprine and 6-mercaptopurine are mainly utilized for maintenance therapy in IBD
- Infliximab, which inhibits tumor necrosis factor, is increasingly utilized to induce and maintain therapy for Crohn's disease; this agent is less well studied with regard to safety in pregnancy, but it has been used for patients who are refractory to other agents
- Mode of delivery should be dictated by disease activity; no substantial data exist to recommend a cesarean section in patients without a history of perianal disease; however, in patients with Crohn's disease and a history of active perianal disease, a cesarean section should be considered; consultation with a gastroenterologist and colorectal surgeon is advisable to assist in determining the route of delivery on a case-by-case basis

Bariatric Surgery

CLINICAL PROFILE

- Obesity is an epidemic in the United States; 66% of adults are either overweight or obese; 29% of women of reproductive age are obese as defined as a body mass index of over 30
- Obesity is associated with reduced fertility, mainly secondary to oligo and anovulation
- Obese patients have increased risks of gestational diabetes, preeclampsia, cesarean delivery, and peripartum infectious and thromboembolic morbidity; there is also an increased fetal risk of congenital anomalies, growth abnormalities, and stillbirth
- Bariatric surgery may be indicated for an individual having a BMI of >40 (or 30 if other comorbidities are present)
- More than 100,000 bariatric procedures are performed in the United States annually, half of which are performed on women of reproductive age
- Two types of procedures are commonly performed: restrictive (most notably lap banding) and a combination of restrictive and malabsorptive operations such as Roux-en-Y; both techniques can be performed laparoscopically

UPDATE #3

Bariatric surgery procedures are of two main categories: restrictive (banding) and bypass. The obstetrical consequences may differ. For example, patients with bypass procedures are more prone to nutritional deficiencies including Vitamin B_{12} and iron. Both procedures, however, carry these risks. The obstetrician should have an increased awareness of surgical complications that may occur in these patients (Kirshtein et al, 2010; Wax et al, 2007).

MANAGEMENT

- Authorities have suggested waiting 12 to 24 months after bariatric surgery before conceiving so the fetus is not exposed to a rapid weight loss environment
- Nutritional deficiencies are more common after Roux-en-Y procedures and include iron, vitamin B_{12}, folate, vitamin D, calcium, and protein; assessment and replacement of these deficiencies are paramount
- Bariatric surgery complications (anastomotic leaks, bowel obstructions, internal hernias, ventral hernias, band erosion, and band migration) may be more difficult to assess in pregnancy; all gastrointestinal problems—including nausea, vomiting, and abdominal pain—should be thoroughly evaluated in these patients, and liberal consultation with a general surgeon familiar with bariatric procedures should be obtained; delay in diagnosis has been associated with maternal death
- Patients with adjustable gastric bands may benefit from consultation with a bariatric surgeon, particularly if there are increased symptoms of nausea and vomiting
- Dumping syndrome can occur after gastric bypass procedures; patients with dumping syndrome may not tolerate a 50-gm glucose challenge used for gestational diabetes screening; an alternative method of screening should be considered, including home glucose monitoring for at least 1 week between 24 and 28 weeks of gestation
- Extended release medications may not be effectively absorbed; instead oral solutions or rapid release medications are preferred
- If utilizing medications where a therapeutic concentration is important, testing maternal drug levels is necessary

Viral Hepatitis

CLINICAL PROFILE

- Most common cause of jaundice during pregnancy
- Six primary subtypes (Table 23-4), with various routes of infection and incubation periods; hepatitis A (HAV) and hepatitis E (HEV) exhibit no risk of chronic maternal disease; vertical transmission is potentially possible in all viruses except HAV

TABLE 23-4   Infectious Hepatitis Subtypes

Type	Transmission	Acute Disease Mortality	Chronic Disease Potential	Vaccination	Comments
HAV	Fecal-oral	Low ~ 1%	None	Indicated for high-risk groups and postexposure prophylaxis Immune globulin available	Children are often asymptomatic and may be a potential source of infection in women Rare vertical transmission risk if mother acutely ill at delivery
HBV	Parenteral Sexual contact	Low ~ 1%	10%-15%	Indicated for high-risk groups and postexposure prophylaxis Immune globulin available Pregnancy is not a contraindication to vaccination	Risk of transmission via blood products estimated at 1/137,000 screened units Risk of vertical transmission
HCV	Transfusion of blood products Intravenous drug use	Indolent infection initially	50% Associated increased risk of lymphoma and cryoglobulinemia Coexistent HIV infection reported to accelerate the progression and severity of hepatic injury	No	Risk of vertical transmission approximately 5% Risk of vertical transmission is much higher in the presence of coinfection with HIV
HDV	Blood		70%-80% patients with chronic HB+D develop cirrhosis Disease progression is much faster than HBV	No	Infection occurs simultaneously with HBV (coinfection) or after HBV (super infection) Risk of vertical transmission
HEV	Waterborne	Higher risk of fulminant infection in pregnant women		No	HIV-infected women with HEV have a high mortality rate Risk of vertical transmission

TABLE 23-5   Infectious Hepatitis Diagnostic Criteria

Feature	Hepatitis A	Hepatitis B	Hepatitis C	Hepatitis D	Hepatitis E
Incubation	14-50 days	30-80 days	30-160 days	30-180 days	14-63 days
Symptoms	Malaise, anorexia, nausea, vomiting, diarrhea, cholestasis, jaundice, acholic stools, dark urine	Insidious onset, anorexia, malaise, nausea, vomiting, abdominal pain, jaundice	Most asymptomatic		
Diagnosis	IgM anti-HAV Ab	HBsAg, anti-HBs, anti-HBc, HBeAg, HBV DNA	HC antibody	Delta Ag, IgM specific Ab	IgM anti-HEV Ab

DIAGNOSIS (Table 23-5)

- Risk factors warranting hepatitis C screening (Centers for Disease Control and Prevention guidelines; American College of Obstetricians and Gynecologists, ACOG Practice Bulletin No. 86, 2007)
  - Individuals who should be screened routinely:
    - Persons who ever injected illegal drugs (even once)
    - Persons notified that they received blood products before 1987 or from a donor who later tested positive for hepatitis C virus (HCV)
    - Recipients of transfusions or organ transplants, particularly if received before July 1992

- Persons ever on long-term hemodialysis
- Persons with persistently elevated alanine aminotransferase (ALT) or other evidence of liver disease
- Persons seeking evaluation or care for a sexually transmitted infection, including human immunodeficiency virus
- Individuals for whom routine testing is of uncertain need:
  1. Recipients of tissue transplants (e.g., cornea, skin, sperm, ova)
  2. Users of intranasal cocaine or other illegal noninjected drugs

3. Persons with a history of tattooing or body piercing
4. Persons with a history of sexually transmitted diseases or multiple sexual partners
5. Long-term steady sex partner of an HCV-infected individual

UPDATE #4

Routine prenatal screening of all pregnant women by HbsAg testing is recommended to identify those at risk of perinatal transmission and thus appropriately provide prophylaxis to the newborn (American College of Obstetricians and Gynecologists, ACOG Practice Bulletin No. 86, 2007).

MANAGEMENT

- For acute hepatitis, supportive care
- Hepatitis A vaccination and immune globulin appear to be safe in pregnancy and should be considered for those postexposure or if traveling to endemic areas
- All pregnant women should be tested for HbsAg; infants born to women who are positive or of unknown status should receive a hepatitis B vaccine and hepatitis B immune globulin (HBIG) within 12 hours of birth
- Infants of mothers who are HBsAg negative should receive hepatitis B vaccine before 2 months of age; preterm infants less than 2000 gm should have their first vaccine delayed until 1 month after birth
- At present, there is no consensus as to whether the route of delivery influences vertical transmission risk for hepatitis B or C; however, it seems prudent to avoid procedures that break the fetal skin barrier such as scalp electrodes
- The risk of transmission of hepatitis B associated with amniocentesis is low
- Patients with hepatitis C should be screened for human immunodeficiency virus (HIV) given the increased risk of vertical transmission if both infections are present
- Breast-feeding is not contraindicated with HAV with appropriate hygienic precautions, in those chronically infected with HBV providing the infant receives vaccine and HBIG, or in women with hepatitis C (HC)

Gallbladder Disease

CLINICAL PROFILE

- Cholelithiasis is common in the adult population; obesity and parity appear to increase the frequency of gallstones
- Complications of gallstones are the second most common nongynecologic condition requiring surgery during pregnancy; gallbladder disease is the most common nonobstetric cause of hospital admission in the first year after delivery
- Pregnancy appears to also increase the incidence of gallstones, presumably because of the elevated levels of sex steroid hormones resulting in biliary stasis and increased cholesterol saturation of bile
- Disorders associated with gallstones include biliary colic, acute cholecystitis, common bile duct obstruction, ascending cholangitis, gallstone ileus, and pancreatitis

DIAGNOSIS

- Biliary colic may be associated with anorexia, nausea and vomiting, and upper quadrant pain; infectious complications usually have leukocytosis and fever
- Laboratory abnormalities include elevated bilirubin levels, aspartate aminotransferase (AST), alamine aminotransferase (ALT), and alkaline phosphatase; however, the latter is commonly elevated in normal pregnancies due to the placental production
- Ultrasound is accurate in diagnosing gallstones; to evaluate for extra hepatic ductal stones, other modalities of imaging may be necessary (see the Pancreatitis section)

MANAGEMENT

- Conservative management of biliary colic and acute cholecystitis includes withdrawal of food and liquids, the application of intravenous fluids, pain control, and possibly nasogastric suction and antibiotics
- The choice between medical and surgical management during pregnancy is somewhat controversial; there is a significant relapse rate when medical management is used, but this has to be balanced against the potential risks of surgery; Lu et al. (2004) suggested that surgical management is safe and is associated with decreased days in the hospital, reduced rates of labor induction, and preterm deliveries; a decision analysis by Jelin et al. (2008) concluded that laparoscopic cholecystectomy was superior to nonoperative management for pregnant women presenting in the first or second trimester with biliary tract disease

Intrahepatic Cholestasis of Pregnancy (ICP)

CLINICAL PROFILE

- Affects approximately 1% of Caucasians, 2% of South Asians, and up to 5% of Chilean women
- There is a high recurrence risk in subsequent pregnancies
- Etiology is complex, with genetic, environmental, and hormonal factors; sisters of affected women have a high risk of developing ICP; there are known mutations in genes that code for bile salt transporters and hepatic bile salt receptors that may be seen in some affected women
- Women with hepatitis C and selenium deficiency are more likely to develop ICP; incidence is higher during winter months, in twins, and in cases of in vitro fertilization
- Fetal complications that occur more frequently in affected patients include preterm labor, asphyxia, meconium-stained amniotic fluid, and fetal death; pathogenesis is not fully understood but theorized because of the elevated bile acid levels

UPDATE #5

There is debate in the literature about the extent of ICP-associated fetal risk secondary to most studies are not large enough to quantify the frequency of complications. Geenes et al. (2009) reviewed a number of series reporting adverse outcomes. One study attempted to correlate the risk with the degree of bile acid elevation and suggested a 1% to 2% increase for every additional μmol/L of maternal bile acids (Glantz et al, 2004).

TABLE 23-6 **Hepatic Diseases Unique to Pregnancy**

	ICP	HELLP	AFLP
% Pregnancies	0.1%	0.2%-0.6%	0.005%-0.01%
Onset/trimester	25-32 weeks	3 or postpartum	3 or postpartum
Family history	Often	No	Occasionally
Presence of preeclampsia	No	Yes	50%
Typical clinical features	Pruritus, mild jaundice, elevated bile acids, ↓ vitamin K	Hemolysis, thrombocytopenia	Liver failure, coagulopathy, encephalopathy, hypoglycemia, disseminated intravascular coagulation (DIC)
Aminotransferases	Mild to 10-20 fold elevation	Mild to 10-20 fold elevation	300-500 typical but variable
Bilirubin	<5 mg/dL	<5 mg/dL unless massive necrosis	Often <5 mg/dL, higher if severe
Hepatic imaging	Normal	Hepatic infarcts, hematomas, rupture	Fatty infiltration
Histology	Normal-mild cholestasis, no necrosis	Patchy/extensive necrosis and hemorrhage	Microvesicular fat in zone 3
Maternal mortality	0%	1%-25%	7%-18%
Fetal/perinatal mortality	0-1.4%	11%	9%-23%
Recurrence in subsequent pregnancies	45%-70%	4%-19%	LCHAD defect—yes, no fatty acid oxidation defect—rare

Adapted from Hay JE: Liver disease in pregnancy, *Hepatology* 47:1067-1076, 2008.

DIAGNOSIS

- Symptoms include pruritus without a rash; this is usually generalized but can affect the palms and soles
- Laboratory workup includes serum bile acids and liver transaminases (refer to Table 23-6, which compares the three hepatic disorders unique to pregnancy)
- If diagnosis is uncertain, a liver ultrasound should be performed to rule out gallstones or biliary obstruction
- Other conditions that may be associated with ICP include hepatitis C, autoimmune hepatitis, and primary biliary cirrhosis; these should be considered, particularly if the symptoms present early in pregnancy

MANAGEMENT

- Ursodeoxycholic acid (UDCA) is the mainstay of maternal symptom relief; it usually will improve the biochemical abnormalities as well; there are no data powered sufficiently to assess whether correction of the bile acids will reduce the fetal risks associated with ICP
- Strategies for fetal surveillance with electronic fetal monitoring or biophysical profile may be helpful, but there is no guarantee that they will reduce the risk of adverse perinatal outcome
- Given the increased fetal risk, management strategies may include delivery by 38 weeks' gestation or consideration of delivery after 36 weeks (with confirmation of fetal pulmonary maturity)

Acute Fatty Liver of Pregnancy (AFLP)

UPDATE #6

The pathophysiology of acute fatty liver of pregnancy (AFLP) may involve defects in mitochondrial fatty acid beta-oxidation. Under nonpregnant conditions, an individual who is heterozygous for these enzyme mutations will be asymptomatic. However, if a heterozygous woman is carrying a homozygous fetus, fetal fatty acids may accumulate in the maternal circulation, accumulate in the maternal liver, and ultimately lead to hepatic dysfunction (Lee et al, 2009). Care providers of the neonate should be informed of this potential mutation to allow screening.

CLINICAL PROFILE

- Rare third-trimester disorder associated with significant perinatal and maternal mortality
- Etiology is unknown; however, in approximately 20% of cases there are disorders of fatty acid β-oxidation; a woman who is heterozygous for long-chain-3-hydroxyacyl-coenzyme A dehydrogenase (LCHAD) carrying a fetus with a homozygous deficiency for this enzyme may be unable to metabolize the increased amounts of fatty acids; the increased metabolic load may result in hepatotoxicity
- Increased frequency in twins
- Symptoms are usually nonspecific including nausea, vomiting, anorexia, and upper quadrant pain
- There is a significant overlap with Lemolysis, elevated liver function tests, low platelets (HELLP) syndrome

DIAGNOSIS

- The diagnosis is suggested by clinical manifestations; rarely liver biopsy is performed
- Distinguishing features
- Disease is usually associated with coagulopathy, disseminated intravascular coagulation, elevated bilirubin, liver function tests including bilirubin; metabolic acidosis, renal dysfunction, and elevated ammonia may also be seen
- Imaging studies, particularly computerized tomography, may be helpful but inconsistent; therefore, diagnosis is usually made on clinical evaluation

MANAGEMENT

- Maternal stabilization followed by expeditious delivery of the fetus
- Multidisciplinary team management in an intensive care unit setting
- Serial laboratory studies including complete blood count, prothrombin time (PT), partial thromboplastin time (PTT), fibrinogen, blood urea nitrogen (BUN), creatinine, liver function tests, blood gases, and ammonia levels every 6 hours
- Patients usually have profound hypoglycemia and require intravenous glucose infusions
- If evidence of multisystem failure is present, ventilation and dialysis may be required
- N-acetylcysteine may be helpful
- Involve a liver team to assist in the evaluation and potential management of fulminant liver failure
- Notify the pediatricians of the potential deficiency of LCHAD in the neonate
- The affected patient should be screened for defects in fatty acid oxidation to determine possible recurrence risk

Pregnancy after Liver Transplantation

CLINICAL PROFILE

- There are approximately 3000 female liver transplant recipients of childbearing age
- Patients transplanted for biliary atresia have a higher graft survival and overall survival when compared to those with hepatitis C and cirrhosis
- Pregnancies are usually successful, but there is a higher rate of hypertensive disorders, growth restriction, prematurity, and antepartum bleeding when compared to matched controls

UPDATE #7

A recent series of 206 patients with liver transplants were compared to controls matched by age, hospital, and year (Coffin et al, 2010). Significant odds ratios (in parentheses) in the study population included increased fetal mortality (3.23), prematurity (3.13), intrauterine growth restriction (2.25), and hypertensive disorders of pregnancy (4.23).

- The use of conventional immunosuppressive agents at present does not seem to increase the risk of fetal malformations; the most commonly used agents include cyclosporine A, prednisolone, and tacrolimus; the Food and Drug Administration currently classifies cyclosporine and tacrolimus as category C in terms of their risk in pregnancy
- The current data regarding breast-feeding is not definitive; the American Association of Pediatrics supports breast-feeding by those taking prednisone but advises against it in women taking cyclosporine and provides no information on tacrolimus

MANAGEMENT (Table 23-7)

- Optimal timing between transplant and conception has not been established; it is suggested that 1 year is reasonable to allow graft function to stabilize and for immunosuppressant medication to reduce to basal levels
- Summary of management options

Pancreatitis

CLINICAL PROFILE

- Incidence is approximately 3 in 10,000 pregnancies
- The etiology is more likely due to gallstones in pregnancy, whereas alcohol is the most common causative agent in nonpregnant adults
- Occurs more commonly in the third trimester and puerperium
- Symptoms include epigastric pain radiating to the flanks and shoulders and usually accompanied by abdominal tenderness

DIAGNOSIS

- Serum amylase; rapid, but nonspecific test, usually increases at least three times normal
- Serum lipase; more specific for pancreatitis
- Abdominal ultrasound to assess for biliary pathology
- Magnetic resonance cholangiopancreatography (MRCP) is a preferred method of evaluating the common bile duct; however, it may miss small stones in the distal common bile duct
- Endoscopic ultrasound is a semi-invasive procedure requiring sedation, but it can be helpful detecting common bile duct stones; this modality is more sensitive than MRCP

MANAGEMENT

- General principles of management are not different than those used in nonpregnant women
- Bowel rest with or without nasogastric suction
- Fluid and electrolyte replacement
- Antibiotic usage is controversial but likely not needed in the presence of mild disease, normal common bile duct size, and no evidence of cholangitis
- Patients with gallstones need to be evaluated for early cholecystectomy to prevent recurrence
- Endoscopic retrograde cholangiopancreatography (ERCP) may be indicated in patients with severe acute pancreatitis, who show evidence of biliary obstruction, or who are postcholecystectomy; ERCP requires fluoroscopy and may be complicated by hemorrhage, cholangitis, and perforation
- Endoscopic sphincterotomy (ES) may be an alternative when common bile duct stones are present, but cholecystectomy needs to be delayed

TABLE 23-7   **Management Considerations for Patients with Solid Organ Transplants**

Prepregnancy

1. Patients should defer conception for at least 1 year with adequate contraception.
2. Assessment of graft function:
   A. Recent biopsy
   B. Liver function tests
   C. Renal function tests including creatinine and proteinuria
3. Hepatitis B and C, cytomegalovirus, toxoplasmosis, and herpes simplex status.
4. Maintenance immunosuppressant options:
   A. Azathioprine (D)
   B. Cyclosporine (C)
   C. Tacrolimus (C)
   D. Corticosteroids (B)
   E. Mycophenolate mofetil (D)
   F. Sirolimus (C)
5. The effect of comorbid conditions (e.g., diabetes, hypertension) should be considered and their management optimized.
6. Vaccinations should be given, if needed (e.g., hepatitis, tetanus, pneumococcal, human papillomavirus, and influenza).
7. Explore the cause of the original disease; discuss genetic factors if relevant.
8. Discuss the effect of pregnancy on allograft function.
9. Discuss the risks of intrauterine growth restriction, prematurity, and low birth weight.

Prenatal

1. Accurate and early diagnosis and dating of pregnancy.
2. Clinical and laboratory monitoring of the functional status of the transplanted organs and immunosuppressive drug levels:
   A. Every 4 weeks until 32 weeks
   B. Then every 2 weeks until 36 weeks
   C. Then weekly until delivery

3. Monthly urine culture.
4. Surveillance for rejection, with biopsy considered if it is suspected.
5. Surveillance for bacterial or viral infections (e.g., cytomegalovirus, toxoplasmosis, hepatitis in the first trimester, and repeat if signs of rejection or tenderness over the graft site).
6. Fetal surveillance after 32 weeks (e.g., nonstress tests, ultrasonographic evaluation).
7. Monitoring for hypertension and nephropathy.
8. Surveillance for preeclampsia.
9. Screening for gestational diabetes.

Labor and Delivery

1. Cesarean delivery for obstetric reasons:
   A. Vigilance for location of transplanted organ prenatally
2. For heart, lung or heart-lung recipients:
   A. Continuous cardiac monitoring
   B. Vigilance for poor or absent cough reflex and the need for airway protection because of denervation
   C. Attention to unpredictable response to vasoactive medications
   D. Judicious use of intravenous fluids

Postpartum

1. Monitor immunosuppressive drug levels for at least 1 month postpartum and adjust as needed.
2. Surveillance for rejection, with biopsy considered if it is suspected.
3. Breast-feeding may be appropriate; monitor neonatal drug levels.
4. Contraception counseling.

Adapted from Mastrobattista JM, Gomez-Lobo V: Pregnancy after solid organ transplantation, *Obstet Gynecol* 112:119-132, 2008.

SUGGESTED READINGS

Nausea and Vomiting

American College of Obstetrics and Gynecology: ACOG practice bulletin no. 52: nausea and vomiting of pregnancy, *Obstet Gynecol* 103(4):803–814, 2004.

Gastrointestinal Reflux Disease

Cappell MS: Gastric and duodenal ulcers during pregnancy, *Gastroenterol Clin North Am* 32(1):263–308, 2003.
Kelly TF, Savides TJ: Gastrointestinal disease in pregnancy. In Creasy RK, Resnik R, Iams JD, et al: *Creasy & Resnik's maternal-fetal medicine, principles and practice*, ed 6, Philadelphia, 2009, Saunders Elsevier, pp 1041–1057.

Appendicitis

Basaran A, Basaran M: Diagnosis of acute appendicitis during pregnancy: a systematic review, *Obstet Gynecol Surv* 64(7):481–488, 2009.
Brown JJS, Wilson C, Coleman S, Joypaul BV: Appendicitis in pregnancy: an ongoing dilemma, *Colorectal Dis* 11(2):116–122, 2009.
Kelly TF, Savides TJ: Gastrointestinal disease in pregnancy. In Creasy RK, Resnik R, Iams JD, et al: *Creasy & Resnik's maternal-fetal medicine, principles and practice*, ed 6, Philadelphia, 2009, Saunders Elsevier, pp 1041–1057.
Pedrosa I, Levine D, Eyvazzadeh AD, et al: MR imaging evaluation of acute appendicitis in pregnancy, *Radiology* 238(3):891–899, 2006.

Irritable Bowel Syndrome

Mayer EA: Clinical practice: irritable bowel syndrome, *N Engl J Med* 358(16):1692–1699, 2008.

Inflammatory Bowel Disease

Cassina M, Fabris L, Okolicsanyi L, et al: Therapy of inflammatory bowel diseases in pregnancy and lactation, *Expert Opin Drug Saf* 8(5):695–707, 2009.
Dignass AU, Hartmann F, Sturm A, Stein J: Management of inflammatory bowel diseases during pregnancy, *Dig Dis* 27(3):341–346, 2009.
Dubinsky M, Abraham B, Mahadevan U: Management of the pregnant IBD patient, *Inflam Bowel Dis* 14(12):1736–1750, 2008.
Mahadevan U, Sandborn WJ, Li D, et al: Pregnancy outcomes in women with inflammatory bowel disease: a large community-based study from Northern California, *Gastroenterology* 133(4):1106–1112, 2007.

Bariatric Surgery

American College of Obstetricians and Gynecologists: ACOG practice bulletin no. 105: bariatric surgery and pregnancy, *Obstet Gynecol* 113(6):1405–1413, 2009.
Kirshtein B, Lantsberg L, Mizrahi S, Avinoach E: Bariatric emergencies for non-bariatric surgeons: complications of laparoscopic banding, *Obes Surg* 20(11):1468–1478, 2010.

Maggard MA, Yermilov I, Zhaoping L, et al: Pregnancy and fertility following bariatric surgery, *JAMA* 300(19):2286–2296, 2008.

Wax JR, Pinette MG, Cartin A, Blackstone J: Female reproductive issues following bariatric surgery, *Obstet Gynecol Surv* 62(9):595–604, 2007.

Hepatitis

American College of Obstetricians and Gynecologists: ACOG practice bulletin no. 86: viral hepatitis in pregnancy, *Obstet Gynecol* 110(4):941–956, 2007.

Jonas MM: Hepatitis B and pregnancy: an underestimated issue, *Liver Int* 29(Suppl 1):133–139, 2009.

Lee NM, Brady CW: Liver disease in pregnancy, *World J Gastroenterol* 15(8):897–906, 2009.

Sinha S, Kumar M: Pregnancy at chronic hepatitis B virus infection, *Hepatol Res* 40(1):31–48, 2010.

Gallbladder Disease

Jelin EB, Smink DS, Vernon AH, Brooks DC: Management of biliary tract disease during pregnancy: a decision analysis, *Surg Endosc* 22(1):54–60, 2008.

Lu EJ, Curet MJ, El-Sayed YY, Kirkwood KS: Medical versus surgical management of biliary tract disease in pregnancy, *Am J Surg* 188(6): 755–759, 2004.

Williamson C, Mackillop L: Diseases of the liver, biliary system and pancreas. In Creasy RK, Resnik R, Iams JD, et al: *Creasy & Resnik's maternal-fetal medicine, principles and practice*, ed 6, Philadelphia, 2009, Saunders Elsevier, pp 1059–1077.

Intrahepatic Cholestasis of Pregnancy

Geenes V, Williamson C: Intrahepatic cholestasis of pregnancy, *World J Gastroenterol* 15(17):2049–2066, 2009.

Glantz A, Hanns-Ulrich M, Lars-Åke M: Intrahepatic cholestasis of pregnancy: relationships between bile acid levels and fetal complication rates, *Hepatology* 40(2):467–474, 2004.

Acute Fatty Liver of Pregnancy

Hay JE: Liver disease in pregnancy, *Hepatology* 47(3):1067–1076, 2008.

Ibdah JA: Acute fatty liver of pregnancy: an update on pathogenesis and clinical implications, *World J Gastroenterol* 12(46):7397–7404, 2006.

Lee NM, Brady CW: Liver disease in pregnancy, *World J Gastroenterol* 15(8):897–906, 2009.

Liver Transplantation

Coffin CS, Shaheen AA, Burak KW, Myers RP: Pregnancy outcomes among liver transplant recipients in the United States: a nationwide case-control analysis, *Liver Transpl* 16(1):56–63, 2010.

Heneghan MA, Selzner M, Yoshida EM, Mullhaupt B: Pregnancy and sexual function in liver transplantation, *J Hepatology* 49(4):507–519, 2008.

Mastrobattista JM, Gomez-Lobo V: Pregnancy after solid organ transplantation, *Obstet Gynecol* 112(4):119–132, 2008.

McKay DB, Josephson MA: Pregnancy in recipients of solid organs: effects on mother and child, *N Engl J Med* 354(12):1281–1293, 2006.

Nagy S, Bush MC, Berkowitz R, et al: Pregnancy outcome in liver transplant recipients, *Obstet Gynecol* 102:121–128, 2003.

Pancreatitis

Eddy JJ, Gideonsen MD, Song JY, et al: Pancreatitis in pregnancy, *Obstet Gynecol* 112(5):1075–1081, 2008.

Pitchumoni CS, Yegneswaran B: Acute pancreatitis in pregnancy, *World J Gastroenterol* 15(45):5641–5646, 2009.

Tang S, Mayo MJ, Rodriguez-Frias E, et al: Safety and utility of ERCP during pregnancy, *Gastrointest Endosc* 69(3 Pt 1):453–461, 2009.

Chapter 24

Preeclampsia

TANIA F. ESAKOFF • MARI-PAULE THIET

KEY UPDATES

1 There does not appear to be an association between inherited thrombophilia and increased risk of preeclampsia.

2 Fetal survival appears to have improved in preeclamptic pregnancies since the late 1970s, whereas the relative risk of neonatal death following a preeclamptic pregnancy has not changed.

3 Twelve hours of postpartum magnesium sulfate for mild preeclampsia appears to have a clinical course similar to that of 24-hour therapy and infrequently leads to disease progression.

4 Systolic hypertension, not diastolic hypertension, appears to carry an increased risk of stroke in patients with preeclampsia and eclampsia.

5 Hemolysis elevated liver enzymes low platelets (HELLP) syndrome is associated with high perinatal morbidity and mortality. The role of expectant management remote from term and use of corticosteroids for improving maternal outcome are still experimental.

Background

- Preeclampsia remains a leading cause of maternal and neonatal morbidity in the United States and worldwide
- Preeclampsia, defined as new onset hypertension (usually after 20 weeks' gestation) in the presence of new onset proteinuria, complicates 2% to 8% of pregnancies

Etiology/Pathophysiology

GENETICS

- Women with family history of preeclampsia as well as women and their male partners who themselves were products of pregnancies complicated by preeclampsia are more likely to have pregnancies complicated by preeclampsia
- The degree of trophoblastic invasion into maternal spiral arteries is thought to be associated with parental genetic factors; suboptimal trophoblastic invasion may be related to the vascular deficiency that leads to preeclampsia

ENDOTHELIAL DYSFUNCTION

- Poor control of diseases with endothelial dysfunction, such as hypertension and diabetes, appears to increase risk of preeclampsia
- Women with history of preeclampsia are more likely to develop subsequent cardiovascular disease, renal disease, and insulin resistance later in life—diseases that all involve endothelial dysfunction

IMMUNE-MEDIATED INVASION

- Placenta has a key role in the pathogenesis of preeclampsia as evidenced by the fact that delivery of the fetus alone is not sufficient to lead to a resolution of preeclampsia
- Pregnancies with increased trophoblastic tissue load such as molar pregnancies and multiple gestations have an even higher risk of developing preeclampsia
- Women exposed to the same paternal semen in prior pregnancies ("seminal priming") may be less likely to mount an immune response during the trophoblast invasion stage and thus are less likely to develop preeclampsia

PATHOPHYSIOLOGY (TWO-STAGE PROCESS)

- Extravillous cytotrophoblast invades the endometrium in normal pregnancy
- Invasion promoted by maternal natural killer cells (NK cells)
- Stage I (<20 weeks)
  - Inadequate invasion by extravillous cytotrophoblast causes vascular remodeling and angiogenesis
- Stage II (>20 weeks)
  - Placenta exhibits a generalized inflammatory response in the setting of placental hypoxia
  - Oxidative stress within the placenta leads to a release of multiple factors including sFlt-1 (an antiangiogenic factor that antagonizes vascular endothelial growth factor, VEGF), soluble endoglin (which functions synergistically with sFlt-1), proinflammatory cytokines, and trophoblast debris, resulting in a generalized maternal inflammatory response

- Maternal inflammatory response leads to decreased vasodilatory capacity and hypertension; increased permeability leads to proteinuria and pulmonary edema

Risk Factors

PRECONCEPTIONAL FACTORS

- Nulliparity, primipaternity, and initial or novel sperm exposure
- Previous history of preeclampsia
- History of severe preeclampsia in the first pregnancy may increase risk of recurrence by 45%
- Severe preeclampsia in the midtrimester carries a recurrence rate as high as 65%
- Family history of preeclampsia carries a threefold increased risk of preeclampsia and a fourfold increased risk of severe preeclampsia
- Risk increased by underlying maternal diseases such as chronic hypertension, obesity, and insulin resistance/diabetes mellitus among others
- Stress and work-related strain appear to increase risk
- Smoking appears to decrease risk

UPDATE #1

A recent large multicenter cohort study showed that although preeclampsia is associated with placental underperfusion, this does not appear to be a result of thrombophilia (Kahn et al, 2009).

PREGNANCY-ASSOCIATED FACTORS

- Multiple gestation significantly increases the incidence and severity of preeclampsia
- Fetal structural congenital anomalies, chromosomal anomalies, and hydatidiform moles all increase risk

Evaluation and Diagnosis

- Requires new onset hypertension and proteinuria
- Hypertension
  - New onset of systolic blood pressure of at least 140 mmHg or a diastolic blood pressure of at least 90 mmHg recorded on two occasions at least 6 hours but no more than 7 days apart
  - Diagnosed after 20 weeks in a previously normotensive patient
- Severe preeclampsia defined by sustained elevations in systolic blood pressure of at least 160 mmHg systolic or at least 110 mmHg diastolic for at least 6 hours
- Proteinuria defined as greater than or equal to 300 mg in 24 hours for mild preeclampsia and greater than or equal to 5 g in 24 hours for severe preeclampsia
- When 24-hour urine collection not available, urine dipstick can be used and proteinuria defined as at least 1+ on at least two different specimens 6 hours apart
- A spot urine protein to creatinine ratio of greater than or equal to 0.2 suggests mild preeclampsia
- Urine dipstick values should not be used to diagnose severe proteinuria

- Symptoms of severe preeclampsia include persistent cerebral symptoms such as headache or vision changes, epigastric or right upper quadrant pain
- Laboratory abnormalities of severe preeclampsia include abnormal liver enzymes and thrombocytopenia with platelets less than 100,000/mm^3
- End-organ involvement such as oliguria, pulmonary edema, and fetal intrauterine growth restriction are diagnostic of severe preeclampsia
- Table 24-1 lists the features distinguishing between mild and severe preeclampsia
- Coexisting chronic hypertension (defined as hypertension diagnosed before pregnancy) complicates the diagnosis of preeclampsia
  - Superimposed preeclampsia is diagnosed in a woman with no previous proteinuria who develops proteinuria (at least 300 mg in 24 hours)
  - Superimposed preeclampsia is diagnosed in a woman with preexisting proteinuria before 20 weeks' gestation with new exacerbation of previously well-controlled hypertension with a systolic blood pressure of 180 mmHg or more or diastolic blood pressure of 110 mmHg or more
  - Headache, vision changes or epigastric pain, elevations in liver enzymes, or a decrease in platelets to less than 100,000/mm^3 lead to the diagnosis of superimposed preeclampsia
- Hemolysis elevated liver enzymes low platelets (HELLP) syndrome is in the spectrum of severe preeclampsia
  - Hemolysis—microangiopathic hemolytic anemia—presents with an abnormal peripheral smear, elevated indirect serum bilirubin, low serum haptoglobin levels, elevated lactate dehydrogenase (LDH) levels (usually over 600 U/L), and a significant drop in hemoglobin levels

Maternal and Perinatal Outcomes

- Outcome depends on gestational age at onset of preeclampsia, gestational age at the time of delivery, severity of disease, the presence of multifetal gestation,

TABLE 24-1 Criteria for Diagnosis of Mild Preeclampsia versus Severe Preeclampsia

	Mild Preeclampsia	Severe Preeclampsia
Blood pressure	≥ 140/90	≥160/110
Proteinuria	≥300 mg/24 hours	≥5 g/24 hours
Symptoms: headache, vision changes, right upper quadrant (RUQ)/epigastric pain	Absent	Present
Laboratory abnormalities: thrombocytopenia, elevated liver enzymes, elevated creatinine	Absent	Present
Maternal end organ effects: pulmonary edema, oliguria	Absent	Present
Fetal effects: intrauterine growth restriction	Absent	Present

and the presence of preexisting conditions such as pregestational diabetes or renal disease
- Mild preeclampsia outcomes tend to be similar to normotensive pregnancies
- Rate of eclampsia (convulsions) is less than 1%
- Cesarean delivery rate is increased, associated with increased labor induction
- Rates of all complications are increased in women with severe preeclampsia
  - Maternal mortality is 0.2%
  - Increased morbidity includes convulsions, pulmonary edema, acute renal failure, acute liver failure, liver hemorrhage, stroke, and disseminated intravascular coagulopathy

UPDATE #2

In Norway, a large population-based observational study demonstrated that although fetal survival in preeclamptic pregnancies has vastly improved since the 1970s, possibly because of aggressive clinical management, the relative risk of neonatal death after a preeclamptic pregnancy has not changed (Basso et al, 2006).

Management

Goal: minimize risk to maternal health while taking into account fetal gestational age and the risk for perinatal complications

MILD PREECLAMPSIA

- At term (at least 37 weeks of gestational age), delivery procedures should be initiated
- If the maternal status is stable and the fetus cephalic, vaginal delivery can be safely attempted
- Mildly elevated blood pressures (<160 mmHg systolic) do not need treatment

- Management of mild preeclampsia before 37 weeks' gestational age:
  - Usually managed expectantly until signs of severe preeclampsia, fetal maturity is documented, or 37 weeks
  - Inpatient and outpatient management in reliable patients are options
  - There is no evidence for the efficacy of bed rest
  - Daily fetal movement counting and twice weekly nonstress tests or weekly biophysical profiles until delivery
  - Assessment of fetal growth every 3 to 4 weeks
  - Frequent assessment of symptoms, blood pressure monitoring, and at least weekly laboratory evaluation

SEVERE PREECLAMPSIA (Figure 24-1)

- For those at 34 weeks or more in gestation, delivery procedures should be initiated
- Proceed with delivery regardless of gestational age when eclampsia is imminent as indicated by persistent somatic symptoms (headache or abdominal pain) or if there is multiorgan dysfunction, severe fetal growth restriction, suspected placental abruption, or nonreassuring fetal testing
- Management under 34 weeks of gestational age depends on maternal condition, fetal biophysical status, and the level of perinatal care available at the inpatient facility
- Administer antenatal steroids for women with preeclampsia under 34 weeks of gestational age to enhance fetal pulmonary maturity, even if only as few as 4 hours are expected from the first dose until delivery
- Magnesium sulfate for seizure prophylaxis is administered on admission to patients at 34 weeks or greater and continued until 24 hours postpartum
  - In patients under 34 weeks, magnesium sulfate is administered until the decision regarding candidacy for expectant management as an inpatient is made

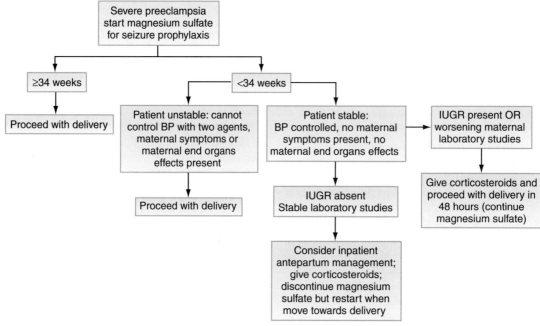

Figure 24-1. Algorithm for management of severe preeclampsia.

- Severe hypertension (greater than or equal to 160 mmHg systolic or greater than or equal to 90 mmHg diastolic) requires aggressive treatment with antihypertensives
- Persistent severe range blood pressures despite maximum treatment or persistent cerebral symptoms as well as thrombocytopenia (platelets less than 100,000/fl), elevated liver enzymes, epigastric pain, or serum creatinine ≥2.0 mg/dL typically necessitate delivery within 24 to 48 hours irrespective of fetal gestational age
- Preeclampsia occurs rarely before 24 weeks, but if diagnosed, pregnancy termination should be offered given the maternal risks involved

IMPORTANT INTRAPARTUM CONSIDERATIONS

- Continuous fetal and maternal monitoring of vital signs and laboratory values is essential
- Adequate pain control may improve blood pressure control
- When administered appropriately, regional anesthesia is considered to be the analgesia and anesthesia method of choice for women with preeclampsia
- General anesthesia carries significantly increased risks associated with airway and blood pressure management
- Magnesium sulfate is the agent of choice for prevention of seizures in severe preeclampsia (50% reduction from 1.9 to 0.8%)
- Efficacy of magnesium sulfate in management of mild preeclampsia is unclear

UPDATE #3

Twelve hours of postpartum magnesium sulfate therapy for mild preeclampsia was associated with infrequent disease progression. Patients with chronic hypertension and insulin-requiring diabetes are at risk of progressing to severe preeclampsia postpartum (Ehrenberg et al, 2006).

- Goal of antihypertensive therapy is to decrease central nervous and cardiovascular system complications
- Appropriate medications should be administered to achieve reduction of systolic blood pressure below 160 mmHg and diastolic blood pressure below 110 mmHg or greater

UPDATE #4

A recent study demonstrated that unlike the development of severe diastolic hypertension, the development of severe systolic hypertension appears to carry an increased risk of stroke in patients with preeclampsia and eclampsia. This suggests that systolic pressure should be the trigger for antihypertensive therapy (Martin et al, 2005).

- IV hydralazine in doses of 5 to 10 mg given every 15 to 20 minutes for a maximum dose of 30 mg is the most commonly used agent for control of severe hypertension
  - IV labetalol can be administered at 20 to 40 mg every 10 to 15 minutes for a maximum of 220 mg
  - Oral nifedipine given at 10 to 20 mg every 30 minutes for a maximum of 50 mg
- Beware of effects of calcium channel blockers used with IV magnesium sulfate, which may lead to maternal hypotension

MODE OF DELIVERY

- Presence of severe preeclampsia is not an indication for cesarean delivery
- However, cervical Bishop score and the estimated duration of induced labor should be considered together with the trend of maternal vital signs and systemic complications; in cases where rapid maternal or fetal deterioration is noted, cesarean delivery should be undertaken

POSTPARTUM CONSIDERATIONS

- Continue frequent assessment of symptoms, blood pressures, urinary output, and oral/intravenous intake
- Preeclamptic patients are particularly at risk for developing pulmonary edema, for the following reasons:
  - Increased IV fluid hydration during labor and during preparation for regional anesthesia
  - Increased capillary leak present in preeclampsia
- Hypertension may persist for weeks if not months, and if the blood pressure is persistently elevated in the severe range, oral antihypertensives should be initiated
- Preeclampsia may develop for the first time in the postpartum period

MANAGEMENT OF HELLP SYNDROME

- Tends to be on the more morbid end of the preeclampsia spectrum, with a perinatal mortality rate of 7% to 20%
- Delivery should be expedited if the patient is at least 34 weeks
- Under 34 weeks' gestational age, expectant management should be attempted only in a high-risk center with frequent monitoring
- The presence of other diseases with similar symptoms as HELLP should be excluded, such as acute fatty liver of pregnancy (AFLP), thrombotic thrombocytopenic purpura (TTP), hemolytic uremic syndrome (HUS), immune thrombocytopenic purpura (ITP), systemic lupus erythematosus (SLE), antiphospholipid antibody syndrome (APS), cholecystitis, fulminant viral hepatitis, and acute pancreatitis
- Platelet transfusion is indicated in patients with active bleeding or a platelet count less than 20,000/mm^3 or in advance of a cesarean with platelet count less than 50,000/mm^3
- Though most patients resolve their symptoms within 48 hours of delivery, some will experience significant deterioration of their disease over as long as 2 weeks.
- The use of high-dose corticosteroids (10 mg of dexamethasone administered intravenously every 6 to 12 hours for two doses followed by 5 to 6 mg intravenous doses given 6 to 12 hours later for two additional doses) for postpartum HELLP syndrome is of disputed efficacy
- Recurrence risk of HELLP syndrome is between 2% and 19%

UPDATE #5

HELLP syndrome is associated with life-threatening complications for both the mother and the fetus. Despite the large amount of literature on this subject, the potential benefits of pursuing expectant management remote from term and of using corticosteroids to improve maternal outcomes remain experimental (Sibai, 2004).

Prediction of Preeclampsia

BIOCHEMICAL MARKERS

- Preeclampsia appears to arise from an imbalance of circulating angiogenic factors, which predates the onset of clinical preeclampsia
  - Reduced serum placental growth factor (PIGF) and elevated soluble FMS-like tyrosine kinases (sFLt)-1 and endoglin are associated with preeclampsia
- Novel biomarkers such as dimethylarginine and placental protein-13 are not yet clearly associated with preeclampsia

BIOPHYSICAL MARKERS

- Increased uterine artery blood flow resistance as evidenced in Doppler ultrasound measurements in the early second trimester have been correlated with later appearance of preeclampsia
- Combined biophysical and biochemical markers for prediction of preeclampsia may be useful in the future.

Prevention of Preeclampsia

PRIMARY

- Normalization of body fat, blood pressure and glucose profile if diabetic may have a beneficial effect

SECONDARY

- Antihypertensives may reduce the risk of severe hypertension, but do not appear to decrease the risk of developing preeclampsia or proteinuria
- Fish oil supplementation
  - Is based on the observation that fish oil causes inhibition of platelet thromboxane A2 production without affecting prostacyclin
  - However, it has not been shown to be efficacious and may actually increase the risk of developing hypertensive disorders of pregnancy
- Calcium supplementation has not been shown to have a benefit for preventing recurrent preeclampsia
- Vitamin C and E supplementation
  - Is based on the hypothesis that an imbalance between oxidant and antioxidant activity in placental and maternal lipid peroxidation and unregulated free radical production leads to the observed endothelial damage
  - However, these vitamins have not been shown to be beneficial
- Antithrombotic agents: low-dose aspirin
  - Is based on the assumption that vasospasm and activation of the coagulation-hemostasis systems in preeclampsia are due to an imbalance in the thromboxane A2-to-prostocycline ratio
  - Low dose aspirin (LDASA) inhibits biosynthesis of platelet thromboxane A2 with little effect on vascular prostacyclin production thus favoring vasodilation
    - There is no evidence that LDASA prevents iatrogenic premature birth in nulliparous women; there may be a role for LDASA in preventing or reducing the severity of preeclampsia
    - Number needed to treat is 114

A Suggested Algorithm for Evaluation of a Patient with a History of Preeclampsia

- Before conception
  - Identify risk factors for preeclampsia, and review the outcomes of the previous pregnancy
  - Optimize maternal health
  - Begin folic acid supplementation
- In the first trimester
  - Obtain ultrasound for dating and fetal number
  - Obtain baseline metabolic profile, complete blood count, baseline urinalysis, and baseline 24-hour urine for protein
  - Continue folic acid supplementation
  - In patients with antiphospholipid antibody syndrome, start low-dose aspirin and heparin
  - In patients without antiphospholipid antibodies, consider offering low-dose aspirin therapy at 12 weeks' gestation
- In the second trimester
  - Monitor for signs and symptoms of preeclampsia
  - Evaluate for fetal anomalies with ultrasound at 18 to 20 weeks
- In the third trimester
  - Continue monitoring for symptoms, blood pressure changes, and laboratory changes
  - Consider serial ultrasounds for growth
  - Begin antenatal testing with twice weekly nonstress tests and amniotic fluid checks or biophysical profiles at 32 weeks

Summary

- Preeclampsia is a common and often morbid disease
- Identify high-risk patients before pregnancy if possible
- Once preeclampsia is diagnosed, close monitoring with blood pressure assessment, symptom assessment, laboratory evaluation, and fetal well-being evaluation are necessary
- Administer magnesium sulfate for seizure prophylaxis
- All patients with preeclampsia under 34 weeks' gestational age should be given antenatal corticosteroids for fetal lung maturity
- HELLP syndrome is in the spectrum of preeclampsia and should be managed similarly to severe preeclampsia
- Low-dose aspirin is the only intervention that is possibly helpful to decrease the risk of recurrent preeclampsia

SUGGESTED READINGS

Background and Epidemiology

ACOG Committee on Practice Bulletins–Obstetrics: ACOG practice bulletin: diagnosis and management of preeclampsia and eclampsia, *Obstet Gynecol* 99(1):159–167, 2002.
Report of the National High Blood Pressure Education Program Working Group on High Blood Pressure in Pregnancy, *Am J Obstet Gynecol* 183(1):S1–S22, 2000.

Etiology/Pathophysiology

Barton J, Sibai B: Prediction and prevention of recurrent preeclampsia, *Obstet Gynecol* 112(2 Pt 1):359–372, 2008.
Cudihy D, Lee RV: The pathophysiology of pre-eclampsia: Current clinical concepts, *J Obstet Gynaecol* 29(7):576–582, 2009.

Esplin M, Fausett M, Fraser A, et al: Paternal and maternal components of the predisposition to preeclampsia, *N Engl J Med* 344(12):867–872, 2001.

Harkskamp R, Zeeman G: Preeclampsia: at risk for remote cardiovascular disease, *Am J Med Sci* 334(4):291–295, 2007.

Redman C, Sargent I: Latest advances in understanding preeclampsia, *Science* 308(5728):1592–1594, 2005.

Risk Factors

Kahn SR, Platt R, McNamara H, et al: Inherited thrombophilia and preeclampsia within a multicenter cohort: the Montreal Preeclampsia Study, *AJOG* 200(2):151 e1-5, 2009.

Sibai BM: Chronic hypertension in pregnancy, *Obstet Gynecol* 100(2): 369–377, 2002.

Perinatal Outcomes

Basso O, Rasmussen S, Weinberg CR, et al: Trends in fetal and infant survival following preeclampsia, *JAMA* 296(11):1357–1362, 2006.

Buchbinder A, Sibai BM, Caritis S, et al: Adverse perinatal outcomes are significantly higher in severe gestational hypertension than in mild preeclampsia, *Am J Obstet Gynecol* 186(1):66–71, 2002.

Hauth JC, Ewell MG, Levine RL, et al: Pregnancy outcomes in healthy nulliparas women who subsequently developed hypertension: Calcium for Preeclampsia Prevention Study Group, *Obstet Gynecol* 95(1):24–28, 2000.

Sibai BM: Diagnosis, controversies, and management of the syndrome of hemolysis, elevated liver enzymes, and low platelet count, *Obstet Gynecol* 103(5 Pt 1):981–991, 2004.

Management

Altman D, Carroli G, Duley L, et al: Do women with preeclampsia, and their babies, benefit from magnesium sulfate? The Magpie trial: a randomized placebo-controlled trial, *Lancet* 359(9321):1877–1890, 2002.

Chames MC, Haddad B, Barton JR, et al: Subsequent pregnancy outcome in women with a history of HELLP syndrome at 28 weeks of gestation, *Am J Obstet Gynecol* 188(6):1504–1548, 2003.

Duley L, Henderson-Smart DJ: Drugs for rapid treatment of very high blood pressure during pregnancy (Cochrane Review), *Cochrane Library* 2, 2002.

Ehrenberg HM, Mercer BM: Abbreviated postpartum magnesium sulfate therapy for women with mild preeclampsia: a randomized controlled trial, *Obstet Gynecol* 108(4):833–838, 2006.

Martin JN Jr, Thigpen BD, Moore RC, et al: Stroke and severe preeclampsia: a paradigm shift focusing on systolic blood pressure, *Obstet Gynecol* 105(2):246–254, 2005.

Martin JN Jr, Thigpen BD, Rose CH, et al: Maternal benefit of high-dose intravenous corticosteroid therapy for HELLP, *Am J Obstet Gynecol* 189(3):830–834, 2003.

O'Brien JM, Milligan DA, Barton JR: Impact of high-dose corticosteroid therapy for patients with HELLP (hemolysis, elevated liver enzymes, and low platelet count) syndrome, *Am J Obstet Gynecol* 183(4):921–924, 2000.

van Pampus MG, Wolf H, Mayruhu G, et al: Long-term follow-up in patients with a history of (H)ELLP syndrome, *Hypertens Pregnancy* 20(1):15–23, 2001.

Prediction and Prevention of Preeclampsia

Abalos E, Duley L, Steyn DW, Henderson-Smart DJ: Antihypertensive drug therapy for mild to moderate hypertension during pregnancy, *Cochrane Database Syst Rev*(1):CD002252, 2007.

Barton JR, Sibai BM: Prediction and prevention of recurrent preeclampsia, *Obstet Gynecol* 112(2 Pt 1):359–372, 2008.

Chien PF, Arnott N, Gordon A, et al: How useful is uterine artery Doppler flow velocimetry in the prediction of preeclampsia, intrauterine growth retardation and prenatal death? An overview, *BJOG* 107(2):196–208, 2000.

Espinoza J, Romero R, Nien JK, et al: Identification of patients at risk for early onset and/or severe preeclampsia with the use of uterine artery Doppler velocimetry and placental growth factor, *Am J Obstet Gynecol* 196(4), 2007. 326 e1-13[Published erratum appears in Am J Obstet Gynecol 196(4):614, 2007].

Hofmeyr GJ, Duley L, Atallah A: Dietary calcium supplementation for prevention of pre-eclampsia and related problems: a systematic review and a commentary, *BJOG* 114(8):933–943, 2007.

Levine RJ, Lam C, Qian C, et al: Soluble endoglin and other circulating antiangiogenic factors in preeclampsia, *N Engl J Med* 355(10):992–1005, 2006. [Published erratum appears in N Engl J Med 355(10):1840, 2006].

Olsen SF, Secher NJ, Tabor A, et al: Randomized clinical trials of fish oil supplementation in high risk pregnancies. Fish Oil Trials in Pregnancy (FOTIP) Team, *BJOG* 107(3):382–395, 2000.

Poston L, Briley AL, Seed PT, et al: Vitamins in Preeclampsia (VIP) Trial Consortium: vitamin C and vitamin E in pregnant women at risk for preeclampsia (VIP trial): randomized placebo-controlled trial, *Lancet* 367(9517):1145–1154, 2006.

Sergio F, Maria Clara D, Gabriella F, et al: Prophylaxis of recurrent preeclampsia: low-molecular-weight heparin plus low-dose aspirin versus low-dose aspirin alone, *Hypertens Pregnancy* 25(2):115–127, 2006.

Spinnato JA 2nd, Freire S, Pinto e Silva JL, et al: Antioxidant therapy to prevent preeclampsia: a randomized controlled trial, *Obstet Gynecol* 110(6):1311–1318, 2007.

Stepan H, Unversucht A, Wessel N, Faber R: Predictive value of maternal angiogenic factors in second trimester pregnancies with abnormal uterine perfusion, *Hypertension* 49(4):818–824, 2007.

Villar J, Purwar M, Merialdi M, et al: WHO randomized trial of supplementation with Vitamins C and E among pregnant women at high risk for pre-eclampsia in populations of low nutritional status from developing countries, *BJOG* 116(6):780–788, 2009.

Widmer M, Villar J, Benigni A, et al: Mapping the theories of preeclampsia and the role of angiogenic factors: a systemic review, *Obstet Gynecol* 109(1):168–180, 2007.

Yu CK, Papageorghiou AT, Parra M, et al: Fetal Medicine Foundation Second Trimester Screening Group: Randomized controlled trial using low-dose aspirin in the prevention of preeclampsia in women with abnormal uterine artery Doppler at 23 weeks' gestation, *Ultrasound Obstet Gynecol* 22(3):233–239, 2003.

Chapter 25

Endocrine Disorders in Pregnancy

GLADYS A. RAMOS • INDER J. CHOPRA • SHANNON R. BALES

KEY UPDATES

1 The American Diabetes Association has added a hemoglobin A1c of ≥6.5 to the diagnostic criteria for type 2 diabetes mellitus (DM).

2 There are no significant differences in pregnancy outcomes or glycemic control when pregestational diabetes is treated with subcutaneous insulin or insulin pump.

3 Two trials have now demonstrated that treating gestational diabetes is associated with improved outcomes.

4 The recent Hyperglycemia and Adverse Pregnancy Outcomes (HAPO) study described a continuous association between maternal glucose concentrations and increasing birth weight, cord c peptide levels, and other markers of perinatal morbidity.

5 In secondary analysis of their randomized control trial, Langer and colleagues found that glyburide and insulin were equally efficacious in the treatment of gestational diabetes mellitus (GDM) in all severity levels.

6 Metformin is an option for the treatment of gestational diabetes but is associated with a failure rate of 46%.

7 Normograms of thyroid stimulating hormone (TSH) are needed based on gestational age and number of fetuses to adequately diagnose thyroid disease in pregnancy.

8 Propylthiouracil (PTU) may rarely be associated with liver toxicity; therefore, liver function tests must be monitored during pregnancy.

9 Levothyroxine requirements have been seen to increase as early as the fifth week of gestation. Given the importance of thyroid hormone for cognitive development of the fetus, it is recommended that doses of levothyroxine be increased 30% upon a positive pregnancy test.

Pregestational Diabetes in Pregnancy

CLINICAL PROFILE

- Currently, 17 million people in the United States have some form of diagnosed diabetes
- The data from 2003 to 2006 indicate that approximately 10.2% (11.5 million) of women older than 20 years of age have diabetes
- Ethnic predisposition: American Indian, African American, Asian, and Latino
- An epidemic of childhood obesity is currently under way in the United States, with approximately 30% of children and youth (23 million) overweight

DIAGNOSIS

- Patients with type 1 diabetes (formerly termed "juvenile-onset diabetes") typically present with hyperglycemia, ketosis, and dehydration in childhood or adolescence
  - The diagnosis is often made during a hospital admission for diabetic ketoacidosis and coma

- Rarely is the diagnosis of type 1 diabetes first made during pregnancy
- Women diagnosed early in pregnancy with gestational diabetes are later found to have overt, type 2 diabetes after delivery
- The American Diabetic Association has outlined four criteria for the diagnosis of type 2 diabetes in nonpregnant subjects; they include the following:
  - Finding of a casual plasma glucose of ≥200 mg/dL
  - A fasting plasma glucose of ≥126 mg/dL
  - A 2-hour glucose value of ≥200 mg/dL on a 75-g, 2-hour glucose tolerance test (GTT), or
  - a hemoglobin A1C ≥6.5%, was recently added to the diagnostic criteria (Executive Summary, 2010)

UPDATE #1

The American Diabetes Association has added a hemoglobin A1C of ≥6.5 to the diagnostic criteria for type 2 DM (Executive Summary, 2010).

MANAGEMENT

- Preconception management
- The important elements to be considered are the patient's level of glycemic control; the current status of the patient's retinal and renal health; and any medications being taken, especially antihypertensive or thyroid medications
- Assessment of the patient's risk of complications during pregnancy, including worsening of renal or ophthalmologic function
- Congenital anomalies
  - The risk of a fetal structural anomaly is fourfold to eightfold higher
  - The major congenital anomalies occurred in 4.8% for type 1 diabetes and 4.3% for type 2 diabetes
  - Neural tube defects in insulin-dependent diabetics increased 4.2-fold, and congenital heart disease increased 3.4-fold
  - Prenatal diagnosis of these anomalies was accomplished in 65% of neonates
  - The typical defects and their frequency of occurrence was noted in a prospective study of infants with major malformations (Table 25-1)
  - Pathogenesis
    - Fetal hyperglycemia may promote excessive formation of oxygen radicals in the mitochondria of susceptible tissues, leading to the formation of hydroperoxides, which inhibit prostacyclin
    - The resulting overabundance of thromboxanes and other prostaglandins may then disrupt vascularization of developing tissues
- Preconception management—glucose control:
  - Establishing a regimen of frequent, regular monitoring of capillary blood glucose levels
  - Adopting an insulin dosing regimen that results in smooth interprandial glucose profile (fasting blood glucose value 90 to 99 mg/dL, 1-hour postprandial glucose level of <140 mg/dL, or 2-hour postprandial glucose level <120 mg/dL, no reactions between meals or at night)
  - Bringing HbA_{1c} level into the normal range
  - Developing family, financial, and personal resources to assist the patient if pregnancy complications require that she lose work time or assume total bed rest

TABLE 25-1 Congenital Malformations in Infants of Insulin-Dependent Diabetic Mothers

Anomaly	Appropriate Risk Ratio	Percent Risk
All cardiac defects	18×	8.5
All central nervous system anomalies	16×	5.3
Anencephaly	13×	
Spina bifida	20×	
All congenital anomalies	8×	18.4

Data from Becerra JE, Khoury MJ, Cordero JF, et al: Diabetes mellitus during pregnancy and the risks for specific birth defects: a population based case control study, *Pediatrics* 86(1): 1990.

- This preconception care has been shown to decrease congenital anomalies and result in fewer hospitalizations, fewer infants requiring intravenous glucose after delivery, and a substantial reduction in total costs
- Glycemic control during pregnancy
  - The Fifth International Workshop Conference on Gestational Diabetes currently recommends the following:
    - Fasting plasma glucose below 90 to 99 mg/dL (5.0 to 5.5 mmol/liter) and
    - 1-hour postprandial plasma glucose below 140 mg/dL (7.8 mmol/liter) or
    - 2-hour postprandial plasma glucose below 120 to 127 mg/dL (6.7 to 7.1 mmol/liter)
  - Postprandial values must be assessed because they have the strongest correlation with fetal growth
  - A typical schedule involves performing blood glucose checks upon rising in the morning, 1 or 2 hours after breakfast, before and after lunch, before and after dinner, and before bedtime
  - The goal of physiologic glycemic control in pregnancy, however, is not met by simply avoiding hypoglycemia
- Principles of dietary therapy
  - Three major meals and three snacks are prescribed
  - Nutritional therapy should be supervised by a trained professional who performs formal dietary assessment and counseling at several points during the pregnancy
  - Moderate restriction of dietary carbohydrate intake to 35% to 40% of calories has been shown to reduce maternal glucose levels and improve maternal and fetal outcomes
- Principles of insulin therapy
  - No available insulin delivery method approaches the precise secretion of the hormone from the human pancreas
  - The therapeutic goal of exogenous insulin therapy during pregnancy is to achieve diurnal glucose excursions similar to those of nondiabetic pregnant women
  - Normal pregnant women maintain postprandial blood glucose excursions within a relatively narrow range (70 to 120 mg/dL)
  - Use of regular insulin before each major meal helps limit postprandial hyperglycemia
  - To provide basal insulin levels between feedings, a longer-acting preparation is necessary, such as isoprostane insulin (NPH) or insulin zinc (Lente)
  - Typical subcutaneous insulin dosing regimens are two thirds of total insulin in the morning, of which two thirds are intermediate-acting and one third is regular insulin; the remaining one third of the total insulin dose is given in the evening: 50% is short-acting insulin given prior to dinner, and 50% is intermediate-acting insulin given at bedtime
  - The use of an insulin pump for type 1 diabetes mellitus during pregnancy has become more widespread; an advantage of this approach is the more physiologic insulin release pattern that may be achieved with the pump

UPDATE #2
A recent meta-analysis of six randomized controlled trials comparing subcutaneous insulin to the insulin pump didn't find any significant differences in pregnancy outcomes or glycemic control (Mukhopadhyay et al, 2007).

- Prenatal obstetric management
  - Periodic biophysical testing of the fetus
- Testing should be initiated early enough to avoid significant risk of stillbirth but not so early that the risk of a false-positive result is high
- In patients with poor glycemic control or significant hypertension, testing should begin as early as 28 weeks of gestation
- In lower-risk patients, most centers begin formal fetal testing by 34 to 36 weeks
- Counting of fetal movements is performed in all pregnancies from 28 weeks of gestation onward
  - Choosing the timing and route of delivery
    - Timing of delivery should be selected to minimize maternal and neonatal morbidity and mortality
    - Delaying delivery to as near as possible to the estimated date of confinement maximizes cervical ripeness and improves the chances of spontaneous labor and vaginal delivery
    - Optimal time for delivery of most diabetic pregnancies is between 39 and 40 weeks
    - Delivery of a diabetic patient before 39 weeks of gestation without documentation of fetal lung maturity should be performed only for compelling maternal or fetal reasons
    - Fetal lung maturity should be verified in such cases from the presence of more than 3% phosphatidyl glycerol or the equivalent in amniotic fluid as ascertained from an amniocentesis specimen
    - A policy of elective cesarean section for suspected fetal macrosomia (ultrasonographically estimated fetal weight of greater than 4500 g) would require 443 cesarean deliveries to avoid one permanent brachial plexus injury
  - Intrapartum glycemic management
    - Maintenance of intrapartum metabolic homeostasis is essential to avoid fetal hypoxemia and promote a smooth postnatal transition
    - Strict maternal euglycemia during labor does not guarantee newborn euglycemia in infants with macrosomia and long-established islet cell hypertrophy
    - Combined insulin and glucose infusion during labor to maintain maternal blood glucose in a narrow range (80 to 110 mg/dL) during labor is a common and reasonable practice
    - Typical infusion rates are 5% dextrose in lactated Ringer's solution at 100 mL/hr and regular insulin at 0.5 to 1.0 U/hr
    - Capillary blood glucose levels are monitored hourly in such patients
  - Neonatal morbidity
    - Neonatal hypoglycemia
      - Neonatal hypoglycemia occurs in up to 20% of infants born to mothers with diabetes

- It is related to the level of maternal glycemic control over the 6 to 12 weeks before birth
- It most commonly occurs between 1 and 5 hours after birth, as the rich supply of maternal glucose stops with ligation of the umbilical cord and the infant's levels of circulating insulin remain elevated
- These infants therefore require close monitoring for blood glucose concentration during the first hours after birth
- Hyperbilirubinemia
  - The risk of hyperbilirubinemia is higher in IDMs than in normal infants
  - Prematurity and polycythemia are the primary contributing factors
  - Increased destruction of red blood cells contributes to the risks of jaundice and kernicterus
  - This complication is usually treated with phototherapy, but exchange transfusions may be necessary for marked bilirubin elevations
- Polycythemia and hyperviscosity
  - Polycythemia (defined as central venous hemoglobin concentration >20 g/dL or hematocrit >65%) is not uncommon in IDMs and is related to glycemic control
  - Hyperglycemia is a powerful stimulus to fetal erythropoietin production, probably mediated by decreased fetal oxygen tension
  - Untreated, neonatal polycythemia may promote vascular sludging, ischemia, and infarction of vital tissues, including the kidneys and central nervous system
- Hypertrophic and congestive cardiomyopathy
  - Prevalence of myocardial hypertrophy in IDMs may exceed 30% at birth; almost all cases resolve by 1 year of age
  - The pathogenesis of hypertrophic cardiomyopathy in IDMs is unclear, although it is recognized to be associated with poor maternal metabolic control
  - There is evidence that the fetal myocardium is particularly sensitive to insulin during gestation, and in fetal rhesus monkeys it has been reported that there is a doubling of cardiac mass with hyperinsulinemia
  - Halse et al (2005) noted that B-type natriuretic protein (BNP), a marker for congestive cardiac failure, is elevated in neonates whose mothers had poor glycemic control during the third trimester
  - IDMs may also have congestive cardiomyopathy without hypertrophy; echocardiography shows the myocardium to be overstretched and poorly contractile
  - This condition is often rapidly reversible with correction of neonatal hypoglycemia, hypocalcemia, and polycythemia; it responds to digoxin, diuretics, or both
- Respiratory distress syndrome (RDS)
  - Surfactant production occurs late in diabetic pregnancies
  - The near-term infant of a mother with poorly controlled diabetes is more likely to have neonatal RDS than the infant of a nondiabetic mother at the same gestational age

- The nondiabetic fetus achieves pulmonary maturity at a mean gestational age of 34 to 35 weeks
- By 37 weeks, more than 99% of normal newborn infants have mature lung profiles as assessed by phospholipid assays
  - The risk of respiratory distress has passed until after 38.5 weeks of gestation
  - Any delivery contemplated before 38.5 weeks for other than the most urgent fetal and maternal indications should be preceded by documentation of pulmonary maturity through amniocentesis
- Birth injury
  - Shoulder dystocia, defined as difficulty in delivering the fetal body after expulsion of the fetal head, is an obstetric emergency that places the fetus and mother at great risk
  - Shoulder dystocia occurs in 0.3% to 0.5% of vaginal deliveries among normal pregnant women; the incidence is twofold to fourfold higher in women with diabetes, probably because the hyperglycemia of diabetic pregnancy causes the fetal shoulder and abdominal widths to become massive
  - Athukorala et al (2007) investigated this relationship and found a strong association with fasting hyperglycemia such that with each 1 mmol increase in the fasting value in the oral glucose-tolerance test, there was an increasing relative risk (RR) of 2.09 (95% confidence interval [CI] 1.03 to 4.25)
- Obstetric complications
  - Preeclampsia
    - Preeclampsia is more common among women with diabetes, occurring two to three times more frequently in women with pregestational diabetes than in nondiabetic women
    - Preeclampsia develops in more than one third of women who have had diabetes for more than 20 years
    - Renal function assessment (creatinine, blood urea nitrogen [BUN], uric acid, and 24-hour urine collection) should be performed each trimester in women with evidence of pregestational diabetes and vascular disease
  - Polyhydramnios
    - Polyhydramnios is usually diagnosed when any single vertical pocket of amniotic fluid is deeper than 8 cm (equivalent to the 97th percentile) or when the sum of four pockets, one from each quadrant of the uterus (amniotic fluid index), exceeds approximately 24 cm (the 95th percentile)
    - The principal causes of hydramnios in diabetic pregnancy are fetal gastrointestinal anomalies (e.g., esophageal atresia) and poor glycemic control
    - The main clinical problems associated with hydramnios are fetal malposition and preterm labor

Gestational Diabetes

CLINICAL PROFILE

- Gestational diabetes mellitus (GDM) is defined as glucose intolerance that begins or is first recognized during pregnancy

- GDM complicates no more than 2.55% to 6% of pregnancies in the United States (>135,000 cases annually)
- Several risk factors significantly increase the likelihood of GDM, including a maternal age of 35 years or more; a body mass index (BMI) higher than 22 kg/m²; and Asian, Latin, or "other" ethnicity

UPDATE #3

Two trials have now demonstrated that treating gestational diabetes is associated with improved outcomes:
- In 2005, a randomized control trial in Australian—in which women with GDM diagnosed at 24 to 34 weeks were randomized to treatment versus no intervention—demonstrated decreased perinatal complications among infants born to mothers who were treated (Crowther et al, 2005).
- A randomized trial by the maternal fetal medicine units was performed, in which 958 women with gestational diabetes were randomized to usual prenatal care or treatment (Landon et al, 2007).
- Women randomized to treatment underwent nutritional counseling, diet therapy, and insulin treatment if indicated. Among those who underwent treatment, there were lower mean birthweight, neonatal fat mass, rates of large for gestational age, and macrosomic (>4000 g) infants.
- There was also a trend toward lower cord c peptide in the treatment group.
- Maternal outcomes were significant for lower rates of cesarean delivery, preeclampsia, and shoulder dystocia.

DIAGNOSIS

- Screening should be performed with the use of 50 g of glucose at 26 to 28 weeks of gestation
- Various threshold levels for the 50-g glucose challenge are in use, including 140 mg/dL, 135 mg/dL, and 130 mg/dL; the sensitivity of the GDM testing regimen depends on the threshold value used
- Definitive diagnosis of gestational diabetes is made with a 100 g GTT; two or more values must be met or exceeded for the diagnosis of GDM to be made
- A GTT should be performed after an overnight fast and with modest carbohydrate loading before the test (Table 25-2)
- Hypoglycemia during the 100-g oral glucose tolerance test (OGTT) occurs in 6.3% of patients; these women have a significantly lower risk of developing GDM and have lower birth weights

TABLE 25-2 **Criteria for Gestational Diabetes: Venous Plasma Glucose Level**

	With 100-g Glucose Load		With 75-g Glucose Load	
	mg/dL	mmol/L	mg/dL	mmol/L
Fasting value	95	5.3	95	5.3
1-hr value	180	10.0	180	10.0
2-hr value	155	8.6	155	8.6
3-hr value	140	7.8	—	—

UPDATE #4

The recent Hyperglycemia and Adverse Pregnancy Outcomes (HAPO) study described a continuous association between maternal glucose concentrations and increasing birth weight, cord c peptide levels, and other markers of perinatal morbidity as glucose levels below those used to diagnose GDM (HAPO Study Cooperative Research Group et al, 2008).

MANAGEMENT

- Please see pregestational diabetes section for the following:
  - Glycemic control during pregnancy
  - Principles of dietary therapy
  - Principles of insulin therapy
- Oral hypoglycemic therapy
- Glyburide
  - Glyburide, a second-generation sulfonylurea, has been shown to cross the placenta minimally in both laboratory studies and a large clinical trial
  - The prospective randomized trial, conducted by Langer and associates (2000), compared glyburide and insulin in 404 women with gestational diabetes and showed equivalently excellent maternal glycemic control and perinatal outcomes
  - Following the publication of the randomized control trial, several retrospective series have been published comprising 504 glyburide-treated patients
  - Jacobson et al. performed a retrospective cohort comparison of glyburide and insulin treatment of gestational diabetes
  - There were no statistically significant differences in gestational age at delivery, mode of delivery, birthweight, large for gestational age (LGA), or percentage of macrosomia
  - Women in the glyburide group also had significantly lower posttreatment fasting and postprandial blood glucose levels
  - The glyburide group was also superior in achieving target glycemic levels (86% versus 63%, P < 0.001)
  - The failure rate (transfer to insulin) was 12%
  - Conway et al (2004) reported a retrospective cohort of 75 glyburide-treated GDM patients
  - Good glycemic control was achieved by 84% of the subjects with glyburide, and 16% were switched to insulin
  - The rate of fetal macrosomia was similar between women successfully treated with glyburide and those who converted to insulin (11.1% versus 8.3%; p = 1.0); mean birth weight was also similar
  - A nonsignificantly higher proportion of infants in the glyburide group required intravenous glucose infusions because of hypoglycemia (25% versus 12.7%, p = 0.37)

UPDATE #5

In a secondary analysis of their randomized control trial, Langer and colleagues found that glyburide and insulin were equally efficacious in the treatment of GDM in all severity levels, when a fasting glucose on oral glucose challenge test was between 95 and 139 mg/dL. Eighty percent of women treated with glyburide will obtain glycemic control goals (Langer et al, 2005).

- Metformin
  - Metformin is frequently employed in patients with polycystic ovary syndrome and type 2 diabetes to improve insulin resistance and fertility
  - Metformin therapy has been demonstrated to improve the success of ovulation induction and may reduce first-trimester pregnancy loss in women with polycystic ovary syndrome
  - Older studies evaluating the efficacy and safety of the treatment of pregestational and gestational diabetics with metformin raised concerns regarding a higher perinatal mortality, higher rate of preeclampsia, and failure of therapy; however, the metformin-treated women were older, more obese, and treated later in pregnancy

UPDATE #6

Recently a large randomized controlled trial was performed comparing metformin to insulin for the treatment of gestational diabetes:
- This study was powered to rule out or detect a 33% increase in composite outcome (neonatal hypoglycemia, respiratory distress, need for phototherapy, birth trauma, 5-minute Apgar of less than 7 or prematurity) in neonates born to mothers treated with metformin.
- Seven hundred and fifty-one women with gestational diabetes between 20 and 30 weeks of gestation were randomized to metformin or insulin. Of these, 363 women were assigned to metformin and 370 to insulin.
- Forty-six percent of women receiving metformin required the addition of insulin to obtain adequate glycemic control; there were no differences in the rate of the primary composite outcome.
- There was a lower rate of severe neonatal hypoglycemia in the metformin-treated group and no differences in neonatal anthropometric measurement.
- There was, however, a higher rate of prematurity in the metformin-treated group (12.1%) versus the insulin group (7.6%) (Rowan et al, 2008).

Maternal Thyroid Diseases

MATERNAL THYROID FUNCTION IN PREGNANCY

- Physiologic changes
  - Estrogen-dependent increase in thyroid-binding globulin
  - This results in an increase in total thyroxine (TT_4) and total triiodothyronine (TT_3) levels throughout pregnancy
  - Human chorionic gonadotropin (hCG) has a stimulatory effect on the thyroid such that thyroid stimulating hormone (TSH) can be normal or decreased in the first trimester and early second trimester

UPDATE #7

The decrease in TSH hormone seen in the first trimester appears to be greater in twins than it is in singleton pregnancies. Therefore, nomograms are needed based on gestational age and number of fetuses to adequately diagnose disease in pregnancy (Dashe et al, 2005).

FETAL THYROID FUNCTION

- The fetal thyroid actively concentrates iodide after 10 weeks, releases T4 after 12 weeks, and becomes responsive to pituitary TSH at 20 weeks of gestation
- Maternal TSH does not cross the placenta
- Maternal thyroid hormones and thyrotropin-releasing hormone (TRH) are transferred to the fetus throughout gestation
- Recent studies show that by 4 weeks after conception, very small amounts of T4 and T3 from the maternal origin are found in the fetal compartment with T4 levels increasing throughout gestation; free T4 levels reach concentrations of biologic significance in the adult by midgestation
- Studies using rat models have demonstrated that this thyroid hormone is important for corticogenesis very early in the pregnancy
- Transplacental transfer of thyroid-stimulating immunoglobulin (TSI) may occur, causing fetal thyrotoxicosis
- Other substances that may be transferred from the maternal compartment to the fetal compartment and affect fetal thyroid function are iodine, a radioactive isotope of iodine, propylthiouracil (PTU), and methimazole

Hyperthyroidism

CLINICAL PROFILE

- Hyperthyroidism occurs in approximately 0.2% of pregnancies
- Results in a significant increase in the prevalence of both low-birth-weight delivery and a trend toward higher neonatal mortality
- The most common cause of thyrotoxicosis (85% of cases) in women of child-bearing age is Graves' disease
  - Other causes are acute (or subacute) thyroiditis (transient), Hashimoto disease, hydatidiform mole, choriocarcinoma, toxic nodular goiter, and toxic adenoma
- Graves' disease has a peak incidence during the reproductive years, but patients with the disorder may actually have remissions during pregnancy, followed by postpartum exacerbations

DIAGNOSIS

- Signs and symptoms: intolerance to heat, nervousness, irritability, emotional lability, and increased perspiration, along with tachycardia and anxiety
- Laboratory data are difficult to evaluate because total serum thyroxin values are normally elevated during pregnancy as a result of estrogen-induced increases in thyroxine-binding globulin
- Low TSH with an elevated free thyroxin level is diagnostic

MANAGEMENT

- Radioactive iodine therapy is contraindicated during pregnancy
- Treatment of the pregnant woman with thyrotoxicosis involves a choice between antithyroid drugs and surgery
- The therapeutic goal is to achieve a euthyroid, or perhaps slightly hyperthyroid, state in the mother while preventing hypothyroidism and hyperthyroidism in the fetus
- Either PTU or methimazole may be used to treat thyrotoxicosis during pregnancy
- Methimazole therapy was thought to be associated with aplasia cutis in the offspring of treated women; however, this causal relationship hasn't been proved
- PTU crosses the placenta more slowly than methimazole and has become the drug of choice for use during pregnancy; ordinarily, thyrotoxicosis can be controlled with doses of 300 mg per day

> **UPDATE #8**
>
> PTU may rarely be associated with liver toxicity; therefore, monitor liver function tests during pregnancy (Bahn et al, 2009).

- Once the disorder is under control, however, it is important to keep the dose as low as possible, preferably less than 100 mg daily, because this drug does cross the placenta and blocks fetal thyroid function, possibly producing hypothyroidism in the fetus
- In women with cardiovascular effects, the use of beta-blockers may be appropriate to achieve rapid control of thyrotoxicosis
- Iodides have also been used, particularly in combination with beta-blocking agents, to control thyrotoxicosis; long-term iodide therapy, however, presents a risk to the fetus; because of the inhibition of the incorporation of iodide into thyroglobulin, a large, obstructive goiter can develop in the fetus
- Surgery during pregnancy is best reserved for cases in which the mother is hypersensitive to antithyroid drugs, compliance with medication is poor, or in rare cases in which drugs are ineffective in controlling the disease
- Effects on the newborn
  - Approximately 1% of infants born to mothers with some level of thyrotoxicosis themselves have thyrotoxicosis
  - Assessment of fetal risk in utero includes measurement of TSIs, with the expectation that if the titers are high, there is a higher risk of thyrotoxicosis
  - Additional assessment of the fetus should pay particular attention to elevated resting heart rate and poor fetal growth
- Pathogenesis of Graves' disease
  - Thyroid-stimulating immunoglobulins (TSI), which appear to be immunoglobulin G (IgG), are present in pregnant women with Graves' disease and cross the placenta easily to cause neonatal hyperthyroidism in some infants
  - The clinical spectrum of Graves' disease in utero is quite broad and may result in stillbirth or preterm delivery
  - Some affected infants have widespread evidence of autoimmune disease, including thrombocytopenic purpura and generalized hypertrophy of the lymphatic tissues
  - Thyroid storm can occur shortly after birth, or the infant may have disease that is transient in nature, lasting from 1 to 5 months

- Infants born to mothers who have been treated with thioamides may appear normal at birth but demonstrate signs of thyrotoxicosis at 7 to 10 days of age, when the effect of thioamide suppression of thyroxine synthesis is no longer present; the measurement of thyroid-stimulating antibodies (TSAbs) is useful in predicting whether the fetus will be affected

Hypothyroidism

CLINICAL PROFILE

- Hypothyroidism complicates about 1 to 3 per 1000 pregnancies
- The leading cause of hypothyroidism in pregnancy is Hashimoto's thyroiditis, which is a chronic autoimmune thyroiditis characterized by painless inflammation and enlargement of the thyroid gland
- Other causes of primary hypothyroidism include iodine deficiency, thyroidectomy, or ablative radioiodine therapy for hyperthyroidism
- Secondary causes of hypothyroidism include Sheehan's syndrome caused by obstetric hemorrhage leading to pituitary ischemia, necrosis, and abnormalities in all pituitary hormones, lymphocytic hypophysitis, and hypophysectomy
- Women with hypothyroidism are at increased risk of pregnancy complications such as a higher rate of miscarriage, preeclampsia, placental abruption, growth restriction, and stillbirth

DIAGNOSIS

- The finding of a goiter may be associated with cases of Hashimoto's thyroiditis or due to iodine deficiency
- The signs and symptoms of hypothyroidism are usually insidious and easily confused with those of normal pregnancy including fatigue, cold intolerance, cramping, constipation, weight gain, hair loss, insomnia, and mental slowness
- In the classic definition of hypothyroidism the serum TSH is elevated and the free T4 is low
- Other forms of hypothyroidism have also been described, including subclinical hypothyroidism, defined as an elevated TSH with a normal free T4, or hypothyroxinemia, defined as a normal TSH but a low free T4; these have no clinical significance to the mother but may be associated with neonatal effects discussed later

MANAGEMENT

- Levothyroxine is the treatment of choice
- Adults with complete hypothyroidism require approximately 1.7 micrograms/kg of body weight and should be initiated on full replacement
- The goal of therapy is normalization of the TSH level; therefore, the TSH is checked at 4- to 6-week increments and the dose of levothyroxine adjusted by 25 to 50 microgram increments
- Neonatal neurologic development
  - In humans, early epidemiologic data from iodine-deficient areas of Switzerland suggested a link between mental retardation in the children of women with abnormal thyroid function

- Studies performed by Haddow et al. found that in women with overt, untreated hypothyroidism, the IQ points of children aged 7 to 9 years utilizing the Wechsler Intelligence Scale IQ test were 7 points lower in cases than in controls (p = 0.005) (Haddow et al, 1999; the percentage of children with IQ scores less than 85% was higher in the cases than in controls (19% versus 5%, p = 0.007)
- Early in human development there is expression of nuclear thyroid receptors that are already occupied by T3, suggesting that normal maternal T4 levels are necessary for normal cortical development

UPDATE #9
Levothyroxine requirements have been seen to increase as early as the fifth week of gestation, and given the importance for cognitive development of the fetus, it is recommended that doses of levothyroxine are increased 30% upon a positive pregnancy test (Alexander et al, 2004).

- Controversy exists as to whether subclinical hypothyroidism (defined as an elevated TSH but normal free T4) and hypothyroxinemia (defined as a normal TSH but a low free T4) warrant treatment in pregnancy
- Studies performed by Pop et al. in the iodine deficient areas of the Netherlands have shown that free T4 levels below the 10th percentile at 12 weeks of gestation were associated with lower scores on the Dutch version of the Bayley Scale of Infant Development at 10 months (1999); in their study they included women with a low free T4 (hypothyroxinemia) and excluded women with elevated TSH; a follow-up study on these same infants, tested in both motor and mental scores at 1 and 2 years of age, found significantly lower scores in infants born to mothers with low free T4 levels (Pop et al, 2003)
- Casey et al. performed a study on patients at Parkland Hospital with subclinical hypothyroidism defined as a TSH at >97.5th percentile and a normal free T4; approximately 2.3% of women screened (404 women) were identified as having subclinical hypothyroidism, and when compared to normal controls, they had a higher incidence of placental abruption (RR 3.0, 95th CI 1.1 to 8.2) and preterm birth at <34 weeks' gestation (RR 1.8, 95th CI 1.1 to 2.9); the authors concluded that the reduction in IQ in children born to women with subclinical hypothyroidism may be due to prematurity (Casey et al, 2006)
- The American College of Obstetricians and Gynecologists (ACOG) does not recommend universal screening given that decision and cost-effectiveness studies on the impact of such a strategy are currently lacking
- Data on therapy dosing, efficacy, or if medication should be stopped after pregnancy in otherwise asymptomatic women with subclinical hypothyroidism and hypothyroxinemia are lacking
- Currently under way is a multicenter randomized trial to examine whether screening and treatment

of hypothyroxinemia or subclinical hypothyroidism have a long-term effect on neurodevelopment of offspring (clinicaltrials.gov identifier NCT00388297)

Hyperparathyroidism

CLINICAL PROFILE

- Primary hyperparathyroidism usually presents after childbearing
- Incidence is about 8 in 100,000 women of childbearing age
- May be caused by adenomas or hyperplasia
- Hypercalcemia is hallmark of diagnosis but may be masked in pregnancy
  - Pregnancy is characterized by increased demands of calcium and increased urinary loss of calcium
  - There is a vitamin D–mediated increase in calcium absorption in the gut
  - Vitamin D levels increase in pregnancy
  - In pregnancy there is a decrease in total calcium concentration, whereas free ionized calcium concentrations are unchanged
- Hypercalcemia may improve during pregnancy
- There is increased risk of pancreatitis and hypercalcemic crisis in the postpartum period
- Associated with an increased risk of miscarriage, fetal demise, growth restriction, and premature labor
- Risk of miscarriage increases significantly if the calcium level is >11.4 mg/dL
- Fetal parathyroid hormone suppression by high maternal calcium levels leads to neonatal tetany, convulsions, and hypocalcemia
- Neonatal hypocalcemia usually presents from 5 to 14 days after delivery but may be delayed up to 1 month in breast-fed infants

DIAGNOSIS

- Symptoms include fatigue, thirst, hyperemesis, depression, constipation, muscle weakness, mental changes, or patients may be asymptomatic
- Patients have a higher incidence of renal calculi and pancreatitis
- Parathyroid hormone levels increase
- Hypercalcemia is hallmark of diagnosis but may be masked in pregnancy
- Ultrasound of the neck may detect parathyroid adenomas

MANAGEMENT

- Surgical treatment is the mainstay outside of pregnancy
- Patients with mild disease can be treated with low-calcium diet and oral phosphate
- If the calcium level is >11.4 mg/dL, surgical treatment can be considered in the first and second trimester of pregnancy

VII. Hypoparathyroidism

CLINICAL PROFILE

- Most commonly as a result of thyroid surgery
- May be caused by autoimmune disease

- Untreated hypocalcemia in pregnancy is associated with fetal demise, fetal hypocalcemia, secondary hyperparathyroidism, bone demineralization, and neonatal rickets
- Neonatal hypocalcemic seizures may be noted shortly after delivery

DIAGNOSIS

- Low free calcium levels
- Elevated parathyroid hormone levels

MANAGEMENT

- Normalization of calcium levels with vitamin D and calcium supplements
- Levels of vitamin D increase two- to threefold during the course of pregnancy
- Calcium and albumin should be measured monthly
- Vitamin D is supplemented with calcitriol (1,25-dihydroxycholecalciferol) and alfacalcidol (1alpha-hydroxycholecalciferol)
- Excessive supplementation can be associated with maternal hypercalcemia and overmineralization of fetal bones
- Postpartum vitamin D levels need to be decreased

SUGGESTED READINGS

Pregestational Diabetes

ACOG Committee on Practice Bulletins: ACOG practice bulletin: clinical management guidelines for obstetricians-gynecologists no. 60, 2005. Pregestational diabetes mellitus, *Obstet Gynecol* 105(3):675–685, 2005.

Executive summary: standards of medical care in diabetes—2010, *Diabetes Care* 33(Suppl 1):S4–S10, 2010.

Gabbe SG, Holing E, Temple P, et al: Benefits, risks, costs, and patient satisfaction associated with insulin pump therapy for the pregnancy complicated by type 1 diabetes mellitus, *Am J Obstet Gynecol* 182(6): 1283–1291, 2000.

Langer O, Conway D, Berkus M, et al: A comparison of glyburide and insulin in women with gestational diabetes mellitus, *N Engl J Med* 343(16): 1134–1138, 2000.

Moore TR: Glyburide for the treatment of gestational diabetes: a critical appraisal, *Diabetes Care* 30(Suppl 2):S209–S213, 2007.

Mukhopadhyay A, Farrell T, Fraser RB, Ola B: Continuous subcutaneous insulin infusion vs intensive conventional insulin therapy in pregnant diabetic women: a systematic review and metaanalysis of randomized, controlled trials, *Am J Obstet Gynecol* 197(5):447–456, 2007.

Gestational Diabetes

Crowther CA, Jiller JE, Moss JR, et al: Effect of treatment of gestational diabetes mellitus on pregnancy outcomes, *N Engl J Med* 352(24): 2477–2486, 2005.

Ecker JL, Greene MF: Gestational diabetes—setting limits, exploring treatments (editorial), *N Engl J Med* 358(19):2061–2063, 2008.

HAPO Study Cooperative Research Group: Hyperglycemia and Adverse Pregnancy Outcome (HAPO) Study: associations with neonatal anthropometrics, *Diabetes* 58(2):453–459, 2009.

HAPO Study Cooperative Research Group, et al: Hyperglycemia and adverse pregnancy outcomes, *N Engl J Med* 358(19):1991–2002.

Jacobson GF, Ramos GA, Ching JY, et al: Comparison of glyburide and insulin for the management of gestational diabetes in a large managed care organization, *Am J Obstet Gynecol* 193(1):118–124, 2005.

Landon MB, Thom E, Spong CY, et al: National Institute of Child Health and Human Development Maternal Fetal Medicine Unit Network randomized clinical trial: Standard therapy versus no therapy for mild gestational diabetes, *Diabetes Care* 30(Suppl 2):S194–S199, 2007.

Langer O, Yogev Y, Xenakis EM, Rosenn B: Insulin and glyburide therapy: dosage, severity level of gestational diabetes, and pregnancy outcome, *Am J Obstet Gynecol* 192(1):134–139, 2005.

Moore TR: Glyburide for the treatment of gestational diabetes: a critical appraisal, *Diabetes Care* 30(Suppl 2):S209–S213, 2007.

Rowan JA, Hague WM, Gao W, et al: MiG Trial Investigators: Metformin versus insulin for the treatment of gestational diabetes, *N Engl J Med* 358(19):2003–2015, 2008.

Thyroid Disorders

Alexander EK, Marqusee E, Lawrence J, et al: Timing and magnitude of increases in levothyroxine requirements during pregnancy in women with hypothyroidism, *N Engl J Med* 351(3):241–249, 2004.

American College of Obstetricians and Gynecologists: ACOG practice bulletin: clinical management guidelines for obstetrician-gynecologists no. 37, August 2002 (replaces practice bulletin no. 32, November 2001): thyroid disease in pregnancy, *Obstet Gynecol* 100(2):387–396, 2002.

Bahn RS, Burch HS, Cooper DS, et al: The role of propylthiouracil in the management of Graves' Disease in adults: report of a meeting jointly sponsored by the American Thyroid Association and the Food and Drug Administration, *Thyroid* 19(7):673–674, 2009.

Casey BM, Leveno KJ: Thyroid disease in pregnancy, *Obstet Gynecol* 108(5):1283–1292, 2006.

Dashe JS, Casey BM, Wells CE, et al: Thyroid-stimulating hormone in singleton and twin pregnancy: importance of gestational age-specific reference ranges, *Obstet Gynecol* 106(4):753–757, 2005.

Gyamfi C, Wapner R, D'Alton ME: Thyroid dysfunction in pregnancy, the basic science and clinical evidence surrounding the controversy in management, *Obstet Gynecol* 113(3):702–707, 2009.

Haddow JE, Palomaki GE, Allan WC, et al: Maternal thyroid deficiency during pregnancy and subsequent neuropsychological development of the child, *N Engl J Med* 341(8):549–555, 1999.

Pop VJ, Browthers EP, Vader HL, et al: Maternal hypothyroxinaemia during early pregnancy and subsequent child development: a 3 year follow up study, *Clin Endocrinol (Oxf)* 59(3):282–288, 2003.

Pop VJ, Kuijpens JL, Van Baar AL, et al: Low maternal free thyroxine concentrations during early pregnancy are associated with impaired psychomotor development in infancy, *Clin Endocrinol (Oxf)* 50(2):149–155, 1999.

Parathyroid Disorders

Norman J, Politz D, Politz L: Hyperparathyroidism during pregnancy and the effect of rising calcium on pregnancy loss: a call for earlier intervention, *Clin Endocrinol* 71(1):104–109, 2009.

Schnatz PF, Curry SL: Primary hyperparathyroidism in pregnancy: evidence-based management, *Obstet Gynecol Surv* 57(6):365–376, 2002.

References

Please go to expertconsult.com to view references.

Chapter 26

Perinatal Substance Abuse

J. SETH HAWKINS

KEY UPDATES

1 Perinatal substance abuse is common and confers substantial risks in pregnancy, but intervention for perinatal substance abuse during prenatal care decreases these risks.

2 Screening and intervening for alcohol use can reduce drinking during pregnancy.

3 Multimodal interventions for smoking, such as counseling, pharmacotherapy, and supportive care, confer pregnancy benefits, including higher birth weights and greater likelihood of quitting.

4 Cocaine use during pregnancy imparts significant risks of adverse pregnancy outcomes and may affect cognitive function in children and adolescents.

5 Methamphetamine use during pregnancy has increased dramatically and is associated with lower maternal quality of life and numerous adverse obstetrical and neonatal outcomes.

6 Recent data indicate that marijuana may have adverse effects on neurobehavioral measures in the neonatal period and on IQ in childhood.

7 Methadone maintenance provides benefits in opioid-dependent pregnant women, but opioid detoxification during pregnancy, and the relationship of maternal methadone dose to the development of Neonatal Abstinence Syndrome, remains controversial.

Perinatal Substance Abuse in Broad Context

- Perinatal substance abuse encompasses the use of illicit substances during pregnancy, as well as the use of legal drugs such as tobacco and alcohol
  - Overall, alcohol use occurs in approximately 1 in 10 pregnancies
  - Binge drinking and illicit drug use occurs in approximately 1 in 20 pregnancies (Substance Abuse and Mental Health Services Administration, 2009)
- The rate of illicit drug use is higher in younger pregnant women
  - For women ages 18 to 25 years, the rate of illicit drug use is 7.1% during pregnancy (compared to 16.2% in nonpregnant women)
  - For the youngest cohort, ages 15 to 17 years, the rate of illicit drug use during pregnancy exceeds the rate in nonpregnant patients at 21.6% versus 12.9% (Substance Abuse and Mental Health Services Administration, 2009)
- Of the illicit drug use during pregnancy, marijuana use accounts for approximately two thirds, whereas cocaine accounts for 10%
  - Of those pregnant women who use illicit drugs, more than 50% also use tobacco and alcohol (Ebrahim et al, 2003)

- Women who abuse substances during pregnancy have a significantly higher risk of abusing more than one substance
- Perinatal substance abuse increases the risk of being diagnosed with a sexually transmitted disease (STD), acquiring hepatitis or the human immunodeficiency virus (HIV) via needle use, and being hospitalized because of violence (Bauer et al, 2002)

UPDATE #1

Prenatal care itself has been shown to reduce the risks of preterm birth, low birth weight, and small-for-gestational age in mothers using drugs (El-Mohandes et al, 2003). The addition of substance abuse intervention to prenatal care confers substantial benefits on pregnancy outcomes. A large study of Kaiser Permanente members indicated that drug-abusing women who received such care, and control women who screened negative for drugs, delivered babies with similar rates of assisted ventilation, low birth weight, and prematurity (Armstrong et al, 2003). Another study of Kaiser Permanente members reported that drug-abusing women who received intervention had significantly lower rates of preterm delivery, placental abruption, and fetal demise, as compared to women who screened positive but did not participate in the prenatal care substance abuse program (Goler et al, 2008). Prenatal care programs that incorporate substance abuse interventions have the potential for substantial cost savings to the health care system (Caughey, 2008).

ALCOHOL USE DURING PREGNANCY

- Although public health efforts have emphasized that no amount of alcohol is considered safe in pregnancy, the use of alcohol during pregnancy is nonetheless widespread
  - The Centers for Disease Control and Prevention (CDC) reported that the use of alcohol and the prevalence of binge drinking during pregnancy did not change significantly from 1991 to 2005
    - Average annual percentage of pregnant women using alcohol was 12.2%
    - Binge drinking occurred in 1.9% of pregnancies on average
      - In this report, the CDC defined binge drinking as ≥ five drinks on any one occasion
      - In 2006, the CDC changed its definition of binge drinking to ≥ four drinks on any one occasion
  - For 2008, 10.6% of pregnant women ages 15 to 44 reported alcohol use in the month prior to the National Survey on Drug Use and Health (Substance Abuse and Mental Health Services Administration, 2009)
    - About 4.1% of pregnant women reported binge drinking in this survey, which was higher than the average rate (1.9%) reported by the CDC from 1991 to 2005
      - Both surveys used a definition of ≥ five drinks on any one occasion
      - It is unknown if this is a true increase in the rate of binge drinking or if the different rates are due to different survey methodologies
  - These numbers represent overall use within the United States and may differ in specific populations
    - In a Danish study, more than 50% of women reported at least one episode of binge drinking during the first 20 weeks of gestation (Kesmodel, 2001)
  - In women with heavy alcohol use during pregnancy, it is also necessary to screen for other drugs of abuse
    - Shor et al. (2010) reported that neonates with heavy in utero alcohol exposure had odds ratios of 1.90 (95% confidence interval [CI], 1.13 to 3.20) for narcotic opioid exposure and 3.30 (95% CI, 1.06 to 10.27) for amphetamine exposure when compared with neonates with no alcohol exposure
- The relatively common use of alcohol during pregnancy has important short- and long-term implications for the fetus
  - Both heavy and binge drinking are associated with increased risks of stillbirth and infant mortality according to the Danish National Birth Cohort
    - The risk of stillbirth was studied in 89,201 women (Strandberg-Larsen et al, 2008), and women with three or more binge drinking episodes had an adjusted hazard ratio of 1.56 (95% CI, 1.01 to 2.40) for stillbirth relative to nondrinkers
    - An increased risk of infant mortality among term births relative to nondrinkers was documented among 79,215 women, particularly in the postneonatal period (Strandberg-Larsen et al, 2009)
      - The hazard ratios for infant mortality:
        - For more than four drinks of alcohol per week: 2.71 (95% CI 1.35 to 5.45)
        - For binging on three or more occasions: 1.97 (95% CI 1.10 to 3.54)
      - The hazard ratios for postneonatal mortality:
        - For more than four drinks of alcohol per week: 3.25 (95% CI 1.25 to 8.47)
        - For binging on three or more occasions: 2.41 (95% CI 1.06 to 5.46)
  - Binge or heavy drinking is associated with dysmorphia as well as negative cognitive and behavioral outcomes in children (Bailey et al, 2004)
    - The most severe manifestation is fetal alcohol syndrome (FAS; Table 26-1)
      - Fetal alcohol spectrum disorder (FASD) represents a continuum of adverse congenital outcomes that do not meet the criteria of FAS
      - The prevalence of FAS varies according to different surveys
        - Occurs in 0.2 to 1.5 cases per 1000 live births, accounting for 1000 and 6000 yearly cases within the United States (Bertrand et al, 2005)
        - The prevalence is higher among African Americans and Native Americans compared to Caucasians (Russo et al, 2004)
          - The prevalence is sevenfold higher in African Americans after controlling for frequency of maternal drinking, chronic alcohol problems, and age
          - The rate of FAS per 1000 live births in southwestern Native American communities ranges from 1.3 to 10.6, with an average of 6.1 for FAS and 17.9 for FASD
          - Twenty-five percent of Native American women who deliver a baby with FASD will deliver a second affected baby
          - Genetic polymorphisms, nutritional factors, and other unknown factors may account for these disparities
    - Not all features of FAS diminish as the child matures into adulthood (Spohr et al, 2007)
      - Microcephaly, a smooth philtrum, and thin upper lip do not diminish
      - Short stature and underweight persist in males
      - Affected females tend to have higher body weight in adulthood
      - Behavioral problems, intellectual disability, and dependent living are all significantly increased in adulthood
  - There is no known threshold dose for which the effect of alcohol on the developing fetus is clearly manifest

---

TABLE 26-1   Diagnosis of Fetal Alcohol Syndrome

Fetal alcohol syndrome (FAS) is diagnosed after birth with documentation of:

1. Three facial abnormalities: smooth philtrum, thin vermilion border and small palpebral fissures (all must be present)
2. Central nervous system abnormalities (either structural, neurologic, or functional deficits)
3. Deficit in growth (height or weight less than 10th percentile) identified at least once and adjusted for age, sex, gestational age, race, and ethnicity

Children who do not meet the full criteria for FAS should be considered for fetal alcohol disorder spectrum (FADS).

- Because alcohol use during pregnancy, including binge drinking, is common, alcohol is an important preventable cause of birth defects

UPDATE #2

To reduce the prevalence of alcohol use during pregnancy and its sequelae, efforts have been made to screen and educate women about alcohol use during pregnancy (Floyd et al, 2005). Recent evidence suggests that screening and brief interventions may be beneficial. Chang et al. (2005) conducted a randomized trial of a single session brief intervention among 304 women and their partners. These women had an affirmative response to at least two of four questions encompassing the T-ACE alcohol screen (Table 26-2) while initiating prenatal care at a clinic, faculty, or private group practice affiliated with the Brigham and Women's Hospital in Boston. Both the women and their partners received separate interventions. For the women, the single session brief intervention included three short assessments: (1) to estimate daily alcohol intake during the 6 previous months, (2) to assess the temptation to drink and ability to abstain when presented with 20 common situations, and (3) to ask participants to answer "true" or "false" on seven statements about healthy habits during pregnancy. Their partners received a single-session brief intervention comprising four short assessments: (1) a survey about healthy habits, (2) nine questions by the National Institute on Alcohol Abuse and Alcoholism about use of alcohol in the previous 30 days, (3) questions about the partner's alcohol consumption over the previous 90 days, and (4) a survey asking participants to answer "true" or "false" on seven statements about healthy habits during pregnancy. Notably, pregnant women with the highest alcohol intake reduced their drinking most significantly, and this effect was significantly enhanced with partner participation. A study by Rayburn et al. emphasized that maternal awareness of pregnancy itself was insufficient to limit alcohol consumption among women who drank frequently or in binges. Among such women, more than half (52.3%) continued to drink beer, even after they had recognized their own pregnancies (Rayburn et al, 2006).

SMOKING DURING PREGNANCY

- Tobacco smoke increases the risks of poor fetal growth and preterm birth
  - A study of 7098 pregnancies in The Netherlands (Jaddoe et al, 2008) reported that smoking was associated with low birthweight (aOR 1.75, 95% CI 1.20, 2.56) and preterm birth (aOR 1.36, 95% CI 1.04, 1.78)
    - Smoking more than nine cigarettes per day after 25 weeks' gestation was associated with an even greater risk of low birthweight (aOR 3.39, 95% CI 1.45, 7.91) and preterm birth (aOR 2.52, 95% CI 1.36, 4.67)
    - Passive smoking of >3 hours per day was associated with a significantly elevated risk of low birthweight (4.10, 95% CI 1.81, 9.27] but not preterm birth
- Bernstein et al. (2005) reported that smoking during the third trimester was the strongest predictor of birth weight percentile
  - The marginal effect on fetal growth for each additional daily cigarette was a 27-gram reduction in birth weight
- The negative impact on fetal growth contributes to the increased incidence of fetal growth restriction among women who smoke
  - Bada et al. (2002) reported an attributable risk of approximately 14% for smoking on fetal growth restriction
- The degree of fetal growth deficit is not only influenced by the amount of smoking, but also by the fetal genotype
  - Fetuses with the GSTT1 deletion in the *CYP1A1 gene* had a significantly greater reduction in birth weight compared to fetuses without the GSTT1 deletion, among which the effect of smoking was not significant (Aagaard-Tillery et al, 2010)
- Smoking increases the risk of wound complications after cesarean delivery (Avila et al, 2006)
- Quitting smoking reduces the risks of delivering a preterm or small for gestational age (SGA) infant (Polakowski et al, 2009)
  - Quitting during the first trimester reduced the risks to levels that were statistically insignificant from the levels of pregnant women who did not smoke
    - Preterm birth aOR 0.69 (95% CI 0.65 to 0.74)
    - SGA infant aOR 0.47 (95% CI 0.40 to 0.55)
    - The risk reductions for smoking cessation during the second trimester were less remarkable compared to the effects of stopping in the first trimester, but they were nonetheless significant
- The American College of Obstetricians and Gynecologists (ACOG) encourages the use of the five "A's" as an initial intervention (Table 26-3)
  - This counseling intervention works best with women smoking fewer than 20 cigarettes a day (American College of Obstetricians and Gynecologists, 2005)
- Counseling alone may not be completely effective in 80% of pregnant women who smoke (Crawford et al, 2008)
- ACOG recommends that pharmacotherapy be considered when nonpharmacologic methods have been unsuccessful (American College of Obstetricians and Gynecologists, 2005)
- Multimodal pregnancy interventions can reduce smoking among pregnant women better than a single intervention
- Cochrane Database Systematic Review of 72 trials involving interventions to promote quitting smoking during pregnancy (Lumley et al, 2009):
  - Low birth weight, relative risk of 0.83 (95% CI 0.73 to 0.95)
  - Preterm birth, relative risk of 0.86 (95% CI 0.74 to 9.98)

TABLE 26-2   T-ACE Screening Instrument for Alcohol Use during Pregnancy

A number of screening instruments exist, but the T-ACE screen was designed for use in pregnant women (Chiodo et al, 2010). The T-ACE screen encompasses four questions:

1. T (tolerance): How many drinks does it take to make you feel high?
2. A (annoyed): Have people annoyed you by criticizing your drinking?
3. C (cut-down): Have you ever felt you ought to cut down on your drinking?
4. E (eye-opener): Have you ever had a drink first thing in the morning to steady your nerves or to get rid of a hangover?

Two points are assessed if the answer to "T" is more than two drinks, whereas one point is assessed for an affirmative response to "A," "C," or "E." A total score of two points or more is considered positive.

UPDATE #3

A recent randomized controlled trial of a 6-week treatment plan with 2 mg of nicotine gum or placebo, followed by a 6-week taper period, resulted in significantly fewer cigarettes smoked per day (−5.7 versus −3.5, p = 0.035) and greater birth weights (3267 grams versus 2950 grams, p < 0.001), even though quit rates were not increased (Oncken et al, 2008). Unfortunately, recent data indicate that pregnant women are reluctant to try smoking cessation medications, especially if they lack health insurance (Rigotti et al, 2008). In the study by Rigotti et al., 29.3% reported that their obstetric provider discussed a cessation medication during pregnancy, but only 10.8% used either nicotine replacement (7.4%) or bupropion (3.4%) during pregnancy. Additionally, of the 29.4% of women who received counseling about smoking cessation medication at their postpartum visit, fewer than half actually used the medication postpartum. Cessation rates have been reported to be higher (14% versus 5%, p < 0.0001) when patients are invited to join a multimodal smoking cessation program, which included nicotine replacement therapy as one option, as compared to controls who received standard counseling as part of prenatal care (Hegaard et al, 2003).

COCAINE USE DURING PREGNANCY

- Cocaine is the hydrochloride salt of the benzoylmethylecgonine alkaloid and is inhaled
- "Crack" is a lower-purity derivative that is usually smoked after rederiving the alkaloid
  - A rock of impure cocaine is dissolved in water in the presence of heat and a base, such as baking soda
    - "Crack" refers to the sound made during the heating process
- Purity varies greatly and impurities pose additional toxicity risks
  - Cocaine is "cut" with adulterants in order to increase profit margins
    - Adulterants include other medications, chemicals or household products
    - A study in France showed that the median cocaine content in samples obtained from users was only 22% (Evrard et al, 2010)
- Cocaine prevents presynaptic reuptake of sympathomimetic neurotransmitters such as norepinephrine, dopamine, and serotonin
  - Stimulation of the central nervous and cardiovascular systems leads to the following:
    - Euphoria or agitation
    - Hyperactivity
    - Mydriasis
    - Tachycardia
    - Hypertension
  - Toxicity may manifest as follows:
    - Chest pain
    - Arrhythmias
    - Myocardial infarction
    - Seizures
    - Stroke
    - The risk of maternal death is more than doubled (Wolfe et al, 2005)
- Maternal vasoconstriction and hypertension are associated with placental abruption
  - The risk of abruption is increased 5- to 10-fold among cocaine users (Oyelese et al, 2006)
  - Abruption is related to the increased risk of stillbirth
- Cocaine readily crosses the placenta and has a direct fetal vasoactive effect, leading to vascular disruptions that may affect fetal growth and development
  - Prenatal cocaine use has been associated with intrauterine growth deficits (Bada et al, 2002; Bandstra et al, 2001)
  - The effect on growth has been detectable as late as 7 to 10 years of age (Richardson et al, 2007)

TABLE 26-3 The Five "A's" for Screening for Tobacco in Pregnancy

A (Ask): Inquire about smoking using a multiple-choice question:
1. "I have NEVER smoked or have smoked FEWER THAN 100 cigarettes in my lifetime."
2. "I stopped smoking BEFORE I found out I was pregnant, and I am not smoking now."
3. "I stopped smoking AFTER I found out I was pregnant, and I am not smoking now."
4. "I smoke some now, but I have cut down on the number of cigarettes I smoke SINCE I found out I was pregnant."
5. "I smoke regularly now, about the same as BEFORE I found out I was pregnant."
If the patient answers affirmatively to statement B or C, reinforce this decision by congratulating her and encouraging her to avoid smoking. However, if statement D or E is chosen, document this in the record and proceed to the next question.

A (Advise): Clearly and strongly counsel the patient to quit by personalizing the benefits this decision will have for the woman and her baby, both before and after birth.

A (Assess): Determine the patient's willingness to quit within the next 30 days. If she is unwilling to quit, provide information to motivate her to quit and revisit her decision at subsequent prenatal care visits. If she is willing to cut down, encourage this decision but emphasize that stopping completely will maximize the benefits for pregnancy. If she is willing to quit, proceed to Assist.

A (Assist): During this 3-minute intervention, pregnancy-specific, self-help smoking cessation information is provided to the patient, as well as social support emphasizing assistance in helping her to quit smoking. Also help to identify social support within the patient's group, including family and friends, to act as allies in her goal of stopping smoking. Problem-solving tactics for smoking cessation are also encouraged, such as identifying stressful situations associated with smoking, as well as how to cope with such stress.

A (Arrange): Determine whether the patient remains smoke-free at follow-up prenatal visits. Always encourage her to avoid tobacco.

Adapted from Melvin CL, Dolan-Mullen P, Windsor RA, et al: Recommended cessation counseling for pregnant women who smoke: a review of the evidence. *Tobacco Control* 9(Suppl III):iii80-iii84, 2009.

- The bulk of studies appear to indicate little if any increased risk for congenital anomalies
  - A meta-analysis from 2001 of 33 studies (Addis et al, 2001) found significance only for placental abruption and premature rupture of membranes, but not major malformations
  - A prospective, longitudinal cohort reported that cocaine-exposed babies were significantly more likely to be premature and have smaller birth weights, lengths, and head circumferences, but there were no difference in rates of congenital malformations (Behnke et al, 2001)
- The differential diagnosis for any pregnant woman who presents with hypertension must include stimulant (cocaine or methamphetamine) intoxication
  - Hydralazine or labetalol can be used to treat cocaine-induced hypertension that is severe (Kuczkowski, 2007)
- Depletion of catecholamine neurotransmitters results in a "crash" on withdrawal, as well as the subsequent psychological manifestations
  - The crash is marked by increasing depression and somnolence
  - Psychological manifestations during late withdrawal include the following:
    - Severe agitation or psychosis
    - Paranoia
    - Formication

UPDATE #4

Recent data suggest that cognitive deficits and neurobehavioral defects may be detectable into childhood. A review of the effects of prenatal cocaine exposure from 32 studies reported significant negative associations with sustained attention and behavioral control, after controlling for potential confounders (Ackerman et al, 2010). Effects on executive function (Warner et al, 2005) and IQ have also been reported. In particular, 9-year-olds with prenatal cocaine exposure had poorer perceptual reasoning IQ that was related to birth head circumference at birth (Singer et al, 2008). Even in adolescence, subjects with prenatal cocaine exposure were reported to show significantly reduced global cerebral blood flow by functional magnetic resonance imaging (MRI) compared to matched controls (Rao et al, 2007).

METHAMPHETAMINE USE DURING PREGNANCY

- Signs and symptoms of methamphetamine intoxication and withdrawal are similar to those of cocaine
- Methamphetamine is an N-methylated amphetamine, remarkable for its increased lipid-solubility and ease in crossing the blood-brain barrier
  - Approximately 75% of women smoke the crystal form, whereas 20% use methamphetamine intravenously and 5% take oral forms
  - MDMA (3,4-methylenedioxy-N-methylamphetamine) is an oral methamphetamine analogue also called "Ecstasy"

It is reputed to enhance empathy and friendliness

- The prevalence of methamphetamine use by pregnant women has increased dramatically

- Methamphetamine use accounted for 24% of pregnant women admitted in 2006, up from 8% in 1994 (Terplan et al, 2009)
  - Methamphetamine is now the primary substance used by pregnant women who were in treatment for substance abuse
- Cox et al. (2008) used the Nationwide Inpatient Sample to show that the hospitalization rate for amphetamine use doubled from 1998 to 2004
- Methamphetamine use adversely affects fetal growth and neonatal neurobehavioral measures
  - The risk of delivering a small for gestational age (SGA) neonate is 3.5 times greater with methamphetamine use (Smith et al, 2006)
  - Newborns assessed with the NICU (neonatal intensive care unit) Network Neurobehavioral Scale showed increased physiologic stress, poorer quality of movement, and decreased arousal, with a dose response for stress correlating with values for a methamphetamine metabolite in their meconium (Smith et al, 2008)

UPDATE #5

Pregnant women who use methamphetamine are more likely to be of a lower socioeconomic status and to experience higher rates of pregnancy complications and adverse outcomes. In 2006, 33% of pregnant women using methamphetamine and seeking treatment were in supervised living situations, 16% were homeless, 88% were unemployed, 16% had psychiatric disorders, and 41% were under criminal justice system referral (Terplan et al, 2009). Compared to pregnant women without a substance abuse diagnosis, women using amphetamines were significantly more likely to have medical or obstetrical complications (Table 26-4). A prospective longitudinal study of methamphetamine use in pregnancy indicated that affected pregnant women were more likely to have tenuous social support and lower quality of life (Derauf et al, 2007). Women who use MDMA (Ecstasy) are more often younger with an unintended pregnancy. MDMA users are also more likely to smoke, drink heavily, and use other drugs of abuse during pregnancy (Ho et al, 2001), and although they tend to stop using MDMA by the second trimester, nearly two thirds continue to drink and nearly half continue to use tobacco and marijuana throughout pregnancy (Moore et al, 2010).

MARIJUANA USE DURING PREGNANCY

- Marijuana is the most commonly used illicit drug during pregnancy
  - A perception that marijuana is a "soft" or safer drug contributes to its relatively high use (Substance Abuse and Mental Health Services Administration, 2009)
  - Estimates of its prevalence during pregnancy vary by trimester (Substance Abuse and Mental Health Services Administration, Office of Applied Studies, 2009)
    - 4.6% during the first trimester
    - 2.9% in the second trimester
    - 1.4% during the third trimester
    - Use rises to 3.8% within 3 months of delivery
      - Women resume using marijuana soon after giving birth

TABLE 26-4 **Adjusted Prevalence Ratios for Women Who Abuse Amphetamines during Pregnancy Compared to Non-Substance-Abusing Pregnant Women**

Select Medical Conditions among Nondelivery Hospitalizations	Prevalence Ratio	95% Confidence Interval
Psychiatric disorders	22.04	18.28-26.56
Hepatitis	19.59	13.75-27.91
Epilepsy, convulsions	4.54	3.20-6.45
Injury	2.98	2.16-4.10
Cardiovascular disorders	2.91	2.21-3.82
Anemia	2.32	1.85-2.92
Hypertension complicating delivery	1.71	1.35-2.17
Urinary tract infections	1.66	1.37-2.01

Select Obstetrical Conditions among Delivery Hospitalizations	Prevalence Ratio	95% Confidence Interval
Placental abruption	4.48	3.94-5.09
Preterm birth	2.45	2.26-2.65
Fetal demise	2.24	1.66-3.01
Precipitous labor	2.15	1.89-2.46
Hypertension complicating pregnancy	1.62	1.45-1.79
Placenta previa	1.58	1.10-2.27
Premature rupture of membranes	1.35	1.18-1.55
Poor fetal growth	1.30	1.05-1.60

Data from Cox S, Posner SF, Kourtis AP, Jamieson DJ: Hospitalizations with amphetamine abuse among pregnant women, *Obstet Gyncol* 111: 341-347, 2008.

- Education level and being in a relationship with a substance abuser are significant risk factors for maternal use in pregnancy (El Marroun et al, 2008; van Gelder et al, 2010)
  - Use of marijuana by the father of the fetus (OR 38.56, 95% CI 26.14 to 58.88) was the most significant risk factor for use during pregnancy (El Marroun et al, 2008)
  - Continued use during pregnancy was primarily determined by a low education level (OR 3.22, 95% CI 1.54 to 6.74) (El Marroun et al, 2008)
  - Other risk factors identified include the following:
    - Unemployed with low income; underweight; concurrent use of alcohol, tobacco, or both (van Gelder et al, 2010)
    - Childhood trauma and delinquency (El Marroun et al, 2008)
    - Use was not associated with maternal age in El Marroun et al. (2008), but younger age was associated with marijuana use in van Gelder et al. (2010)
    - Bessa et al. (2010) reported that the use of marijuana by younger pregnant women is thought to be underreported
- Marijuana is usually smoked for its hallucinogenic properties
- The clinical presentation may be complex because of the propensity of marijuana users to use other substances during pregnancy (Kuczkowski, 2007)
  - Signs of acute marijuana use include the following:
    - Euphoria or anxiety
    - Tachycardia
    - Conjunctival congestion

OPIOID ABUSE DURING PREGNANCY

- Opioid abuse during pregnancy comprises both the abuse of prescription medication as well as the use of illicit forms, such as heroin
  - "Opioid" is the more general term and includes synthetic forms
  - "Opiate" generally implies forms derived from the alkaloid of opium poppy, such as opium, morphine, and heroin (Trescot et al, 2008)

UPDATE #6

Although the lipid-soluble active ingredient (δ9-tetrahydrocannabinol) easily crosses the maternal-fetal interface, most studies show no effect on obstetric and neonatal outcomes (Schempf, 2007). A recent case-control study of data from the National Birth Defects Prevention Study involving 15,208 mothers showed no significant associations between marijuana and malformations (van Gelder et al, 2009), nor was there an association with low birth weight or preterm birth among women from the same study who were interviewed regarding substance use (van Gelder et al, 2010). However, neonates born to women using only marijuana during pregnancy have been reported to show neurobehavioral changes with increased excitability and arousal compared to non-exposed newborns (Carvalho de Moraes Barros M et al, 2006). The effect of marijuana may even persist into childhood. In one study, schoolchildren at 6 years of age who were born to women who smoked one or more marijuana cigarettes in the first trimester were significantly more likely to have lower verbal reasoning scores on the Stanford-Binet Intelligence Scale. Babies born to second-trimester users had lower composite, short-term memory, and quantitative scores, whereas third-trimester use was associated with lower quantitative scores (Goldschmidt et al, 2008).

- Opioid intoxication is indicated by the following:
  - Decreased consciousness leading to coma
  - Respiratory depression
  - Pupillary miosis
  - Euphoria
  - Conjunctival injection
  - Severe intoxication may lead to arrhythmias and seizures
- Withdrawal begins within approximately 12 hours for short-acting opioids and 30 hours for methadone
  - Early symptoms of withdrawal include the following:
    - Agitation
    - Anxiety
    - Diaphoresis
    - Lacrimation
    - Insomnia
    - Yawning
  - Late symptoms of withdrawal include the following:
    - Abdominal cramping
    - Diarrhea
    - Nausea and vomiting
    - Goose bumps
    - Pupillary dilation
- Adverse health and social consequences of illicit opioid use include the following:
  - Viral and bacterial infections (hepatitis, soft tissue, endocarditis, tuberculosis, STDs)
  - Concurrent abuse of other substances

TABLE 26-5   Protocol for Initiation of Methadone Maintenance Therapy

1. Pregnant women desiring methadone maintenance therapy are admitted to the hospital.
2. Patients are thoroughly assessed, and an ultrasound examination is performed to confirm gestational age.
3. Fetal surveillance is performed once the gestation reaches viability.
4. Methadone is initiated at a usual initial dosage of 10 to 30 mg, divided into two daily doses. The lower dose is appropriate for short-acting oral opioids (codeine, hydrocodone, oxycodone).
5. Only methadone is approved for use in pregnancy; therefore, buprenorphine-maintained pregnant patients who do not refuse methadone can be transferred to methadone (for 2 to 4 mg buprenorphine, begin 20 mg of methadone; for 6 to 8 mg buprenorphine, begin 30 mg of methadone; for 8 mg of buprenorphine or more, begin 40 mg of methadone).
6. The methadone dosage is increased by 5 mg every 6 hours as needed, based on symptoms at peak methadone levels (2 to 4 hours after a dose).
7. Steady-state levels require 4 to 5 days to be reached, so the dose should be increased gradually to prevent overdose and the patient monitored at least 7 days to ensure she is not overmedicated.
8. The optimal dose is where there are no withdrawal or overmedication symptoms for at least 24 hours after a dose, and the woman uses no other opioid and feels minimal or no cravings.
9. A urinary toxicologic screen is performed every morning or if there is suspicion of illicit drug use or evidence of intoxication.
10. Patients are discharged with follow-up support services and a urinary toxicologic screen at each prenatal care visit.

Adapted from Jones HE, Martin PR, Heil SH, et al: Treatment of opioid-dependent pregnant women: clinical and research issues, *J Subst Abuse Treat* 35:245-259, 2008.

- An increased maternal mortality rate
- Higher rates of unemployment, prostitution, and criminal activity leading to criminal justice system referral
- Tendency to progress from intermittent use to dependence, notable for tolerance and the development of withdrawal symptoms
- Risks specific to pregnancy include the following:
  - Inadequate prenatal care (Kaltenbach et al, 1998)
  - Greater rates of obstetrical and fetal complications including the following (Bell et al, 2008):
    - Placental abruption
    - Preterm birth
    - Small for gestational age
    - Prolonged neonatal stay
    - Stillbirth
    - Neonatal death
  - Fetal withdrawal, marked by hyperadrenergic excitation and elevated amniotic fluid norepinephrine levels (Zuspan et al, 1975)
- In an effort to ensure more stable serum levels in the opioid-dependent mother, avoid withdrawal in the fetus, and reduce adverse outcomes, methadone maintenance therapy (MMT) has become widely employed (Table 26-5)
  - In nonpregnant adults, MMT reduces the rates of adverse health and social consequences described earlier
  - The NIH National Consensus Development Panel on Effective Medical Treatment of Opioid Addiction (1999) noted that MMT had been shown to decrease obstetrical and fetal complications
    - Specific benefits of MMT during pregnancy include the following:
      - Increased duration of gestation
      - Higher birth weight
      - Facilitation of prenatal care via participation in a methadone program
    - It is recommended that opioid-dependent pregnant women be offered MMT
- Some studies have compared methadone maintenance to maintenance with buprenorphine, but the Cochrane

Database concludes that more studies are needed (Minozzi et al, 2008)
- Several studies suggest that methadone detoxification in pregnancy may be safely performed, but detoxification during pregnancy remains controversial
  - Opioid detoxification during pregnancy was first reported in the 1960s (Blinick et al, 1969); however, it fell out of favor after Zuspan et al. (1975) associated withdrawal with elevated amniotic fluid catecholamines
  - Maas et al. (1990) reported on a maternal detoxification program in which 17 of 75 women in a methadone program underwent successful detoxification prior to delivery, which was associated with longer duration of pregnancy, normal birth weights, normal head circumferences, and a lower incidence of neonatal abstinence syndrome (NAS) (55% versus 88%, $p < 0.05$)
  - Dashe et al. (1998) reported the results of a trial for methadone detoxification in pregnancy, in which patients admitted to an intensive inpatient program safely underwent methadone detoxification in pregnancy
  - Luty et al. (2003) reported that methadone detoxification during pregnancy is not associated with an increased risk of second-trimester miscarriage or third-trimester preterm delivery
  - Some authorities caution against reducing the methadone dose during pregnancy given the clear benefits of MMT and the lack of a dose-response relationship between methadone and NAS reported in some studies (Berghella et al, 2003); thus, opioid detoxification during pregnancy remains controversial
- In labor, patients should continue MMT if possible; however, this is insufficient for pain relief (Jones et al, 2008)
  - Women on MMT may receive an epidural, but nalbuphine (Nubain) and butorphanol (Stadol) may precipitate withdrawal and are avoided
  - Postdelivery, pain is managed with opioids in combination with acetaminophen and a nonsteroidal anti-inflammatory drug (NSAID)

- Postcesarean patients on MMT required 70% higher doses of opioids compared to nondependent controls, especially in the first 24 hours, but opioid utilization after vaginal delivery was similar to controls despite higher pain scores (Meyer et al, 2007)
- Breast-feeding is recommended in postpartum women maintained on methadone (Jansson, 2008)

UPDATE #7

Since the 1970s, some authors have associated the development or severity of neonatal withdrawal (called neonatal abstinence syndrome [NAS]) with the maternal methadone dose, whereas other authors have found no correlation. Review of the literature published since the early 2000s indicates that this controversy remains unresolved. Dashe et al. (2002) reported that maternal methadone dosage was associated with the duration of neonatal hospitalization, NAS scores, and need for neonatal treatment. Reducing the methadone dosage as part of a methadone detoxification program decreased the incidence and severity of neonatal withdrawal. However, Berghella et al. (2003) and McCarthy et al. (2005) did not find a correlation between maternal dose and the need for treatment for NAS, nor was a correlation found between maternal dose and NAS scores or length of neonatal treatment (Berghella et al, 2003). To explain these discrepant findings, Dashe et al. (2004) theorized that at lower maternal methadone doses there is a positive correlation between dose and neonatal withdrawal, but above a certain threshold there is no longer a dose-response relationship. As Dashe et al. (2004) described, some older data support this theory. In several of these older studies, in which pregnant women were on relatively lower doses of methadone (<40 mg per day), a positive association between increasing methadone dose and NAS was reported. More recent studies have made comparisons using even higher doses, and the controversy remains unresolved. Lim et al. (2009) reported that higher doses (71 to 139 mg per day and ≥140 mg per day) actually correlated with significantly increased rates of treatment for NAS and length of hospital stay, with every 5.5 mg increase of methadone dose statistically associated with one additional day of neonatal treatment for NAS. In another study of a maternal population taking an average methadone dose of 64 mg per day, Wouldes et al. (2010) found that methadone doses of less than 59 mg per day correlated with need for treatment and the duration of neonatal hospitalization. These two studies contrast with two other studies in maternal populations taking average doses of 90 mg and 127 mg per day (Bakstad et al, 2009, and Seligman et al, 2008, respectively), which reported that methadone dose at delivery did not correlate with duration of treatment for NAS. In yet

another study (Velez et al, 2009) of a population with a mean methadone dose of 75.6 mg per day, maternal methadone dose did not correlate with NAS scores. However, 27.3% of mothers in this study were also taking selective serotonin reuptake inhibitor (SSRI) medications, potentially affecting neonatal neurobehavioral measures. Thus, confounding and conflicting data make interpretation of these various studies difficult.

SUGGESTED READINGS

Perinatal Substance Abuse

Substance Abuse and Mental Health Services Administration: *Results from the 2008 national survey on drug use and health: national findings, Office of Applied Studies,* Rockville, MD, 2009, National Survey on Drug Use and Health (NSDUH) Series H-36, HHS Publication No. SMA 09-4434).

Alcohol Use

Centers for Disease Control: Alcohol use among pregnant and nonpregnant women of childbearing age: United States, 1991-2005, *MMWR* 58(19): 529–532, 2009.
Chang G, McNamara TK, Orav EJ, et al: Brief intervention for prenatal alcohol use: A randomized trial, *Obstet Gynecol* 105(5 Pt 1):991–998, 2005.
Floyd RL, O'Connor MJ, Sokol RJ, et al: Recognition and prevention of fetal alcohol syndrome, *Obstet Gynecol* 106(5 Pt 1):1059–1064, 2005.

Smoking

American College of Obstetricians and Gynecologists: ACOG committee opinion no. 316, October 2005. Smoking cessation during pregnancy, *Obstet Gynecol* 106(4):883–888, 2005.

Cocaine Use

Bada HS, Das A, Bauer CR, et al: Gestational cocaine exposure and intrauterine growth: maternal lifestyle study, *Obstet Gynecol* 100(5 Pt 1):916–924, 2002.

Methamphetamine Use

Cox S, Posner SF, Kourtis AP, et al: Hospitalizations with amphetamine abuse among pregnant women, *Obstet Gynecol* 111(2 Pt 1):341–347, 2008.

Marijuana Use

Schempf AH: Illicit drug use and neonatal outcomes: a critical review, *Obstet Gynecol Surv* 62(11):749–757, 2007.
Substance Abuse and Mental Health Services Administration, Office of Applied Studies: *The NSDUH [National Survey on Drug Use and Health] Report: substance use among women during pregnancy and following childbirth,* Rockville, MD, May 21, 2009.

Opioid Abuse

Jones HE, Martin PR, Heil SH, et al: Treatment of opioid-dependent pregnant women: clinical and research issues, *J Subst Abuse Treat* 35(3):245–259, 2008.

References

Please go to expertconsult.com to view references.

Chapter 27

Neoplasia in Pregnancy

KRISHNANSU S. TEWARI

KEY UPDATES

1   Cervical neoplasia remains the most common malignancy diagnosed in pregnancy.

2   In 2006, the American Society for Colposcopy and Cervical Pathology (ASCCP) updated its recommendations for cervical cancer screening in pregnancy and management of cervical intraepithelial neoplasia (CIN) and adenocarcinoma in situ (AIS) in pregnancy.

3   The safe performance of CO_2 laser cervical conization for CIN3/carcinoma in situ (CIS) and microinvasive carcinoma during the second trimester has been reported.

4   Vaginal delivery may result in a regression of CIN.

5   A deliberate delay in therapy to permit gestational advancement is acceptable for most cases of pregnancy complicated by early-stage cervical carcinoma with no evidence of nodal involvement.

6   Radical trachelectomy with or without laparoscopic pelvic lymph node dissection has been safely performed during pregnancy for early-stage cervical carcinoma.

7   Neoadjuvant chemotherapy may be administered during the second trimester and early third trimester to control tumor spread in cases of locally advanced cervical carcinoma.

8   Because of the risks of obstructed labor, hemorrhage, possible lymphatic dissemination of tumor, and tumor implantation in the episiotomy site, vaginal delivery is contraindicated in patients diagnosed with invasive cervical cancer.

9   Cesarean section with radical hysterectomy and bilateral pelvic lymphadenectomy remains the treatment of choice with documented fetal pulmonary maturity between 34 and 36 weeks' gestational age.

10   Most adnexal masses in pregnancy do not require antepartum surgical intervention.

11   Laparoscopic evaluation of adnexal masses may be safely performed between 16 and 20 weeks of gestation.

12   Serum CA-125 is elevated during the first trimester but may be useful in evaluating an adnexal mass or the response to therapy for ovarian cancer during the second and third trimesters.

13   The chemotherapy regimen consisting of bleomycin, etoposide, and cisplatin (BEP) may be used after the first trimester to treat patients with malignant germ cell tumors of the ovary.

14   Platinum- and taxane-based chemotherapy regimens may be used after the first trimester to treat patients with epithelial ovarian carcinoma.

15   Sentinel lymph node biopsy may be carried out safely in patients with pregnancy-associated breast cancer (PABC) after the first trimester when performed with a low-dose lymphoscintigraphic technique.

16   The FAC regimen (5-fluorouracil, doxorubicin, cyclophosphamide) and taxanes have been administered during the second and third trimesters for patients with PABC and have been generally well tolerated with no significant adverse fetal/neonatal effects.

17   The use of targeted agents such as trastuzumab has been associated with congenital anomalies in the fetus, and its elective use is discouraged.

18 Tamoxifen has documented teratogenic effects when used during pregnancy, and its elective use is discouraged.

19 The two main anthracyclines used to treat acute leukemias, daunorubicin and idarubicin, have both been associated with a high incidence of fetal malformations, even if given after the first trimester, and should be avoided; doxorubicin could serve as an alternative.

20 Patients with Hodgkin's lymphoma (HL) and non-Hodgkin lymphoma (NHL) can be electively treated with the ABVD (doxorubicin, bleomycin, vinblastine, and dacarbazine) or CHOP (cyclophosphamide, doxorubicin, vincristine, and prednisone) regimens after the first trimester; the addition of rituximab for pregnant women with B-cell lymphomas can also be considered.

21 Although no reported adverse fetal effects have been associated with interferon therapy for melanoma during the second trimester, experience with this drug in pregnancy is limited.

22 When melanoma involves the placenta, the risk for fetal metastases is approximately 22%.

23 In cases of twin pregnancy with a complete hydatidiform mole and coexisting live fetus, continuation of pregnancy is acceptable with a normal fetal karyotype, no anomalies, no early preeclampsia, and declination of hCG levels; the risk of persistent trophoblastic disease may rise to 30%.

Abnormal Cervical Cytology

CLINICAL PROFILE

- Pregnancy represents an ideal period during which cervical cancer screening can occur, as women in childbearing age are often healthy and may not undergo regular screening because they may not have annual well-woman visits
- Approximately 5% of Papanicolaou tests performed during pregnancy are abnormal
- The majority of patients with abnormal cervical cytology are asymptomatic

UPDATE #1
Cervical neoplasia remains the most common malignancy diagnosed in pregnancy (Tewari, 2011).

DIAGNOSIS

- Papanicolaou screening is performed as in the nonpregnant patient
- Liquid-based or conventional Pap tests are appropriate in pregnancy
- Reflex high-risk human papilloma virus (HR-HPV)testing can be performed for atypical cells of undetermined significance (ASCUS) Pap tests
- Co-testing with HR-HPV can be performed for women over age 30
- Human papilloma virus (HPV) genotyping may be performed for women with normal Pap tests who are found to be HR-HPV positive
- Patients infected with the human immunodeficiency virus (HIV) should undergo more frequent screening (e.g., every 6 months) as in the nonpregnant state
- Patients should undergo Pap testing during their prenatal visit and at 6 weeks postpartum

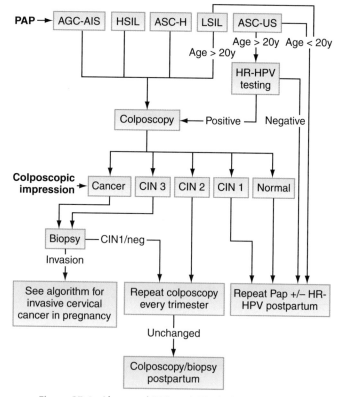

Figure 27-1. Abnormal PAP and CIN during pregnancy.

MANAGEMENT OF ABNORMAL CERVICAL CYTOLOGY (Figure 27-1)

- HPV negative ASCUS may have repeat screening postpartum
- HPV positive/normal Pap with negative HPV 16/18 genotyping may undergo repeat testing postpartum or in 1 year

- HPV positive-normal Pap with positive HPV 16/18 genotyping should undergo colposcopy
- HPV positive ASCUS should undergo colposcopy
- Patients with low-grade squamous intraepithelial lesions (LSIL), high-grade squamous intraepithelial lesions (HSIL), or cytologic findings suggestive of CIS or squamous cell carcinoma should undergo colposcopy
- Patients with atypical glandular cells (AGUS) or cytologic findings suggestive of AIS or adenocarcinoma should undergo colposcopy (see the section on AIS and Cervical Carcinoma)
- Colposcopy in pregnancy is best performed by an expert colposcopist familiar with the physiologic changes that occur in the pregnant cervix

UPDATE #2

In 2006, the American Society for Colposcopy and Cervical Pathology (ASCCP) updated its recommendations for cervical cancer screening in pregnancy and management of cervical intraepithelial neoplasia (CIN) and adenocarcinoma in situ (AIS) in pregnancy (Wright et al, 2007).

Cervical Intraepithelial Neoplasia (CIN)

CLINICAL PROFILE OF CIN

- Median age is similar as in nonpregnant populations (i.e., 29 years for CIN 3)
- Usually asymptomatic
- Risk factors include early onset of sexual activity, multiple sexual partners, promiscuous partner, history of sexually transmitted diseases (STDs), tobacco use, immunosuppression
- HPV 16 and HPV 18 are most common

DIAGNOSIS OF CIN

- Colposcopic findings suggestive of CIN1-3 may include raised, irregular acetowhite epithelium, punctuation, mosaicism, and abnormal vessels
- Lugol's solution may be helpful in delineating lesions
- The single most concerning area/lesion identified should be biopsied with alligator jaw (gold handle) forceps
- Random biopsies for patients with negative findings on colposcopy as well as for those in whom the colposcopy is considered inadequate are not indicated
- Endocervical curettage is contraindicated during pregnancy

MANAGEMENT OF CIN (See Figure 27-1)

- Expectant management during pregnancy is acceptable for CIN1-3 and CIS
- In patients for whom there is no concern for microinvasion, serial colposcopy during pregnancy (e.g., every trimester) is not necessary
- Definitive management of CIN/CIS should be deferred to the postpartum period in most cases
- Local excision (e.g., wedge excision or shallow "coin" biopsy) can be performed for patients with CIN3 or CIS for whom there is a concern for microinvasion based on either colposcopic or pathologic findings

UPDATE #3

The safe performance of CO_2 laser cervical conization for CIN3/CIS and microinvasive carcinoma during the second trimester has been reported (Tsuritani et al, 2009).

- Cervical conization by the "cold knife" technique is contraindicated in pregnancy
- Vaginal delivery is not contraindicated in patients with CIN1-3 or CIS

UPDATE #4

Vaginal delivery may result in regression of CIN (Ueda et al, 2009).

Adenocarcinoma in Situ (AIS)

CLINICAL PROFILE OF AIS

- Usually asymptomatic
- AGUS Pap may suggest diagnosis
- Risk factors similar to those for CIN and also include possible estrogen exposures
- HPV 16 and HPV 18 are most common

DIAGNOSIS OF AIS

- Colposcopic-directed biopsy for AGUS or other abnormal Pap/HR-HPV testing
- Other procedures performed in the nonpregnant state for evaluation of atypical glandular cells of undetermined significance (AGUS) Pap are contraindicated during pregnancy (e.g., endocervical curettage (ECC), cold knife conization, large loop excision of the transformation zone (LLETZ), hysteroscopy, dilation and curettage [D&C])
- Differential diagnosis includes the following:
  - Adenocarcinoma in situ of the uterine cervix
  - Adenocarcinoma of the uterine cervix (usual type)
  - Adenocarcinoma of the uterine cervix (variant types, e.g., clear cell, adenoma malignum)
  - Clear cell adenocarcinoma of the vagina
  - Bartholin's gland adenocarcinoma
  - Endometrial hyperplasia with or without atypia
  - Endometrial adenocarcinoma (endometrioid type or nonendometrioid type)
  - Adenocarcinoma of the fallopian tube
  - Adenocarcinoma of the ovary

MANAGEMENT OF AIS

- Expectant management during pregnancy is acceptable for AIS
- In patients for whom there is no concern for microinvasion, serial colposcopy during pregnancy (e.g., every trimester) is not necessary
- Definitive management of AIS should be deferred to the postpartum period
- Local excision (e.g., wedge excision or shallow "coin" biopsy) can be performed for patients with AIS for whom there is a concern for microinvasion based on either colposcopic or pathologic findings
- Laser conization has been safely reported during pregnancy and may be considered for patients in whom there is a concern for microinvasion

- Cervical conization by the "cold knife" technique is contraindicated in pregnancy
- Vaginal delivery is not contraindicated in patients with AIS

Invasive Cancer of the Cervix

CLINICAL PROFILE

- Median age similar to nonpregnant (i.e., 45 years)
- Squamous histology 70% to 75%, adenocarcinoma (usual type) 20% to 25%; others 5% (small cell neuroendocrine carcinoma, villoglandular adenocarcinoma, primary cervical lymphoma, etc.)
- Risk factors similar to those for CIN/CIS and AIS
- Symptoms as in nonpregnant state; in one study, the presenting symptoms of invasive disease among pregnant women included abnormal vaginal bleeding (63%), vaginal discharge (13%), postcoital bleeding (4%), and pelvic pain (2%)
  - Early-stage disease: asymptomatic or abnormal vaginal discharge or bleeding (e.g., intermenstrual, postcoital, postmenopausal)
  - Locally advanced disease: as stated earlier, plus pelvic pain, lower extremity swelling, leg pain, blocked kidney, hematuria, rectal bleeding, vesicovaginal or rectovaginal fistulae
  - Metastatic disease: all of the symptoms previously stated plus hemoptysis, supraclavicular adenopathy, bone pain

DIAGNOSIS AND CLINICAL STAGING OF CERVICAL CARCINOMA

- International Federation of Gynecology and obstetrics (FIGO) staging system also applies in pregnancy
  - Cervical biopsy, history, and physical examination (including bimanual and rectovaginal pelvic examination), serum chemistry, urinalysis, cystoscopy, proctoscopy, and chest radiograph with abdominal shielding are appropriate during pregnancy
- To avoid risks of ionizing radiation exposure to the fetus, ultrasonography may be used to evaluate the kidneys for hydronephrosis, and magnetic resonance imaging (MRI) of the pelvis can be used to assess parametrial extension of the tumor

MANAGEMENT (Figure 27-2)

- Multidisciplinary team should be assembled: gynecologic oncologist, perinatologist, obstetrician, anesthesiologist, neonatologist, pathologist, radiologist, labor and delivery nurse, others as needed (medical social worker, hospital ethics committee representative, etc.)
- FIGO stage IA1 (early stromal invasion): pregnancy may proceed safely to term with route of delivery determined by obstetric indications

> **UPDATE #5**
>
> A deliberate delay in therapy to permit gestational advancement is acceptable for most cases of pregnancy complicated by early-stage cervical carcinoma without evidence of nodal involvement (Morice et al, 2009).

- FIGO stage IA2-IB1: pregnancy may proceed and corticosteroids administered to enhance fetal pulmonary maturation; at approximately 34 to 35 weeks' gestational age, with a mature fetal lung profile on amniocentesis, a cesarean section (C/S) with immediate radical hysterectomy and bilateral pelvic lymphadenectomies is recommended; the surgical option is preferred over pelvic radiation therapy because of the overall result, which includes

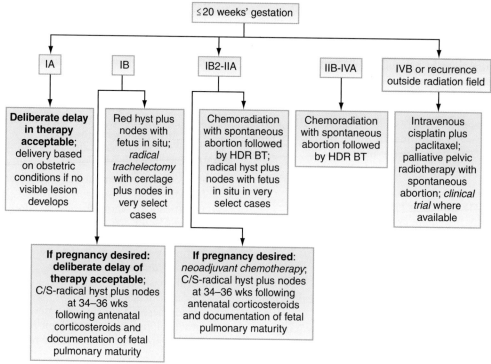

Figure 27-2. Invasive cervical carcinoma under 20 weeks' gestation.

ovarian preservation, improved sexual function, and elimination of unnecessary delays in treatment

UPDATE #6
Radical trachelectomy with or without laparoscopic pelvic lymph node dissection has been safely performed during pregnancy for early-stage cervical carcinoma (van de Nieuwenhof et al, 2008).

UPDATE #7
Neoadjuvant chemotherapy may be administered during the second trimester and early third trimester to control tumor spread in cases of locally advanced cervical carcinoma (Karam et al, 2007; Tewari et al, 1998).

- FIGO stage IB2-IVA: C/S with radical surgery is an option for IB2 and IIA lesions, but the probability of needing adjuvant pelvic radiation or chemoradiation therapy is high; for patients with FIGO stage IIB-IVA, chemoradiation is standard of care and should be started without regard to the pregnancy if the fetus is previable (a viable fetus may be delivered via hysterotomy at the earliest time when pulmonary maturation can be documented)
- Following the onset of radiotherapy, spontaneous abortion occurs at about 35 days in the first trimester and at approximately 45 days in the second trimester

UPDATE #8
Because of the risks of obstructed labor, hemorrhage, possible lymphatic dissemination of tumor, and tumor implantation in the episiotomy site, vaginal delivery is contraindicated in patients diagnosed with invasive cervical cancer (Baloglu et al, 2007).

UPDATE #9
Cesarean section with radical hysterectomy and bilateral pelvic lymphadenectomy remains the treatment of choice with documented fetal pulmonary maturity between 34 to 36 weeks' gestational age (Hunter et al, 2008).

- Recurrence at the episiotomy site is associated with a poor prognosis, which is another reason why C/S delivery is indicated if the diagnosis (FIGO stage IA2 and above) is made antenatally; patients diagnosed with cervical cancer during the postpartum period should have vigilant examination of the episiotomy and any vaginal laceration sites
- Patients with advanced disease (i.e., FIGO stage IB2 and above) should be offered immediate therapy; those who refuse may be treated with neoadjuvant chemotherapy (vincristine 1 mg/m2 plus cisplatin 50 mg/m2) during the second and early third trimesters in an effort to control the cancer and possibly even shrink the primary lesion
- Overall prognosis for all stages of cervical cancer in pregnancy is similar to that in nonpregnant women; the favorable overall prognosis for pregnant patients is related to a greater proportion of pregnant patients with stage I disease
- Clinical stage remains the most important determinant of prognosis

Ovarian Cancer

CLINICAL PROFILE
- Median age (nonpregnant): 65 (epithelial malignancies); 19 (malignant germ cell tumors)
- No screening test in the general population
- Symptoms: bloating with abdominal/pelvic discomfort/pressure/pain

Shortness of breath, bowel/bladder dysfunction in some
- Etiology unknown
- Breast cancer (BRCA) gene and MSH/MLH mutations account for up to 10% (epithelial cancers)
- Oral contraceptives (OCPs), pregnancy, lactation protective (epithelial cancers)

DIFFERENTIAL DIAGNOSIS (TEWARI ET AL, 1998)
- Luteoma of pregnancy
- Theca-lutein cyst
- Dermoid cyst (most common neoplasm)
- Other benign: Brenner tumor, fibrothecoma, ovarian pregnancy
- Tumor of low malignant potential
- Sex cord-stromal tumors (granulosa cell tumor, Sertoli-Leydig cell tumor)
- Malignant germ cell tumor of the ovary

Dysgerminoma (most common malignant neoplasm)
- Epithelial carcinoma

DIAGNOSIS
- Epithelial carcinomas: most present with advanced stage disease (FIGO III/IV)
- Malignant germ cell tumors: majority FIGO stage I
- Dysgerminoma most common in pregnancy
- Tumor markers: CA-125, carcinoembryonic antigen (CEA) (epithelial); human chorionic Gonadotropin (hCG), alpha fetoprotein (AFP) (malignant germ cell tumors)
- Preoperative imaging: abdominal and pelvic ultrasonography, magnetic resonance imaging (MRI), chest radiograph (CXR), with abdominal shielding

MANAGEMENT (Figure 27-3)
- Size of the adnexal mass at time of diagnosis is inversely related to the likelihood of spontaneous regression
- Adnexal masses greater than 6 cm that persist into the second trimester may warrant removal at approximately 18 weeks' gestational age if there are associated maternal symptoms or suspicious findings on ultrasonography (e.g., solid components, excrescences, abnormal blood flow, nodules), development of metastases (e.g., ascites, omental caking), or significant elevations in serum tumor markers

UPDATE #10
Most adnexal masses in pregnancy do not require antepartum surgical intervention (Leiserowitz, 2006).

- Exploratory surgery around the 18th week of gestation has minimal associated fetal wastage
- Whenever exploration is conducted, the uterus should not be manipulated during surgery ("hands off the uterus" approach) in an effort to minimize its irritability

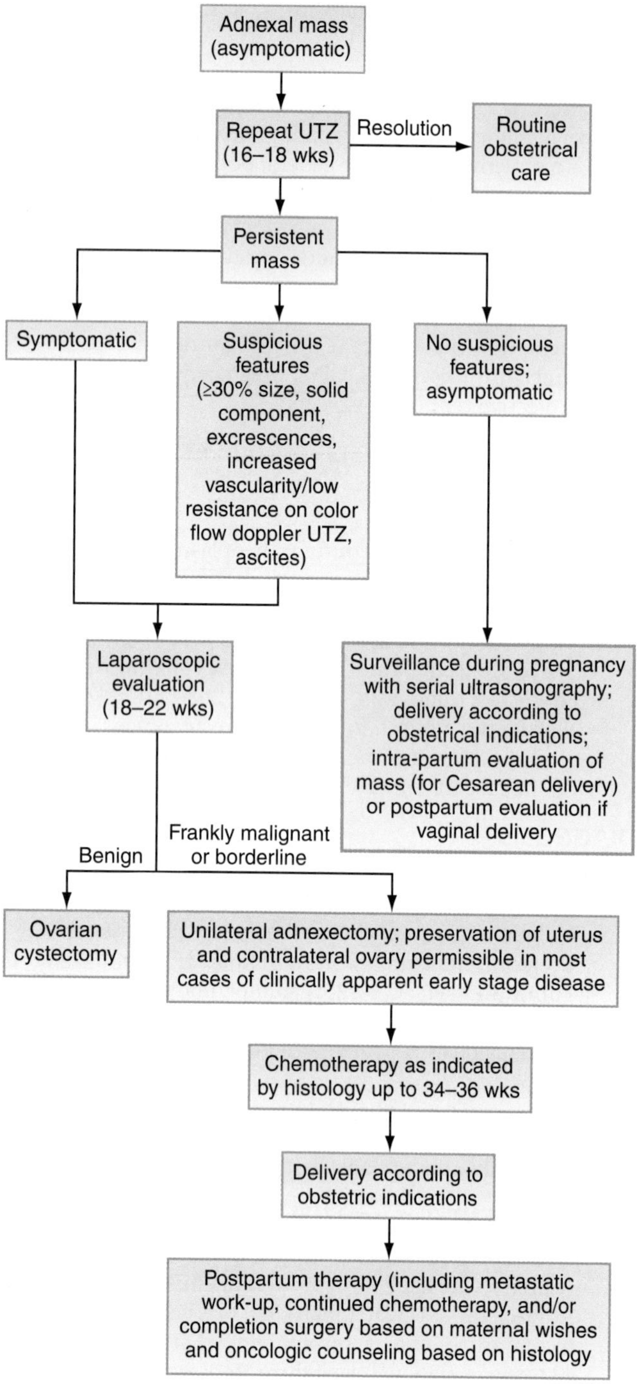

```
        Adnexal mass
        (asymptomatic)
             │
             ▼
      ┌──────────────┐   Resolution   ┌──────────┐
      │  Repeat UTZ  │ ─────────────▶ │ Routine  │
      │  (16–18 wks) │                │obstetrical│
      └──────────────┘                │   care   │
             │                        └──────────┘
             ▼
        Persistent
          mass
```

Figure 27-3. Pelvic mass and ovarian cancer during pregnancy.

- Use of tocolytics such as indomethacin may be useful in reducing the risk of miscarriage

UPDATE #11

Laparoscopic evaluation of adnexal masses may be safely performed between 16 to 20 weeks of gestation (Whiteside et al, 2009).

- Laparoscopic evaluation
- Sixteen to 20 weeks
- Tilt table to left or right with patient supine to move uterus away from site of trocar insertion

- Left upper quadrant or subxyphoid insertion of trocar with at least 6 cm from point of entry and top of fundus
- Open Hasson technique preferred
  - Veress technique has been used successfully (ultrasound guidance; elevation of abdominal wall during insertion)
  - Intra-abdominal pressure kept below 15 mmHg with patient in Trendelenburg position to ensure adequate venous return and uteroplacental blood flow during surgery
  - Positive pressure ventilation to maintain adequate lung volumes as needed
  - Fetal monitoring if indicated

UPDATE #12

Serum CA-125 is elevated during the first trimester, but it may be useful in evaluating an adnexal mass or the response to therapy for ovarian cancer during the second and third trimesters (Marret et al, 2010).

- If a malignant ovarian neoplasm is found at the time of abdominal exploration, the surgeon's first obligation is to properly stage the disease, allowing for preservation of the uterus and contralateral ovary (if these structures do not appear to be involved by the cancer) in most cases
  - In presumed clinical stage I disease:
    - Unilateral adnexectomy
    - Infracolic omentectomy
    - Pelvic and para-aortic lymph node sampling
    - Abdominal and pelvic peritoneal biopsies
    - Four-quadrant abdominal and pelvic washings
    - Appendectomy (for mucinous lesions)
- Malignant germ cell tumors of the ovary

UPDATE #13

The chemotherapy regimen consisting of bleomycin, etoposide, and cisplatin (BEP) may be used after the first trimester to treat patients with malignant germ cell tumors of the ovary (Ghaemmaghami et al, 2009).

- Combined chemotherapy has improved survival markedly for malignant germ cell ovarian tumors and can permit preservation of childbearing capacity as well as maintenance of the existing pregnancy (stage I and most cases > stage I)
- Sex cord-stromal tumors
- Adjuvant chemotherapy during pregnancy not indicated
- Behave as they do in nonpregnant women, presenting with early-stage disease and having a slow, low-grade, and indolent course
- Epithelial tumors
- Borderline tumors (low malignant potential [LMP]): cystectomy/unilateral salpingo-oophorectomy (USO) only
- Epithelial carcinomas
  - Once the diagnosis of epithelial ovarian cancer (i.e., carcinoma) is made during pregnancy, appropriate therapy should not be withheld

- Patients remote from term (e.g., during the first trimester) with metastatic disease should be advised to undergo hysterectomy with the fetus in situ in conjunction with tumor debulking

UPDATE #14

Platinum- and taxane-based chemotherapy regimens may be used after the first trimester to treat patients with epithelial ovarian carcinoma (Modares Gilani et al, 2007).

- Because there does not appear to be any significant risk to the fetus when ovarian cancer chemotherapy drugs (e.g., platinum and taxanes) are used in the second and third trimesters, pregnant patients diagnosed during these periods should be offered the opportunity to receive platinum-based therapy without terminating their pregnancy, even in the setting of advanced-stage disease
- Pregnancy does not alter the prognosis of most ovarian malignant neoplasms, but complications such as torsion and rupture may increase the incidence of spontaneous abortion or preterm delivery

Breast Cancer

CLINICAL PROFILE

- Pregnancy-associated breast cancer (PABC) is defined as breast cancer diagnosed during pregnancy or lactation up to 12 months postpartum
- PABC is the second most common malignancy to complicate pregnancy but, unlike cervical cancer, it is not screened for during pregnancy, and because delays in diagnosis are common and the diagnosis itself is elusive, oftentimes patients are diagnosed with advanced tumors for which prognosis is poor
- A delay of 2 to 15 months longer from manifestation of the first symptoms to the diagnosis of cancer occurs in PABC most commonly
- Hormonal factors to be taken into consideration when dealing with PABC include the effect of a recent antecedent pregnancy on prognosis, influence on breast-feeding, estrogen receptor and progesterone receptor status, tamoxifen use, prophylactic oophorectomy, and pregnancy termination
- PABC has been considered an ominous diagnosis, but when age and stage are taken into account there is no difference in the survival of PABC cases as compared with non-PABC cases

DIFFERENTIAL DIAGNOSIS

- Lactating adenoma
- Fibroadenoma
- Fibrocystic disease
- Lobular hyperplasia
- Galactocele
- Abscess
- Lipoma
- Hamartoma
- Carcinoma

DIAGNOSIS AND STAGING

- Ultrasonography is the preferred imaging modality because of the radiodensity of the breast in the pregnant or lactating patient
- Approximately 75% to 90% of PABCs are ductal carcinomas, mirroring what is observed in the nonpregnant population
- Clinicopathologic factors
  - Estrogen receptor and progesterone receptor status
  - Human epidermal growth factor receptor-2 (Her-2)/neu
  - Oncotype Dx
  - Serum tumor markers: CA 27-29, CEA
- Magnetic resonance imaging (MRI)
  - Preferred to ultrasonography for hepatic imaging
- Safest and most sensitive imaging modality to study the brain

MANAGEMENT (Figure 27-4)

- Therapeutic abortion is not currently believed to be an essential component of effective treatment for early disease, despite the theoretic advantage of removing the source of massive estrogen production
- Lumpectomy or partial mastectomy is more commonly used, especially when the lesion is not large, although the preferred surgical treatment for stage I, stage II, and some stage III tumors involves mastectomy, thus avoiding the need for adjuvant radiotherapy in most cases (i.e., early-stage breast cancer)
- Circumareolar incisions are associated with diminished ability to lactate because such incisions interrupt a large number of major milk ducts; radial incisions in the breast interrupt fewer ducts but may be cosmetically inferior
- To avoid the development of a hernia in the abdominal wall at the donor site, an interval of at least 12 months between breast reconstruction with a transverse rectus abdominis myocutaneous (TRAM) flap and pregnancy is recommended

UPDATE #15

Sentinel lymph node biopsy may be carried out safely in patients with pregnancy-associated breast cancer (PABC) when performed with a low-dose lymphoscintigraphic technique (Gentilini et al, 2010).

- Most reports of chemotherapy use during pregnancy for PABC are associated with favorable neonatal outcomes, provided that it is administered after the first trimester

UPDATE #16

The FAC regimen (5-fluorouracil, doxorubicin, cyclophosphamide) and taxanes have been administered during the second and third trimesters for patients with PABC and have been generally well tolerated with no significant adverse fetal/neonatal effects (Azim et al, 2010).

UPDATE #17

The use of targeted agents such as trastuzumab has been associated with congenital anomalies in the fetus, and its elective use is discouraged (Beale et al, 2009).

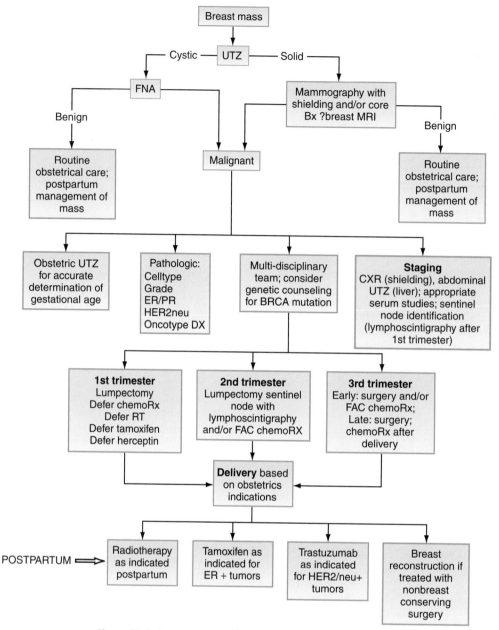

Figure 27-4. Breast mass and breast cancer during pregnancy.

- Trastuzumab use during pregnancy has been associated with oligohydramnios/anhydramnios, fetal renal/respiratory failure, and neonatal death

UPDATE #18

Tamoxifen has documented teratogenic effects when used during pregnancy, and its elective use is discouraged (Tewari et al, 1997).

- Tamoxifen use during pregnancy has been associated with ambiguous genitalia and Goldenhar syndrome (deformities of the face)
- Women treated with adjuvant radiation during the postpartum period will not be able to lactate from the irradiated breast
- For those who continue to ovulate and who desire future childbearing, it has been common practice to recommend a waiting period of 2 years following the diagnosis of breast cancer before attempting to conceive, as most recurrences take place within the first 2 years of diagnosis
- It would appear that future pregnancies are safe for the mother unless she has an estrogen receptor-positive tumor and has not been placed into remission; conversely, if a pregnancy occurs, there appears to be no justification for recommending its termination in patients without evidence of recurrence
- Women with PABC have the same survival stage for stage as do nonpregnant women with breast cancer

Leukemia

CLINICAL PROFILE

- Acute leukemia: 1 in every 10,000 pregnancies
- Acute myeloid leukemia (AML): 60%

- Acute lymphoblastic leukemia (ALL)
- Acute promyelocytic leukemia (APL)
- In pregnancy, persistent fever, weight loss, lymphadenopathy, or an abnormal differential on the complete blood count should raise suspicion for leukemia

MANAGEMENT

- High risk of pregnancy-associated complications because of the high risk of bleeding and infection

UPDATE #19

The two main anthracyclines used to treat acute leukemias, daunorubicin and idarubicin, have both been associated with a high incidence of fetal malformations, even if given after the first trimester, and should be avoided; doxorubicin could serve as an alternative (Azim et al, 2010).

- Patients with acute leukemia are often very ill, and the primary concern is to save the mother's life through induction of chemotherapy or radiotherapy
- Early pregnancy diagnosis: should counsel for immediate termination
- Later in pregnancy: may be offered chemotherapy if willing to keep the pregnancy

Hodgkin's Disease

CLINICAL PROFILE

- The nodular sclerosis subtype of Hodgkin's disease is the most common subtype encountered in pregnancy and carries a favorable prognosis
- Pregnancy does not appear to adversely affect the course of the disease, and interruption of pregnancy is not indicated in most cases
- Pregnant women with Hodgkin's lymphoma present with typical manifestations, with painless enlargement of lymph nodes above the diaphragm (e.g., cervical, submaxillary, or axillary nodes)

MANAGEMENT

- Single agent vinblastine can be used to control the disease and is associated with a 7% anomaly rate when administered during the first trimester; it should be continued until significant disease progression

UPDATE #20

Patients with Hodgkin's lymphoma (HL) and non-Hodgkin's lymphoma (NHL) can be electively treated with the ABVD (doxorubicin, bleomycin, vinblastine, and dacarbazine) or CHOP (cyclophosphamide, doxorubicin, vincristine, and prednisone) regimens after the first trimester; the addition of rituximab for pregnant women with B-cell lymphomas can also be considered (Azim et al, 2010).

- Delivery should be delayed as long as possible after the last dose of chemotherapy (before the next dose) to decrease the risk of marrow suppression in the neonate
- Umbilical cord blood should be collected at delivery and stored as a possible source of human leukocyte antigen-compatible stem cells

- If treatment is necessary during the second and third trimesters of pregnancy, the standard ABVD regimen (doxorubicin, bleomycin, vinblastine, dacarbazine) should be used
- The inverted Y field for radiation therapy is not an option at any time during pregnancy
- When evaluating young women with Hodgkin's disease for whom preservation of ovarian function is desired and pelvic irradiation is planned, surgical oophoropexy can be performed at the time of staging laparotomy
- The ovaries can be brought as close to the midline as possible behind the uterus where they can be shielded underneath a protective block placed between the two arms of the Y during radiation therapy following delivery

Non-Hodgkin's Lymphoma

CLINICAL PROFILE

- In NHL, the high incidence of breast, uterine, cervical, and ovarian involvement noted among pregnant women has been attributed to hormonal influences and increased blood flow to those organs

MANAGEMENT

- When NHL complicates pregnancy, a delay in treatment cannot be justified, and a woman who has not completed the first half of pregnancy should be advised to undergo therapeutic abortion unless she is willing to expose herself and her fetus to the risks of combination chemotherapy
- Because high-dose methotrexate is an integral component of many effective regimens for Burkitt lymphoma, therapeutic abortion for women diagnosed in the first trimester is essential

Melanoma

CLINICAL PROFILE

- The incidence of melanoma is rising with approximately 10,000 cases occurring annually among women aged 20 to 40 years
- The Clark microstaging classification provides a histologic staging scheme for classifying melanomas on the basis of level of penetration of the melanoma under the dermis
- The average age of the patient with melanoma is 45 years, and 35% of women will be diagnosed during childbearing years
- Myths about melanoma in pregnancy include the beliefs that pregnancy increases the risk of developing melanoma, pregnancy worsens prognosis, future pregnancies adversely affect prognosis and risk of recurrence, and oral contraceptives and hormone replacement therapy in women with a history of melanoma are contraindicated—none of these claims are substantiated by the medical literature

MANAGEMENT

- A changing skin lesion should be subjected to excisional biopsy
  - Early diagnosis of stage I disease will often lead to curative therapy

- Irrespective of pregnancy, treatment of melanoma is related to depth of invasion and stage
- Lesions less than 1 mm in thickness usually require a wide deep excision with a 1-cm margin, and those between 1 and 4 mm need a 2-cm margin
- Wide, deep local excision can be performed safely under 30 weeks' gestation, and for those beyond 30 weeks' gestation, sentinel node identification can be offered after delivery
- Melanomas constitute nearly 50% of all tumors that metastasize to the placenta and account for nearly 90% of those that metastasize to the fetus

UPDATE #21

Although no reported adverse fetal effects have been associated with interferon therapy for melanoma during the second trimester, experience with this drug in pregnancy is limited (de Carolis et al, 2006).

- Pregnant women with advanced or recurrent disease should undergo ultrasound examination during pregnancy for assessment of any obvious fetal tumor masses
- Attention should be directed to placental thickness as well as to the fetal liver and size of the fetal spleen
- Contemporary studies note no survival difference in patients with melanoma who are pregnant compared with nonpregnant patients
- Multivariate analyses demonstrated that the stage of diseased at diagnosis, and not the pregnancy, is the only consistent finding that influences prognosis
- Pregnancy does not confer a worse prognosis for melanoma when matched for stage of disease
- At delivery, cord blood should be examined for malignant cells and the placental tissue should be sent for detailed pathologic evaluation

Placental and Fetal Metastases

CLINICAL PROFILE

- Melanoma is the most common cancer to metastasize to the placenta and fetus

UPDATE #22

When melanoma involves the placenta, the risk for fetal metastases is approximately 22% (Alexander et al, 2003).

- In order of frequency: melanomas (30%), breast cancer (18%), other hematologic malignancies (13%)
- In the setting of confirmed placental metastases or in cases of maternal breast cancer, hematopoietic malignancy, or melanoma concomitant with pregnancy, an MRI of the brain and postpartum computed tomography (CT) scans of the chest, abdomen, and pelvis are advisable
- Metastatic disease to the products of conception predicts an ominous course for the mother
- The prognosis for the infant has been excellent with 53 of the reported cases revealing no evidence of disease in the baby

MANAGEMENT

- Any child born to a mother with active or suspected malignancy should initially have a thorough physical examination with a complete blood count, comprehensive metabolic panel, liver function tests, coagulation battery, serum lactate dehydrogenase (LDH), and uric acid levels, and urinalysis
- The placenta should be macroscopically and microscopically examined for tumor involvement

Gestational Trophoblastic Disease

CLINICAL PROFILE

- Presenting symptoms of a complete hydatidiform mole with coexisting fetus is similar to that which is seen with complete hydatidiform moles alone (i.e., size greater than dates, abnormal vaginal bleeding)
- A twin pregnancy with a complete hydatidiform mole and coexisting fetus may be diagnosed later in gestational age (e.g., 20 weeks versus 13 weeks), have a higher preevacuation β-hCG level, and have a greater propensity to develop persistent gestational trophoblastic neoplasia necessitating chemotherapy

MANAGEMENT

- Once fetal anomalies and an abnormal karyotype are excluded, the literature supports continuing the pregnancy provided there is no evidence of preeclampsia and the mother strongly wishes to do so

UPDATE #23

In cases of twin pregnancy with a complete hydatidiform mole and coexisting live fetus, continuation of pregnancy is acceptable with a normal fetal karyotype, no anomalies, no early preeclampsia, and declination of hCG levels; the risk of persistent trophoblastic disease may rise to 30% (Dolapcioglu et al, 2009).

- The overall risk of developing persistent gestational trophoblastic neoplasia (GTN) is 33% irrespective of whether the pregnancy is terminated or carried to viability or term
- The major obstacles to continuing the pregnancy are the development of a paraneoplastic medical complication, catastrophic vaginal hemorrhage, and formation of metastatic foci antenatally

SUGGESTED READINGS

General

Amant F, van Calsteren K, Vergote I, et al: Gynecologic oncology in pregnancy, *Crit Rev Oncol Hematol* 67(3):187–195, 2008.

Azim HA Jr, Peccatori FA, Pavlidis N: Treatment of the pregnant mother with cancer: a systematic review on the use of cytotoxic, endocrine, targeted agents and immunotherapy during pregnancy. Part I: solid tumors, *Cancer Treat Rev* 36(2):1010–1019, 2010.

Berman ML, Di Saia PJ, Tewari KS: Pelvic malignancies, gestational trophoblastic neoplasia, and nonpelvic malignancies. In Creasy RK, Resnik R, editors: *Maternal-fetal medicine: principles and practice*, ed 5, Philadelphia, 2004, Saunders, pp 1213–1242.

Doyle S, Messiou C, Rutherford JM, et al: Cancer presenting during pregnancy: radiological perspectives, *Clin Radiol* 64(9):857–871, 2009.

Luis A, Christie DR, Kaminski A, et al: Pregnancy and radiotherapy: management options for minimizing risk, case series and comprehensive literature review, *J Med Imaging Radiat Oncol* 53(6):559–568, 2009.

Oto A, Ernst R, Jesse MK, et al: Magnetic resonance imaging of the chest, abdomen, and pelvis in the evaluation of pregnant patients with neoplasms, *Am J Perinatol* 24(4):243–250, 2007.

Tewari KS: Cancer in pregnancy. In Di Saia PJ, Creasman WT, editors: *Clinical gynecologic oncology*, ed 8, St. Louis, 2011, Mosby Elsevier, 405–478.

Cervical Cancer

Baloglu A, Uysal D, Aslan N, Yigit S: Advanced stage of cervical carcinoma undiagnosed during antenatal period in term pregnancy and concomitant metastasis on episiotomy scar during delivery: A case report and review of the literature, *Int J Gynecol Cancer* 17(5):1155–1159, 2007.

Hunter MI, Monk BJ, Tewari KS: Cervical neoplasia in pregnancy. Part 1: screening and management of preinvasive disease, *Am J Obstet Gynecol* 199(1):3–9, 2008.

Hunter MI, Tewari K, Monk BJ: Cervical neoplasia in pregnancy. Part 2: current treatment of invasive disease, *Am J Obstet Gynecol* 199(1):10–18, 2008.

Karam A, Feldman N, Hoschneider CH: Neoadjuvant cisplatin and radical cesarean hysterectomy for cervical cancer in pregnancy, *Nat Clin Pract Oncol* 4(6):375–380, 2007.

Morice P, Narducci F, Mathevet P, et al: French recommendations on the management of invasive cervical cancer during pregnancy, *Int J Gynecol Cancer* 19(9):1638–1641, 2009.

Tewari K, Cappuccini F, Gambino A, et al: Neoadjuvant chemotherapy in the management of locally advanced cervical carcinoma in pregnancy: a report of two cases and review of issues specific to the management of cervical cancer in pregnancy, including, planned delay of therapy, *Cancer* 82(8):1529–1534, 1998.

Tsuritani M, Watanabe Y, Kotani Y, et al: Retrospective evaluation of CO_2 laser conization in pregnant women with carcinoma in situ or microinvasive carcinoma, *Gynecol Obstet Invest* 68(4):230–233, 2009.

Ueda Y, Enomoto T, Miyatake T, et al: Postpartum outcome of cervical intraepithelial neoplasia in pregnant women determined by route of delivery, *Reprod Sci* 16(11):1034–1039, 2009.

van de Nieuwenhof HP, van Ham MA, Lotgering FK, et al: First case of vaginal radical trachelectomy in a pregnant patient, *Int J Gynecol Cancer* 18(6):1381–1385, 2008.

Wright TC Jr, Massad LS, Dunton CJ, et al: 2006 consensus guidelines for the management of women with abnormal cervical screening tests, *J Low Genit Tract Dis* 11(4):201–222, 2007.

Wright TC Jr, Massad LS, Dunton CJ, et al: 2006 consensus guidelines for the management of women with cervical intraepithelial neoplasia or adenocarcinoma in situ, *J Low Genit Tract Dis* 11(4):223–239, 2007.

Ovarian Cancer

Ghaemmaghami F, Abbasi F, Abadi AG: A favorable maternal and neonatal outcome following chemotherapy with etoposide, bleomycin, and cisplatin for management of grade 3 immature teratoma of the ovary, *J Gynecol Oncol* 20(4):257–259, 2009.

Marret H, Lhomme C, Lecuru F, et al: Guidelines for the management of ovarian cancer during pregnancy, *Eur J Obstet Gynecol Reprod Biol* 149(1):18–21, 2010.

Modares Gilani M, Karimi Zarchi M, Behtash N, et al: Preservation of pregnancy in a patient with advanced ovarian cancer at 20 weeks' gestation: case report and literature review, *Int J Gynecol Cancer* 17(5):1140–1143, 2007.

Leiserowitz GS, Zing G, Cress R, et al: Adnexal masses in pregnancy: how often are they malignant? *Gynecol Oncol* 101(2):315–321, 2006.

Whiteside JL, Keup HL: Laparoscopic management of the ovarian mass: a practical approach, *Clin Obstet Gynecol* 52(3):327–334, 2009.

Breast Cancer

Beale JM, Tuohy J, McDowell SJ: Herceptin (trastuzumab) therapy in a twin pregnancy with associated oligohydramnios, *Am J Obstet Gynecol* 201(1):e13–e14, 2009.

Gentilini O, Cremonesi M, Toesca A, et al: Sentinel lymph node biopsy in pregnant patients with breast cancer, *Eur J Nucl Med Mol Imaging* 37(1):78–83, 2010.

Tewari K, Bonebrake RG, Asrat T, Shanberg AM: Ambiguous genitalia in infant exposed to tamoxifen in utero secondary to inflammatory breast cancer during pregnancy, *Lancet* 350(9072):183, 1997.

Leukemia and Lymphoma

Azim HA Jr, Pavlidis N, Peccatori FA: Treatment of the pregnant mother with cancer: a systematic review on the use of cytotoxic, endocrine, targeted agents and immunotherapy during pregnancy. Part II: hematological tumors, *Cancer Treat Rev* 36(2):110–121, 2010.

Melanoma

de Carolis S, Grimolizzi F, Garofalo S, et al: Cancer in pregnancy: results of a series of 32 patients, *Anticancer Res* 26(3B):2413–2418, 2006.

Placental and Fetal Metastases

Alexander A, Samlowski WE, Grossman D, et al: Metastatic melanoma in pregnancy: risk of transplacental metastases in the infant, *J Clin Oncol* 21(11):2179–2186, 2003.

Gestational Trophoblastic Neoplasia

Dolapcioglu K, Gungoren A, Hakverdi S, et al: Twin pregnancy with a complete hydatidiform mole and co-existent live fetus: two case reports and review of the literature, *Arch Gynecol Obstet* 279(3):431–436, 2009.

References

Please go to expertconsult.com to view references.

Chapter 28

Obesity and Pregnancy

D. YVETTE LACOURSIERE

KEY UPDATES

1   New Institute of Medicine (IOM) weight gain recommendations have lowered the recommended weight gain in obese pregnant women to 11 to 20 pounds.

2   Obesity increases the risk of fetal neural tube, cardiac, and cleft palate defects.

3   Labor induction, duration of labor, oxytocin requirement, cesarean delivery, and failed vaginal birth after cesarean (VBAC) is increased in obese women.

4   Obese women are more likely to experience mood disturbances during and after pregnancy.

5   Obesity is not an absolute contraindication to physical activity during pregnancy.

6   Bariatric surgery may decrease gestational diabetes, hypertension, pregnancy weight gain, cesarean delivery, and macrosomia.

7   Case reports of gastrointestinal obstruction, hernias, and bleeding, as well as erosion and migration of the band during pregnancy, have been reported in women who have had bariatric surgery. Thus, abdominal pain in this group of women warrants prompt attention.

Obesity and Pregnancy

DIAGNOSIS

- Two thirds of American women are overweight or obese
- The World Health Organization defines normal body mass index (BMI) as between 18.5 and 24.9, overweight as from 25 to 29.9, and obesity as ≥30 (Figure 28-1). Obesity is further classified by severity: class 1 (30 to 34.9), class 2 (35 to 39.9), and class 3 (≥40)
- BMI is reported as kg/m^2 and can be converted by a simple formula (Figure 28-2)
- Weight during pregnancy is described in terms of prepregnancy BMI and gestational weight gain, both of which exert untoward influences on outcomes; maternal obesity is defined as a prepregnancy BMI of ≥30

UPDATE #1

The new Institute of Medicine (IOM) recommendations for weight gain during pregnancy were released in 2009 (Institute of Medicine, 2009). The IOM decreased the recommended amount of weight gained by obese women (Table 28-1) and made no changes in the other categories. These guidelines have elicited some controversies, with prominent clinician researchers suggesting that the decrease in weight gain is insufficient (Artal et al, 2010).

CLINICAL PROFILE

- Obesity increases the risk of multiple obstetric and neonatal complications (Table 28-2), even after controlling for diabetes and hypertension
- Obese women of reproductive age who are considering pregnancy should be advised of the risks of obesity

and encouraged to decrease weight prior to attempting conception

UPDATE #2

Fetal anomalies, particularly neural tube, cardiac, and cleft palate defects, are more common and the ability to detect anomalous fetuses on ultrasound is decreased by at least 20% (Dashe et al, 2009).

UPDATE #3

Labor induction, duration of labor, oxytocin requirement, and cesarean delivery is increased in obese women (Pevzner et al, 2009). Cesarean deliveries occur in up to half of obese women, a rate that increases as BMI increases. VBAC success rate decreases by 20% to 50% in obese women, and a weight gain of over 40 pounds decreases success by 40% (Durnwald et al, 2004).

- Excess weight gain during pregnancy and postpartum retention lead to long-term obesity and related morbidity. Nearly 70% of incident obesity can be prevented with decreasing weight gain during pregnancy

UPDATE #4

Obesity has been associated with psychosocial stressors outside of pregnancy including the following:
- Early traumatic events
- Socioeconomic
- Anxiety, depression, and suicide
- Stigmatization

More recent data suggest that psychosocial stressors also are associated with maternal obesity; specifically depressive symp-

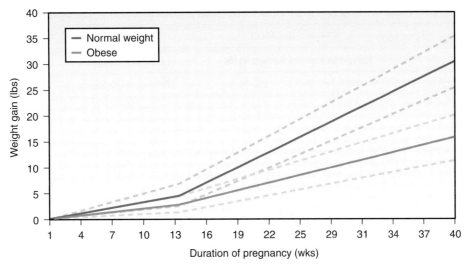

Figure 28-1. Weight gain comparison between normal weight and obese BMI categories. The differences between the median *(solid lines)* and range *(dotted lines)* of recommended weight gain for pregnant women within normal weight (BMI 18.5 to 24.9 kg/m²) and obese (BMI >30 kg/m² categories is shown in this figure. (Data from the Institute of Medicine. Adapted from *Weight gain during pregnancy: reexamining the guidelines. Resource Sheet, 2009* (website). www.iom.edu/~/media/Files/Report%20Files/2009/Weight-Gain-During-Pregnancy-Reexamining-the-Guidelines/Resource%20Page%20-%20Weight%20Gain%20During%20Pregnancy.ashx. Accessed August 2010.)

Pounds/inches calculation:

$$BMI = \frac{Weight\ (lbs.) \times 703}{Height\ (in.)^2}$$

Figure 28-2. BMI is reported as kg/m² and can be converted by this simple formula.

toms during and after pregnancy are more common in obese women (LaCoursiere et al, 2010; Laraia et al, 2009).

- Obesity and breast-feeding discontinuation interact to increase childhood obesity

MANAGEMENT

- Preconceptional counseling for weight loss and increased physical activity are encouraged
- Obtain an early assessment of glucose tolerance (1 hour GTT or fasting plasma glucose with a hemoglobin A1C) and if normal repeat a glucose tolerance test at 24 to 28 weeks (1 hour with subsequent 3 hour GTT if abnormal or 2 hour GTT)
- Consider thyroid stimulating hormone (TSH) and electrocardiogram (EKG) if warranted by clinical symptoms or physical finding
- Screen for depression in the first trimester
- Monitor weight gain and set weight gain goals with the patient

UPDATE #5

Encourage physical activity. Obesity itself is not an absolute contraindication to exercise in pregnancy. Women should be assessed for significant cardiac and pulmonary comorbidities and orthopedic limitations, especially if BMI >40 (Table 28-3). If there are no contraindications, then moderate physical activity of 30 minutes or more, nearly each day of the week, is recommended (American College of Obstetricians and Gynecologists, ACOG Committee Opinion No. 267, 2002). Physical activity has been shown to improve glycemic control in gestational diabetics.

- Avoid labor induction if the woman has an unfavorable cervix
- Obtain anesthesia consult, antepartum, or in early labor
- Close the subcutaneous layer at cesarean delivery, and consider doubling the preoperative antibiotics in women with a BMI >35 or who are >220 lbs
- Apply pneumatic compression devices or heparin for prolonged bed rest and after surgery
- Screen for postpartum depression and breast-feeding difficulties

Impact of Gastric Bypass on Pregnancy Outcomes

- Women should be cautioned to avoid pregnancy in the rapid-weight-loss phase (first 1 to 2 years) after bariatric surgery
- Additional attention should be paid to contraception as conception increases; the effectiveness of the oral contraceptive pill has been reported to decline, possibly secondary to malabsorption; nonoral methods of contraception are preferred after bariatric surgery

UPDATE #6

Overall lower pregnancy complication rates are seen in women who have had bariatric surgery compared to obese women without a history of weight reduction surgery. A decrease is seen in the likelihood of gestational diabetes, hypertension, pregnancy weight gain, cesarean delivery, and macrosomia. In a recent study, the gestational diabetes mellitus (GDM) rates were 22% in obese women and 0% in the post-bariatric-surgery group. Preeclampsia rates were likewise lower, 3% compared to 0%, and no additional risk of low birth weight or premature delivery was identified (Maggard et al, 2008).

UPDATE #7

Exercise caution in women with a history of bariatric surgery and abdominal pain. Early consultation with a bariatric surgeon is warranted. At least 20 reports of pregnancy complications after

TABLE 28-1   New Recommendations for Total and Rate of Weight Gain during Pregnancy, by Pregnancy BMI

Prepregnancy BMI	Total Weight Gain		Rates of Weight Gain*Second and Third Trimester	
	Range in kg	Range in lbs	Mean (range) in kg/week	Mean (range) in lbs/week
Underweight (< 18.5 kg/m²)	12.5-18	28-40	0.51 (0.44-0.58)	1 (1-1.3)
Normal weight (18.5-24.9 kg/m²)	11.5-16	25-35	0.42 (0.35-0.50)	1 (0.8-1)
Overweight (25.0-29.9 kg/m²)	7-11.5	15-25	0.28 (0.23-0.33)	0.6 (0.5-0.7)
Obese (≥ 30.0 kg/m²)	5-9	11-20	0.22 (0.17-0.27)	0.5 (0.4-0.6)

*Calculations assume a 0.5-2 kg (1.1-4.4 lbs) weight gain in the first trimester (based on IOM and NRCC, 2009).
From Institute of Medicine (US) and National Research Council (US) Committee to Reexamine IOM Pregnancy Weight Guidelines: *Weight gain during pregnancy: reexamining the guidelines*, Washington, DC, 2009, National Academics Press.

TABLE 28-2   Maternal and Neonatal Outcomes Associated with Obesity

Preconceptional/Early Antepartum	Postpartum
Decreased fertility(oligo/ anovulation)	Postpartum endometritis
Spontaneous abortion	Depression
Antepartum	
Gestational diabetes	Breast-feeding
Gestational hypertension/ preeclampsia	discontinuation
	Fetal/neonatal
Deep vein thrombosis/ pulmonary emboli	Fetal anomalies (neural tube, cardiac, cleft)
Indicated preterm birth (↓ spontaneous PTB)	Inaccurate ultrasonographic imaging
Intrapartum	Stillbirth
Cesarean delivery	Macrosomia
Failed vaginal birth after cesarean	Childhood obesity
Excess blood loss	
Prolonged operative time	
Wound complications (infection, separation)	
Chorioamnionitis	
Difficult to obtain anesthesia (regional/general endotracheal anesthesia [GETA])	
Anesthesia complications	

TABLE 28-3   Contraindications to Aerobic Exercise during Pregnancy

Absolute	Relative
Hemodynamically significant cardiac disease	Severe anemia
Restrictive lung disease	Unevaluated maternal arrhythmia
Incompetent cervix	Chronic bronchitis
Multiple gestation at risk for premature labor	Poorly controlled type 1 diabetes, seizure disorder, hypertension, hyperthyroidism
Persistent bleeding after the first trimester	
Previa after 26 weeks	Class 3 obesity
Preterm labor (PTL), rupture of membranes (ROM), preeclampsia, gestational hypertension in the current pregnancy	History of extremely sedentary lifestyle
	Orthopedic limitations
	Heavy smoker
Warning signs: vaginal bleeding, dyspnea prior to exertion, dizziness, headache, chest pain, muscle weakness, calf pain and swelling, preterm labor, decreased fetal movement, loss of amniotic fluid	

From American College of Obstetricians and Gynecologists: ACOG committee opinion no. 267: exercise during pregnancy and the postpartum period, *Obstet Gynecol* 99:171-173, 2002.

bariatric surgery have been described, including anastomotic leaks, intestinal obstruction, internal hernias, gastrointestinal bleeding, and erosion and migration of the band. Exploratory surgery is more common in post-bariatric-surgery patients, and it is often associated with a delay in diagnosis (American College of Obstetricians and Gynecologists, Practice Bulletin No. 105, 2009; Kirshtein, 2010).

- Although uncommon, women with a history of bariatric surgery (primarily malabsorptive procedures) are at increased risk of iron deficiency anemia and may be deficient in vitamin B_{12}, calcium, and folic acid. They should be screened each trimester for these insufficiencies and supplemented as needed.

- Rapid release and oral solutions are preferred for supplementation and other medications. Extended release medications should be avoided.

- Secondary to dumping syndrome women may not tolerate a 1-hour glucose test with 50-gram oral load. Alternatively, women can check fasting and postprandial glucoses for 1 to 2 weeks at 24 to 28 weeks for evaluation of glucose tolerance.

- Breast-feeding after bariatric surgery has been associated with nutritional defects in the infant.

SUGGESTED READINGS

Management of Obese Pregnant [Women] (Trends, Gestational Weight Gain, Labor Management)

American College of Obstetricians and Gynecologists: ACOG committee opinion no. 315: obesity in pregnancy, *Obstet Gynecol* 106(3):671–675, 2005.

Artal R, Lockwood CJ, Brown HL: Weight gain recommendations in pregnancy and the obesity epidemic, *Obstet Gynecol* 115(1):152–155, 2010.

Catalano P: Management of obesity in pregnancy, *Obstet Gynecol* 109(2 Pt 1): 419–433, 2007.

Durnwald CP, Ehrenberg HM, Mercer BM: The impact of maternal obesity and weight gain on vaginal birth after cesarean section success, *Am J Obstet Gynecol* 191(3):954–957, 2004.

Flegal KM, Carroll MD, Ogden CL, Curtin LR: Prevalence and trends in obesity among US adults, 1999-2008, *JAMA* 303(3):235–241, 2010.

Institute of Medicine (US) and National Research Council (US) Committee to Reexamine IOM Pregnancy Weight Guidelines: *Weight gain during pregnancy: reexamining the guidelines*, Washington, DC, 2009, National Academies Press.

Juhasz G, Gyamfi C, Gyamfi P, et al: Effect of body mass index and excessive weight gain on success of vaginal birth after cesarean delivery, *Obstet Gynecol* 106(4):741–746, 2005.

Olson CM, Strawderman MS, Hinton PS, Pearson TA: Gestational weight gain and postpartum behaviors associated with weight change from early pregnancy to 1 y postpartum, *Int J Obes Relat Metab Disord* 27(1):117–127, 2003.

Pevzner L, Powers BL, Rayburn WF, et al: Effects of maternal obesity on duration and outcomes of prostaglandin cervical ripening and labor induction, *Obstet Gynecol* 114(6):1315–1321, 2009.

Rooney BL, Schauberger CW, Mathiason MA: Impact of perinatal weight change on long term obesity and obesity related illnesses, *Obstet Gynecol* 106(6):1349–1356, 2005.

Walsh C, Scaife C, Hopf H: Prevention and management of surgical site infections in morbidly obese women, *Obstet Gynecol* 113(2 Pt 1):411–415, 2009.

Obesity and Fetal Anomalies

Dashe JS, Mcintire DD, Twickler DM: Effect of maternal obesity on the ultrasound detection of anomalous fetuses, *Obstet Gynecol* 113(5):1001–1007, 2009.

Obesity and Mood

LaCoursiere DY, Barrett-Connor E, O'Hara MW, et al: The association of obesity and screening positive for postpartum depression, *BJOG* 117(8):1011–1018, 2010.

Laraia BA, Siega-Riz AM, Dole N, London E: Pregravid weight is associated with prior dietary restraint and psychosocial factors during pregnancy, *Obesity* 17(3):550–558, 2009.

Obesity and Physical Activity

American College of Obstetricians and Gynecologists: ACOG committee opinion. no. 267, January 2002: exercise during pregnancy and the postpartum period, *Obstet Gynecol* 99(1):171–173, 2002.

Pregnancy after Bariatric Surgery

American College of Obstetricians and Gynecologists: ACOG practice bulletin no. 105: bariatric surgery and pregnancy, *Obstet Gynecol* 113(6):1405–1413, 2009.

Kirshtein B, Lantsberg L, Mizrahi S, Avinoach E: Bariatric emergencies for non-bariatric surgeons: complications of laparoscopic gastric banding, *Obes Surg* 20(11):1468–1478, 2010.

Maggard MA, Yermilov I, Li Z, et al: Pregnancy and fertility following bariatric surgery, *JAMA* 300(19):2286–2296, 2008.

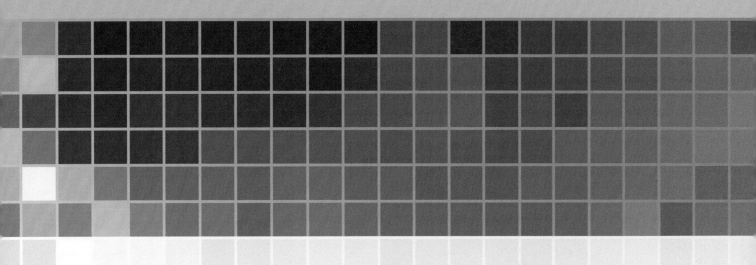

SECTION 7

Reproduction and Fertility

Chapter 29

Management of the Infertile Couple

AMANDA SKILLERN • MARCELLE I. CEDARS

KEY UPDATES

1. Infertility affects approximately one twelfth of couples and is increasingly a problem for older, nulligravid women.

2. Anti-Müllerian hormone (AMH) is the best serum marker of ovarian reserve (or the number of follicles/oocytes available in a given month).

3. Clomiphene citrate is first-line treatment for ovulation induction in anovulatory patients with polycystic ovary syndrome (PCOS).

4. Women with PCOS, and all obese patients, should be encouraged to lose weight prior to attempting fertility.

5. There is no strong evidence to support a relationship between the use of fertility drugs and either breast or ovarian cancer.

6. Submucosal leiomyomata may have a negative impact on implantation, pregnancy rates, and ongoing pregnancy rates. The case is less well documented for intramural myomas.

7. Laparoscopy is no longer part of the standard infertility evaluation. Chlamydia antibody (CAT) and hysterosalpingogram (HSG) should be integrated into the diagnostic evaluation.

8. Male-factor infertility may be impacted by environmental insults.

9. CC-IUI is the first treatment for unexplained infertility. Following failure with clomiphene citrate and intrauterine insemination (CC-IUI), in vitro fertilization (IVF) should be the next step in women <40 years of age to limit risks of multiple gestations and cost.

10. Obesity, for both men and women, may be an important factor negatively affecting spontaneous conception and treatment outcome.

Introduction and Definitions

- Infertility is the inability to achieve a pregnancy in 1 year or 12 ovulatory, exposed, cycles
- Infertility may be primary, with no prior conceptions, or secondary, following a prior conception whether delivered or not
- The inability to carry a pregnancy, pregnancy loss, is a different disease and is covered in the chapter on repetitive pregnancy loss
- Infertility is common, affecting approximately one twelfth of couples; the rate of infertility has not increased and, in fact, may be decreasing (Figure 29-1); the rate of primary infertility (infertility without a prior pregnancy) and the percentage of couples seeking care for infertility have increased
- The increased rate of primary infertility (Figure 29-2) may be due to two factors: a delay in the start of childbearing commensurate with an increase in the rate of infertility with age; these factors may also be contributing to the apparent increase in impaired fecundity (see Figure 29-1), but this finding needs to be further explored

UPDATE #1

Infertility affects approximately one twelfth of couples and is increasingly a problem for older, nulligravid women (Centers for Disease Control and Prevention, 2011). Infertility may be due to abnormalities in ovulation (oocyte production), uterine/tubal/pelvic anatomy, or abnormalities in sperm production.

Ovarian Function

OVARIAN AGING

Chronologic age is the strongest determinant of success for both spontaneous pregnancy and active management in fertility. But within a given age group, individual variability exists, and it has long been a goal to be able to better advise patients as to their likelihood for success and the potential need for more aggressive management.

1. Anti-Müllerian hormone (AMH) as a measure of ovarian aging
   - Menstrual cyclicity and follicle-stimulation hormone (FSH) have traditionally been used as measures of ovarian aging (Soules et al, 2001)

- Elevated FSH alone, however, has been shown to be a poor predictor of future pregnancy, spontaneous or assisted, in younger (<36 years old) women (van Rooij et al, 2004)
- It is unclear how women with signs of diminished ovarian reserve (elevated FSH) who do not meet strict criteria for primary ovarian insufficiency (i.e., amenorrhea plus FSH >40 mIU/nL) should be counseled with regard to fertility treatment
- Novel ovarian markers may be a more sensitive measurement of ovarian reserve (fertility capacity)
- Anti-Müllerian hormone (AMH) is produced by the granulosa cells of the preantral and early antral follicles (Durlinger et al, 2002)
- Unlike FSH, E2, and InhibinB, AMH levels have limited inter- and intracycle variability (La Marca et al, 2006)

UPDATE #2

AMH has been shown to be superior to other hormonal markers of ovarian reserve. There is evidence that AMH levels are significantly more associated with egg numbers retrieved following stimulation from in vitro fertilization (IVF) than other serum markers (Broer et al, 2009; Hazout et al, 2004). Studies have demonstrated low or undetectable AMH levels in patients with hypergonadotropic secondary amenorrhea (de Koning et al, 2008) and premature ovarian failure (La Marca et al, 2006). Additionally AMH is highly correlated with the antral follicles count (AFC) (Figure 29-3, Rosen unpublished). In predictive models, both AMH and AFC have been shown to correlate with the onset of menopause. However, though both markers of ovarian reserve (AMH and AFC) correlate well with the number of oocytes retrieved during an IVF cycle, they do not appear to predict successful pregnancy.

POLYCYSTIC OVARIAN SYNDROME (THESSALONIKI)

PCOS is characterized by two of the following: oligo-amenorrhea, hyperandrogenism/hyperandrogenemia, or polycystic ovaries; for conception, the most critical of these factors is the irregular cycles with anovulation; ovulation induction should be safe and effective

1. Clomiphene citrate as first-line fertility treatment for PCOS
   - Clomiphene citrate (CC) alone is superior to metformin alone in achieving conception, pregnancy, and live birth in patients with PCOS
   - The addition of metformin to clomiphene citrate conferred no additional benefit with respect to conception, pregnancy, or live birth rate in the general PCOS population (Legro et al, 2007)
   - Although both clomiphene citrate and metformin can induce ovulation, a pregnancy was almost twice as likely when ovulation occurred as a result of CC (21.7% versus 39.5%, p = 0.002), (Legro et al, 2007)

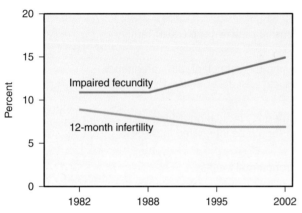

Figure 29-1. Percentage of married women—ages 15 to 44 years—with impaired fecundity or infertility 1982 to 2002. Impaired fecundity includes the inability to carry a pregnancy to term, and thus pregnancy loss. (Adapted from Centers for Disease Control and Prevention, National Survey of Family Growth: *Cycle 6 [2002] reports* [website]. www.cdc.gov/nchs/nsfg/nsfg_products.htm #cycle6. Accessed June 28, 2011.)

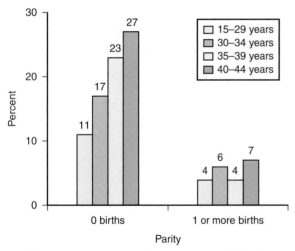

Figure 29-2. Percentage of married women—ages 15 to 44—with 12 months of infertility by parity and age in 2002. (Adapted from Centers for Disease Control and Prevention, National Survey of Family Growth: *Cycle 6 [2002] reports* [website]. www.cdc.gov/nchs/nsfg/nsfg_products.htm#cycle6. Accessed June 28, 2011.)

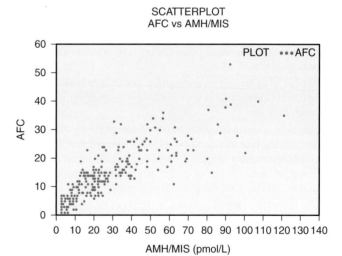

Figure 29-3. Correlation between AFC as assessed by vaginal ultrasound (2 to10 mm follicles) compared with serum AMH.

Clomiphene citrate is the recommended first-line therapy for ovulatory dysfunction/infertility in women with PCOS (Legro et al, 2007). Recommended second-line treatment includes exogenous gonadotropins with intense monitoring or laparoscopic ovarian surgery. Third-line treatment for infertility in PCOS is in vitro fertilization (IVF). Metformin use in PCOS should be restricted to those women with impaired glucose tolerance and is not recommended for ovulation induction (Thessaloniki ESHRE/ASRM-Sponsored PCOS Consensus Workshop Group, 2008).

2. Letrozole in ovulation induction
   - Because of the antiestrogenic effects of CC on endometrium and cervical mucus, recent research has been conducted on an alternative medication for ovulation induction
   - Aromatase inhibitors such as letrozole act by inhibiting the conversion of androgens into estrogens; thus, estrogen feedback to the pituitary is decreased and endogenous gonadotropin release is increased
   - A review of the literature on the use of letrozole for ovulation induction reported ovulation rates of 70% to 84%, pregnancy rates of 20% to 27% per cycle, and mean endometrial thickness of 7 to 9 mm (Holzer et al, 2006)
   - The addition of letrozole to exogenous gonadotropin cycles (so-called flare cycles) decreases gonadotropin requirements without a negative effect on pregnancy rates (Holzer et al, 2006)

Letrozole appears to be as effective as clomiphene citrate in ovulation induction, without the associated negative effects on the endometrium. Letrozole can be considered an efficacious alternative to clomiphene citrate for ovulation induction (Holzer et al, 2006).

3. Clinical features of PCOS are predictive of reproductive outcomes
   - Hirsutism scores have been shown to predict conception, pregnancy, and live birth, but not ovulation. Specifically, women with a normal Ferriman-Galway score (<8) were significantly more likely to conceive and achieve live birth than those with a score of ≥16 (Rausch et al, 2009)
   - Baseline free androgen index ([total testosterone/SHBG] × 100), baseline proinsulin level, and duration of attempting conception are significant predictors of ovulation, conception, pregnancy, and live birth; specifically, lower free androgen index, lower proinsulin levels, and shorter duration of attempting conception are associated with more favorable outcomes in all parameters (Rausch et al, 2009)

As opposed to obesity or insulin resistance, the extent of clinical and biochemical hyperandrogenism appears to be the strongest negative predictor of successful ovulation induction and conception for women with PCOS.

4. Impact of lifestyle modification on PCOS
   - Several investigators have demonstrated improvements in metabolic and endocrine parameters after lifestyle modification in women with PCOS (Hoeger, 2006)
   - Improvement in insulin sensitivity has been shown after weight loss in women with PCOS; euglycemic clamp studies (Moran et al, 2010) as well as studies of glucose tolerance tests (Kiddy et al, 1992) and fasting insulin parameters (Moran et al, 2003) have shown improvement in insulin sensitivity after weight loss in women with PCOS
   - Weight reduction, in some studies as little as 5% of total body weight, has been associated with increase in SHBG and decrease in free testosterone (Hoeger, 2006)
   - Improvement in hirsutism (40%) has also been shown with weight reduction in this population (Hoeger, 2006)
   - Many nonrandomized studies have suggested an improvement in reproductive parameters with weight reduction in women with PCOS
   - Menstrual cyclicity, ovulation, and spontaneous pregnancy have all been shown to improve in women with PCOS who reduce their body weight, even losing 5% to 10% of total body weight (Hoeger, 2006)
   - There have been no randomized studies to date on the impact of modest weight reduction on live birth rate, either spontaneous or assisted, in women with PCOS (Hoeger, 2006)

Weight loss is a key component of treatment for anovulatory infertility in women with PCOS.

5. PCOS and complications of pregnancy
   - According to a recent meta-analysis, women with PCOS are at increased risk of pregnancy and neonatal complications (Boomsma et al, 2006)
   - Women with PCOS demonstrated a significantly higher likelihood of developing gestational diabetes, OR 2.94 (95% confidence interval [CI]: 1.70 to 5.08), pregnancy-induced hypertension, OR 3.67 (95% CI: 1.98 to 6.81), and preeclampsia, OR 3.47 (95% CI:1.95 to 6.17) (Boomsma et al, 2006)
   - The chance of premature delivery, neonatal intensive care unit (ICU) admission, and perinatal mortality were all found to be increased in women with PCOS (Boomsma et al, 2006)

Women with PCOS, and all obese patients, should be encouraged to lose weight prior to attempting fertility. Miscarriage rates (Thum et al, 2007) appear to increase with marked obesity (BMI >35) and pregnancy complications increase, making these high-risk pregnancies and potentially affecting childhood health and well-being.

6. Metabolic parameters in daughters of women with PCOS
   - Daughters of women with PCOS ("PCOS daughters") are comparable to daughters of women without PCOS ("control daughters") with respect to body mass index (BMI) and waist circumference (Sir-Petermann et al, 2007)
   - During the prepubertal period, PCOS daughters had levels of fasting glucose, insulin, lipids, leptin, homeostasis model of assessment-insulin resistance (HOMA-IR), testosterone, and SHBG that were not different from control daughters
   - However, prepubertal PCOS daughters had significantly lower adiponectin levels as well as higher poststimulated insulin levels than did control daughters (Sir-Petermann et al, 2007)
   - In the pubertal period, PCOS daughters had levels of fasting glucose, insulin, leptin, adiponectin, and

HOMA-IR that were not different from control daughters
- Triglycerides and poststimulated insulin levels were significantly higher in pubertal PCOS daughters than in control daughters
- Testosterone levels were significantly higher, and SHBG levels significantly lower in pubertal PCOS daughters than in their control counterparts (Sir-Petermann et al, 2007)
- Adiponectin may be an early marker of metabolic derangement in prepubertal daughters of women with PCOS, and it appears to be independent of body weight

OVULATION INDUCTION AND INCIDENCE OF CANCER

1. Incidence of breast cancer
   - Epidemiologic studies have suggested an association between fewer lifetime ovulatory events and decreased risk of breast cancer (e.g., late menarche, early menopause)
   - Previous small studies have raised the suggestion that ovulation induction could be linked to increased breast cancer risk by increasing the number of lifetime ovulatory events
   - Among women who participated in the Nurses Health Study II (Terry et al, 2006), the presence of infertility resulting from an ovulatory defect was associated with a lower risk of breast cancer; additionally, treatment with ovulation induction did not increase cancer risk; in fact, the incidence of breast cancer was lowest in those women who had ever been treated with ovulation induction therapy
2. Incidence of ovarian cancer
   - The theory of "incessant ovulation" as the etiology of ovarian cancer has led to the concern that use of fertility drugs, with the induction of multiple ovulatory sites, may increase ovarian cancer risk
   - Since 1992, small studies have suggested such an increased risk; however, recent large studies, including a study of more than 50,000 infertility patients from a Danish registry (Jensen et al, 2009) and a recent critical review of the literature (Vlahos et al, 2010), have not been able to identify an increased risk independent of the risk associate with infertility and nulliparity

UPDATE #5
There is no strong evidence to support a relationship between the use of fertility drugs and either breast or ovarian cancer (Vlohos et al, 2010). Ongoing studies aimed at early detection of malignancy and identification of subgroups that may be at higher risk should continue. Additionally, large cohorts, such as the Danish registry should continue through the age at which ovarian and breast cancer risk peaks.

Uterine Factor

LEIOMYOMATA AND FERTILITY

1. Submucosal leiomyomata
   - Several small studies have demonstrated an association between submucosal leiomyomata

and decreased implantation, decreased ongoing pregnancy rates, and increased miscarriage rates (Casini et al, 2006; Eldar-Geva et al, 1998; Farhi et al, 1995; Klatsky et al, 2008)
- In subfertile populations, patients with submucosal myomata who have undergone hysteroscopic resection achieve pregnancy rates comparable to control groups without fibroids or previous myomectomies (Klatsky et al, 2008; Narayan et al, 1994; Shokeir, 2005; Surrey et al, 2005)

UPDATE #6
Submucosal leiomyomata seem to have an adverse impact on implantation and ongoing pregnancy, based on several small studies (Klatsky, 2008). This has led to the recommendation for resection of submucosal myomata prior to embarking on IVF. The impact on fertility in patients not undergoing IVF has not been documented.

2. Intramural leiomyomata
   - A systematic literature review (Klatsky et al, 2008) revealed disparate findings regarding intramural leiomyomata in the literature; the authors felt that there was insufficient evidence to offer routine resection of intramural myomata for reproductive optimization
   - A recent meta-analysis reviewed 19 observational studies in IVF populations; meta-analysis of the results of these studies revealed a significant decrease in both clinical pregnancy rates and live birth rate following IVF in patients with noncavity distorting intramural leiomyomata (Sunkara et al, 2010)

Data regarding impact of intramural leiomyomata are conflicting, and no randomized trials regarding the removal of intramural myomas are available. Additionally, there have been no studies documenting increased conception or delivery rates following surgery. Further research is needed in this area.

Tubal Factor

DIAGNOSIS

- Mol et al. (2001) performed a cost-effectiveness analysis to determine the best strategy for diagnosing tubal pathology; for young women with a high chance for spontaneous conception, testing for chlamydia antibody (CAT) is the most cost-effective test
- For older women or women with long-term infertility and a lower chance for conception, hysterosalpingogram (HSG) should be a first-line approach
- More recent approaches support this model (den Hartog et al, 2008) and suggest laparoscopy be utilized only when there is a positive history (history of pelvic inflammatory disease or adnexal mass) or when testing with a positive CAT and abnormal HSG findings is present
- Laparoscopy may be indicated in young women when followed by expectant management and no further intervention (Moayeri et al, 2009)

UPDATE #7

Current data do not support the inclusion of laparoscopy as routine in the infertility evaluation. CAT and HSG should be integrated into the diagnostic evaluation (den Hartog et al, 2008; Mol et al, 2001).

Male Subfertility

CIRCULATING HORMONE LEVELS AND SPERM PARAMETERS

- Circulating levels of follicle-stimulating hormone (FSH) and Inhibin B are thought to be reflective of Sertoli cell function and spermatogenesis (Meeker et al, 2007)
- FSH and luteinizing hormone (LH) have been shown to be inversely associated with sperm concentration, motility, and morphology (Meeker et al, 2007)
- Inhibin B and free T4 levels have been shown to be positively associated with sperm concentration (Meeker et al, 2007)
- There is a threshold for increased risk for poor semen parameters at the highest quintile for FSH and the lowest quintile for Inhibin B (Meeker et al, 2007)

Similar to gonadal compromise in women, poor semen parameters are associated with high circulating levels of FSH and LH and low circulating levels of Inhibin B and free T4.

PHTHALATE EXPOSURE AND MALE HORMONE LEVELS

- Phthalates have a wide range of commercial and industrial uses, including the manufacture of plastics and personal care products (e.g., lotion, fragrances); thus, human exposure to phthalates is widespread (Meeker et al, 2009)
- Detectable concentrations of mono (2-ethylhexyl) phthalate (MEHP), the urinary metabolite of di (2-ethylhexyl) phthalate (DEHP), were found in 83% of urinary samples collected at a fertility clinic (Meeker et al, 2009)
- After adjusting for potential confounders, MEHP levels were inversely associated with circulating testosterone, estradiol, and free androgen index in these patients (Meeker et al, 2009)

UPDATE #8

Male factor infertility may be impacted by environmental insults. Exposure to phthalates, specifically DEHP, appears to affect circulating steroid levels in adult men (Meeker et al, 2009).

BISPHENOL A (BPA) EXPOSURE, SEMEN PARAMETERS, AND SPERM DNA DAMAGE

- BPA is a chemical used in the manufacture of polycarbonate plastics, such as water bottles and food packaging
- Increasing urinary BPA concentrations have been shown to be associated with slightly elevated odds for poor sperm motility, concentration, and morphology; however, these results did not reach statistical significance (Meeker et al, 2010)
- Increasing urinary BPA concentrations were associated with increased sperm DNA damage as measured by percentage of DNA in sperm tails; however, there were

no differences in other measures of DNA damage related to BPA concentrations (Meeker et al, 2010)

Although there is some suggestion of an association between BPA exposure and semen parameters, further research is needed in this area.

Unexplained Infertility

Infertility is increasingly "unexplained" for two reasons: (1) couples may be at the lower extreme of the normal distribution for fertility, perhaps related to the age of the female partner or (2) there remains an, as yet, unidentified problem. We have, over time, eliminated many tests from the evaluation of infertile couples, as these tests were not found to be predictive of spontaneous conception (endometrial biopsy, postcoital test). Additionally, there was limited additional conception benefit to laparoscopy solely for infertility (Marcoux et al, 1997; Mol et al, 2001) so it is likely for many couples labeled as "unexplained" that the female partner may have minimal or mild endometriosis.

OVULATION INDUCTION

1. Clomiphene citrate (CC) and intrauterine insemination (IUI)
   - Clomiphene citrate has both estrogenic and antiestrogenic effects, depending on tissue type
   - CC acts as a competitive inhibitor of estrogen feedback at the level of the hypothalamus, increasing the release of gonadotropin-releasing hormone (GnRH) and, as a result, endogenous gonadotropins
   - Clomiphene citrate has been used as a first-line approach in ovulation induction for oligo-anovulatory women for more than 40 years
   - More recently, CC has been used in the initial treatment of unexplained infertility
   - A large retrospective review of 4199 CC-IUI cycles performed in women with either oligo-anovulation or unexplained infertility (ovulatory by history, normal endocrine parameters, semen analysis with at least 5 million total motile count, at least one patent fallopian tube) assessed outcomes (Dovey et al, 2008)
   - Total pregnancies and pregnancy rate per cycle decline with age, such that women aged 43 and older have only a 1% pregnancy rate per cycle of CC-IUI (Dovey ct al, 2008)

UPDATE #9

CC-IUI is the first treatment for unexplained infertility. Following failure with CC-IUI, IVF should be the next step in women <40 years of age to limit risks of multiple gestations and costs (Reindollar et al, 2010). If the mean duration of infertility is <2 years, then pregnancy rates were similar with treatment compared with no treatment, and young women should be encouraged to continue well-timed spontaneous attempts. In trials, looking at CC alone (without insemination), no increase in monthly fecundity is documented over control cycles without treatment. Treatment with CC-IUI lacks direct evidence except for a single study regarding efficacy compared to placebo (Figure 29-4). But, because of its low cost and risk compared with gonadotropin treatment, a short course is indicated. For CC + IUI, with the exception of ages 41 to 42, 90% or more of all pregnancies were initiated in the first three cycles of CC-IUI. In the 41-to-42 age group, 83.3% of all pregnancies initiated

Study name	Comparison	Statistics for each study			Pregnancy/Total		Risk difference and 95% CI
		Risk difference	Lower limit	Upper limit	Treatment	Control	
Hughes 2004	IVF	0.39	0.16	0.62	12/24	3/27	
Bhattacharya 2006	CC	−0.02	−0.09	0.05	28/194	32/193	
Guzick 1999	IUI	0.08	0.02	0.14	42/234	23/233	
Martinez 1990	IUI	0.24	0.03	0.45	5/19	1/20	
Steures 2007	IUI	0.03	−0.13	0.19	11/51	9/48	
Guzick 1999 Pts	SOIUI	0.23	0.16	0.31	77/231	23/233	
Steures 2006 Pts	SOIUI	−0.04	−0.15	0.06	29/127	34/126	
Deaton 1990	CCIUI	0.20	−0.03	0.44	8/23	4/28	
Fisch 1999	CC	0.08	−0.02	0.17	10/76	4/72	
		0.09	0.06	0.12	222/979	133/980	

−0.50   −0.25   0.00   0.25   0.50

Control better   Treatment better

Figure 29-4. Estimates of differences in pregnancy rate per cycle between treatment and control cycles in trials of treatment for unexplained infertility. CC, Clomiphene citrate; duration, duration of infertility; IUI, intrauterine insemination; IVF, in vitro fertilization; SO/IUI, super-ovulation/IUI. (Adapted from Practice Committee of American Society for Reproductive Medicine: Obesity and reproduction: an educational bulletin, *Fertil Steril* 90[5 Suppl]:S21-S299, 2008.)

occurred in the first four cycles. Thus, it appears reasonable to offer a limited number of CC-IUI cycles as an initial approach to subfertility without regard to ovulatory status (Dovey et al, 2008).

2. Letrozole–IUI
   • Pregnancy outcomes after ovulation induction with letrozole are similar to pregnancies achieved via CC or gonadotropins (Gregoriou et al, 2008; Mitwally et al, 2005)
   • Specifically, there has been shown to be no statistically significant difference in the rate of miscarriage or ectopic pregnancy in women treated with letrozole (Mitwally et al, 2005)
   • Letrozole use has been shown to have a significantly lower rate of multiple gestations when compared with clomiphene citrate, exogenous gonadotropins, or both (Casper, 2009; Gregoriou et al, 2008; Mitwally et al, 2005)
   • Concerns raised regarding increased risk of congenital birth defects with letrozole have not been supported (Gill et al, 2008; Tulandi et al, 2006)

Letrozole appears to be as effective as clomiphene citrate in ovulation induction, without the associated negative effects on the endometrium. Letrozole can be considered an efficacious alternative to clomiphene citrate for ovulation induction (Badawy et al, 2009; Holzer et al, 2006).

3. Gonadotropin–IUI
   • Gonadotropin–IUI (controlled ovarian hyperstimulation [COH]-IUI) was thought to enhance pregnancy rate by increasing the number of follicles/oocytes available in a given cycle and allowing more sperm access to the upper reproductive tract
   • However, since the mid-1990s, with the introduction of oral agents for ovulation stimulation in unexplained infertility, 20% to 30% of couples conceive with these simpler modalities;; it is less clear that there remains an increased pregnancy rate with gonadotropin stimulation in this context
   • A recent randomized controlled trial of "conventional arm" (CC-IUI, COH-IUI, IVF) versus

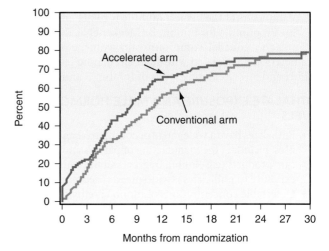

Figure 29-5. Kaplan-Meier estimates of cumulative incidence of pregnancy leading to delivery of a live born. (Adapted from Reindollar, RH, Regan MM, et al: A randomized clinical trial to evaluate optimal treatment for unexplained infertility: the fast track and standard treatment [FASTT] trial, *Fertil Steril* 94[3]:888-899, 2010.)

"accelerated arm" (CC-IUI, IVF) documented a higher pregnancy rate, over a shorter period of time, with less risk of multiple births and less apparent cost (Reindollar et al, 2010) (Figure 29-5)

For couples with unexplained infertility, following failure with oral agents and IUI, IVF is the next treatment strategy.

Assisted Reproductive Technologies

PREIMPLANTATION GENETIC SCREENING (PGS)

   • Traditional morphologic embryo grading does not reflect the genetic complement of the embryo
   • PGS is the assessment of the genetic makeup of an embryo via fluorescence in situ hybridization (FISH) (Donoso et al, 2007)
   • PGS is performed when the couple is known or presumed to be chromosomally normal (Thessaloniki ESHRE/ASRM-Sponsored PCOS Consensus Workshop Group, 2008)

- PGS has been touted as a means to improve the success of IVF by selecting genetically normal embryos, which in theory would have improved implantation rates and reduced miscarriage rates
  1. In advanced maternal age
     - Maternal age is one of the most important factors predicting success in IVF (Hardarson et al, 2008)
     - Increased rates of genetic aneuploidy are seen in the oocytes of women of advanced reproductive age (Hardarson et al, 2008)

In randomized controlled trials, PGS, with embryo biopsy on day 3 and analysis by FISH, has not been shown to confer a benefit in either clinical pregnancy rate or delivery rate in women of advanced maternal age (Hardarson et al, 2008; Mastenbroek et al, 2007; Staessen et al, 2008; Thessaloniki ESHRE/ASRM-Sponsored PCOS Consensus Workshop Group, 2008). In fact, both the clinical pregnancy rate (Hardarson et al, 2008; Mastenbroek et al, 2007; Staessen et al, 2008) and the live birth rate (Mastenbroek et al, 2007) were lower for women who were randomized to PGS in published studies. Newer technologies including trophectoderm biopsy on day 5 and more complete genetic evaluation with complete genomic hybridization (CGH) or microarray technology, are under exploration but await adequate randomized trials.

  2. PGS in recurrent pregnancy loss
     - Recurrent pregnancy loss (RPL) is defined as three or more losses occurring at less than 20 weeks' gestation (Thessaloniki ESHRE/ASRM-Sponsored PCOS Consensus Workshop Group, 2008)
     - PGS of embryos of women with RPL has demonstrated an increased rate of aneuploidy, independent of maternal age (Thessaloniki ESHRE/ASRM-Sponsored PCOS Consensus Workshop Group, 2008)
     - One small randomized controlled trial of 19 patients showed an increased pregnancy rate per transfer in the PGS group (Werlin et al, 2003); however, the subsequent miscarriage rate was not reported, and the small sample size limits the ability to draw definitive conclusions
     - Other studies of PGS in RPL have failed to definitively show a benefit of the technique (Donoso et al, 2007; Thessaloniki ESHRE/ASRM-Sponsored PCOS Consensus Workshop Group, 2008)

Current evidence does not support the use of PGS in RPL, in the absence of an identified parental genetic abnormality (e.g. translocation), as the technique does not appear to improve pregnancy rates or decrease miscarriage rates in this population (Thessaloniki ESHRE/ASRM-Sponsored PCOS Consensus Workshop Group, 2008).

ASSISTED REPRODUCTIVE TECHNOLOGY (ART) AND CHILDHOOD OUTCOME

  1. Imprinting
     - IVF and embryo culture have been shown to affect the methylation status of genes in animals such as mice and sheep; questions whether the same phenomenon in humans may lead to increased incidence of imprinting disorders have been raised in recent years (e.g., Maher, 2005)
     - A Dutch study compared national population data to questionnaire data from parents of children with Angelman syndrome, Beckwith-Wiedemann syndrome, and Prader-Willi syndrome (Doornbos et al, 2007)
     - There was an increased risk of an affected child after the use of ART (ICSI, IVF, IUI, and controlled ovarian hyperstimulation); however, there was an equally increased risk of an affected child if the conception took greater than 12 months of unprotected intercourse (i.e., infertility) without the use of ART (Doornbos et al, 2007)
     - The authors concluded that there was no independent effect of ART over the risk of baseline infertility for a child affected with an imprinting disorder (Doornbos et al, 2007)

Some evidence supports an increased risk for imprinting disorders in children born to couples meeting diagnostic criteria for infertility (>12 months unprotected intercourse) independent of use or type of ART (Doornbos et al, 2007).

ART AND BODY COMPOSITION

- Murine studies have demonstrated detrimental effects of embryo culture on adult body composition and adiposity (Sjoblom et al, 2005)
- It is unclear whether ART affects the trajectory of body composition and adipogenesis in the human
- Children born via IVF, ages 8 to 18, had some significantly increased measures of peripheral body fat, including the sum of peripheral skinfolds; these differences persisted after controlling for current risk factors, early life, and parental factors (Ceelen et al, 2007)
- Measures of total body fat, including dual-energy x-ray absorptiometry (DEXA) measurement of total body fat mass and total sum of skinfolds, were not significantly different in IVF children compared to controls (Ceelen et al, 2007)

INTRACYTOPLASMIC SPERM INJECTION (ICSI) AND MEDICAL OUTCOMES

- Concerns have been raised regarding the long-term outcome of children born via ICSI, as ICSI bypasses the process of natural sperm selection (Belva et al, 2007)
- A prospective study of 8-year-old ICSI children revealed no significant differences between the ICSI children and their spontaneously conceived controls on physical exam; moreover, extensive neurologic exam did not show significant differences between ICSI children and controls (Belva et al, 2007)
- Although minor malformations were similar in ICSI children and spontaneously conceived controls, major malformations were more common in ICSI children (Belva et al, 2007)
- In another study comparing 5- to 8-year-old ICSI children to matched children born after both IVF and spontaneous conception, no differences in malformations were found among the groups (Knoester et al, 2008)
- Although ICSI children had lower mean birth weights, they were of comparable weight to the other groups by the age of 5 to 8 (Knoester et al, 2008)
- Growth parameters such as head circumference were also similar among children born after ICSI, IVF, or spontaneous conception (Knoester et al, 2008)

Physical and neurologic exam parameters and growth appear to be similar in ICSI children and children conceived spontaneously or via IVF. There is conflicting evidence as to whether major congenital malformations are more common in ICSI children.

Obesity and Reproduction

SUBFERTILITY AND OBESITY

- Subfertility in overweight women is typically related to ovulatory dysfunction
- A previously published case-control study demonstrated increased rates of anovulatory subfertility in overweight and obese women; the odds ratio increased as BMI increased (Rich-Edwards et al, 1994)
- A majority of overweight and obese anovulatory women who decrease body weight 5% to 10% experience a return of ovulatory function (Crosignani et al, 2003)
- Increased time to conception has also been shown in women with increased waist-to-hip ratios, independent of BMI or menstrual cyclicity (Zaadstra et al, 1993); this implicates factors beyond ovulatory dysfunction in subfertility in overweight women
- Large population-based studies have demonstrated a dose-response relationship between increasing BMI and time to pregnancy in both sexes (Ramlau-Hansen et al, 2007)
- Couples in which both partners were overweight, or obese, had increased times to pregnancy. This association was independent of other risks factors, as couples with tubal disease, endometriosis, uterine malformations, or known metabolic disorders were excluded from analysis (Ramlau-Hansen et al, 2007)

UPDATE #10

Obesity, for both men and women, may be an important factor negatively affecting spontaneous conception and treatment outcome. Increasing BMI is associated with increasing time to conception in both sexes. Subfertility is more likely when both partners are overweight or obese (Ramlau-Hansen et al, 2007).

MALE SUBFERTILITY AND OBESITY

- Oligospermia and asthenospermia increase with increasing BMI (Hammoud et al, 2008)
- Altered hormonal milieu may be responsible for poor sperm parameters in obese men; specifically, increased conversion of testosterone to estrogen by peripheral adipose cells may reduce both circulating androgens and gonadotropins (Baker, 1998; Bray, 1997; Jarow et al, 1993)
- The scrotum is also closer to the body in obese men, and thus is prone to higher temperatures, which may also adversely affect semen parameters (Jung et al, 2000)

SUGGESTED READINGS

Ovarian Aging

Centers for Disease Control and Prevention, National Survey of Family Growth: *Cycle 6(2002) reports*. www.cdc.gov/nchs/nsfg/nsfg_products.htm #cycle6 Accessed June 28, 2011.
de Koning CH, McDonnell J, Themmen AP, et al: The endocrine and follicular growth dynamics throughout the menstrual cycle in women with consistently or variably elevated early follicular phase FSH compared with controls, *Hum Reprod* 23(6):1416–1423, 2008.

Durlinger AL, Visser JA, Themmen AP: Regulation of ovarian function: the role of anti-Müllerian hormone, *Reproduction* 124(5):601–609, 2002.
Hazout A, Bouchard P, Seifer DB, et al: Serum antimullerian hormone/ mullerian-inhibiting substance appears to be a more discriminatory marker of assisted reproductive technology outcome than follicle-stimulating hormone, inhibin B, or estradiol, *Fertil Steril* 82(5):1323–1329, 2004.
La Marca A, Pati M, Orvieto R, et al: Serum anti-müllerian hormone levels in women with secondary amenorrhea, *Fertil Steril* 85(5):1547–1549, 2006.
van Rooij IA, de Jong E, Broekmans FJ, et al: High follicle-stimulating hormone levels should not necessarily lead to the exclusion of subfertile patients from treatment, *Fertil Steril* 81(6):1478–1485, 2004.

Polycystic Ovary Syndrome

Holzer H, Casper R, Tulandi T: A new era in ovulation induction, *Fertil Steril* 85(2):277–284, 2006.
Legro RS, Barnhart HX, Schlaff WD, et al: Clomiphene, metformin, or both for infertility in the polycystic ovary syndrome, *N Engl J Med* 356(6): 551–566, 2007.

PCOS: Lifestyle

Guzick DS, Wing R, Smith D, et al: Endocrine consequences of weight loss in obese, hyperandrogenic, anovulatory women, *Fertil Steril* 61(4):598–604, 1994.
Hoeger KM: Role of lifestyle modification in the management of polycystic ovary syndrome, *Best Pract Res Clin Endocrinol Metab* 20(2):293–310, 2006.
Moran LJ, Noakes M, Clifton PM, Norman RJ: The effect of modifying dietary protein and carbohydrate in weight loss on arterial compliance and postprandial lipidemia in overweight women with polycystic ovary syndrome, *Fertil Steril* 94(6):2451–2454, 2010.
Thum MY, El-Sheikhah A, et al: The influence of body mass index to in-vitro fertilisation treatment outcome, risk of miscarriage and pregnancy outcome, *J Obstet Gynaecol* 27(7):699–702, 2007.

Fertility Drugs and Cancer Risk

Jensen A, Sharif H, Frederiksen K, Kjaer SK, et al: Use of fertility drugs and risk of ovarian cancer: Danish Population Based Cohort Study, *BMJ* 338:b249, 2009.
Vlahos NF, Economopoulos KP, Creatsas G, et al: Fertility drugs and ovarian cancer risk: a critical review of the literature, *Ann N Y Acad Sci* 1205:214–219, 2010.

Leiomyomata

Klatsky PC, Tran ND, Caughey AB, Fujimoto VY: Fibroids and reproductive outcomes: a systematic literature review from conception to delivery, *Am J Obstet Gynecol* 198(4):357–366, 2008.
Sunkara SK, Khairy M, El-Toukhy T, et al: The effect of intramural fibroids without uterine cavity involvement on the outcome of IVF treatment: a systematic review and meta-analysis, *Hum Reprod* 25(2):418–429, 2010.

Tubal Factor

den Hartog JE, Lardenoije CM, Severens JL, et al: Screening strategies for tubal factor subfertility, *Hum Reprod* 23(8):1840–1848, 2008.
Moayeri SE, Lee HC, Lathi RB, et al: Laparoscopy in women with unexplained infertility: a cost-effectiveness analysis, *Fertil Steril* 92(2):471–480, 2009.
Mol BW, Collins JA, Van Der Veen F, Bossuyt PM: Cost-effectiveness of hysterosalpingography, laparoscopy, and chlamydia antibody testing in subfertile couples, *Fertil Steril* 75(3):571–580, 2001.

Male Factor

Meeker JD, Ehrlich S, Toth TL, et al: Semen quality and sperm DNA damage in relation to urinary bisphenol A among men from an infertility clinic, *Reprod Toxicol* 30(4):532–539, 2010.

Unexplained Infertility

Badawy A, Elnashar A, Totongy M, et al: Clomiphene citrate or aromatase inhibitors for superovulation in women with unexplained infertility undergoing intrauterine insemination: a prospective randomized trial, *Fertil Steril* 92(4):1355–1359, 2009.
Dovey S, Sneeringer RM, Penzias AS: Clomiphene citrate and intrauterine insemination: analysis of more than 4100 cycles, *Fertil Steril* 90(6): 2281–2286, 2008.
Gill SK, Moretti M, Koren G: Is the use of letrozole to induce ovulation teratogenic? *Can Fam Physician* 54(3):353–354, 2008.
Gregoriou O, Vlahos NF, Konidaris S, et al: Randomized controlled trial comparing superovulation with letrozole versus recombinant follicle-stimulating hormone combined with intrauterine insemination for couples with unexplained infertility who had failed clomiphene citrate stimulation and intrauterine insemination, *Fertil Steril* 90(3):678–683, 2008.

Marcoux S, Maheux R, Bérubé S: Laparoscopic surgery in infertile women with minimal or mild endometriosis: Canadian Collaborative Group on Endometriosis, *N Engl J Med* 337(4):217–222, 1997.

Mitwally MF, Biljan MM, Casper RF: Pregnancy outcome after the use of an aromatase inhibitor for ovarian stimulation, *Am J Obstet Gynecol* 192(2):381–386, 2005.

Reindollar RH, Regan MM, Neumann PJ, et al: A randomized clinical trial to evaluate optimal treatment for unexplained infertility: the fast track and standard treatment (FASTT) trial, *Fertil Steril* 94(3):888–899, 2010.

Thessaloniki ESHRE/ASRM-Sponsored PCOS Consensus Workshop Group: Consensus on infertility treatment related to polycystic ovary syndrome, *Hum Reprod* 23(3):462–477, 2008.

ART: PGS

Donoso P, Staessen C, Fauser BC, Devroey P: Current value of preimplantation genetic aneuploidy screening in IVF, *Hum Reprod Update* 13(1):15–25, 2007.

Hardarson T, Hanson C, Lundin K, et al: Preimplantation genetic screening in women of advanced maternal age caused a decrease in clinical pregnancy rate: a randomized controlled trial, *Hum Reprod* 23(12):2806–2812, 2008.

Mastenbroek S, Twisk M, van Echten-Arends J, et al: In vitro fertilization with preimplantation genetic screening, *N Engl J Med* 357(1):9–17, 2007.

Staessen C, Verpoest W, Donoso P, et al: Preimplantation genetic screening does not improve delivery rate in women under the age of 36 following single-embryo transfer, *Hum Reprod* 23(12):2818–2825, 2008.

ART Childhood Outcome

Belva F, Henriet S, Liebaers I, et al: Medical outcome of 8-year-old singleton ICSI children (born > or = 32 weeks' gestation) and a spontaneously conceived comparison group, *Hum Reprod* 22(2):506–515, 2007.

Ceelen M, van Weissenbruch MM, Roos JC, et al: Body composition in children and adolescents born after in vitro fertilization or spontaneous conception, *J Clin Endocrinol Metab* 92(9):3417–3423, 2007.

Doornbos ME, Maas SM, McDonnell J, et al: Infertility, assisted reproduction technologies and imprinting disturbances: a Dutch study, *Hum Reprod* 22(9):2476–2480, 2007.

Knoester M, Helmerhorst FM, Vandenbroucke JP, et al: Perinatal outcome, health, growth, and medical care utilization of 5- to 8-year-old intracytoplasmic sperm injection singletons, *Fertil Steril* 89(5):1133–1146, 2008.

Obesity

Crosignani P, Colombo M, Vegetti W, et al: Overweight and obese anovulatory patients with polycystic ovaries: parallel improvements in anthropometric indices, ovarian physiology, and fertility rate induced by diet, *Hum Reprod* 18(9):1928–1932, 2003.

Hammoud AO, Wilde N, Gibson M, et al: Male obesity and alteration in sperm parameters, *Fertil Steril* 90(6):2222–2225, 2008.

Practice Committee of American Society for Reproductive Medicine: Obesity and reproduction: an educational bulletin, *Fertil Steril* 90(Suppl 5), S21–S299, 2008.

Ramlau-Hansen CH, Thulstrup AM, Nohr EA, et al: Subfecundity in overweight and obese couples, *Hum Reprod* 22(6):1634–1637, 2007.

References

Please go to expertconsult.com to view references.

Chapter 30

Contraception

CAROLYN B. SUFRIN • PHILIP D. DARNEY

KEY UPDATES

1 The Centers for Disease Control's *Medical Eligibility Criteria for Contraceptive Use* provides important recommendations for the safe use of contraceptive methods in women with various health conditions.

2 Depomedroxyprogesterone acetate is not associated with an increase in the incidence of fractures but may cause weight gain in susceptible users.

3 Hormonal contraception is safe and effective in obese women; the contraceptive patch is less effective in women over 80 kg.

4 The most common side effect among women using the subdermal contraceptive implant is unpredictable, though not heavy, bleeding.

5 Intrauterine contraception is safe for both parous and nulliparous women, is as effective as permanent sterilization, and does *not* cause pelvic inflammatory disease or infertility.

6 The absolute risk of a venous thromboembolic event in women using combined hormonal contraception is very low and always lower than in pregnancy, but it is slightly increased for women using the contraceptive patch and pills with third-generation progestins compared to other methods.

7 When choosing an oral contraceptive with a patient, consider the estrogen dose and the progestin type that will minimize the risk of side effects.

8 Extended cycle and immediate start of patch, vaginal ring, and oral contraceptives are effective and acceptable options for hormonal contraceptives.

9 Postpartum contraception should be started by 3 weeks in women who are not exclusively breast-feeding and by 3 months in women who are. All methods are safe, but combined hormonal contraception should be initiated after 3 weeks in non-breast-feeding women and 6 weeks in breast-feeding women.

Context

NEED FOR CONTRACEPTION

- Family planning plays a direct and crucial role in advancing maternal and child health. A recent report by the Guttmacher Institute and the United Nations Population Fund emphasizes the direct health benefits of meeting the needs for family planning, maternal, and newborn health services in developing countries. It is estimated that this would reduce annual maternal deaths by two thirds from 356,000 to 105,000, newborn deaths from 3.2 million to 1.5 million, and unintended pregnancies from 75 million to 22 million. If all unplanned pregnancies could be eliminated, it is estimated that there would be 22 million fewer abortions each year. Unintended pregnancies also cause obstetric fistulae, infertility, septic abortion, and other morbidities that degrade the lives of women in poor countries.

- In the United States, 43 million women are of reproductive age, are sexually active, and do not want to become pregnant. The typical U.S. woman wants only two children. To achieve this goal, she must use contraceptives for roughly three decades.

- Half of all pregnancies in the United States are unintended, and half of those occur among women who were not using a method of contraception in the month they got pregnant. The other half were using a method but experienced a contraceptive failure as a result of either the user or the method.

USE OF CONTRACEPTION

- Overall, 62% of U.S. women ages 15 to 44 are currently using a method of contraception; this is comparable to the global context, where 61% of women use some form of contraception, but is much lower than in Western European countries where contraceptive prevalence approaches 90%

TABLE 30-1 Summary of Contraceptive Efficacy

Method	Percentage of Women Experiencing an Unintended Pregnancy within the First Year of Use		Percentage of Women Continuing Use at 1 Year
	Typical Use	Perfect Use	
No method	85	85	
Spermicides	29	18	42
Withdrawal	27	4	43
Fertility awareness-based methods	25		51
Diaphragm	16	6	57
Condom			
Female	21	5	49
Male	15	2	53
Combined pill and progestin-only pill	8	0.3	68
Contraceptive patch (Ortho Evra)	8	0.3	68
Contraceptive vaginal ring (NuvaRing)	8	0.3	68
Depo-Provera	3	0.3	56
IUD			
Copper T (ParaGard)	0.8	0.6	78
LNG-IUS (Mirena)	0.2	0.2	80
Subdermal implant (Implanon)	0.05	0.05	84
Female sterilization	0.5	0.5	100
Male sterilization	0.15	0.10	100

Adapted from Trussell J: Contraceptive efficacy. In Hatcher RA, Trussell J, Nelson AL, et al: *Contraceptive technology,* ed 19 revised, New York, 2007, Ardent Media.

- Globally and in the United States, poorly educated women, low-income women, and those who suffer from domestic violence experience higher rates of unintended pregnancies, abortions, and teen pregnancies than women who are empowered by education and employment opportunities and who have access to modern contraceptives

Overview

WHICH METHODS ARE COMMONLY USED?

- Among the women using contraception in the United States, oral contraceptive pills (OCPs) are the most common (28%), followed by female tubal sterilization (27%); intrauterine contraception (IUC) use is low, at 5.5%; globally, the most commonly used method is female sterilization (38%), followed by IUC (25%), then OCPs (7.5%)

CONTRACEPTIVE MECHANISMS OF ACTION

- Cervical mucus thickening: progestins
- Ovarian effects: progestins suppress luteinizing hormone (LH) surge, thus inhibit ovulation; estrogens suppress FSH, thus inhibit growth of dominant follicle
- Endometrial effects: progestins cause endometrial atrophy; estrogens prevent breakthrough bleeding from progestin-induced atrophy; copper IUC creates sterile inflammatory reaction in uterine cavity
- Spermicidal: copper ions inhibit sperm motility; films, creams, and foams coat sperm cell membrane to immobilize

APPROACH TO CHOOSING THE BEST METHOD WITH YOUR PATIENT

1. Efficacy
   - The most effective methods are the ones that require least intervention from the patient
     - Long-acting methods reduce gap between typical and perfect use efficacy; "perfect use" efficacy involves consistent and correct use, whereas "typical use" reflects efficacy in real life, outside the context of a clinical trial (Table 30-1)
2. Medical comorbidities
   - Consider risks and benefits of individual methods within the context of any medical conditions your patient may have
   - Use Medical Eligibility Criteria from the Centers for Disease Control (CDC) and World Health Organization (WHO); evidenced-based recommendations on safety of contraception methods with specific coexisting diagnoses (Table 30-2)
   - Estrogen-containing methods (combined OCP, contraceptive patch, contraceptive vaginal ring) should not be used in women with a current or prior venous thromboembolic event, active hepatitis, uncontrolled hypertension, smokers (>15 cigarettes/day) older than 35 years old, diabetes with vascular disease, stroke or ischemic heart disease, or migraine headaches with focal neurologic symptoms
   - Always balance contraception concerns against the risks of pregnancy, which for some women—especially those in poor countries—pose a greater hazard to

TABLE 30-2 **Summary Chart of U.S. Medical Eligibility Criteria for Contraceptive Use, 2010**

Key:

1 No restriction (method can be used)

2 Advantages generally outweigh theoretic or proved risks

3 Theoretic or proved risks usually outweigh the advantages

4 Unacceptable health risk (method not to be used)

This summary sheet only contains a subset of the recommendations from the U.S. MEC. For complete guidance, see www.cdc.gov/reproductivehealth/usmec.

Most contraceptive methods do not protect against sexually transmitted infections (STIs). Consistent and correct use of the male latex condom reduces the risk of STIs and HIV.

Condition	Subcondition	Combined pill, patch, ring		Progestin-only pill		Injection		Implant		LNG—IUD		Copper-IUD	
		I	C	I	C	I	C	I	C	I	C	I	C
Age		Menarche to <40 = 1 ≥40 = 2		Menarche to <18 = 1 18-45 = 1 >45 = 1		Menarche to <18 = 2 18-45 = 1 >45 = 2		Menarche to <18 = 1 18-45 = 1 >45 = 1		Menarche to <20 = 2 ≥20 = 1		Menarche to <20 = 2 ≥20 = 1	
Anatomic abnormalities	a) Distorted uterine cavity									4		4	
	b) Other abnormalities									2		2	
Anemias	a) Thalassemia	1		1		1		1		1		2	
	b) Sickle cell disease‡	2		1		1		1		1		2	
	c) Iron-deficiency anemia	1		1		1		1		1		2	
Benign ovarian tumors	(including cysts)	1		1		1		1		1		1	
Breast disease	a) Undiagnosed mass	2*		2*		2*		2*		2		1	
	b) Benign breast disease	1		1		1		1		1		1	
	c) Family history of cancer	1		1		1		1		1		1	
	d) Breast cancer‡												
	i) Current	4		4		4		4		4		1	
	ii) Past and no evidence of current disease for 5 years	3		3		3		3		3		1	
Breast-feeding	a) < 21 days postpartum	4		2*		2*		2*					
	b) 21-30 days postpartum	3		2		2		2					
	c) 30-42 days postpartum	3		1		1		1					
	i) With other risk factors for VTE (age >35, previous VTE, thrombophilia, immobility, transfusion at delivery, BMI>=30, postpartum hemorrhage, post-cesarean delivery, pre-eclampsia, smoking)												
	ii) Without other risk factors for VTE	2		1		1		1					
	d) >42 days postpartum	2		1		1		1					
Cervical cancer	Awaiting treatment	2		1		2		2		4	2	4	2
Cervical ectropion		1		1		1		1		1		1	
Cervical intraepithelial neoplasia (CIN)		2		1		2		2		2		1	

TABLE 30-2   **Summary Chart of U.S. Medical Eligibility Criteria for Contraceptive Use, 2010—cont'd**

Condition	Subcondition	Combined pill, patch, ring I	C	Progestin-only pill I	C	Injection I	C	Implant I	C	LNG—IUD I	C	Copper-IUD I	C
Cirrhosis	a) Mild (compensated)	1		1		1		1		1		1	
	b) Severe‡ (decompensated)	4		3		3		3		3		1	
Deep venous thrombosis	a) History of DVT/PE, not on anticoagulant therapy												
(DVT) /Pulmonary embolism (PE)	i) Higher risk for recurrent DVT/PE	4		2		2		2		2		1	
	ii) Lower risk for recurrent DVT/PE	3		2		2		2		2		1	
	b) Acute DVT/PE	4		2		2		2		2		2	
	c) DVT/PE and established on anticoagulant therapy for at least 3 months												
	i) Higher risk for recurrent DVT/PE	4*		2		2		2		2		2	
	ii) Lower risk for recurrent DVT/PE	3*		2		2		2		2		2	
	d) Family history (first-degree relatives)	2		1		1		1		1		1	
	e) Major surgery												
	i) With prolonged immobilization	4		2		2		2		2		1	
	ii) Without prolonged immobilization	2		1		1		1		1		1	
	f) Minor surgery without immobilization	1		1		1		1		1		1	
Depressive disorders		1*		1*		1*		1*		1*		1*	
Diabetes mellitus (DM)	a) History of gestational DM only	1		1		1		1		1		1	
	b) Nonvascular disease												
	i) Noninsulin dependent	2		2		2		2		2		1	
	ii) Insulin dependent‡	2		2		2		2		2		1	
	c) Nephropathy/ retinopathy/ neuropathy‡	3/4*		2		3		2		2		1	
	d) Other vascular disease or diabetes of >20 years' duration‡	3/4*		2		3		2		2		1	
Endometrial cancer‡		1		1		1		1		4	2	4	2
Endometrial hyperplasia		1		1		1		1		1		1	
Endometriosis		1		1		1		1		1		2	
Epilepsy‡§	See drug interactions	1*		1*		1*		1*		1		1	
Gallbladder disease	a) Symptomatic												
	i) Treated by cholecystectomy	2		2		2		2		2		1	
	ii) Medically treated	3		2		2		2		2		1	
	iii) Current	3		2		2		2		2		1	
	b) Asymptomatic	2		2		2		2		2		1	

Continued

TABLE 30-2   **Summary Chart of U.S. Medical Eligibility Criteria for Contraceptive Use, 2010—cont'd**

Condition	Subcondition	Combined pill, patch, ring — I	C	Progestin-only pill — I	C	Injection — I	C	Implant — I	C	LNG—IUD — I	C	Copper-IUD — I	C
Gestational trophoblastic disease	a) Decreasing or undetectable ß-hCG levels	1		1		1		1		3		3	
	b) Persistently elevated ß-hCG levels or malignant disease‡	1		1		1		1		4		4	
Headaches	a) Nonmigrainous	1*	2*	1*	1*	1*	1*	1*	1*	1*	1*	1*	
	b) Migraine												
	i) Without aura, age <35	2*	3*	1*	2*	2*	2*	2*	2*	2*	2*	1*	
	ii) Without aura, age ≥35	3*	4*	1*	2*	2*	2*	2*	2*	2*	2*	1*	
	iii) With aura, any age	4*	4*	2*	3*	2*	3*	2*	3*	2*	3*	1*	
History of bariatric surgery‡	a) Restrictive procedures	1		1		1		1		1		1	
	b) Malabsorptive procedures	COCs: 3 P/R: 1		3		1		1		1		1	
History of cholestasis	a) Pregnancy related	2		1		1		1		1		1	
	b) Past COC related	3		2		2		2		2		1	
History of high blood pressure during pregnancy		2		1		1		1		1		1	
History of pelvic surgery		1		1		1		1		1		1	
HIV	High risk or HIV infected‡	1		1		1		1		2	2	2	2
	AIDS (see drug interactions) ‡§	1*		1*		1*		1*		3	2*	3	2*
	Clinically well on ARV therapy§	If on treatment see drug interactions								2	2	2	2
Hyperlipidemias		2/3*		2*		2*		2*		2*		1*	
Hypertension	a) Adequately controlled hypertension	3*		1*		2*		1*		1		1	
	b) Elevated blood pressure levels (properly taken measurements)												
	i) Systolic 140-159 or diastolic 90-99	3		1		2		1		1		1	
	ii) Systolic ≥160 or diastolic ≥100‡	4		2		3		2		2		1	
	c) Vascular disease	4		2		3		2		2		1	
Inflammatory bowel disease	(Ulcerative colitis, Crohn's disease)	2/3*		2		2		1		1		1	
Ischemic heart disease‡	Current and history of	4		2	3	3		2	3	2	3	1	
Liver tumors	a) Benign												
	i) Focal nodular hyperplasia	2		2		2		2		2		1	
	ii) Hepatocellular adenoma‡	4		3		3		3		3		1	
	b) Malignant‡	4		3		3		3		3		1	

TABLE 30-2 Summary Chart of U.S. Medical Eligibility Criteria for Contraceptive Use, 2010—cont'd

Condition	Subcondition	Combined pill, patch, ring I	C	Progestin-only pill I	C	Injection I	C	Implant I	C	LNG—IUD I	C	Copper-IUD I	C
Malaria		1		1		1		1		1		1	
Multiple risk factors for arterial cardiovascular disease	(such as older age, smoking, diabetes, and hypertension)	3/4*		2*		3*		2*		2		1	
Obesity	a) ≥30 kg/m² body mass index (BMI)	2		1		1		1		1		1	
	b) Menarche to <18 years and ≥30 kg/m² BMI	2		1		2		1		1		1	
Ovarian cancer‡		1		1		1		1		1		1	
Parity	a) Nulliparous	1		1		1		1		2		2	
	b) Parous	1		1		1		1		1		1	
Past ectopic pregnancy		1		2		1		1		1		1	
Pelvic inflammatory disease	a) Past (assuming no current risk factors of STIs) i) With subsequent pregnancy	1		1		1		1		1	1	1	1
	ii) Without subsequent pregnancy	1		1		1		1		2	2	2	2
	b) Current	1		1		1		1		4	2*	4	2*
Peripartum cardiomyopathy‡	a) Normal or mildly impaired cardiac function i) <6 months	4		1		1		1		2		2	
	ii) ≥6 months	3		1		1		1		2		2	
	b) Moderately or severely impaired cardiac function	4		2		2		2		2		2	
Postabortion	a) First trimester	1*		1*		1*		1*		1*		1*	
	b) Second trimester	1*		1*		1*		1*		2		2	
	c) Immediately postseptic abortion	1*		1*		1*		1*		4		4	
Postpartum (in non-breast-feeding women)	a) <21 days	4		1		1		1					
	b) ≥21-42 days	1		1		1		1					
	i) With other risk factors for VTE (age >35, previous VTE, thrombophilia, immobility, transfusion at delivery, BMI ≥30, postpartum hemorrhage, postcesarean delivery, pre-eclampsia, smoking)	3		1		1		1					
	ii) without other risk factors for VTE	2		1		1		1					
	c) >42 days	1		1		1		1					

Continued

TABLE 30-2   Summary Chart of U.S. Medical Eligibility Criteria for Contraceptive Use, 2010—cont'd

Condition	Subcondition	Combined pill, patch, ring I	C	Progestin-only pill I	C	Injection I	C	Implant I	C	LNG—IUD I	C	Copper-IUD I	C
Postpartum (in breast-feeding or non-breast-feeding women, including postcaesarean section)	a) <10 minutes after delivery of the placenta									2		1	
	b) 10 minutes after delivery of the placenta to <4 weeks									2		2	
	c) ≥4 weeks									1		1	
	d) Puerperal sepsis									4		4	
Pregnancy		NA*		NA*		NA*		NA*		4*		4*	
Rheumatoid arthritis	a) On immunosuppressive therapy	2		1		2/3*		1		2	1	2	1
	b) Not on immunosuppressive therapy	2		1		2		1		1		1	
Schistosomiasis	a) Uncomplicated	1		1		1		1		1		1	
	b) Fibrosis of the liver‡	1		1		1		1		1		1	
Severe dysmenorrhea		1		1		1		1		1		2	
Sexually transmitted infections	a) Current purulent cervicitis or chlamydial infection or gonorrhea	1		1		1		1		4	2*	4	2*
	b) Other STIs (excluding HIV and hepatitis)	1		1		1		1		2	2	2	2
	c) Vaginitis (including trichomonas vaginalis and bacterial vaginosis)	1		1		1		1		2	2	2	2
	d) Increased risk of STIs	1		1		1		1		2/3*	2	2/3*	2
Smoking	a) Age <35	2		1		1		1		1		1	
	b) Age ≥35, <15 cigarettes/day	3		1		1		1		1		1	
	c) Age ≥35, ≥15 cigarettes/day	4		1		1		1		1		1	
Solid organ transplantation‡	a) Complicated	4		2		2		2		3	2	3	2
	b) Uncomplicated	2*		2		2		2		2		2	
Stroke‡	History of cerebrovascular accident	4		2	3	3		2	3	2		1	
Superficial venous thrombosis	a) Varicose veins	1		1		1		1		1		1	
	b) Superficial thrombophlebitis	2		1		1		1		1		1	
Systemic lupus erythematosus‡	a) Positive (or unknown) antiphospholipid antibodies	4		3		3	3	3		3		1	1
	b) Severe thrombocytopenia	2		2		3	2	2		2*		3*	2*
	c) Immunosuppressive treatment	2		2		2	2	2		2		2	1
	d) None of the above	2		2		2	2	2		2		1	1
Thrombogenic mutations‡		4*		2*		2*		2*		2*		1*	
Thyroid disorders	a) Simple goiter/hyperthyroid/hypothyroid	1		1		1		1		1		1	

TABLE 30-2   **Summary Chart of U.S. Medical Eligibility Criteria for Contraceptive Use, 2010—cont'd**

Condition	Subcondition	Combined pill, patch, ring		Progestin-only pill		Injection		Implant		LNG—IUD		Copper-IUD	
		I	C	I	C	I	C	I	C	I	C	I	C
Tuberculosis‡	a) Nonpelvic	1*		1*		1*		1*		1		1	
	b) Pelvic	1*		1*		1*		1*		4	3	4	3
Unexplained vaginal bleeding	(suspicious for serious condition) before evaluation	2*		2*		3*		3*		4*	2*	4*	2*
Uterine fibroids		1		1		1		1		2		2	
Vaginal bleeding patterns	a) Irregular pattern without heavy bleeding	1		2		2		2		1	1	1	
	b) Heavy or prolonged bleeding	1*		2*		2*		2*		1*	2*	2*	
Valvular heart disease	a) Uncomplicated	2		1		1		1		1		1	
	b) Complicated‡	4		1		1		1		1		1	
Viral hepatitis	a) Acute or flare	3/4*	2	1		1		1		1		1	
	b) Carrier/chronic	1	1	1		1		1		1		1	
Drug Interactions													
Antiretroviral therapy (ARV)	a) Nucleoside reverse transcriptase inhibitors	1*		1		1		1		2/3*	2*	2/3*	2*
	b) Non-nucleoside reverse transcriptase inhibitors	2*		2*		1		2*		2/3*	2*	2/3*	2*
	c) Ritonavir-boosted protease inhibitors	3*		3*		1		2*		2/3*	2*	2/3*	2*
Anticonvulsant therapy	a) Certain anticonvulsants (phenytoin, carbamazepine, barbiturates, primidone, topiramate, oxcarbazepine)	3*		3*		1		2*		1		1	
	b) Lamotrigine	3*		1		1		1		1		1	
Antimicrobial therapy	a) Broad-spectrum antibiotics	1		1		1		1		1		1	
	b) Antifungals	1		1		1		1		1		1	
	c) Antiparasitics	1		1		1		1		1		1	
	d) Rifampicin or rifabutin therapy	3*		3*		1		2*		1		1	

I = initiation of contraceptive method; C = continuation of contraceptive method.
*Please see the complete guidance for a clarification to this classification (www.cdc.gov/reproductivehealth/usmec).
‡Condition that exposes the woman to increased risk as a result of unintended pregnancy.
§Please refer to the U.S. MEC guidance related to drug interactions at the end of this chart.

life and health than any possible contraceptive risks; noncontraceptive benefits (Table 30-3)
- Hormonal contraceptive methods, including the levonorgestrel intrauterine system (IUS) and subdermal implants, have noncontraceptive effects that may be desirable for patients with coexisting gynecologic conditions such as dysmenorrhea, menorrhagia, pelvic pain, fibroids, hirsutism, acne, ovarian cysts, or risk factors for endometrial hyperplasia
- Combined OCPs reduce a woman's lifetime risk of ovarian cancer and, along with progestin-only methods, are protective from endometrial cancer; OCPs *do not* increase a woman's risk of breast cancer
- Methods with a progestin component thicken cervical mucus and thus create a mechanical barrier that may reduce the risk of transmission of some sexually transmitted infections (STIs)
- All methods of contraception reduce the risk of ectopic pregnancy—because they all prevent pregnancy; those that completely suppress ovulation, like OCP, depo medroxyprogesterone acetate (DMPA), and Implanon—provide the greatest protection

TABLE 30-3 Major Methods of Contraception: Safety Concerns, Side Effects, and Noncontraceptive Benefits

Method	Side Effects	Complications (Rare)	Noncontraceptive Benefits
Combined hormonal contraception (pills, patch, ring)	Nausea, vomiting, headaches, mastalgia, spotting and breakthrough bleeding, mood changes	Cardiovascular complications (DVT, PE, MI, hypertension), depression, cholelithiasis	Decreases dysmenorrhea, PMS, and menstrual blood loss, including these symptoms associated with fibroids; reduces risk of ectopic pregnancy and ovarian cysts; reduces acne and hirsutism; protection from ovarian and endometrial cancer; protection from PID
Progestin-only pills	Spotting, breakthrough bleeding, amenorrhea, mood changes, headaches, hot flashes	None	Decreases menstrual pain and blood loss; no effect on lactation
Progestin injection (Depo Provera)	Menstrual changes, weight gain (see Update #2), headaches, hair loss, mood changes	Allergic reaction, excessive weight gain, depression, may increase insulin resistance	Improves dysmenorrhea, endometriosis, menorrhagia; decreases ovarian cyst formation; no effect on lactation; reduces sickle cell crises and seizures in women with these conditions; protection from ovarian and endometrial cancer
Progestin implant (Implanon)	Unpredictable bleeding, headaches, hair loss, mood changes, weight gain or loss	Infection at insertion site; complicated removal; depression	Decreases ovarian cyst formation; less blood loss per cycle; no effect on lactation
LNG-IUS	Irregular bleeding; cramping; headaches; acne	Perforation (1/1000); infection at time of insertion (1/1000)	Improves dysmenorrhea and pelvic pain; treats abnormal uterine bleeding from anovulatory cycles, menorrhagia, adenomyosis, and fibroid-related bleeding (50% amenorrhea by 1 year); protection from endometrial cancer; protection and treatment of endometrial hyperplasia
Copper IUD	Increased menstrual blood flow and cramping	Perforation (1/1000); infection at time of insertion (1/1000)	No effect on lactation
Sterilization	Pain at surgical site; adhesions; regret	Surgical complications; if pregnancy occurs, ectopic pregnancy risk is increased	None
Male condom	Decreased spontaneity or sensation; skin irritation; latex allergy	Anaphylactic reaction to latex	Reduces risk of STIs

Adapted from Trussell J, Kowal D: The essentials of contraception. In Hatcher RA, Trussell J, Nelson AL, et al: *Contraceptive technology,* ed 19 revised, New York, 2007, Ardent Media.

UPDATE#1

Medical Eligibility Criteria: The Centers for Disease Control (CDC) in 2010 released evidence-based guidelines for the use of contraceptive methods in women with a variety of coexisting characteristics or medical conditions. Adapted from the World Health Organization's Medical Eligibility Criteria (MEC) for Contraceptive Use, the CDC MEC are modified for use in the United States. Providers should use this key reference as a guide to safety when counseling patients about contraceptive methods (www.cdc.gov/mmwr/pdf/rr/rr5904.pdf).

INITIATING AND DISCONTINUING METHODS

- Pelvic exam is not necessary prior to initiating contraception, other than before inserting IUC or surgical sterilization

- Check blood pressure if starting combined hormonal contraception
- "Quickstart" is generally preferred: start use on the day the method is selected; rule out pregnancy clinically (within 7 days of first day of menses or no unprotected sexual activity since last menses) or with urine pregnancy test (if patient has had unprotected sex within 10 days of this test, repeat test 1 week later)
- Other than permanent sterilization, no methods affect future fertility; DMPA users may have delayed return to fertility

SPECIAL POPULATIONS

- *Adolescents.* Long-acting, reversible methods are particularly well suited to this group, as they do not require frequent remembering on the user's part. All methods, including intrauterine contraception, are appropriate choices for adolescents.

- *Perimenopausal women.* These women still have a need for contraception, and many methods may also help their perimenopausal symptoms. Vasomotor symptoms respond well to combined hormonal contraception, as does irregular bleeding. The levonorgestrel intrauterine system (Mirena) (LNG-IUS) and DMPA are also helpful with perimenopausal bleeding. Women using hormone replacement therapy can use the LNG-IUS as the progestin component.

- *Postabortion.* Birth control should be started immediately after a woman undergoes an abortion procedure. Placement of intrauterine contraception is safe and effective after dilation and curettage or dilation and evacuation.

- *HIV-positive women.* Contraception is very important for women who have tested positive for the human immunodeficiency virus (HIV), to optimize the planning of their pregnancies and reducing maternal-to-child transmission of HIV. Hormonal contraception does not alter the efficacy of antiretroviral therapy. Although some HIV medications increase clearance of combined oral contraceptive pills there is no effect on efficacy in pregnancy prevention. Intrauterine contraception is safe and effective in HIV-positive women. Some women at high risk of HIV acquisition *may* be at greater risk when they use high-dose progestin methods. Studies are inconclusive.

- *Mentally disabled women.* Contraceptive counseling in this population should pay particular attention to the consensual nature of sexual activity in which a patient is engaged, as developmentally delayed women are more commonly the victims of coerced sex. Select a method that is appropriate to a woman's lifestyle and her capacity to use methods that require varying degrees of patient remembering. Physicians must adhere to the highest ethical standards if considering sterilization for women with developmental disabilities.

- *Incarcerated women.* Most women in jails or prisons are eventually released into the community. Incarceration is an opportunity to provide them with access to contraception counseling and a method for current and future use.

Method Use

LONG-ACTING METHODS

1. Injectable: every 3 months
   - Description
     - Depo medroxyprogesterone acetate (DMPA): 150 mg intramuscularly or 104 mg subcutaneously every 13 weeks
   - Key benefits, ideal candidates, and precautions
     - Long acting (3 months), less to remember than daily or monthly methods, discreet
     - Ideal for women with contraindications to estrogen use
     - Improves endometriosis and dysmenorrhea; 50% are amenorrheic after 1 year of use
     - May have delayed return to fertility, average 10 months after last injection
     - Initiating and continuing method
   - Quick start initiation; if more than 13 weeks since last injection, rule out pregnancy

Depo Medroxyprogesterone Acetate (DMPA) Does Not Increase the Rate of Fractures

Because of the suppression of follicular development, DMPA induces a state of relative estrogen deficiency, similar to lactation. After 2 years of use, bone mineral density, as measured by bone densitometry, decreases by 5.7% to 7.5% in adults (Berenson et al, 2004; Clark et al, 2004) and 5% in adolescents (Scholes et al, 2005). However, bone density is a surrogate marker, and DMPA use has not been shown to increase the risk of actual fractures (Lopez et al, 2009). The changes in BMD are reversible after discontinuing DMPA (Kaunitz et al, 2008). Whereas the Food and Drug Administration (FDA) has issued a black box warning to limit DMPA to 2 years of use, the World Health Organization and the American College of Obstetricians and Gynecologists disagree and support the use of DMPA for as long a duration as women desire to use (American College of Obstetricians and Gynecologists Committee on Gynecologic Practice, ACOG Committee Opinion No. 415, 2008; World Health Organization, 2005). Moreover, long-term DMPA use is not an indication for performing bone densitometry screening.

UPDATE #3

Obesity and Contraception

The growing epidemic of obesity in the United States raises several concerns about the efficacy and safety of contraception among obese women. Overall, although pharmacokinetics may be altered in obese women using hormonal contraception, all methods except the patch appear to have the same efficacy (Lopez et al, 2010). Women who weigh more than 80 kg have an increased risk of contraceptive failure when using the patch, and this method is therefore not recommended for them (Zeiman et al, 2002). Regarding safety, although obesity is an independent risk factor for a venous thromboembolic event (VTE), this additional risk of obesity while using combined OCPs is very small, and is still significantly less than the risk of clot during pregnancy. (Society of Family Planning et al, 2009). Hormonal contraception does not appear to increase the risk of obese women developing type 2 diabetes (Fahmy et al, 1991; Lopez et al, 2009). Women who have undergone bariatric surgery should wait 1 to 2 years before planning a pregnancy (American College of Obstetricians and Gynecologists, ACOG Practice Bulletin No. 105, 2009) and thus require effective contraception. Oral absorption of pills is decreased, and thus nonoral methods of birth control are recommended (Mehri, 2007).

Some studies of hormonal contraceptive use report weight gain, whereas others do not. Most of these studies do not use an appropriate comparison group and thus it is difficult to conclude whether they actually affect weight. Among a cohort of adolescents using hormonal contraception, DMPA users gained 4 kg more in a 5-year time period than OCP users or non users of contraception; there was no difference among obese versus nonobese teens (Beksinska et al, 2010). The amount of weight gain with DMPA is variable, ranging from 3 kg at 1 year to 5 kg at 18 months. Recent evidence suggests that most DMPA users who experience 5% weight gain within 6 months of starting DMPA will continue to have excessive weight gain during use. Pre-depo obesity does not appear to predict weight gain (Le et al, 2009).

2. Subdermal implant (Implanon): every 3 years
   - Description
     - Etonogestrel 68 mg, slow continuous release for 3 years (60 mcg/day, 25 to 30 mcg/day by year 3)

from a 4 cm × 2 mm ethylene vinylacetate (EVA) rod; placed subdermally in the upper, inner arm
- Other implants available in many countries (progestin release, efficacy, and side effects similar to Implanon)
  - Norplant: six silastic capsules releasing levonorgestrel; effective 7 years
  - Jadelle or Sinoplant: two Silastic rods releasing levonorgestrel; effective 5 years
- Key benefits, ideal candidates, and precautions
  - Long acting, nothing to remember
  - Easy insertion and removal
  - Highly effective and rapidly reversible
  - Good for women with contraindications to estrogen
  - Many women experience unpredictable bleeding
- Insertion and removal
  - May be inserted during an office visit, postabortion, or postpartum
  - Insert within 7 days of menses or if pregnancy can be ruled out clinically (see Overview if nonmenstrual start, use a backup method for 7 days
  - FDA requires taking company-sponsored course in order to provide Implanon
  - Insertion done under local anesthetic in the office and takes 1 to 2 minutes; with local anesthetic, patients experience virtually no pain
  - Implant is inserted with a self-contained insertion needle and obturator: no incision required
  - Removal in office with local anesthesia and small incision (2 to 3 mm), average time 3 minutes

UPDATE #4

Subdermal Implants and Bleeding Patterns

Although 18% to 27% of women experience unpredictable bleeding while using Implanon (Mansour et al, 2008), only 10.4% (Blumenthal et al, 2008) to 14.4% (Darney et al, 2009) actually discontinue the method for this reason. In pooled analyses of 11 clinical trials and 942 women, the most common bleeding pattern during a 90-day reference period was amenorrhea (21%). Women experienced an average of 13 to 18 bleeding or spotting days in 3-month reference periods throughout the 3 years of use (Darney et al, 2009; Mansour et al, 2008). Prolonged bleeding was the most commonly reported pattern, at 17%. Although few data exist thus far to guide symptom management, bothersome episodes of prolonged bleeding can be managed with nonsteroidal anti-inflammatory drugs (NSAIDs), with a short course of estrogen (1.25 mg conjugated equine estrogen × 7 days). Pilot data suggest that the combination of mifepristone and estrogen may be of benefit (Weisberg et al, 2009).

3. Intrauterine contraception: every 5 to 10 years
   - Description
     - T-shaped, flexible device placed into the uterine cavity; two types of devices are available in the United States with many other varieties used worldwide
     - Levonorgestrel Intrauterine System (LNG-IUS) (Mirena): releases 20 mcg of levonorgestrel per day (14 mcg/day by 5 years) into the uterine cavity; minimal systemic absorption (0.1 to 0.2 ng/ml) (Nilsson, 1980); approved for 5 years of use, effective for up to 7 years

- T 380A Intrauterine Copper IUC (ParaGard): polyethylene frame wrapped in copper wire; approved for 10 years of use, effective for at least 12 years
- Key benefits, ideal candidates, and precautions
  - Long acting, nothing to remember
  - Highly effective and rapidly reversible
  - Easy to insert and remove
  - Good for women with contraindications to estrogen (LNG-IUS and Copper) or women who want a hormone-free method (Copper)
  - Copper IUC can be used as emergency contraception within 8 days of ovulation after unprotected intercourse
  - LNG-IUS is especially good for women with oligomenorrhea or anovulatory bleeding who need exogenous progestin for endometrial protection; women with menorrhagia; and women on anticoagulation; has been used to treat endometrial hyperplasia
  - Can be used in nulliparous women; adolescents; women with a history of prior ectopic, STI or pelvic inflammatory disease (PID); women not in a monogamous relationship; women with fibroids that do not distort the uterine cavity; immediately postpartum (within 48 hours) or postabortion
  - Avoid Copper IUC in women with anemia or menorrhagia and women with Wilson's disease or copper allergy
  - Risk of expulsion is ~4% to 5%, declines over time

UPDATE #5

IUCs Do Not Cause PID or Infertility

Intrauterine device (IUD) use in the United States remains limited, despite it being a highly effective, reversible, well-tolerated method. This is likely because of persistent myths associating IUC use with PID, myths that were based on earlier, poorly designed studies and on IUDs that are no longer in use. Numerous well-designed trials have confirmed that there is no association between IUC use and PID. The largest of these studies was a multicenter WHO trial of 22,908 IUC insertions. The risk of PID in the 3 weeks immediately after insertion was 9.7/1000 women, but after this time period it was 1.4/1,000, similar to the baseline risk (Farley, 1992). Despite this insertion risk, prophylactic antibiotics at the time of IUC insertion are of no benefit (Grimes et al, 1999). Screening for gonorrhea and chlamydia should be performed when indicated at the time of insertion, and those with positive results should be treated in a timely fashion, without removal of the IUC. Similarly, if PID is diagnosed and treated in someone with an IUC in place, the IUD should not be removed, unless the woman has not responded to parenteral therapy.

A well-designed case-control study of women with tubal factor primary infertility found no association between previous IUC use and infertility (Hubacher et al, 2001).

- Insertion and removal
  - If indicated, screen women for gonorrhea and chlamydia on the same day as their IUD insertion (following CDC screening recommendations for STI screening: annual screening if younger than 26 or if risk factors such as new partner or multiple sexual partners); do not insert in women with current evidence of active cervicitis or PID
  - Timing can occur at any point in menstrual cycle, as long as pregnancy can be ruled out

- Follow standard insertion procedures, including pelvic examination, betaine prep of cervix, no-touch technique using tenaculum on the cervix, uterine sound (uterus should be 6 to 10 cm), followed by IUD inserter; trim strings 2 to 3 cm in length from the external os
- NSAIDs may reduce procedure pain; most women will not require local cervical anesthetic
- Easy removal by grasping and pulling strings with ring forceps; if strings not visible on examination, try to locate them within the endocervical canal using a Cytobrush; if still not seen, localize IUD with ultrasound and, if not seen in the uterus, with an abdominal flat plate film

4. Permanent sterilization:
   - Description
     - Permanent contraception through surgical sterilization and disruption of the fallopian tubes either by occlusion or ligation
     - May be performed immediately postpartum (within 48 hours) or as an interval procedure either hysteroscopically or laparoscopically
     - Hysteroscopic sterilization (Essure) places nickel-titanium coils in the proximal segment of the tubes and induces a scarring reaction over 3 months, leading to permanent, irreversible tubal occlusion; occlusion must be confirmed radiographically before relying on this method
     - Laparoscopic methods use bands, clips, or electrocautery to occlude tubes permanently
     - Male sterilization is simple, safe, and effective, particularly with the "no-scalpel" vasectomy technique
   - Key benefits, ideal candidates, and precautions
     - Offers permanent contraception; counseling must emphasize the permanent nature of this method
     - Ideal for women who are certain that they do not desire future fertility; women younger than 25 are more likely to regret their sterilization decision later in life
     - Hysteroscopic sterilization is a particularly good choice for obese women because it avoids the need to access the peritoneal cavity
     - Although highly effective, contraceptive failures do occur, and the risk does not decrease over time; the 10-year cumulative incidence of pregnancy ranges from 0.5% to 1.8% depending on which method is used; of pregnancies that occur after tubal sterilization, one third are ectopic; bipolar cautery is associated with a higher rate of ectopic pregnancy than other techniques
   - Techniques
     - *Postpartum salpingectomy.* Accomplished through small periumbilical incision or at the time of cesarean delivery. Multiple techniques, the most frequently used ones (Pomeroy method and Parkland method) involving ligation of a portion of the tube with catgut suture and excising a 2 to 3 cm segment of the fallopian tube.
     - *Laparoscopic tubal sterilization.* Single or double puncture to access the tubes laparoscopically. Titanium clips (Filshie), silicone bands (Fallope), or electrosurgical desiccation (bipolar cautery) used to occlude tubes bilaterally. Commonly done under general anesthesia in United States, but with conscious sedation in much of Asia.
     - *Hysteroscopic, transcervical tubal sterilization.* Can be done in office setting with local anesthesia, with or without sedation. Administer NSAID within 30 minutes of procedure to reduce tubal spasm. Hysteroscopic placement of coils in the proximal portion of the fallopian tubes. Successful bilateral placement rate is 92% to 96%. Women must use another method of contraception until hysterosalpingogram (HSG), performed at 3 months, confirms bilateral tubal occlusion. Bilateral occlusion rate at 3 months is 92% to 99%, and 99% to 100% at 12 months.

MONTHLY CONTRACEPTION

1. Contraceptive vaginal ring: NuvaRing
   - Description
     - Flexible, combined hormonal contraceptive 2-inch ring, easily inserted by patient
     - Releases ethinyl estradiol 15 mcg per day and etonogestrel 120 mcg per day, absorbed systemically through vaginal mucosa
   - Key benefits, ideal candidates, and precautions
     - Convenient, monthly self-administration of effective and reversible contraceptive method; less to remember than daily pills or episodic methods
     - Noncontraceptive benefits of other combined hormonal contraceptives, with lowest overall estrogen exposure and therefore fewer estrogen-related side effects
     - Avoid in women with contraindications to estrogen (Table 30-2)
   - Initiation and continuation
     - Quick start initiation preferred (see Overview) use a backup method for 7 days unless first ring was inserted within 5 days of start of menses
     - Traditional instructions are to leave the ring in place for 3 weeks, and remove for 1 week to induce a withdrawal bleed
     - Ring may be used continuously for 4 weeks with no hormone-free interval; alternatively, you can instruct patients to always insert a new ring on the same day each month; if they wish to have a withdrawal bleed, they can remove the ring 4 to 5 days before their designated "new ring" day; it should be noted that these are both off-label, but effective uses, as the ring releases hormone for 35 days while in place
     - If ring falls out, the same ring should be replaced immediately; if it has been out of the vagina for more than 3 hours, a backup method must be used for 7 days

2. Injectable
   - Although not available in the United States, monthly, combined hormonal contraception is used in other countries

WEEKLY CONTRACEPTION

1. Transdermal contraceptive patch: Ortho Evra
   - Description
     - Square patch, 4.5 cm, applied to skin on lower abdomen, upper torso, or upper outer arm
     - Releases ethinyl estradiol 20 mcg per day and 150 mcg of norelgestromin per day

- Key benefits, ideal candidates, and precautions
  - Convenient, weekly self-administration of effective and reversible contraceptive method; less to remember than daily pills or episodic methods
  - Noncontraceptive benefits of other combined hormonal contraceptives
  - Avoid in women with contraindications to estrogen (see Table 30-2); higher overall estrogen exposure than combined OCP or vaginal ring
- Initiation and continuation
  - Quick start initiation preferred (see Overview) use backup for 7 days, unless initiated within 5 days of start of menses
  - Patch is changed once a week for 3 consecutive weeks, followed by a 7-day hormone-free interval; patch should not be used continuously because of the higher estrogen exposure
  - If more than 9 days since a new patch applied, woman should use a backup method for 7 days
  - Safe to shower, swim, and exercise with patch in place

UPDATE #6

The Patch, Third-Generation Progestins, Drospirenone, and Risk of Venous Thromboembolic Events (VTE)

The use of any combined hormonal contraceptive method increases a woman's risk of a VTE, such as pulmonary embolus or deep vein thrombosis, relative to nonpregnant women not using hormonal contraception. This risk was initially attributed solely to the estrogen component of combined hormonal contraception (CHC), but numerous case-control and cohort studies have investigated the role of the third-generation progestins desogestrel and gestodene, and of drospirenone. A meta-analysis of 12 case-control studies showed increased odds of nonfatal VTE in women using third-generation desogestrel OCPs versus second-generation levonorgestrel OCPs, with an adjusted odds ratio of 1.5 (95% confidence interval [CI] 1.2 to 1.4) (Kemmeren et al, 2001). These results were replicated in a subsequent, large case-control study of 1.3 million women (Jick et al, 2006). For pills containing drospirenone, the European Active Surveillance Study (EURAS) found no increased risk of VTE in 142,475 women-years of exposure. However, a recent cohort study 10.4 million women-years of exposure did find an increased risk of nonfatal VTE in women using drospirenone OCPs compared to levonorgestrel OCPs, with an adjusted relative risk of 1.6 (1.3 to 2.1) (Lindegaard et al, 2009). In summary, although desogestrel and drospirenone appear to increase the risk of clot relative to levonorgestrel OCPs, *the absolute risk remains low and is lower than the risk of a clot in pregnancy.* The risk of VTE among nonpregnant women not on OCPs is 4.4 per 10,000 ♀-years; with desogestrel OCPs the risk is 6.5 per 10,000 ♀-years, and with drospirenone OCPs the risk is 7.8 per 10,000 ♀-years; in pregnancy, the risk is 29 per 10,000 ♀-years (Heinemann et al, 2007; Lindengaard et al, 2009).

A similar story exists for the risk of VTE in women using the contraceptive patch. Pharmacokinetics studies showed that women using the patch are exposed to significantly more estrogen than women using OCPs or the ring (van den Heuvel et al, 2005). Two case-control studies showed conflicting results, one with no increased risk of VTE in women using the patch (Jick et al, 2007) and another demonstrating a 2.4 times greater odds of VTE in patch users (95% CI 1.1 to 5.5) (Cole et al, 2007), compared to second-generation OCPs. In both studies, new users of hormonal contraception did not have an increased

risk of VTE. If use of the patch is associated with an increased risk of VTE, the absolute risk, again, remains low and is lower than in pregnancy.

DAILY CONTRACEPTION

1. Combined oral contraceptive (COC) pill
   - Description
     - Pill taken every day at the same time; hormonally active pills are followed by placebo pills with no hormones
     - Each hormonally active pill contains ethinyl estradiol and a progestin; the combination of the dose of estrogen and the type of progestin varies among different OCPs

---

UPDATE #7

Choosing a COC

1. *Choose estrogen dose.* Any pill with less than 50 mcg of ethinyl estradiol is considered "low dose." Among those, the ultra-low dose 20 mcg has the fewest estrogen-related side effects (nausea, breast tenderness, headaches) but increased breakthrough bleeding (Gallo et al, 2011).
2. *Choose progestin type.* Third-generation progestins and drospirenone are associated with an increased relative risk of VTE, though the absolute risk remains low (see Update #6). Some OCPs are approved to treat acne, hirsutism, and pre-menstrual dysphoric disorder, but all COCs usually provide relief of these symptoms; their superiority relative to other COCs has not been adequately demonstrated in rigorous trials (American College of Obstetricians and Gynecologists, ACOG Practice Bulletin No. 110, 2010; Wong et al, 2009).
3. *Make other adjustments based on woman's side effects.* That is, lower the estrogen dose if mastalgia or raise the estrogen dose if breakthrough bleeding.

Ethinyl Estradiol Dose	Progestin Type
20 mcg	"Second generation" (norethindrone, levonorgestrel, norgestimate)
30 mcg	"Third generation" (desogestrel, etonogestrel, gestodene)
35 mcg	Antimineralocorticoid (drospirenone)
50 mcg	(rarely used)

- Key benefits, ideal candidates, and precautions
  - Self-administration of effective and reversible contraceptive method
  - Noncontraceptive benefits of other combined hormonal contraceptives
  - Avoid in women with contraindications to estrogen (see Table 30-2)
- Initiation and continuation
  - Quick start initiation preferred (see Overview) use a backup method for 7 days, unless initiated within 5 days of start of last menses
  - Successful pill use requires individualized systems for remembering daily, timely dosing
  - Traditional use instructs women to take one hormonally active pill daily for 21 days followed by a 7-day placebo, hormone-free interval, during which a withdrawal bleed occurs

- Women may skip the placebo pills and use hormonally active OCPs continuously; several extended-cycle OCPs are available in special packaging
- Missed pill instructions
  - If during week 1 of pill pack and one or more pills are missed: take one active pill as soon as possible, and continue taking one pill daily until the end of the pack; use backup method × 7 days and emergency contraception if indicated
  - If during week 2 or 3 of pill pack and one or two pills are missed: take the active, forgotten pill as soon as possible, and continue taking 1 pill daily until end of pack; skip placebo pills; no need for backup
  - If during week 2 or 3 of pill pack and three or more pills are missed: take the active, forgotten pill as soon as possible, continue taking one pill daily until the end of pack, skip placebo pills, and use backup method × 7 days; use emergency contraception if indicated

UPDATE #8

Extended Cycle COCs

Variations of the traditional 21-7 formulation of COCs exist, in an attempt to improve contraceptive efficacy and to decrease withdrawal bleeds. By day 7 of the hormone-free interval with OCPs, 47% of women will have developed a dominant follicle (Baerwald et al, 2004). Two OCPs (Yaz and Loestrin 24 Fe) have 23 or 24 hormonally active pills, with a shorter hormone-free interval. There is no increase in breakthrough bleeding (Bachman et al, 2004; Endrikat et al, 2001; Spona et al, 1996). Women can also choose 12 weeks of continuous, hormonally active pills followed by one placebo week, either with or without a small dose of ethinyl estradiol (Seasonale or Seasonique, respectively). During the first 3-month cycle, women experience an average of 12 bleeding or spotting days, which decreases to 4 days after 1 year of use (Anderson et al, 2003). Finally, a 1-year continuous OCP (Lybrel) shows high user acceptability and a 72% amenorrhea rate (Foidart et al, 2006; Miller et al, 2003). Although perfect use efficacy is high with these formulations, it is not clear that they offer benefit for improved typical use efficacy compared to traditional COCs.

2. Progestin-only pill
   - Description
     - Pill taken every day at the same time; all pills contain hormone, with no placebo or hormone-free interval
     - Each tablet contains 35 mcg of norethindrone
   - Key benefits, ideal candidates, and precautions
     - Ideal for women who want to use a daily oral method but who have contraindications to estrogen
     - Rapidly reversible
   - Initiation and continuation
     - Quick start preferred (see Overview); use backup for 2 days
     - Must be taken at the same time every day; if a woman is more than 3 hours late taking the pill, she should take it as soon as possible and use backup for 2 days

UPDATE #9

Contraception in Breast-Feeding Women

Ovulation occurs as early as 3 weeks postpartum in women who are partially or not breast-feeding, and 3 months in women who are exclusively breast-feeding (Darney et al, 2005). Combined hormonal contraception can be initiated at 6 weeks postpartum, without effect on milk production or infant growth. For women needing contraception sooner, progestin-only methods can be started without any effect on infant feeding, growth, or breast-feeding continuation. DMPA can be given immediately postpartum, but for breast-feeding women with reliable follow-up, it is reasonable to delay injection 2 to 3 weeks. The subdermal implant does not appear to affect breast-feeding or infant growth (Brito et al, 2009; Taneepanichskul et al, 2006). Intrauterine contraception can be safely inserted within 48 hours postpartum but should be delayed until 4 weeks postpartum in women with puerperal infection (Grimes et al, 2010). The lactational amenorrhea method provides effective contraception but only for women who are exclusively breast-feeding, on infant demand, who are not experiencing cyclic bleeding, and whose infants are less than 6 months old (see the IMAP Statement on Postpartum Contraception and Breast-feeding Women, International Planned Parenthood Federation, 2008).

EPISODIC CONTRACEPTION

1. Emergency contraception (EC) pills
   - Pills taken within 120 hours of unprotected intercourse to prevent pregnancy
   - Not an abortifacient and does not disrupt an already implanted pregnancy
   - Progestin-only EC contains levonorgestrel 150 mcg, taken in one dose, and is available as Plan B (two tablets) or Plan B One Step; it is more effective than the "Yuzpe regimen" of taking high doses of COCs (to total 200 mcg of ethinyl estradiol, divided into two doses 12 hours apart) and has fewer side effects
   - Levonorgestrel EC reduces the risk of pregnancy by 89%
   - Advance provision of EC results in greater use of EC, with no increased risk of STIs
   - Available from pharmacies without a prescription for women 17 years of age and older
   - Ulipristal acetate, a selective progesterone receptor modulator, is also effective and well-tolerated as emergency contraception up to 5 days after unprotected intercourse. It appears to have slightly higher efficacy than levonorgestrel in the 72-120 hour time period. The dose is 30mg, and it is currently available only by prescription.
2. Barrier methods
   - Significant discrepancy between perfect use efficacy and typical use efficacy exists for barrier methods, because of the need for correct use with every act of intercourse; should be coupled with advance provision of emergency contraception pills
   - Male condoms
     - Single-use sheath of latex, polyurethane, or natural membranes worn over the penis prior to contact and until after ejaculation when the penis is removed from vagina, mouth, or anus
     - Effective and important in the prevention of sexually transmitted infections, including HIV; the small HIV can pass through natural membrane condoms but not through latex or plastic ones
   - Female condoms
     - Single use, polyurethane sheath placed into vagina up to 8 hours before intercourse

- Remove from vagina immediately after penis is withdrawn
- Diaphragm
  - Reusable latex rubber dome device placed into vagina to cover cervix 3 hours prior to intercourse
  - Not shown to protect against HIV infection; may reduce risk of gonorrhea and chlamydia
  - Women need to be fitted by doctor for appropriately sized diaphragm
  - More effective when combined with spermicide
- Cervical cap
  - Reusable latex or Silastic dome, which fits over the cervix
  - May be left in place for several days, washed, and reinserted
  - Efficacy is similar to the diaphragm
  - Used with or without spermicide
  - Several brands marketed worldwide (Prentif, Lea's Shield, Femcap, CerCap)
3. Spermicide
   - Gels, creams, foams, film, suppositories, or tablets that contain spermicidal detergent (nonoxynol-9), which immobilize sperm
   - Inserted into the vagina within 15 minutes (gels, creams, foams) or 1 hour (tablets, film, suppository) of intercourse
   - Should not be used by women who are at high risk for acquiring HIV or who are already HIV positive
4. Fertility awareness methods
   - These methods require women to have regular menstrual cycles and entail various ways of close monitoring to determine the infertile and fertile times in the cycle, such as use of "cycle beads" to count days, manual or device analysis of cervical mucous, or basal temperature fluctuations
   - Women avoid intercourse during the fertile phase of their cycle or use a barrier method during this time
   - Efficacy depends on specialized teaching and strict adherence to abstinence or barrier use

Summary

- Unintended pregnancies have a major impact on maternal morbidity and mortality worldwide
- The most effective contraceptive is the one that is easiest for a woman to use
- For most women, the health benefits of contraception outweigh the risks
- The Centers for Disease Control (CDC) and World Health Organization (WHO) Medical Eligibility Criteria (MEC) for Contraceptive Use each provide an evidence-based guide to balancing benefits and risks for women with various health conditions
- Contraceptives have important health benefits, including a reduction in risk of certain cancers, ectopic pregnancy, and pelvic infection, as well as in the management of pelvic pain and abnormal uterine bleeding
- Contraceptives, except for IUDs and sterilization, can be safely provided without a pelvic examination

SUGGESTED READINGS

General

ACOG Committee on Practice Bulletins—Gynecology: ACOG practice bulletin no. 73: use of hormonal contraception in women with coexisting medical conditions, *Obstet Gynecol* 107(6):1453–1472, 2006.

American College of Obstetricians and Gynecologists: ACOG practice bulletin no. 110: noncontraceptive uses of hormonal contraceptives, *Obstet Gynecol* 115(1):206–218, 2010.

Division of Reproductive Health: National Center for Chronic Disease Prevention and Health Promotion: *U.S. medical eligibility criteria for contraceptive use, 2010.* www.cdc.gov/mmwr/pdf/rr/rr5904.pdf. Accessed July 23, 2011.

Society of Family Planning: Edelmen A: Contraceptive considerations in obese women, SFP Guideline 20091, *Contraception* 80(6):583–590, 2009.

Depo Medroxyprogesterone Acetate

American College of Obstetricians and Gynecologists Committee on Gynecologic Practice: ACOG committee opinion no. 415: Depo medroxyprogesterone acetate and bone effects, *Obstet Gynecol* 112(3):727–730, 2008.

Kaunitz AM, Arias R, McClung M: Bone density recovery after depot medroxyprogesterone acetate injectable contraception use, *Contraception* 77(2):67–76, 2008.

Subdermal Implant

Darney P, Patel A, Rosen K, et al: Safety and efficacy of a single-rod etonogestrel implant (Implanon): results from 11 international clinical trials, *Fertil Steril* 91(5):1646–1653, 2009.

Intrauterine Contraception

American College of Obstetricians and Gynecologists: ACOG committee on practice bulletins—gynecology: ACOG practice bulletin: clinical management guidelines for obstetrician-gynecologists no. 59, January 2005: intrauterine device, *Obstet Gynecol* 105(1):223–232, 2005.

American College of Obstetricians and Gynecologists: ACOG committee opinion no. 392, December 2007: intrauterine device and adolescents, *Obstet Gynecol* 110(6):1493–1495, 2007.

Hubacher D, Lara-Ricalde R, Taylor DJ, et al: Use of copper intrauterine devices and the risk of tubal infertility among nulligravid women, *N Engl J Med* 345(8):561–567, 2001.

Lyus R, Lohr P, Prager S, et al: Use of the Mirena™ LNG-IUS and Paragard™ CuT380A intrauterine devices in nulliparous women, *Contraception* 81(5):367–371, 2010.

Female Sterilization

Peterson HB: Sterilization, *Obstet Gynecol* 111(1):189–203, 2008.

Peterson HB, Xia Z, Hughes JM, et al: The risk of ectopic pregnancy after tubal sterilization, U.S. Collaborative Review of Sterilization Working Group, *N Engl J Med* 336(11):762–767, 1997.

Oral Contraceptives

Kemmeren JM, Algra A, Grobbee DE: Third generation oral contraceptives and risk of venous thrombosis: meta-analysis, *BMJ* 323(7305):131–134, 2001.

Lidegaard O, Lokkegaard E, Svendsen AL, Agger C: Hormonal contraception and risk of venous thromboembolism: national follow-up study, *BMJ* 339: b2890, 2009.

Emergency Contraception

American College of Obstetricians and Gynecologists: ACOG practice bulletin no. 112: emergency contraception, *Obstet Gynecol* 115(5):1100–1109, 2010.

Glasier AF, Cameron ST, Fine PM, et al: Ulipristal acetate versus levonorgestrel for emergency contraception: a randomised non-inferiority trial and meta-analysis, *The Lancet* 375(9714):555–562, 2010.

USEFUL WEBSITES

CDC Medical Eligibility Criteria: www.cdc.gov/reproductivehealth/unintendedpregnancy/USMEC.htm

WHO Medical Eligibility Criteria: http://www.who.int/reproductivehealth/publications/family_planning/9789241563888/en/index.html

Association for Reproductive Health Professionals, Association for Reproductive Health Professionals: http://arhp.org.

Guttmacher Institute, Guttmacher Institute: www.guttmacher.org.

References

Please go to expertconsult.com to view references.

Chapter 31

Abortion

CARON KIM • ERICA OBERMAN • ANGELA Y. CHEN

KEY UPDATES

1 Approximately 1.2 million abortions occur each year, making it the second most common surgery in the reproductive-age woman after cesarean delivery.

2 Almost 90% of abortions occur in the first trimester, and the overall complication rate of induced abortion is less than 1%.

3 As gestation increases, however, difficulty increases and the risks of abortion start to rise. Women seeking later second trimester care experience great difficulty with logistical factors that subsequently expose the woman to greater risk at later gestation. Any means of allowing greater access to care earlier would allow care to shift to the lower-risk gestational age group.

4 First-trimester medical abortion regimens using a combination of mifepristone and misoprostol are more successful than those using misoprostol as a single agent.

5 Despite case reports of *Clostridium sordellii* infection following medical abortion, infection remains <1%, comparable to spontaneous abortion and early surgical abortion.

6 Manual aspiration as well as electric vacuum aspiration can effectively be used for first-trimester abortion without a difference in complications. The difference can allow for lower cost and resources to be expended while offering the same quality care.

7 An ultrasound can be used for intraoperative guidance and is a good tool for teaching in a training facility.

8 Many pain management options exist to allow safe and comfortable early surgical abortion in the office setting.

9 For induction of labor in the second trimester, use of mifepristone in combination with misoprostol shortens time to delivery and decreases the need for subsequent instrumentation when compared to use of misoprostol alone.

10 There are various options for pain control for both medical induction of labor and surgical abortions performed in the midtrimester.

11 In the second trimester, complications such as retained products and perforation are reduced considerably with the use of cervical preparation and ultrasound guidance.

12 Inducing fetal demise can be a useful adjunct to midtrimester abortion.

13 Immediate postabortion initiation of contraception is a critical time to prevent recurrence of unintended pregnancy.

Context

UPDATE #1

The Alan Guttmacher Institute estimates that approximately 1.2 million abortions were performed in the United States in 2005. Eighty-seven percent of these abortions were performed in the first trimester (Gamble et al, 2008). Women seeking abortions in the second trimester are more likely to have experienced delay in identification of the pregnancy, experienced logistical challenges in finding an appropriate provider, and noted challenges in obtaining public insurance.

UPDATE #2

The overall complication rate of induced abortion is less than 1%. The risk of mortality associated with induced abortion increases with increasing gestational age, ranging from 1 death per million procedures performed at less than 8 weeks, to 1 in 29,000 for procedures performed from 16 to 20 weeks, to 1 in 11,000 for procedures performed at 21 weeks and greater (Drey et al, 2006).

Preprocedure counseling: Once a woman has decided to proceed with an induced abortion, all options based on gestational age should be thoroughly explained, clearly outlining available procedures for each individual patient. Both surgical and medical methods of abortion are safe and effective. The decision is personal based on timing, affordability, and recovery from the process (Drey et al, 2006).

Occasionally there are psychosocial advantages of one method:

- Early medical abortion allows a woman to return to her usual functions without interruption and without surgical instrumentation; some women equate it to having a heavy menses or miscarriage and are able to carry on their usual daily routines without significant interruption
- Medical abortion in the mid-trimester may require hospitalization on an obstetric floor, where a woman may not want to be with other laboring women
- During the mid-trimester, a healthy woman can choose from a medical induction or a surgical dilation and evacuation; a thorough examination and workup for an unexplained fetal demise or anomalies may be made possible via both procedures; however, a patient who finds it important to grieve and mourn or who has a complex social situation may benefit from an induction of labor; appropriate counseling with social work can be arranged while the patient is in the hospital

Some women may prefer the predictability of an outpatient surgery instead of awaiting completion of medical abortion. In some settings where surgical methods are not available, modern medical abortion regimens represent safe alternatives for abortion that any general obstetrician-gynecologist can provide.

First-Trimester Abortion

UPDATE #4
In medical abortion, misoprostol is used alone or in conjunction with a second agent: mifepristone or methotrexate (Kulier et al, 2004).

MEDICAL ABORTION

1. Mifepristone and misoprostol
   - Mifepristone is a progesterone antagonist that causes decidual necrosis in a pregnant uterus, softens the cervix, and increases prostaglandin sensitivity; when combined with a prostaglandin analogue, it is effective for medical abortion
   - Mifepristone has additional potential applications for emergency contraception, cervical ripening for labor induction, and treatment of uterine fibroids, endometriosis, Cushing's syndrome, breast cancer, and glaucoma, currently under investigation
   - Regimen approved by the Food and Drug Administration (FDA) (recommended for use up to 49 days gestation)
     - Day 1: mifepristone 600 mg orally administered in medical setting
     - Day 2: misoprostol 400 mcg orally administered in medical setting
     - Day 14: follow-up to ensure completion of abortion; aspiration of gestational sac is performed if still present
     - Efficacy 92%, which decreases with advancing gestational age
       - Evidence-based alternative regimen (recommended for use up to 63 days gestation)
     - Day 1: mifepristone 200 mg orally administered in medical setting
     - Day 1 to day 3: misoprostol 800 mcg vaginally or buccally (may be self-administered by patient outside of medical setting)
     - Day 7 to day 14: follow-up to ensure completion of abortion
     - Compared to FDA regimen
       - Increased efficacy to 98%
       - Lower rate of continuing pregnancies
       - Shorter time to expulsion
       - Fewer side effects
       - Improved complete abortion rate
       - Lower cost
2. Misoprostol alone
   - Misoprostol is an inexpensive prostaglandin analogue that has been approved by the FDA for the prevention and treatment of gastric ulcers caused by nonsteroidal anti-inflammatory drugs (NSAIDs)
   - Off-label uses include medical abortion, cervical ripening before surgical abortion, evacuation of uterus in cases of embryonic or fetal death, induction of labor, and prevention of postpartum hemorrhage (Goldberg et al, 2001)
   - Misoprostol is effective, heat stable, and low cost, and thus is on the World Health Organization's Model List of Essential Drugs for the induction of labor and abortion (Weeks et al, 2007)
   - Multiple regimens exist with repeated dosing of misoprostol 800 mcg
   - Misoprostol can be taken via oral, buccal, sublingual, vaginal, rectal routes; for first-trimester abortions, it has been determined that the vaginal route has better efficacy (Blanchard et al, 2005; Kulier et al, 2004); however, a recent study compared serum concentration and uterine contraction effects between vaginal and buccal misoprostol; similar uterine tone and activity were noted between the vaginal and buccal routes (Meckstroth et al, 2006)
   - Studies have shown its efficacy as the sole abortifacient; therefore, it can be used as a single agent in settings where mifepristone or methotrexate is not available; in pregnancies up to 12 weeks, misoprostol alone is given as 800 mg per vagina every 3 to 12 hours for up to three doses (Blanchard et al, 2005; Carbonell et al, 1999); success rates have ranged from 83% to 97% (Carbonell et al, 2003; Creinin et al, 1994; Jain et al, 2002)
3. Methotrexate and misoprostol
   - Methotrexate blocks dihydrofolate reductase required for DNA synthesis
   - Methotrexate is commonly available to treat neoplastic disorders, multiple rheumatologic disorders, asthma,

Crohn's disease, and ectopic pregnancies; hence, it is easily available in regions where there is no access for mifepristone for medical abortion

- For medical abortion up to 49 days gestation, low-dose methotrexate is sufficient; the methotrexate destabilizes the pregnancy by interfering with cytotrophoblastic DNA synthesis and requires the additional effect of misoprostol to expel the pregnancy
- A dose of 50 mg/m^2 of methotrexate given intramuscularly followed by 800 mcg of misoprostol vaginally, 3 to 7 days later; 50 mg oral methotrexate appears to be as effective as the 50 mg/m^2 IM
- Repeat 800 mcg misoprostol dosing can be administered until expulsion of the persistent gestational sac
- Efficacy approaches that of mifepristone with misoprostol regimens but requires greater time to completion, up to 4 weeks in 15% to 25% of users of this regimen, with multiple interval visits
- It is also important to note the teratogenicity of methotrexate, and therefore close follow-up is required for women who have failed the methotrexate-misoprostol regimen

4. Special precautions for medical abortion
   - Inability to comply with medication instructions or planned follow-up
   - Known allergy to medications
   - Long-term steroid use or adrenal insufficiency if using mifepristone
   - Renal or liver disease (applicable to methotrexate)
   - Intrauterine device (IUD) in situ should be removed before initiation of medical abortion
   - Confirmed or suspected ectopic (extrauterine) pregnancy
   - Coagulopathy or current use of anticoagulants
   - Inherited porphyria if using mifepristone
   - Breast-feeding mothers can pump and discard breast milk during medication abortion
   - Lack of access to a provider for expeditious uterine aspiration in the event of excess bleeding or persistent gestational cardiac activity at 2 weeks after onset of medical abortion

UPDATE #5

Infection is a rare complication of medical abortion, <1%, such that few data support antibiotic prophylaxis or change in dosing regimen. *Clostridium sordellii* was identified in three of the five cases of death in North American women who used mifepristone. However, the death rate associated with medical abortion remains at less than 1/100,000, comparable to early surgical abortion and spontaneous abortion (American College of Obstetricians and Gynecologists, ACOG Practice Bulletin No. 67, 2005; Centers for Disease Control and Prevention, 2005; Fjerstad et al, 2009; Grimes, 2005; Kapp et al, 2009).

5. Side effects and complications of medical abortion
   - Common side effects of all regimens can include vaginal bleeding, abdominal cramping, nausea, vomiting, diarrhea, flushing, or chills
   - Vaginal bleeding can vary significantly in both duration and severity, and many report that the bleeding resembles a heavy period or a spontaneous miscarriage
   - Light bleeding and spotting can last for 1 to 3 weeks; reported median bleeding times range from 9 to 13 days; the heaviest period of bleeding typically occurs when the abortion is occurring and persists for 1 to 4 hours
   - Pain of medical abortion is usually described as cramping; treatment with anticipatory guidance, symptomatic relief with heating pad to abdomen or low back, reduced activity, and aggressive oral analgesics result in satisfactory outpatient control
   - Approximately 1% of women experience uterine bleeding that requires uterine aspiration and about 0.1% to 0.4% require transfusion
   - Temperature elevation (defined as more than 100.4° F or 38° C) that is sustained (more than 4 hours) or begins more than 6 to 8 hours after misoprostol administration warrants clinical assessment
   - In the less than 1% there is ongoing gestational growth 2 weeks after onset of medication abortion, and suction curettage is recommended to terminate pregnancy; overall, in 2% to 5% of cases, patients may require vacuum aspiration to resolve an incomplete abortion, end a continuing pregnancy, or control bleeding
   - To date, there is no evidence that mifepristone has teratogenic effects on the fetus; several case reports have associated misoprostol use with cranial and limb defects and Möbius syndrome; methotrexate is known to cause embryopathy
   - Ultrasound evaluation of the endometrium is not predictive of clinical intervention after medical abortion (Ben-Hava et al, 2001; Cowitt et al, 2004; Harwood et al, 2001; Reeves et al, 2009)
   - Ultrasound is, however, useful to detect ongoing pregnancy (1%) so that expeditious surgical treatment can be offered; it is especially useful in pretreatment screening to determine gestational age if discrepant from exam or history and also to identify potential ectopic pregnancies (American College of Obstetricians and Gynecologists, ACOG Practice Bulletin No. 67, 2005)

UPDATE #6

Electric and manual aspirators are similar in completed abortion rates, complication rates, and patient satisfaction. Manual aspirators are low-cost, hand-operated 50- to 60-mL modified syringes that attach directly to the cannula. As the name implies, manual aspirators can be used in settings where electricity or the vacuum aspirator and the associated supplies are not available (Goldberg et al, 2010; Wen et al, 2008). While cervical preparation with laminaria or pharmacologic agents reduces the need for intraoperative mechanical dilation, reduces surgery time and occurrence of lacerations, its utility is limited in first trimester abortion, when dilation is safe and rarely complicated. The patient discomfort, cost, and time required for cervical priming may be worthwhile in the patient at risk for complications or difficult dilation (Allen et al, 2007; Kapp et al, 2010; Schulz et al, 1983; Stubblefield et al, 2004).

SURGICAL ABORTION, SUCTION CURETTAGE

1. Vacuum curettage, uterine aspiration, or suction curettage
   - The most common form of abortion before 13 menstrual weeks
   - Dilation of the cervix can be achieved with mechanical dilators, hygroscopic dilators, such as laminaria, or by prostaglandins such that a cannula of the appropriate size can be inserted into the uterine cavity
   - Cannula size is chosen to match diameter in millimeters with gestational age in weeks +/− 1 mm
2. Complications of surgical abortion
   - Failed or incomplete abortion (0.29% to 1.96% of first-trimester cases) can result in ongoing pregnancy or retained products with subsequent infection; inspection of the tissue and use of intraoperative ultrasound guidance or confirmatory ultrasound after the procedure is a critical step to prevent this complication
   - Perforation
     - Incidence of 0.09 to 2.8/1000
     - Increases with increasing gestational age and teaching settings
   - Hemorrhage related to uterine atony, cervical laceration, incomplete evacuation, coagulopathy, or placental abnormalities
   - Infection
     - Decreased with use of antibiotic prophylaxis (Sawaya et al, 1996)
3. Posttissue examination
   - To be performed immediately following procedure to identify need for reaspiration
   - Imperative to identify gestational sac in addition to villi in early pregnancy to prevent ongoing pregnancy
   - A decrease in quantitative serum beta hCG by at least 50% within 24 to 72 hours following abortion indicates procedure completion in situations in which tissue is insufficient or the examination inconclusive; if levels continue to rise, then further evaluation is needed to distinguish between ectopic pregnancy and persistent intrauterine pregnancy (Creinin et al, 1997)
   - Fetal anomalies, molar pregnancies, and choriocarcinomas can be identified on pathologic examination
4. Perioperative antibiotics
   - Universal prophylaxis has been shown to decrease postabortal infection in extensive meta-analysis (Sawaya et al, 1996)
   - Doxycycline or its analogues such as tetracycline or minocycline has been used for its broad spectrum coverage
   - Metronidazole if allergic, breast-feeding, or otherwise ineligible for doxycycline

UPDATE #7

Ultrasound is useful to detect ongoing pregnancy (1%) so that expeditious surgical treatment can be offered. It is especially useful in pretreatment screening to determine the gestational age if discrepant from exam or history, and also to identify potential ectopic pregnancies (American College of Obstetricians and Gynecologists, ACOG Practice Bulletin No. 67, 2005).

Use of Ultrasound

- Can be used as intraoperative guidance and postoperative confirmation of completion
- May be especially useful as a teaching tool in a training facility
- Associated with decreased complication rates
- Particularly helpful in the challenging body habitus, uterine or cervical anomalies, and to determine completion of the evacuation, especially in the early pregnancy or where tissue examination shows inadequate products were retrieved

UPDATE #8

Pain management for first-trimester surgical abortion is dependent on the resources available and ultimately patient preference. Local anesthesia can be used alongside a variety of other agents (Allen et al, 2009).

- Lidocaine has been described intracervically, paracervically, in the deep low uterine field block, as well as with intrauterine instillation for the purpose of first-trimester abortion; in general, 1% lidocaine is limited at 4.5 mg/kg maximum; the addition of vasopressin into the lidocaine paracervical block reduces blood loss; the addition of ketorolac into the lidocaine paracervical block augments the pain control (Cansino et al, 2009; Edelman et al, 2006; Mankowski et al, 2009; Schulz et al, 1985; Stubblefield et al, 2004)
- Oral NSAIDS, narcotic analgesics, and short-acting oral anxiolytics are useful adjuncts in first-trimester pain management
- Intravenous (IV) conscious sedation, moderate sedation with short-acting intravenous agents, such as fentanyl and midazolam, can improve patient satisfaction with intraoperative pain control when compared with local anesthesia alone; NPO status, staffing, and monitoring, as well as recovery time, may limit the provision of sedation services
- Deep sedation and general anesthesia are limited by the availability of anesthesia providers, resources, staffing, and monitoring; may be indicated for the patient who has exceptional anxiety or pain control issues and who needs monitored anesthesia care in the operating room
- Verbal reassurance, focused breathing, guided imagery, and other nonpharmacologic methods are commonly used as an adjunct for anxiolysis on the awake patient

Second-Trimester Abortion

MEDICAL INDUCTION OF LABOR IN THE SECOND TRIMESTER

UPDATE #9

In combination with misoprostol induction, mifepristone can reduce the abortion interval by 50%. The median time of induction abortion with misoprostol only is 10 to 19 hours. When mifepristone is added to the regimen, the median time is reduced to below 10 hours (Ashok et al, 2004; Goh et al, 2006; Kapp et al, 2007).

1. Mifepristone and misoprostol
   - Mifepristone counters the progesterone effect of uterine relaxation on the gravid uterus; once antagonized, this allows uterine contractions to occur with dilation and softening of the cervix
   - Additionally, mifepristone causes decidual necrosis with increased sensitivity to prostaglandin by fivefold within 24 to 48 hours; subsequent administration of prostaglandins such as misoprostol then affects successful induction without increasing abortion time and without increasing side effects
   - Mifepristone 200 mg is given orally; the patient is typically admitted to the hospital 24 to 48 hours later to start the prostaglandin induction
   - In combination with misoprostol induction, mifepristone can reduce the abortion interval by 50%; median time of induction abortion with misoprostol only is 10 to 19 hours; when mifepristone is added to the regimen, the median time is reduced to below 10 hours (Ashok et al, 2004; Goh et al, 2006; Kapp et al, 2007)
   - Induction protocols vary starting with a misoprostol load of 400 to 800 mcg followed by repeated dosing of misoprostol 200 mcg to 600 mcg every 3 to 12 hours; higher dosage and frequent intervals are associated with greater side effects
   - The vaginal and buccal routes of administration appear to be most effective and equivalent, followed by sublingual and oral routes with higher rates of gastrointestinal (GI) side effects; patients may prefer nonvaginal routes while undergoing medical abortion and having bleeding
2. Misoprostol alone
   - Systemic prostaglandins such as carboprost and dinoprostone have been largely replaced by misoprostol for its favorable side effect profile, lower cost, and efficacy; original studies comparing misoprostol vaginally to dinoprostone demonstrated that misoprostol had fewer side effects and was just as effective
   - The pharmacokinetics of the various routes in which misoprostol can be administered is important to understand in relation to dosing; oral dosing is rapidly absorbed, and plasma concentrations peak at 30 minutes and then decline; this route does have increased GI side effects, compared to other routes
   - The peak in plasma concentration for vaginal routes is approximately 1 to 2 hours and declines slowly, increasing the overall exposure time to the medication
   - When given buccally, the plasma peak concentration is anywhere from 15 to 120 minutes, also with a slow decline similar to the vaginal route; this method has the added advantage of being less invasive in administration
   - Rectal administration has demonstrated rapid peak serum levels (time) similar to that of oral with rapid decline afterward
   - The side effects are dose dependent; presently doses ranging from 200 to 600 mcg every 3 to 12 hours × five doses, dependent on gestational age and rate of absorption are being used; the provider should be cautioned that there is still a risk of uterine rupture in high doses, short interval regimens
   - Misoprostol 400 mcg q 6 hr more effective than q 12 hr
   - Caution is also advised when using misoprostol in patients with previous uterine scar; several examples of midtrimester ruptured uterus with previous scar have been described with misoprostol 200 to 400 mcg at interval of 4 to 6 hours; the risk of cesarean scar rupture is estimated at 0.3% during misoprostol induced abortion; several series have demonstrated safety of misoprostol medical abortion with prior cesarean scar; use of mifepristone potentially can reduce the time required to abort and lessen exposure to uterotonic agents (Dickinson, 2005; Goyal, 2009)
3. High-dose oxytocin
   - Uterine sensitivity to oxytocin increases with increasing gestational age
   - Oxytocin can be used once patient is closer to 20 to 24 weeks, because presence of oxytocin receptors increases with gestational age
   - Recommended dose is 50 units in 500cc D5NS over 3 hours, 1 hour rest, then 100 units in 500cc over 3 hours, then 1 hour rest, then 150 units in 500cc D5NS to a maximum of 300 units in 500cc of D5NS (Williams Obstetrics)
4. Historic methods: hypertonic saline, urea, and intraamniotic prostaglandins
   - Thought to be the most effective method of labor induction prior to the 1970s to 1980s; however, the use of hypertonic instillation has been largely replaced by newer methods with faster expulsion times and better side effect profiles
   - Hypertonic solutions, such as saline or urea, were considered safer because it is less worrisome if there is an inadvertent injection intravascularly
   - Typically 90cc of 24% NaCl or 200 ml or 20% NaCl can be injected intra-amniotically; this method of induction was replaced secondary to the long induction to abortion time and other safety concerns such as high rate of curettage after expulsion of fetus; administered alone, the induction to abortion time on average is 22 to 25 hours (Stubblefield et al, 2004)
   - Intra-amniotic instillation of 80 to 90 g of hypertonic urea is an effective abortifacient; the injection to abortion time remains prolonged, so augmentation with other means such as IV oxytocin or prostaglandins is often implemented
   - 2 mg of the 15-methyl analogue, carboprost tromethamine, can be injected intra-amniotically to induce abortion; often a second injection and transient fetal survival resulted along with significant GI side effect, and in the primigravida, risk for cervical laceration; overnight treatment with laminaria reduced the mean time from instillation to abortion from 29 hours to 14 hours, reduced risk for cervical injury, and reduced the need for second injection
   - The modern addition of misoprostol, mifepristone, and laminaria can be used to expedite expulsion when using these historic methods

SURGICAL ABORTION, DILATION, AND EVACUATION

1. Cervical preparation
   - Dilation and evacuation is the process of removing the uterine contents after surgical dilation of the cervix; this can be done under intraoperative ultrasound guidance, which was found to decrease the incidence of perforation from 1.4% to 0.2% (Darney et al, 1989)
   - The first step is cervical preparation either through medications, laminaria, or both, or via mechanical dilation at the beginning of the procedure; slow, gradual dilation can be achieved through the use of hydroscopic/osmotic dilators, laminaria, Dilapan, and Lamicel, which have been shown to decrease risk of injury to the cervix; laminaria japonica and digitata can be found in various lengths and sizes from 2 to 10 mm in diameter; they are placed in their dehydrated form and after absorption of fluid within the cervix; maximum dilation is achieved in 12 to 24 hours (Hayes et al, 2009)
   - Dilapan-S is available in 3- and 4-mm diameter dilators; most of the dilation occurs in 4 to 6 hours; however, it continues to dilate for up to 24 hours
   - Laminaria and Dilapan both swell to three to four times their original size; in one study, the use of mechanical dilators was associated with the rate of cervical laceration requiring repair from 5% to 0.6% and 10% to 1.2% for procedures between 18 and 20 weeks and between 20 and 26 weeks, respectively (Hayes et al, 2009); preoperative preparation with osmotic dilators can assist with cervical dilation as needed with increasing gestational age
   - There is a small risk in the use of laminaria, such as overdilation leading to labor and untimely delivery, rupture of membranes, and infection; clinical judgment dictates if one or two sets of laminaria placement is needed based on gestational age, parity, and appearance of the cervix; cervical preparation can be augmented with misoprostol or mifepristone when insufficient hygroscopic dilators are able to be inserted or if the patient is a particular risk for complication
   - Osmotic dilators were found to be superior to prostaglandins with respect to cervical dilation throughout the second trimester and with respect to procedure time within the early second trimester; the addition of prostaglandins to osmotic dilators was not found to increase cervical dilation, except after 19 weeks' gestation; however, no impact was seen on procedure time; the addition of mifepristone to misoprostol was found to improve cervical dilation yet increase procedure time and the frequency of preprocedural expulsions; a 2-day cervical preparation was found to produce greater cervical preparation than a 1-day preparation, but it had no impact on procedure time; serious complication rates or ability to complete the procedure did not differ significantly between any of the preparation methods reviewed (Newman et al, 2010)
2. Intraoperative management
   - On the day of the procedure, the laminaria will be removed to allow for the passage of the appropriate instruments; for example, large ovum forceps such as Bierer forceps, used in later procedures, are approximately 2 cm in diameter; therefore, dilating to 2 centimeters is necessary for their passage
   - Evacuation of the uterus done under ultrasound guidance decreases the incidence of retained tissue and perforation (Darney et al, 1989)
   - After all products are removed, systemic uterotonics, such as oxytocin, can be administered along with methylergonovine maleate (Methergine, Novartis Pharmaceuticals) in order to promote uterine tone and involution and to prevent postprocedure hemorrhage
   - A paracervical block with the addition of vasopressin prior to instrumentation of the uterus can also assist in stopping excessive blood loss during and after the procedure
   - Current ACOG practice guidelines recommend the use of prophylactic antibiotics in surgical abortion in the second trimester (D&Es) in preventing perioperative infection

UPDATE #10

Pain control options in the second trimester take into account the higher analgesic needs experienced at higher gestational age, at longer induction intervals, in younger women, in lower-parity women, and in those with a higher level of anxiety and history of dysmenorrhea (Wiebe, 2001).

PAIN CONTROL OPTIONS IN THE SECOND TRIMESTER

- Determined by resources available and patient preference
- Oral NSAIDs with narcotics such as oxycodone or codeine may be used for pain relief
- However, IV medications may be more effective with more rapid onset
- Patient-controlled analgesia (PCA) for IV administration of fentanyl, Dilaudid, or morphine may be used while in the inpatient setting
- Regional anesthesia can also be useful in settings where a provider is available for administration
- Laminaria placement: local anesthesia at the tenaculum site
- Complete cervical block for the insertion and also during the D+E is commonly performed
- Moderate to deep sedation is usually required for the D+E
- Ultimately patient satisfaction and experience of pain can be affected by the duration of the abortion interval

UPDATE #11

Modern methods of midtrimester medical abortion have reduced inpatient length of stay and surgical instrumentation. Surgical abortion in the second trimester (D&Es) has revealed a 1% major complication rate (Diedrich et al, 2009).

COMPLICATIONS

1. Medical induction of labor in the second trimester
   - Compared with historic methods of medical abortion, modern regimens of misoprostol or misoprostol with mifepristone induction reveal that expectant management for the retained placenta is not correlated with adverse outcome

- Rates of instrumentation for the retained placenta range from 2.5% to 10%; most women experience spontaneous placenta expulsion shortly after abortion; intervention to remove the placenta is indicated in the event of excess bleeding or fever (Dickinson et al, 2009; Green et al, 2007)
- Additional medical management with bimanual massage, oxytocin, carboprost, or misoprostol may be appropriate to assist in placenta expulsion
- Rupture of previous uterine scar is rare with medication abortion; medication abortion can be safely accomplished even with history of uterine scar
2. Surgical abortions in the second trimester
   - D+E is a safe procedure and is associated with a 1% major complication rate; however, when a complication occurs, it can be quite serious
   - The history of two or more cesarean deliveries is associated with a sevenfold increase in the odds for a major complication, including an abnormal placentation
   - Hemorrhage, defined as excess blood loss >500 cc, can result from multiple causes:
     - Uterine atony
     - Perforation
     - Cervical laceration
     - Retained products of conception
     - Coagulopathy
     - Abnormal placentation
   - Treatment of atony includes bimanual massage, uterotonic medications, intrauterine balloon tamponade, uterine artery embolization, and the rare incidence of hysterectomy
   - UAE has been demonstrated to be useful for management of postabortion bleeding because of atony, abnormal placentation, and high cervical laceration
   - Cervical laceration can usually be repaired with suture ligation of the descending cervical branches of the uterine artery; rarely a high cervical laceration will require UAE if refractory to tamponade with intrauterine balloon
   - Uterine perforation
     - Associated with greater gestational age, multiparity, and provider inexperience
     - May consider expectant management in cases of small fundal perforation in stable patient without severe pain, excessive bleeding, evidence of adipose or intraabdominal contents in the uterus, and if removal of products of conception complete
     - Laparoscopy or laparotomy for abdominal exploration may be indicated for investigation of vascular or visceral injury or to assist in completion of the abortion
     - Postabortal syndrome or hematometra is treated with prompt reaspiration for the reaccumulated blood distending the uterus; rarely are retained products found; the addition of vasopressin into the paracervical block reduces the frequency of hematometra
     - Disseminated intravascular coagulation (DIC) will ultimately ensue if massive hemorrhage goes uncorrected; be prepared with a prompt set of coagulation studies including fibrinogen and INR to guide therapeutic decisions; in the high-risk patient, be prepared in advance with cross-matched blood products
   - Although the occurrence of complications for surgical abortion is only 1% overall, each subsequent week is associated with a dramatic increase in risk

UPDATE #12

The induction of fetal demise, feticide or fetocide, has been performed with both surgical and medical abortion, especially at gestations nearing viability to avoid transient signs of life after expulsion or extraction (Diedrich et al, 2010).

INDUCTION OF FETAL DEMISE

- Providers often cite that the demised fetus results in more macerated tissues with subsequent faster expulsion or surgical extraction and associated with less blood loss; however, studies have not supported this assertion
- The practice of inducing fetal demise was developed with the advent of multifetal reductions after ART-induced multiple gestations; many pharmacologic agents can be used – hypertonic solutions, lidocaine, digoxin, and potassium chloride; however, digoxin and potassium chloride are now more frequently used for fetal demise in the United States
- Digoxin, whether used, intra-amniotically, intrafetally, or intrathoracically at doses ranging from 1.0 to 2.0 mg, has been found to be highly effective, with a failure rate of around 8%; toxic doses of digoxin in previously healthy adults are greater than 10 mg or a steady-state serum concentration of 10 ng/mL, which will lead to cardiac arrest; when given intrafetally, digoxin induced demise in approximately 4 hours, and when given intra-amniotically fetal demise was noted between 4 hours after the injection and time to procedure the following day (Borgatta et al, 2010; Nucatola et al, 2010)
- Caution should be used in giving digoxin to a patient with hypersensitivity to digoxin products, cardiac conditions including conduction disorders, severe pulmonary disease, electrolyte imbalances, renal disease, and thyroid disorders (Kwon, 2010)
- Hypertonic solutions, such as 90 cc of 24% NaCl or 200 mL of 20% NaCl, injected intra-amniotically is a method of causing demise given their availability and favorable side effect profile
- Lidocaine, when injected via cordocentesis is lethal for the fetus; Senat et al. (2003) described an average 30-mL dose of 1% lidocaine, which was found to be effective for inducing fetal demise
- Fetal intracardiac kCi is also highly effective with immediate cessation of cardiac activity noted shortly after placement and a failure rate of 0%; 5 to 10 mL of 2mEq/mL of kCi via intracardiac injection immediately ceases the fetal heart (Fletcher et al, 1992); the lethal dose of kCi is approximately 2500 mg/kg; intrafetal kCi has almost no side effects; however, inadvertent placement into the maternal intravascular space could be lethal, causing cardiac arrest

Immediate Postabortal Contraception

UPDATE #13

Return to ovulation can occur as early as day 8 after abortion. Given the poor attendance rate at the postoperative visit, contraception should be initiated at the time of abortion when motivation is high to prevent a repeated unintended pregnancy (Madden et al, 2009).

INTRAUTERINE DEVICE INSERTION

- Advantages of certainty of pregnancy absence at initiation, high user motivation
- Perforation and infection risks equal to interval insertion
- Expulsion rate increased after second trimester procedures to approximately 20%, versus 2% to 5% for interval insertions

HORMONAL METHODS CONTRACEPTION

- U.S. medical eligibility criteria for contraceptive use: classifies both combined hormonal contraceptive methods (combined oral contraceptives, vaginal contraceptive ring, and contraceptive patch) and progesterone-only contraception (injection, subdermal implant, progesterone-only pill) as category 1 for immediate postabortion initiation (Centers for Disease Control and Prevention, 2010)

SUGGESTED READINGS

Introduction

Drey EA, Foster DG, Jackson RA, et al: Risk factors associated with presenting for abortion in the second trimester, *Obstet Gynecol* 107(1):128–135, 2006.

Gamble SB, Strauss LT, Parker WY, et al: Abortion surveillance: United States, 2005, *MMWR Surveill Summ* 56(13):1–32, 2008.

First Trimester: Medical Methods

American College of Obstetricians and Gynecologists: ACOG practice bulletin: clinical management guidelines of obstetrician-gynecologists no. 67, October 2005: medical management of abortion, *Obstet Gynecol* 106(4):871–882, 2005.

Carbonell JL, Rodriguez J, Velazco A, et al: Oral and vaginal misoprostol 800 microg every 8 h for early abortion, *Contraception* 67(6):457–462, 2003.

Comparison of two doses of mifepristone in combination with misoprostol for early medical abortion: a randomized trial. World Health Organisation Task Force on Post-ovulatory Methods of Fertility Regulation, *BJOG* 107(4):524–530, 2000.

Creinin M, Fox M, Teal S, et al: A randomized comparison of misoprostol 6 to 8 hrs versus 24 hours after mifepristone for abortion, *Obstet Gynecol* 103 (5 Pt 1):851–859, 2004.

Fischer M, Bhatnagar J, Guarner J, et al: Fatal toxic shock syndrome associated with Clostridium sordellii after medical abortion, *N Engl J Med* 353(22):2352–2360, 2005.

Fjerstad M, Trussell J, Sivin I: Rates of serious infection after changes in regimens for medical abortion, *N Engl J Med* 361(2):145–151, 2009.

Jain JK, Dutton C, Harwood B, et al: A prospective randomized, double-blinded, placebo-controlled trial comparing mifepristone and vaginal misoprostol to vaginal misoprostol alone for elective termination of early pregnancy, *Hum Reprod* 17(6):1477–1482, 2002.

Kruse B, Poppema S, Creinin MD, Paul M: Management of side effects and complications in medical abortion, *Am J Obstet Gynecol* 183:S65–S75, 2000.

Weeks A, Faúndes A: Misoprostol in obstetrics and gynecology, *Int J Gynaecol Obstet*(99 Suppl 2):S156–S159, 2007.

Winikoff B, Dzuba IG, Creinin MD, et al: Two distinct oral routes of misoprostol in mifepristone medical abortion: a randomized controlled trial, *Obstet Gynecol* 112(6):1303–1310, 2008.

First Trimester: Surgical Methods

Acharya G, Morgan H, Paramanantham L, Fernando R: A randomized clinical trial comparing surgical termination of pregnancy with and without ultrasound guidance, *Eur J Obstet Gynecol Reprod Biol* 114(1):69–74, 2004.

Cansino C, Edelman A, Burke A, Jamshidi R: Paracervical block with combined ketorolac and lidocaine in first-trimester surgical abortion: a randomized controlled trial, *Obstet Gynecol* 114(6):1220–1226, 2009.

Goldberg AB, Dean G, Kang MS, et al: Manual versus electric vacuum aspiration for early first-trimester abortion: a controlled study of complication rates, *Obstet Gynecol* 103(1):101–107, 2004.

Kapp N, Lohr PA, Ngo TD, Hayes JL: Cervical preparation for first trimester surgical abortion, *Cochrane Database Syst Rev*(2)CD007207, 2010.

Sawaya GF, Kerlikowske K, Grimes DA: Antibiotics at the time of induced abortion: the case for universal prophylaxis based on a meta-analysis, *Obstet Gynecol* 87(5 Pt 2):884–890, 1996.

Schulz KF, Grimes DA, Cates WJ Jr: Measures to prevent cervical injury during suction curettage abortion, *Lancet* 1(8335):1182–1185, 1983.

Schulz KF, Grimes DA, Christensen DD: Vasopressin reduces blood loss from second trimester dilatation and evacuation abortion, *Lancet* 2(8451):353–356, 1985.

Wen J, Cai QY, Deng F, Li YP: Manual versus electric vacuum aspiration for first-trimester abortion: a systematic review, *BJOG* 115(1):5–13, 2008.

Second Trimester

Goldberg AB, Greenberg MB, Darney PD: Misoprostol and pregnancy, *N Engl J Med* 344(1):38–47, 2001.

Hammond C: Recent advances in second-trimester abortion: an evidence based review, *Am J Obstet Gynecol* 200(4):347–356, 2009.

Hayes JL, Fox MC: Cervical dilation in second trimester abortion, *Clin Obstet Gynecol* 52(2):171–178, 2009.

Stubblefield PG, Carr-Ellis S, Borgatta L: Methods for induced abortion, *Obstet Gynecol* 104(1):174–185, 2004.

Vargas J, Diedrich J: Second-trimester induction of labor, *Clin Obstet and Gynecol* 52(2):188–197, 2009.

References

Please go to expertconsult.com to view references.

Chapter 32

Recurrent Pregnancy Loss and Thrombophilia

HEATHER HUDDLESTON

KEY UPDATES

1 Miscarriage rates increase with age and number of prior miscarriages.

2 Forty percent of couples with recurrent pregnancy loss (RPL) will have an evidenced-based etiology identified.

3 Preimplantation genetic diagnosis has been successfully used to treat patients with RPL and a structural chromosomal rearrangement.

4 Congenital anomalies of the uterus are identified at higher frequency in women with RPL.

5 Some inherited thrombophilias are associated with pregnancy loss, particularly those occurring after 10 weeks.

6 Heavy caffeine intake may associate with pregnancy loss.

7 Being overweight or obese is a risk factor for pregnancy loss.

Introduction and Definitions

SPORADIC PREGNANCY LOSS

- Sporadic pregnancy loss is common, occurring in 10% to 25% of clinically recognized pregnancies
- Risk of miscarriage increases with age: varying from less than 10% at age 20 to more than 50% by age 40 (Figure 32-1)
- Risk of miscarriage increases as the number of prior miscarriages increases (Figure 32-2)
- Numerical chromosomal abnormalities explain more than half of clinically recognized pregnancy loss
  - Trisomies are most common
  - Likelihood of finding an abnormal fetal karyotype increases with maternal age

RECURRENT PREGNANCY LOSS

- Repetitive pregnancy loss (RPL) has been defined as three pregnancy losses and occurs in approximately 1% of couples
- RPL can be either primary (no prior live birth) or secondary (prior live birth)
- Chance of fetal aneuploidy in patients with RPL is lower than in patients experiencing a sporadic loss
- Pregnancy loss is a distressing event for couples, and typically there is increasing psychological burden when this event happens in a repetitive fashion

UPDATE #1

In a large population-based registry linkage study of 634,272 women with 1,221,546 pregnancies in Denmark in 1978-1992, the risk of fetal loss leading to an admission to the hospital was calculated according to maternal age (see Figure 32-1). The risk of loss increased with maternal age with a sharp increase starting at age 35: 20 to 24: 10%, 25 to 29: 11%, 30 to 34: 15%, 35 to 39: 25%, 40 to 44: 51%, >45: 75%. This study also demonstrated increasing rates of fetal loss with increasing numbers of prior miscarriages (see Figure 32-2) (Nybo Andersen et al, 2000).

Etiologies of Recurrent Pregnancy Loss

- Five etiologies of RPL are supported by current evidence
  - Genetic
  - Autoimmune: antiphospholipid antibody syndrome (APS)
  - Anatomic
  - Endocrine
  - Inherited thrombophilia
- Approximately 60% of couples with RPL will have no identified cause
- Evaluation of a couple following two losses is acceptable, as the chance of finding a cause is equal whether there are two or three losses (Table 32-1)

UPDATE #2

A single center retrospective cohort study of 1020 patients with history of two or more spontaneous abortions were evaluated for evidence-based causes of recurrent pregnancy loss. A potential etiology was identified in 40% of patients. An abnormality in parental genetics (karyotype) was identified in 4.4%, uterine anatomy in 18.1%, antiphospholipid antibody syndrome in 16.8%, factor V Leiden in 6.8%, and endocrine in 7.5%. The chance of identifying an abnormal result was not different depending on whether there were two, three, or four losses (Jaslow et al, 2010) (Figure 32-3).

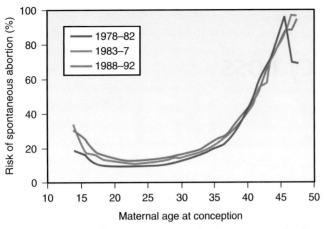

Figure 32-1. **Rates of spontaneous abortion increase steeply after age 35.** (Adapted from Nybo Andersen AM, Wohlfahrt J, Christens P, et al: Maternal age and fetal loss: population based register linkage study, *BMJ* 320[7251]:1708-1712, 2000.)

NULLIPAROUS WOMEN

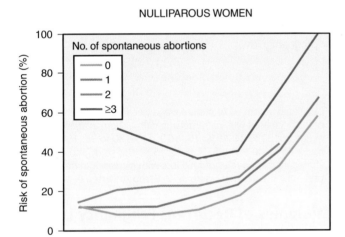

PAROUS WOMEN

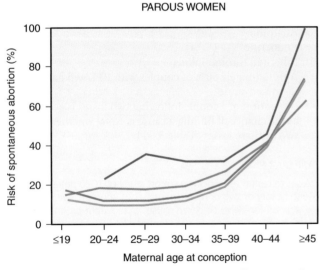

Figure 32-2. **Rates of spontaneous abortion in nulliparous and parous women.** (Adapted from Nybo Andersen AM, Wohlfahrt J, Christens P, et al: Maternal age and fetal loss: population based register linkage study, *BMJ* 320[7251]:1708-1712, 2000.)

TABLE 32-1   Evidence-Based Workup for Recurrent Pregnancy Loss by Etiology

Etiology	Diagnostic Evaluation
Genetic	Parental karyotype
Autoimmune	Anticardiolipin antibody
	Lupus anticoagulant
	Anti-beta-2 glycoprotein antibody
Anatomic	Office hysteroscopy or saline infusion hysterosonography or 3D ultrasound
Endocrine	TSH, fasting glucose, prolactin,
Inherited thrombophilia	Factor V Leiden, prothrombin gene mutation, protein S deficiency
	Possibly: Protein C deficiency, antithrombin III deficiency
Lifestyle	BMI, caffeine intake, cigarette smoking, alcohol consumption

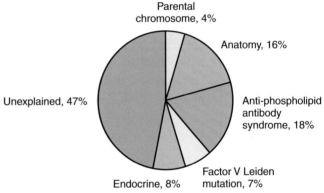

Figure 32-3. **Factors identified in a population of women with recurrent pregnancy loss.** (Data from Jaslow CR, Carney JL, Kutteh WH: Diagnostic factors identified in 1020 women with two versus three or more recurrent pregnancy losses, *Fertil Steril* 93[4]:1234-1243, 2010.)

Parental Genetic Causes of RPL

CLINICAL PROFILE

- Three percent to 5% of couples with RPL will have evidence of a major structural abnormality
- Most common: balanced reciprocal or Robertsonian translocations
- Other less common karyotypic abnormalities: inversions, insertions, and mosaicism
- Rate of chromosomal abnormalities in couples with RPL is five to six times higher than found in the general population

EVALUATION

- Detection of structural chromosomal abnormalities requires a high-resolution karyotype of peripheral blood
- Recommended for both partners

MANAGEMENT

- Begin with referral to genetic counselor to assess future risk of miscarriage and of bearing a chromosomally abnormal offspring with phenotypic anomalies

- Prognosis depends on specific type of translocation, the chromosome involved, and the gender of partner
- Expectant management (no intervention) may lead to reasonable live-birth rates but is accompanied by a high rate of miscarriage and potential for offspring bearing an unbalanced karyotype
- Use of donor gametes may be acceptable option for some couples
- Preimplantation genetic diagnosis (PGD)
  - Screen for embryos that are not affected by a chromosomal rearrangement
  - May decrease the chance of miscarriage

UPDATE #3

Our understanding of the management of the couple with RPL and a structural chromosomal rearrangement has been evolving. Recently, PGD has been proposed as a treatment strategy. A retrospective review of 192 patients with a history of three or more losses undergoing in vitro fertilization (IVF) with PGD for either a reciprocal translocation or Robertsonian translocation reported a pregnancy rate per cycle of 25%. Of pregnancies achieved, the live-birth rate was 87% with a 13% miscarriage rate (Fischer et al, 2009).

In contrast, several authors have demonstrated acceptable pregnancy outcomes for patients with recurrent pregnancy loss and a structural rearrangement when no intervention is taken. In a retrospective series of couples with RPL (n = 1892), 51 couples (2.7%) with a structural chromosome rearrangement were identified. Following evaluation and treatment of concomitant factors, there were 58 monitored pregnancies, with a live-birth rate of 71%. The follow-up time for the study was 4.2 years. Amniocentesis was performed on 22% of the ongoing pregnancies; all were diploid or balanced structural chromosome rearrangements. Thirty-six percent of the miscarriages were found to have an unbalanced structural chromosome rearrangement (Stephenson et al, 2006). In a series of 1324 Dutch couples with a history of RPL, 51 couples (2.5%) were identified as carriers of a structural chromosome rearrangement. Of the 41 carriers with complete miscarriage data, there were 26 (63%) carriers of a reciprocal translocation (18 females and 8 males), 3 (7%) carriers of a Robertsonian translocation, 9 (22%) carriers of an inversion, and 3 others. Following ascertainment of carrier status, 43 pregnancies in 25 carrier couples were documented, of which 30 (70%) were live births. Amniocentesis was performed in 26 of these pregnancies; 58% were diploid, and 42% were balanced structural chromosome rearrangements (Goddijn et al, 2004). Similarly, in a large series of 46 couples with reciprocal translocations who went on to become pregnant, 63% had a live birth with no infant found to be unbalanced (Sugiura-Ogasawara et al, 2004).

Taken together these results suggest that for the couple with RPL and a structural rearrangement, PGD leads to a reasonable live-birth rate with a significant reduction in the rate of miscarriage. In contrast, couples opting for no intervention may obtain acceptable live-birth rates as well, though time, additional miscarriages, and the expenditure of emotional energy may be required.

Autoimmune Causes of RPL: The Antiphospholipid Antibody Syndrome

CLINICAL PROFILE

- Acquired autoimmune disorder
- Associated with pregnancy and thrombotic complications
- Approximately 16% to 20% of cases of recurrent pregnancy loss
- Characterized by antibodies directed against either phospholipids or plasma proteins that are bound to phospholipids
- Mechanism by which these autoantibodies lead to thrombosis or pregnancy loss is incompletely understood but may involve the following:
  - Interference with the signal transduction mechanisms controlling endometrial cell decidualization
  - Promotion of trophoblast apoptosis
  - Impairment of trophoblast fusion and invasion

DIAGNOSIS

- Requires both clinical and laboratory criteria (Table 32-2)
- Laboratory criteria must be measured on two occasions 12 weeks apart

TABLE 32-2 **Antiphospholipid Antibody Syndrome (APS) Is Present If at Least One of the Clinical Criteria and One of the Laboratory Criteria That Follow Are Met***

Clinical Criteria

One or more unexplained deaths of a morphologically normal neonate, or beyond the 10th week of gestation, with normal fetal morphology documented by ultrasound or by direct examination of the fetus

One or more premature births of a morphologically normal neonate before the 34th week of gestation because of (1) eclampsia or severe preeclampsia defined according to standard definition or (2) recognized features of placental insufficiency

Three or more unexplained consecutive spontaneous abortions before the 10th week of gestation, with maternal anatomic or hormonal abnormalities and paternal and maternal chromosomal causes excluded

Laboratory Criteria

Lupus anticoagulant (LA) present in plasma, on two or more occasions at least 12 weeks apart, detected according to the guidelines of the International Society on Thrombosis and Haemostasis

Anticardiolipin (aCL) antibody of IgG or IgM isotype in serum or plasma, present in medium or high titer (i.e., >40 GPL or MPL, or > the 99th percentile), on two or more occasions, at least 12 weeks apart, measured by a standardized enzyme-linked immunosorbent assay (ELISA)

Anti-β_2 glycoprotein-I antibody of IgG or IgM isotype in serum or plasma (in titer > the 99th percentile), present on two or more occasions, at least 12 weeks apart, measured by a standardized ELISA, according to recommended procedures

Adapted from Myakis S: International consensus statement on an update of the classification criteria for definite antiphospholipid syndrome (APS), *J Thromb Haemost* 4(2):295-306, 2006.

- A history of three first-trimester losses is one of the clinical criteria and thus laboratory testing is indicated for all women with this history

TREATMENT

- During pregnancy: low-dose aspirin and either fractionated or unfractionated heparin
- Live-birth rate with treatment approximates 80% compared to 20% without treatment

Anatomic Causes of RPL

CLINICAL PROFILE

- Anatomic abnormalities of the uterine cavity may explain 18% of cases of RPL
- Specific alterations associated with RPL include the following:
  - Endometrial polyps
  - Submucosal fibroids
  - Intramural fibroids >5 cm
  - Uterine anomalies, particularly septate uterus
  - Asherman's syndrome

DIAGNOSIS

- Uterine cavity evaluation is widely recommended for RPL
- Sonohysterography
- Hysterosalpingogram
- Hysteroscopy

MANAGEMENT

- Congenital anomalies: septate uterus
  - The most common uterine anomaly associated with RPL
  - Pregnancy loss may be related to decreased vascularity with the septum tissue
  - Optimal treatment is hysteroscopic metroplasty
  - Available evidence suggests improved live-birth rates following surgical correction
- Congenital anomalies: bicornuate and unicornuate
  - Strong association with preterm delivery
  - No indication for surgical correction in a patient with RPL
- Polyps
- Fibroids
  - Submucous leiomyomas can impede implantation or result in abnormal implantations in the tissue overlying the myoma
  - Submucosal myomas <2.5 centimeters can be removed hysteroscopically
  - Larger fibroids may require an abdominal approach
  - Large (>5 cm) intramural fibroids or intramural fibroids that alter the contour of the uterine cavity may be a concern, and consideration should be given to their removal

ASHERMAN'S SYNDROME

- Characterized as adhesions within the uterine cavity
- Often associated with amenorrhea or lighter than normal menses

- Primarily iatrogenic
- Risk factors
  - Dilation and curettage, particularly postpartum
  - Infection
  - Multiple uterine surgeries
- Pathophysiology: trauma to basalis layer leading to granulation tissue that ultimately forms adhesive bridges
- Treatment is hysteroscopic lysis of adhesions
- Prognosis after treatment is related to severity of disease at time of diagnosis

UPDATE #4

The role played by the uterus in recurrent pregnancy loss has received increasing attention. In a study of 509 women with a history of unexplained recurrent miscarriage and 1976 low-risk women, the presence of congenital uterine anomalies seen on three-dimensional ultrasound was assessed. The anomalies were classified according to American Fertility Society classification. An anomaly was detected in 23.8% of women in the recurrent miscarriage group compared to 5.3% in low-risk women. There was no significant difference in the relative frequency of various anomalies or depth of fundal distortion between the two groups. However, with both arcuate and subseptate uteri, the length of remaining uterine cavity was significantly shorter and the distortion ratio was significantly higher in the recurrent miscarriage group. This study demonstrated a higher prevalence and severity of uterine anomalies in women with recurrent pregnancy loss compared with control women (Salim et al, 2003). Similar results were seen in a review of several studies, which found congenital uterine anomalies were present in 4.3% (ranging from 2.7% to 16.7%) of the general population of fertile women and in 12.6% (ranging from 1.8% to 37.6%) of patients with recurrent pregnancy loss (two or more consecutive losses). A high incidence of pregnancy loss occurred in patients with septate (44.3%), bicornuate (36.0%), and arcuate (25.7%) uteri. Correction of septate defects in particular may have beneficial effects (n = 366, live-birth rate: 83.2%) (Grimbizis et al, 2001).

Endocrine Causes of RPL

CLINICAL PROFILE

- Endocrine factors account for 8% of cases of recurrent pregnancy loss

DIABETES

- Poorly controlled diabetes is associated with pregnancy loss
- Evaluate with fasting glucose

THYROID

- Poorly controlled thyroid disease is related to infertility and pregnancy loss
- Evaluate with thyroid stimulating hormone (TSH) level

PROLACTIN

- Elevated prolactin levels are associated with irregular menstrual cycles, infertility, and possibly miscarriage
- Evaluate with a prolactin level

LUTEAL PHASE DEFECT

- Progesterone is essential for embryo implantation and maintenance of pregnancy
- Inadequate progesterone production may occur in the setting of poor follicular development or corpus luteum function
- Careful documentation of a short luteal phase (<8 days) or clinical evidence of prolonged spotting may be suggestive
- Endometrial biopsies are not a reliable method of diagnosis of luteal phase defects
- Possible treatment strategies include ovulation induction with oral agents such as Clomid or progesterone supplementation in the luteal phase

Hematologic Causes of RPL: Inherited Thrombophilia

CLINICAL PROFILE

- There is a higher prevalence of RPL in patients with genetic thrombophilias
  - Factor V Leiden
  - Prothrombin gene 20210A mutation
  - Deficiencies in protein C
  - Deficiency in protein S
  - Antithrombin III deficiency
- The available evidence more clearly supports an effect of inherited thrombophilia on second-trimester loss
- Role played in first trimester loss remains controversial
- Current evidence suggests no association between mutations in the methylenetetrahydrofolate reductase (MTHFR) gene and recurrent pregnancy loss

MANAGEMENT

- Treatment with anticoagulants for patients with RPL and an inherited thrombophilia remains experimental

UPDATE #5

The preponderance of evidence currently indicates a small effect of several of the thrombophilic mutations on pregnancy loss, particularly in the late first trimester and second trimester. A case-control study nested in a cohort of 32,683 women analyzed 3496 pairs of women matched for classic confounding factors. The factor V Leiden (FVL) mutation and prothrombin gene 20210A (PTG) mutations were associated with an increased risk of miscarriage in Caucasian women with losses occurring after the 10th week of gestation (odds ratio: 3.5 and 2.6, respectively). Among non-Caucasian women, the mutations were rare and the associations with risk of miscarriage less clear (Lissalde-Lavigne et al, 2005). These results echoed those in a previously reported meta-analysis that indicated that heterozygosity for FVL was significantly associated with recurrent loss in an analysis of three studies (776 patients) that included patients with ≥ three losses with all other causes of RPL. Heterozygosity for the PTG mutation was also found to be significantly associated with pregnancy loss in an analysis of nine studies in 2087 patients with two or more losses with other cause not eliminated. For both FVL and PTG mutations, stronger associations were seen for losses diagnosed at >12 weeks. An association with pregnancy loss and protein S deficiency was observed in two studies of

624 patients. Homozygosity for mutations in the methylenetetrahydrofolate reductase (MTHFR) gene was not significantly associated with recurrent loss (Rey et al, 2003).

The management of the patient with an inherited thrombophilia mutation and RPL has not yet been established, but investigation into the role of anticoagulant treatment has begun. One study compared 160 patients with heterozygous FVL, PTG, or protein S deficiency who were given 5 mg folic acid daily before conception and either low-dose aspirin 100 mg daily or low-molecular-weight heparin (enoxaparin) 40 mg taken from the 8th week. Twenty-three of the 80 patients treated with low-dose aspirin and 69 of the 80 patients treated with enoxaparin had a healthy live birth (odds ratio 15.5; P < 0.0001) (Gris et al, 2004).

Infectious Causes of RPL

- Several infections are associated with sporadic loss
  - *Listeria monocytogenes*
  - *Toxoplasma gondii*
  - Cytomegalovirus
  - Primary genital herpes
- No reported associations of infectious agents and recurrent pregnancy loss
- Currently no role for evaluation or treatment of the asymptomatic patient

Lifestyle and Environmental Factors Associated with RPL

FACTORS POSITIVELY ASSOCIATED WITH PREGNANCY LOSS

- Caffeine
  - Intake >200 mg per day may correlate with miscarriage in a dose-dependent fashion
  - Recommend limiting caffeine intake to one to two cups per day
- Cigarette smoking
  - Associated with infertility, pregnancy loss, pregnancy complications
  - Recommend cessation
- Alcohol consumption
  - Associated with miscarriage when excessive
  - Recommend cessation at onset of pregnancy
- Prepregnancy body mass index above 25 mg/m^2
  - Associated with infertility, miscarriage, complications of pregnancy, and delivery
  - Maintenance of healthy body weight is recommended for all women considering pregnancy

FACTORS NOT ASSOCIATED WITH PREGNANCY LOSS

- Moderate exercise
- Occupational factors
- Stress
- Low-level exposure to most environmental chemicals

UPDATE #6

The association of caffeine and miscarriage has long been controversial, with many studies suffering from methodological flaws, particularly recall bias. Two recent studies sought to circumvent recall bias by conducting interviews of women while pregnant. In a study of 2407 clinically recognized pregnancies resulting in 258 pregnancy losses, no relationship of coffee and caffeine intake and pregnancy loss prior to 20 weeks' completed gestation was observed (Savitz et al, 2008). However, different results were obtained in a similar prospective study of 1063 pregnant women identified in a large hospital system. In this study, an increasing dose of daily caffeine intake during pregnancy was associated with an increased risk of miscarriage, compared with no caffeine intake, with an adjusted hazard ratio of 1.42 for caffeine intake of less than 200 mg/day, and aHR of 2.23 (1.34 to 3.69) for intake of 200 or more mg/day (Weng et al, 2008).

UPDATE #7

Increasing evidence points to the deleterious effect excess body weight may have on reproductive health. A recent meta-analysis examined the association of body mass index (BMI) and miscarriage. Patients with a body mass index of ≥ 25 kg/m^2 had significantly higher odds of miscarriage, regardless of the method of conception (odds ratio: 1.7) (Metwally et al, 2008). In an effort to clarify the mechanisms driving the effect of body weight on pregnancy loss, investigators examined the distribution of abnormal karyotypes among women with miscarriages according to BMI and found a significant increase in normal embryonic karyotypes in the miscarriages of overweight and obese women (BMI ≥25). These results suggest that the excess risk of miscarriages in the overweight/obese population is independent of embryonic aneuploidy and likely related to maternal/host factors (Landres et al, 2010).

SUGGESTED READINGS

General

Jaslow CR, Carney JL, Kutteh WH: Diagnostic factors identified in 1020 women with two versus three or more recurrent pregnancy losses, *Fertil Steril* 93(4):1234–1243, 2010.

Jauniaux E, Farquharson RG, Christiansen OB, Exalto N: Evidence-based guidelines for the investigation and medical treatment of recurrent miscarriage, *Hum Reprod* 21(9):2216–2222, 2006.

Nybo Andersen AM, Wohlfahrt J, Christens P, et al: Maternal age and fetal loss: population based register linkage study, *BMJ* 320(7251):1708–1712, 2000.

Rai R, Regan L: Recurrent miscarriage, *Lancet* 368(9535):601–611, 2006.

Stephenson M, Kutteh W: Evaluation and management of recurrent early pregnancy loss, *Clin Obstet Gynecol* 50(1):132–145, 2007.

Genetic Etiologies

Fischer J, Colls P, Escudero T, Munné S: Preimplantation genetic diagnosis (PGD) improves pregnancy outcome for translocation carriers with a history of recurrent losses, *Fertil Steril* 94(1):283–289, 2010.

Goddijn M, Joosten JH, Knegt AC, et al: Clinical relevance of diagnosing structural chromosome abnormalities in couples with repeated miscarriage, *Hum Reprod* 19(4):1013–1017, 2004.

Hassold T, Chiu D: Maternal age-specific rates of numerical chromosome abnormalities with special reference to trisomy, *Hum Genet* 70(1):11–17, 1985.

Sierra S, Stephenson M: Genetics of recurrent pregnancy loss, *Semin Reprod Med* 24(1):17–24, 2006.

Stephenson MD, Awartani KA, Robinson WP: Cytogenetic analysis of miscarriages from couples with recurrent miscarriage: a case-control study, *Hum Reprod* 17(2):446–451, 2002.

Stephenson MD, Sierra S: Reproduction outcomes in recurrent pregnancy loss associated with a parental carrier of a structural chromosome rearrangement, *Hum Repro* Apr 21(4):1076–1082.

Sugiura-Ogasawara M, Ozaki Y, Sato T, et al: Poor prognosis of recurrent aborters with either maternal or paternal reciprocal translocations, *Fertil Steril* 81(2):367–373, 2004.

Antiphospholipid Antibody Syndrome

Empson M, Lassere M, Craig JC, Scott JR: Recurrent pregnancy loss with antiphospholipid antibody: a systematic review of therapeutic trials, *Obstet Gynecol* 99(1):135–144, 2002.

Miyakis S, Lockshin MD, Atsumi T, et al: International consensus statement on an update of the classification criteria for definite antiphospholipid syndrome (APS), *J Thromb Haemost* 4(2):295–306, 2006.

Noble LS, Kutteh WH, Lashey N, et al: Antiphospholipid antibodies associated with recurrent pregnancy loss: prospective, multicenter, controlled pilot study comparing treatment with low-molecular-weight heparin versus unfractionated heparin, *Fertil Steril* 83(3):684–690, 2005.

Rai R, Regan L: Antiphospholipid syndrome in pregnancy: a randomized, controlled trial of treatment, *Obstet Gynecol* 100(6):1354, 2002.

Anatomic Etiologies

Grimbizis GF, Camus M, Tarlatzis BC, et al: Clinical implications of uterine malformations and hysteroscopic treatment results, *Hum Reprod Update* 7(2):161–174, 2001.

Salim R, Regan L, Woelfer B, et al: A comparative study of the morphology of congenital uterine anomalies in women with and without a history of recurrent first trimester miscarriage, *Hum Reprod* 18(1):162–166, 2003.

Inherited Thrombophilias

Gris JC, Mercier E, Quere I, et al: Low-molecular-weight heparin versus low-dose aspirin in women with one fetal loss and a constitutional thrombophilic disorder, *Blood* 103(10):3695–3699, 2004.

Lissalde-Lavigne G, Fabbro-Peray P, Cochery-Nouvellon E, et al: Factor V Leiden and prothrombin G20210A polymorphisms as risk factors for miscarriage during a first intended pregnancy: the matched case-control "NOHA first" study, *J Thromb Haemost* 3(10):2178–2184, 2005.

Rey E, Kahn SR, David M, Shrier I: Thrombophilic disorders and fetal loss: a meta-analysis, *Lancet* 361(9361):901–908, 2003.

Kutteh WH, Triplett DA: Thrombophilias and recurrent pregnancy loss, *Semin Reprod Med* 24(1):54–66, 2006.

Endocrine

Huang KE: The primary treatment of luteal phase inadequacy: progesterone versus clomiphene citrate, *Am J Obstet Gynecol* 155(4):824–828, 1986.

Pearson DW, Kernaghan D, Lee R, Penney GC: The relationship between pre-pregnancy care and early pregnancy loss, major congenital anomaly or perinatal death in type I diabetes mellitus, *BJOG* 114(1):104–107, 2007.

Lifestyle

Armstrong E, Harris LH, Kukla R, et al: Maternal caffeine consumption during pregnancy and the risk of miscarriage, *Am J Obstet Gynecol* 199(5):e13, 2008. author reply e13–e14.

Landres IV, Milki AA, Lathi RB: Karyotype of miscarriages in relation to maternal weight, *Hum Reprod* 25(5):1123–1126, 2010.

Metwally M, Ong KJ, Ledger WL, Li TC: Does high body mass index increase the risk of miscarriage after spontaneous and assisted conception? A meta-analysis of the evidence, *Fertil Steril* 90(3):714–726, 2008.

Savitz DA, Chan RL, Herring AH, et al: Caffeine and miscarriage risk, *Epidemol* 19(10):55–62.

Weng X, Odouli R, Li DK: Maternal caffeine consumption during pregnancy and the risk of miscarriage: a prospective cohort study, *Am J Obstet Gynecol* 198(3):279.e1–.e8, 2008.

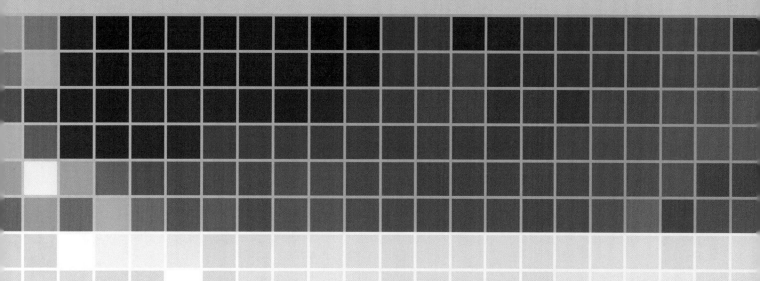

SECTION 8

Gynecologic Health

Chapter 33

Menstrual Disorders

CARRIE M. WAMBACH • CAROLYN J. ALEXANDER

KEY UPDATES

1 Puberty can start as early as 7 years old.

2 Leptin hormone is involved in the initiation of puberty.

3 Depot medroxyprogesterone acetate leads to reversible bone mineral density loss in adolescents.

4 Gonadotropin-releasing hormone antagonists, aromatase inhibitors, and antiprogesterone agents have been shown to rapidly and effectively improve clinical symptoms secondary to fibroids.

5 Polycystic ovary syndrome is associated with metabolic disorders.

6 Premature ovarian failure (POF) is not equivalent with menopause.

7 POF is associated with cardiovascular disease and endothelial dysfunction.

8 Leptin hormone may restore menses in patients with hypothalamic amenorrhea.

The Normal Menstrual Cycle

THE EARLY FOLLICULAR PHASE

- Release of negative feedback from estradiol, progesterone, and inhibin A in the early follicular phase allows an increase in gonadotropin releasing hormone (GnRH) pulse frequency
- Follicle-stimulating hormone (FSH) rises, recruiting one follicle destined for ovulation
- The remainder of primordial follicles recruited each month undergo atresia
- A follicle is surrounded by two types of cells: Granulosa and Theca cells; FSH receptors in the Granulosa cells increase
- Aromatization of androgens in the granulosa cells begins
- Granulosa cells proliferate, and inhibin/activin production (mainly inhibin B) rises
- Increased estrogen from the dominant follicle leads to proliferation of the endometrium and starts to negatively inhibit FSH secretion

THE LATE FOLLICULAR PHASE

- Luteinizing hormone (LH) levels rise, stimulating androgen production in theca cells
- The endometrium continues to thicken
- As levels of estrogen rise, there is a change from the estrogen-mediated negative feedback of gonadotropins to an acute estradiol-mediated positive feedback leading to the LH surge
- GnRH neurons lack estradiol receptors; changes in gonadotropin secretion are likely mediated by other neuronal peptides such as kisspeptin (a product of the kiss1 gene)

OVULATION

- Ovulation occurs 34 to 36 hours after the onset of the LH surge
- In addition to ovulation, the LH surge results in the following:
  - Resumption of meiosis in the oocyte (this is not completed until fertilization has occurred)
  - Luteinization of the granulosa cells
  - Production of prostaglandins and progesterone within the follicle

EARLY SECRETORY (LUTEAL PHASE)

- Progesterone levels rise rapidly, secreted from the newly developed corpus luteum
- With luteinization and the appearance of LH receptors on the corpus luteum, LH directs hormonal synthesis
- Inhibin A production from the corpus luteum increases; inhibin B production falls
- As progesterone and inhibin A increase, gonadotropins are suppressed
- Endometrial angiogenesis begins, mediated by vascular endothelial growth factor (VEGF)
  - Increased expression of VEGF can lead to abnormalities in the menstrual cycle, such as menorrhagia

LATE SECRETORY PHASE

- The corpus luteum degenerates 9 to 11 days after ovulation in the absence of human chorionic growth hormone
- Levels of estradiol, progesterone, and inhibin A decrease significantly, and inhibition is released on the gonadotropins

MENSTRUATION

- Low levels of estrogen and progesterone trigger enzymatic degradation of the functionalis layer of the endometrium, mediated largely by matrix metalloproteinases (MMPs)
  - Abnormally elevated levels of MMPs may play a role in endometriosis
- Progesterone withdrawal stimulates a large inflammatory response in the endometrium
- Degradation occurs from the subsurface capillary system and venous vascular system to the basal arterioles leading to local hemorrhage
- Bleeding is controlled by fibrinolysis and clotting largely mediated by the plasminogen activator inhibitor (PAI-1) and vasoconstriction in the spiral arterioles
- Elevated levels of progesterone allow maximal activity of PAI-1 such that hemostasis and prevention of endometrial breakdown is regulated during pregnancy
- Surface reepithelialization starts by cycle day 5
- Growth of the endometrium is also mediated by several growth factors, including VEGF, TNF-alpha, IGF-1, and TGF-beta

MENSTRUAL CYCLE

- The average adult menstrual cycle lasts 28 days, with a peak length between the ages of 25 and 30 and a shorter cycle after age 40
- Normal cycle length is 24 to 35 days
- Variation in the menstrual cycle is usually secondary to variation in the follicular phase
- The length of the menstrual cycle can be affected by ethnicity, physical activity, smoking, acute stress and alcohol consumption, and disruption in circadian rhythm

Abnormal Bleeding in Adolescents
(Table 33-1)

NORMAL PUBERTY

- Average age of the onset of puberty is 9 to 10 years old

UPDATE #1

Recent studies done by the American Academy of Pediatrics indicate that on average black American girls begin puberty between 8 and 9 years old, and white American girls begin puberty by age 10. However, 15% of girls show signs of puberty at 7 years old. Among them, 10% are white, 15% are of Hispanic, and 23% are African American (Biro et al, 2010).

- On average, puberty follows the sequence of accelerated growth, breast development, adrenarche, then menarche
- In 20% of females, adrenarche is the first sign of puberty
- Typical length of puberty is 4.5 years

UPDATE #2

Prior to the onset of puberty, gradual amplification of gonadotropin-releasing hormone (GnRH) and LH pulses leads to increased levels of gonadotropins and sex steroids. This may be influenced by the leptin hormone. As an adipose tissue hormone, it reflects adequate energy reserves and at a critical body mass can indirectly influence GnRH (Roa et al, 2010).

TABLE 33-1 Cause of Abnormal Vaginal Bleeding in Adolescents

Anatomic	Vaginal anomalies
	Congenital malformation of uterus
	Uterine/cervical polyps
	Endometriosis
Infection	Vaginitis
	Cervicitis
	Endometritis
	Pelvic inflammatory disease
	Human papillomavirus (HPV)
Tumors	Botrytis sarcoma
	Ovarian cyst or ovarian malignancy
	Clear cell carcinoma of the cervix or vagina (consider with diethylstilbestrol exposure)
Complications of pregnancy	Threatened or spontaneous abortion
	Ectopic pregnancy
	Molar pregnancy
	Self or medicated abortion
Coagulopathies	Von Willebrand's disease
	Thrombocytopenia
	Clotting disorders
	Uterine production of menstrual anticoagulants
Variation in menstrual cycle	Midcycle ovulatory bleeding
	Early postmenarcheal anovulation
	Early postmenarcheal estrogen irregularities
	Anovulation
Medications	Danazol
	Spironolactone
	Anticoagulants
	Platelet inhibitors
	Chemotherapy
	Oral contraceptives (breakthrough bleeding or progesterone insufficiency)
	Herbals and supplements
Systemic disease	Thyroid disease
	Adrenal insufficiency
	Cushing's syndrome
	Diabetes mellitus
	Chronic liver disease
	Systemic lupus erythematosus
	Ovarian failure
	Hyperprolactinemia
Androgen excess	Polycystic ovary syndrome
	Exogenous androgens
	Congenital adrenal hyperplasia
Other disorders	Trauma
	Foreign body
	Hypothalamic disorders (stress)

Adapted from Sanfilippo JS, Joesph S, Lara Torre E: Adolescent gynecology, *Obstet Gynecol* 113(4):935-947, 2009.

- Initial low levels of gonadal estrogen lead to increased production of insulin growth factor-1 (IGF-1)
  - Promotes rapid skeletal growth
  - Mutations or deletions of the IGF-1 gene that lead to deficiency of IGF-1 and growth hormone will lead to short stature
- Adrenarche occurs secondary to an increase in adrenal androgens
- Menarche occurs within 2 to 3 years after thelarche, when breast development has reached Tanner stage IV
  - With sufficient levels of estrogen, the endometrial lining thickens and the first menses occurs
  - By age 15, 98% of females will have reached menarche
- At mid-late puberty, maturation of the positive feedback relationship between estradiol and LH occurs and ovulatory cycles begin
  - Most females are anovulatory for the first several months after menarche; for 55% to 82% of adolescents, it will take 24 months to achieve regular ovulatory cycles

EVALUATION

- Although irregular menses are common in adolescents, many presentations require evaluation including the following (from American Academy of Pediatrics Committee on Adolescence, 2006):
  - Menstrual periods that have not started within 3 years of thelarche, or by age 13 with no secondary sexual characteristics, or by age 15
  - Menstrual periods that have not started by age 14 with signs of hirsutism
  - Menses that have not started by age 14 with evidence or suspicion of an anorexia or bulimia
  - Amenorrhea with cyclic monthly pain or abnormal vaginal/uterine exam
  - Irregular menses after a period of normal, regular monthly cycles
  - Menses that occur more frequently than 21 days or less than every 45 days
  - Occur more than 90 days apart even for one cycle
  - Last >7 days
  - Menorrhagia (frequent tampon or pad changes more than q 1 to 2 hours)
- Confirm normal pelvic anatomy with exam and ultrasound
- Basic lab tests include human chorionic gonadotropin (hCG), thyroid-stimulating hormone (TSH), complete blood count, and platelet level
- If menorrhagia is the primary complaint, additional lab work should include fibrinogen, prothrombin time, partial thromboplastin time, bleeding time, Von Willebrand's factor antigen, factor VIII activity, factor XI antigen, ristocetin C cofactor, platelet aggregation studies
- Von Willebrand disease is the most common condition in adolescents with menorrhagia, with a prevalence of 13%

TREATMENT

- Primary goal is to correct the underlying disorder
- Regulate menses:
  - Oral contraceptives (OCs)
  - Cyclic progestins
  - Depot medroxyprogesterone acetate

- Continuous use of oral contraceptives or "no placebo" method may lead to good efficacy and better compliance in adolescents as compared to monthly use
- A possible consequence of starting low-dose OC is a decrease in bone mineral density (BMD)
  - In a review of the literature, Agostino et al. found that adolescents using OC with 20-ug ethinyl estradiol had a lower BMD than untreated controls
  - BMD losses were associated with an earlier age of OC start and treatment duration
  - There is not enough evidence to say if this is completely reversible
- Progesterone-only methods are more difficult for adolescents as progesterone-only pills have to be taken within 3 hours of the same time every day and side effects from the depot medroxyprogesterone acetate (DMPA) include weight gain, moodiness, and irregular bleeding

UPDATE #3

Controversy exists regarding BMD loss in adolescents using DMPA. In a prospective trial evaluating adolescents using DMPA, Norplant, OC, or nothing (controls) age 12 to 21 years old, findings included a significant decrease of BMD after 1 and 2 years of DMPA use as compared to an increase in BMD in Norplant users, OC users, and controls after 1 year. An increase in BMD in Norplant users and controls was also seen after 2 years (Cromer et al, 1996). However, most studies show this loss is reversible after discontinuation and show that there is no increased risk of fracture in users (Beasley, 2010). In 2004, the Food and Drug Administration (FDA) issued a warning regarding BMD loss in users of DMPA and stated that it should be used only by adolescents who have failed other methods. Currently, the World Health Organization (WHO) and the American College of Obstetricians and Gynecologists (ACOG) support its use in adolescents and do not limit its use.

- Adolescents and intrauterine devices
  - WHO supports the use of intrauterine devices from menarche to age 20 as the benefits outweigh the risks
  - Multicenter randomized controlled trials have shown that the risk for pelvic inflammatory disease (PID) with intrauterine device (IUD) insertion is 0 to 2% when no infection is present, and it is 0 to 5% when insertion occurs at the time of documented infection; from 21 days to 8 years after insertion, the risk of PID is 1.4/1000
  - Multicenter randomized controlled trials show that compliance in adolescents is overall high
    - Expulsion may be slightly higher in adolescents

Intermenstrual Bleeding

CAUSES OF INTERMENSTRUAL BLEEDING

- Pregnancy
- Anatomic abnormalities
  - Hysteroscopy done in 370 women with abnormal uterine bleeding unresponsive to progesterone demonstrated an anatomic abnormality in two thirds of women
- Anovulation (discussed later)
- Infection
  - Cervicitis
  - Endometritis

- Malignancy
- Bleeding diathesis
- Hormonal therapy
- Chronic systemic disease
- Cervical or vaginal bleeding

DEFINITIONS

- Menorrhagia: blood loss >80 mL per cycle
- Metrorrhagia: light bleeding from the uterus at irregular intervals
- Menometrorrhagia: heavy bleeding from the uterus at irregular intervals
- Oligomenorrhea: bleeding that occurs at intervals >34 days
- Polymenorrhea: bleeding that occurs at intervals <24 days

FIBROIDS

- Seventy percent of Caucasian women and 80% of black women will have fibroids by age 50
- Submucosal fibroids account for 5% to 10% of abnormal uterine bleeding
- Age is the number one risk factor for the developing fibroids
- Other risk factors include nulliparity, race (black), alcohol, and obesity
- Smoking, multiple full-term pregnancies, and oral contraceptive use may protect against fibroids
- Average growth of a fibroid is 1.2 cm over 2.5 years
- Fibroids are classified depending on location
  - Subserosal: at the serosal surface
  - Intramural: within the uterine myometrium (controversial whether these are 100% contained within the myometrium or can have a submucosal component)
  - Submucosal: sit just beneath the endometrium
  - Submucosal fibroids are further classified by the extension into the myometrium
  - Type 0: completely intracavitary
  - Type I: less than 50% intramural
  - Type II: more than 50% intramural
- Diagnosis
  - Transvaginal ultrasound has 95% to 100% sensitivity for detecting fibroids under the 10-week size
  - Magnetic resonance imaging is the best modality for detecting the absolute number of fibroids and determining the exact location; this can also be used to differentiate between fibroids and adenomyosis
  - Hysterosalpingogram, saline-infused sonography, or hysteroscopy can be used to further determine if a fibroid has a submucosal component or distorts the cavity
  - Differential diagnosis includes adenomyosis, endometriosis, neoplasms (leiomyosarcoma or ovarian tumors), and tubo-ovarian abscess
  - Definitive diagnosis can only be made pathologically
- Medical treatments
  - Nonsteroidal anti-inflammatory drugs
    - Do not decrease menstrual blood loss
    - Decrease painful menses
    - Provide short-term relief

- Estrogen-progesterone contraceptives
  - May control bleeding symptoms without causing further growth of the fibroid
  - May work because of resulting endometrial atrophy
  - Can be first-line treatment
- Progesterone-only therapies (pills, injection, IUD)
  - Controversial data, as progesterone may act as a growth factor for the fibroid while at the same time inducing endometrial atrophy
  - Studies that look at progestin therapy in combination with GnRH agonists show an increase in fibroid volume or uterine volume once the progestins are added
  - Data evaluating levonorgestrel intrauterine devices show that these devices are best used when treating menorrhagia; however, there may be a high failure rate and risk of expulsion if bleeding is very heavy
- Gonadotropin-releasing hormone agonists
  - Most effective treatment for uterine fibroids
  - Provide a 35% to 60% reduction in fibroid volume within 3 months of treatment
  - Most women develop amenorrhea within 1 to 2 months after treatment
  - Works by desensitization and down-regulation of the hypothalamus and pituitary, eventually causing a menopausal state
  - Limited to 6 months or 1 year if hormonal add-back therapy is not given because of the negative impact on bone mineral density
  - Ideally add-back therapy is started after 3 months of use, as the hormones can cause fibroids to regrow and uterine volume to increase
  - Other side effects include vaginal dryness, hot flashes, mood disturbances, and myalgias
  - Resumption of normal menses can lead to rapid regrowth of fibroids
  - GnRH agonists are often used prior to surgery or during the transition from perimenopause to menopause

UPDATE #4

Gonadotropin-releasing hormone antagonists, aromatase inhibitors and antiprogesterone agents are promising, new treatments for fibroids. In one study, a rapid onset of clinical effects with achievement of amenorrhea and reduction in uterine volume was documented within 1 to 2 months' use of GnRH antagonists (Griesinger et al, 2005).

Antiprogesterone agents show a reduction in fibroid size and uterine volume similar to that seen with GnRH agonists. High-dose regimens achieve amenorrhea in most patients, whereas low-dose regimens induce amenorrhea in 40% to 70% of women (Engman et al, 2009). However, major side effects are endometrial hyperplasia (with incident reports of 0 to 63%) and transient elevation in transaminases (4%).

None of these treatments are currently FDA approved for treatment of uterine fibroids.

- Surgical treatments for fibroids
  - Surgery is recommended for the following:
    - Failed medical therapy
    - Persistent and heavy abnormal uterine bleeding
    - Treatment of infertility or recurrent pregnancy loss
    - Rapidly growing pelvic mass in a premenopausal woman or a growing mass in a postmenopausal woman

- Myomectomy
  - An option for women who want to preserve their fertility
  - Data show that 81% of patients have an improvement in menorrhagia after surgery
  - One retrospective study suggested 50% to 60% of women will develop new fibroids within 5 years after surgery and 25% will require a second surgery; a second retrospective series demonstrated a recurrence rate of 11.7% after 1 year and a 33% recurrence rate within 27 months (Yoo et al, 2007)
  - Can be done abdominally, laparoscopically, or robotically
  - Complication rates appear to be similar when hysterectomy and abdominal myomectomy are compared
  - Minimally invasive approaches are recommended if the uterus is 17 weeks or smaller
  - A prospective study compared the laparoscopic removal of fibroids less than and greater than 80 grams; with the exception of a larger blood loss in the greater than 80-gram group, there were no other significant differences in the two groups in terms of surgical complications
  - Randomized controlled trials that have compared laparoscopic approaches to minilaparotomy demonstrate less blood loss, reduced hospital stay, and more rapid recovery with the laparoscopic approach
  - Myometrial infiltration with vasopressin and a tourniquet may be used to decrease intraoperative blood loss
- Hysterectomy
  - Recommended for women who are symptomatic, unresponsive to other treatments, and have no desire for future fertility
  - Thirty percent of all hysterectomies for white women and 50% of all hysterectomies for black women are currently done secondary to symptomatic fibroids
- Hysteroscopic myomectomy
  - Success and complete surgical resection is based on the type of submucosal fibroid and the number of fibroids
  - Successful removal of fibroid at initial hysteroscopy is 85% to 95%
  - Relapse rates are approximately 25% at 5 years
  - Surgical complications include incomplete resection of fibroid, fluid overload, uterine perforation, gas embolism, and infection
- Other treatments
  - Uterine artery embolization (UAE)
    - The American College of Obstetrics and Gynecology considers UAE contraindicated in patients who desire future fertility
    - Uterine arteries are embolized with a polyvinyl alcohol particle of trisacryl gelatin microspheres via the femoral artery
    - Trials demonstrate a 42% reduction in dominant fibroid size in 3 months
    - Most common side effect is postoperative pain
    - The Uterine Artery Embolization in the Treatment of Symptomatic Uterine Fibroid Tumors (EMMY) randomized control trial compared UAE to hysterectomy; results demonstrated less postoperative pain and quicker return to work with UAE; minor complications—including vaginal discharge, hematoma, and fibroid expulsion—were higher in the UAE group; there were similar rates of major complications in both groups
    - Short- and long-term data suggests that overall UAE is safe and effective
    - Successful pregnancies have been reported, although with an increased risk of preterm delivery, postpartum hemorrhage, and abnormal placentation
  - Magnetic resonance imaging-guided focused ultrasound
    - Approved by the FDA in 2004 for treatment of fibroids
    - Uses high-intensity ultrasound waves directed into a focal volume of a fibroid; this energy causes protein denaturation, irreversible cell damage, and coagulative necrosis
    - Contraindicated in fibroids that can be removed hysteroscopically or when intervening bladder or bowel could be damaged in the process
    - Studies show that symptoms improve and uterine size is reduced at 12 months, but more data are needed
- Fertility and fibroids
  - Subserosal fibroids have no impact on fertility
  - Submucosal fibroids appear to decrease the implantation rate and increase the miscarriage rate; the current recommendation is to remove any submucosal fibroid prior to infertility treatment
  - A review of 24 patients in 2008 showed a 72% decrease in implantation rate in women with submucosal fibroids compared to infertile controls
  - Data are more controversial with intramural fibroids, but there appears to be an association with a deceased implantation rate (22% versus 18%) and an increase in the spontaneous abortion rate (8% to 15%) when compared to normal controls
- Fibroids and pregnancy
  - The most common complaint associated with fibroids in pregnancy is pain
  - Short-term pain can be treated with NSAIDs, but caution must be used
  - The most common reason for cesarean section in pregnancy associated with fibroids is malpresentation
  - Regardless of fibroid size, a trial of labor should be encouraged, unless there are other contraindications
  - Postpartum hemorrhage is the most common postpartum complication associated with fibroids secondary to decreased uterine contractility

ENDOMETRIAL POLYPS

- Epidemiology
  - Ten percent to 24% of women are found to have endometrial polyps on endometrial biopsy and hysterectomy specimens
  - Endometrial polyps are responsible for 25% of abnormal bleeding in all women and are a common cause of metrorrhagia
  - Polyps are rare in women younger than 20 years old; incidence peaks in the fifth decade and decreases again after menopause

- Most polyps are benign
  - In a retrospective study of 509 women (most premenopausal) undergoing hysteroscopic polypectomy, 70% were benign, 26% had hyperplasia without atypia, 3% had hyperplasia with atypia, and 0.8% had a malignancy; age, menopausal status, and hypertension increased the risk of premalignant and malignant polyps
  - A second retrospective study evaluated 1242 women who had endometrial polypectomies: 95.2% of polyps were benign, 1.3% were premalignant, and 3.5% were malignant; factors significantly associated with malignancy similarly included age, menopause status, hypertension, and abnormal bleeding
- Diagnosis
  - Saline sonography is the most sensitive method for detecting a polyp with a sensitivity of 93% and a specificity of 94% compared to transvaginal ultrasound that has a sensitivity and specificity of 65% and 76%, respectively
  - Hysteroscopy can also be used as both a diagnostic tool and treatment
- Treatment
  - Polypectomy is recommended for the following patients:
    - Symptomatic women
    - Women at high risk for endometrial hyperplasia
    - Asymptomatic premenopausal women with a polyp larger than 2 cm (no randomized controlled trials)
    - Asymptomatic postmenopausal women with a polyp larger than 1 cm (no randomized controlled trials)
  - Surgical treatment with hysteroscopic polypectomy and dilation and curettage (D&C) is the gold standard
  - Hysterectomy is only recommended if there are multiple recurrent polyps or associated fibroids
  - Recurrence after polypectomy is frequent
- Endometrial polyps and fertility
  - It is recommended to remove endometrial polyps prior to fertility treatments, although there are few trials evaluating this
  - In a prospective randomized trial, 215 infertile women with diagnosed polyps were randomized to hysteroscopic polypectomy or diagnostic hysteroscopy with polyp biopsy (control group); women in the polypectomy group had a 2X better chance of conceiving compared to the control group

Amenorrhea

DEFINITIONS

- Primary amenorrhea
  - Absence of menses by age 15 in the presence of normal secondary sexual development
  - Absence of menses within 5 years after breast development if occurred prior to age 10
- Secondary amenorrhea: absence of menses for greater than three cycles or 6 months in women who have previously had menses
- The World Health Organization separates amenorrheic patients into three groups:
  - WHO I: no evidence of endogenous estrogen, normal or low follicle-stimulating hormone (FSH), normal prolactin, and no evidence of a lesion in the hypothalamus-pituitary region

- WHO II: evidence of estrogen production, normal prolactin and FSH
- WHO III: elevated serum FSH (gonadal failure)

CAUSES OF AMENORRHEA (Table 33-2)

- Anatomic defects
  - All or part of the uterus and vagina are absent in the presence of otherwise normal female sexual characteristics
  - Congenital obstructive defects (transverse vaginal septum, imperforate hymen)
    - Presents with primary amenorrhea and cyclic pelvic pain
- The differential diagnosis of amenorrhea with complete absence of the uterus (diagnosed by exam and magnetic resonance imaging [MRI]) can be divided into two groups based on the presence or absence of breast development
  - Normal breast development
  - Mayer-Rokitansky-Kuster-Hauser syndrome (46 XX)
  - Complete androgen insensitivity syndrome (X-linked recessive disorder, 46 XY)
  - A testosterone level and karyotype will distinguish the two
  - No breast development
    - 5-alpha-reductase-deficiency (46 XY), 17-alpha-hydroxylase deficiency (XY), and XY gonadol dysgenesis
- Asherman's syndrome
  - Secondary amenorrhea that presents most commonly after a procedure (D&C) or episode of endometritis

WHO I Disorders

- Most common diagnosis is hypothalamic amenorrhea
- FSH levels are near normal with a high FSH/LH ratio as seen in prepubertal girls
- Causes of hypothalamic amenorrhea:
  - Stress: increase in corticotrophin-releasing hormone (CRH), which inhibits gonadotropin secretion
  - Anorexia and bulimia: changes in leptin, neuropeptide Y, melanocortins, and CRH lead to low levels of gonadotropins
  - Excessive exercise: women who are in competitive sports have a three-fold higher risk of primary or secondary

TABLE 33-2   Common Causes of Primary Amenorrhea

Cause	Frequency (in Amenorrheic Patients)
Chromosomal abnormalities leading to gonadal dysgenesis	50%
Hypothalamic hypogonadism	20%
Absence of uterus, cervix, vagina, or Müllerian agenesis	15%
Transverse vaginal septum or imperforate hymen	5%
Pituitary disease	5%
Rare disorders including androgen insensitivity syndrome, congenital adrenal hyperplasia, and polycystic ovary syndrome	5%

Adapted from The Practice Committee of the American Society for Reproductive Medicine: Current evaluation of amenorrhea, *Fertil Steril* 82(1):266-272, 2004.

hypothalamic amenorrhea; the highest prevalence is among long-distance runners
- The "female athlete triad" is amenorrhea, abnormal eating, and osteopenia or osteoporosis
- Hypothalamic amenorrhea caused by low body weight can be reversed
  - As patients gain weight and near their ideal body weight, gonadotropin levels return to normal
  - Falsetti et al. demonstrated in a long-term follow-up study of 91 women with functional hypothalamic amenorrhea that 70.7% of women recovered within 9 years; recovery was associated with a higher body mass index (BMI) and a lower cortisol level over time
- Other causes of WHO I disorders:
  - Kallmann syndrome (absence of GnRH and anosmia)
  - Adrenal hypoplasia (adrenal insufficiency, deficient GnRH production, and impaired response to GnRH)
  - Mutations in the GnRH receptor
  - Infiltrative lesions (sarcoidosis, histiocytosis, hemochromatosis)
  - Radiation or chemotherapy
  - Chronic debilitating disease

WHO II Disorders

- Polycystic ovary syndrome
  - Defined differently depending on expert group
  - National Institute of Health Criteria 1990
    a. Clinical or biochemical evidence of hyperandrogenemia
    b. Ovulatory dysfunction (oligomenorrhea or amenorrhea)
    c. Exclusion of other causes of androgen excess or ovulatory dysfunction
    d. Presence of polycystic ovaries on ultrasound not required
  - Rotterdam consensus criteria, 2003
    a. Require two out of the following three criteria: clinical or biochemical evidence of hyperandrogenemia, oligomenorrhea or amenorrhea, or polycystic ovaries by ultrasound
  - Androgen Excess Society, 2006
    a. Requires hyperandrogenemia plus one of the following criteria
    b. Oligomenorrhea/amenorrhea or polycystic ovaries on ultrasound
  - Other androgen excess disorders and disorders of ovulatory dysfunction must be considered and ruled out, including androgen secreting tumors, exogenous androgens, Cushing syndrome, nonclassical congenital adrenal hyperplasia, acromegaly, genetic defects in insulin action, hypothalamic amenorrhea, primary ovarian failure, thyroid disease, and prolactin disorder
  - Polycystic ovary syndrome (PCOS) patients are at increased risk for metabolic disorders

UPDATE #5

PCOS is associated with obesity, diabetes, insulin resistance, hypertension, and hyperlipidemia. In a recent study, the prevalence of the metabolic syndrome among 364 PCOS women was found to be 33.4%. Of those women, 80% had waist circumference >88 cm, 66% had low HDL, 32% had elevated triglycerides, 21% had hypertension, and 5% had elevated fasting glucose (Ehrmann et al, 2006).

- When PCOS is suspected or diagnosed, the workup includes the following:
- Blood pressure
- BMI
- Waist circumference to determine body fat distribution
- Modified Ferriman-Gallwey score
- Androgen levels
- 17-hydroxyprogesterone (to rule out nonclassical congenital adrenal hyperplasia)
- Screening for associated cardiometabolic disorders, including fasting lipids and glucose tolerance test, and pelvic ultrasound
- Treatment for anovulation/PCOS
  - Goal of treatment is to restore normal menstrual cycles and normalize BMI with diet and exercise
  - For patients with PCOS, the 2008 Endocrine Society practice guidelines suggest combined oral contraceptives (OCs) as first-line treatment in patients who are not trying to conceive
    - Act as antiandrogens, as estrogen increases sex hormone binding globulins (SHBGs)
    - Progesterone suppresses LH, which decreases testosterone production
    - Inhibits 5 alpha-reductase activity in skin
    - Regulates menses
  - If hyperandrogenemia is present and is not controlled within 6 months of starting OCs, an antiandrogen can be added
  - Cyclic progesterone therapy (5 to 10 mg of medroxyprogesterone acetate or 200 micrograms of micronized progesterone) 2 weeks every month will also be sufficient for restoring menses and protecting the endometrium if contraception is not desired
  - In addition to stabilizing the endometrium and causing monthly endometrial shedding, progesterone also protects the endometrium
    - It is an anti-estrogen
    - It stimulates 17B-hydroxysteroid dehydrogenase and sulfotransferase activities that convert estradiol to estrone sulfate
    - It antagonizes estrogen's induction of its own receptor and suppresses the estrogen-mediated transcription of oncogenes
  - In cases of hypogonadotropic, hypogonadism anovulatory cycles, use estrogen for 3 weeks, followed by estrogen plus progesterone for 1 to 2 weeks to cycle menses to ensure the endometrial lining is thick enough to shed
  - If contraception is desired, a norethindrone intrauterine device (Mirena IUD), low-dose monophasic combination oral contraceptives, or depot medroxyprogesterone acetate (Depo-Provera) can be used as an alternative to OCs
  - In cases of prolonged heavy bleeding as a result of anovulation, any of the low-dose OCs can be used twice daily for at least 5 to 7 days until bleeding slows, followed by one pill daily
  - Occasionally bleeding is unresponsive to progestins or combination oral contraceptives, as bleeding may be secondary to a very thin or denuded endometrium rather than a thickened, unstable endometrium; in these cases,

high-dose estrogen therapy can be used in both oral and intravenous forms:

- 1.25 mg conjugated estrogens or 2.0 mg micronized estradiol every 4 to 6 hours x24 hours followed by one pill a day for the next 7 to 10 days
- 25 mg conjugated equine estrogens intravenously (IV) every 4 hours for 24 hours until bleeding subsides, followed by oral estrogens 7 to 10 days
- In hemodynamically unstable women, a dilation and curettage is the best option
- Other WHO II disorders: thyroid disorders, diabetes mellitus, exogenous androgens

WHO III Disorders

- Premature ovarian failure:
  - Amenorrhea in the presence of hypergonadotropic hypogonadism prior to the age of 40
  - Pathogenesis
    - Females are born with 1 million to 2 million primordial follicles
    - By puberty, only 300,000 to 500,000 primordial follicles are present
    - Of these, 400 to 500 will ovulate over a lifetime
    - Abnormal recruitment and development of primordial follicles can lead to rapid depletion of follicles and premature ovarian failure or female infertility
    - Other possible causes include chromosome anomalies (45 XO), Fragile X permutation, ovarian toxins, or exposure to radiation or chemotherapy and autoimmune ovarian failure
  - Diagnostic criteria not well defined, but it is generally accepted that 4 months of amenorrhea in addition to two menopausal levels of FSH is sufficient
  - Prevalence of POF is 1/250 by age 35 and 1/100 (1%) by age 40
  - In 90% of women, no etiology is found
  - Significant association with other autoimmune disorders
    - 20% of women will have associated autoimmune hypothyroidism
    - 3% of women will have Addison's disease (adrenal insufficiency)
    - 6% of cases are related to permutations in the *FMR1* gene (gene responsible for Fragile X syndrome)

UPDATE #6

Premature ovarian failure is distinct from menopause, as 50% of women will have recurrent, intermittent resumption of ovarian function after the diagnosis; 5% to 10% of patients will spontaneously conceive after the diagnosis of POF (Nelson et al, 2005).

UPDATE #7

POF is associated with cardiovascular disease. To assess cardiovascular status and endothelial function, Kalantaridou et al. prospectively assessed 18 women with POF before and after 6 months of hormone therapy and compared their endothelial function to 20 age- and BMI-matched premenopausal controls. Results indicated that there is an early onset of endothelial dysfunction with POF; however, this is reversed within at least 6 months of hormone replacement therapy (HRT) (Kalantaridou et al, 2004).

- Turner syndrome
  - 45 XO
  - Associated with short stature, web neck, shield chest, renal abnormalities, autoimmune disorders (50% will present with hypothyroidism), cardiovascular disorders, and hypergonadotropic hypoestrogenic amenorrhea
  - Sixty percent have complete loss of one X chromosome, and 40% are mosaics
  - All patients require an echocardiogram of the aorta, aortic root, and aortic valve at infancy; starting in their teens, a cardiac evaluation (MRI) should be done at 5- to 10-year intervals
  - Additional surveillance includes annual thyroid function testing, thyroid antibodies, intravenous pyelogram or renal ultrasound, audiometry, and annual evaluation of lipid profile and glucose metabolism
  - Estrogen and progesterone replacement at puberty will allow normal pubertal development
- Gonadal dysgenesis associated with 46 XY phenotype (rare disorders):
  - Swyer's syndrome: most cases caused by mutations in the sex-determining region of the Y chromosome (SRY); phenotype includes gonadal dysgenesis, normal Müllerian development, normal female testosterone levels, and lack of secondary sexual development; gonadal streaks should be removed at the time of diagnosis secondary to risk of tumor transformation at any age
  - Vanishing testes syndrome: most common presentation is a phenotypic normal female with lack of progression through puberty; elevated FSH and LH levels are present; the phenotype can be variable depending on the time gonadal failure occurred during development
  - Absent testis determining factor (Ullrich-Turner syndrome): results in absent testes, feminization of the external and internal genitalia in association with primary gonadal failure, and absence of secondary sexual characteristics; Y-DNA hybridization studies demonstrate the abnormality in the short arm of the Y chromosome
- Pituitary disorders
  - Prolactin-secreting adenomas
    - Most common pituitary tumor
    - Diagnosed in 20% of cases of secondary amenorrhea
    - Fifty percent to 60% of women with elevated prolactin will have a pituitary tumor
    - Hyperprolactinemia is associated with decreased suppression of hypothalamic GnRH leading to low estradiol concentrations
  - Sheehan's syndrome: an infarction and necrosis of the pituitary gland after a postpartum hemorrhage; presents with an inability to lactate; deficiencies in growth hormone, gonadotropins, adrenocorticotropic hormone (ACTH), and TSH follow
  - Empty Sella syndrome: congenital or can occur secondary to surgery, radiation, or infarct of the pituitary tumor
  - Infiltrating diseases (hemochromatosis, lymphocytic hypophysitis)
- Evaluation of WHO III disorders
  - Physical exam should be on degree of maturation of secondary sexual features and external genitalia, current

- estrogen status, signs of virilization, and presence or absence of a uterus
- Adequate levels of endogenous estrogen can be assessed using the progesterone withdrawal test
  - Twenty percent of women who have adequate estrogen levels will not have withdrawal bleeding and 40% of women who have low levels of estrogen production will have withdrawal bleeding
- If a uterus is absent on exam, an MRI, karyotype, and serum testosterone level should be done
- If a uterus is present, a pregnancy test should be done first, followed by FSH, prolactin, and TSH
- Elevated FSH consistent with premature ovarian failure
  - A repeat test of FSH and estradiol is necessary to confirm the diagnosis
  - A karyotype should be done in all women who present with elevated gonadotropins prior to the age of 30 or in women who desire to conceive to rule out chromosomal abnormality or presence of a Y chromosome
- When POF presents as primary amenorrhea, 50% of patients will have an abnormal karyotype; when it presents as secondary amenorrhea, nearly 100% of patients will have a normal karyotype
- Karyotypes associated with primary amenorrhea and gonadal failure
  - 45, X0 (Turner syndrome) 50%
  - Mosaics 25%
  - 46, XX 25% (premature ovarian failure)
  - 46, XY-rare
- Karyotypes associated with secondary amenorrhea and gonadal failure (listed in decreasing frequency)
  - 46, XX
  - Mosaics
  - Deletions in X short and long arms
  - 47, XXX
  - 45, X0 (Turner syndrome)
- Screen for Fragile X permutation (FMR1)
- Screen for autoimmune disorders such as thyroid disorders, diabetes mellitus, myasthenia gravis, and Addison's disease
- Dual-energy x-ray absorptometry (DEXA) bone scan at time of diagnosis or after 6 months of amenorrhea; the diagnosis is frequently delayed and many women have been in a prolonged hypoestrogenic state, increasing the risk for osteopenia and osteoporosis
- Testing for ovarian antibodies or ovarian biopsy is not recommended, as there is no clinical utility
- If there are signs of masculinization (hirsutism, acne), evaluate androgen levels to rule out PCOS
- Treatment for WHO III disorders
  - Treatment is aimed at correcting the underlying etiology
  - All women, especially those with premature ovarian failure, Müllerian agenesis, or the presence of a Y chromosome, should be offered psychological counseling
  - If a congenital obstruction is diagnosed, treat surgically
  - In patients with a Y chromosome:
    - Risk of germ cell tumor is high (Table 33-3)
    - Most common tumor is gonadoblastoma
    - Gonadectomy should be performed at time of diagnosis except for androgen insensitivity syndrome, in which the gonads should be left in place until after puberty to allow for a growth spurt and breast development

TABLE 33-3   Prevalence of Tumors with Developmental Sex Disorders

Risk	Type of Developmental Sex Disorder	Prevalence %
High	GD in general	12*
	46XY Gonadal dysgenesis	30
	Frasier syndrome	60
	Denys-Drash syndrome	40
	45 X/46 XY Gonadal dysgenesis	15-40
Immediate	Partial androgen insensitivity syndrome	15
	17-Hydroxysteroid dehydrogenase deficiency	17
Low	Complete androgen insensitivity syndrome	0.8
	Ovotesticular	2.6
Unknown	5-alpha reductase deficiency	
	Leydig cell hypoplasia	

*Might reach more than 30%, if gonadectomy has not been performed.
Adapted from Pleskacova J, Hersmus R, Oosterhuis JW, et al: Tumor risk in disorders of sex development, *Sex Dev* 4(4-5):259-269, 2010.

- If hypothalamic amenorrhea is present, treat with cyclic estrogen and progesterone to prevent bone loss and regulate menses; minimum serum estradiol necessary to protect bone is 40 to 50 pg/mL

UPDATE #8

Welt et al. did a prospective trial evaluating eight women with hypothalamic amenorrhea and demonstrated that with up to 3 months of recombinant human leptin treatment, these women had increased LH levels, LH pulse frequency, an increased number of dominant follicles, increased ovarian volume, and higher estradiol levels as compared to nontreated controls; three eighths of the women treated also achieved ovulatory cycles (Welt et al, 2004).

- Most prolactin adenomas are successfully treated with dopamine agonists
  - In a double-blind, randomized trial involving 459 women comparing bromocriptine and cabergoline, cabergoline had fewer side effects and was more effective at normalizing prolactin levels; prolactin levels normalized in 83% of the patients treated with cabergoline versus 59% of those treated with bromocriptine
  - Surgery is rarely indicated and should be considered only after patients have failed dopamine agonist therapy
- Women with POF should start hormone replacement to prevent bone loss and cardiovascular complications
  - Low-dose estrogen: a 100-ug estradiol patch, 2 mg of oral micronized estradiol, or 1.25 of conjugated equine estradiol is adequate
  - Transdermal estradiol is often the preferred route as it avoids the first pass effect on the liver, is structurally equivalent to 17-beta estradiol produced by the ovary, and is easily measured by serum assays
  - Cyclic progesterone (10 mg of medroxyprogesterone acetate or 200 mg of oral micronized progesterone) should be given for 12 days each month if a uterus is

present; less frequent progesterone use is associated with endometrial hyperplasia
- Oral contraceptives can also be used
- Contraception is not provided by HRT or oral contraceptives in POF patients
- HRT should be continued until at least age 50
- Osteoporosis prevention also includes 1500 mg calcium daily, 1000 mg vitamin D daily, and multivitamins
- Treat other disorders as necessary such as hypothyroidism or adrenal insufficiency

FERTILITY AND GONADAL FAILURE

- There is no proved method of restoring fertility in POF patients
- Ovarian markers such as anti-Müllerian hormone (AMH), inhibin B, and antral follicle count may provide a more accurate assessment of follicular quantity as compared to FSH alone
- Infertility treatments such as gonadotropin stimulation have little if any results
- Donor oocyte in vitro fertilization (IVF) or adoption should be discussed and offered

Chronic Menorrhagia

PHYSIOLOGY AND DEFINITIONS

- Menorrhagia is defined as menstrual blood loss >80 mL or >7 days of bleeding
- In reproductive-age women, the most common causes of menorrhagia include anovulation, endometrial distortion (fibroids, polyps, IUDs, tumors), and adenomyosis

DIAGNOSIS AND EVALUATION FOR ABNORMAL BLEEDING

- A pregnancy test and pelvic ultrasound should be done in everyone who presents with abnormal bleeding: the most common cause of a sudden change from regular menses is a complication of pregnancy
- Determine the amount, duration, and pattern of bleeding
- Check complete blood count (CBC) to rule out anemia
- Check coagulation factors if indicated
- If anovulation is confirmed, additional work-up includes BMI, FSH, prolactin, TSH, and androgens
- Hyperandrogenemia and anovulation should raise suspicion for polycystic ovary syndrome
- An EMB should be performed if a patient is anovulatory and 40 years or older, has had a long duration of exposure to unopposed estrogen regardless of age, or is postmenopausal
  - In a study by Coulam et al., 1270 women with chronic anovulation were followed; 30 patients developed endometrial cancer, with a relative risk (RR) of endometrial cancer of 3.1

ANOVULATION

- Results in amenorrhea in 20% to 50% of cases and menorrhagia in 30% of cases
- Abnormal bleeding results from prolonged exposure to estrogen—in the absence of progesterone, which leads to an unstable endometrium

- The most common causes of adult onset anovulation are ovarian dysfunction (50%), hypothalamic dysfunction (35%), and pituitary disease (15%) (Table 33-4)
- The most common hypothalamic conditions are abnormalities in body composition and weight, stress, and strenuous exercise
- Anovulatory bleeding is often a diagnosis of exclusion, as patients present with irregular and unpredictable menstrual bleeding
- The majority of women with normal monthly cycles (24 to 35 days) who experience premenstrual moliminal symptoms will ovulate
- Methods to detect ovulation (or confirm absence of ovulation):
  - Basal body temperature:
    - Prior to ovulation morning basal body temperature (BBT) <98° F
    - After ovulation BBT is >98° F (sustained a rise in basal body temperature by 0.4° F)
    - A biphasic pattern is almost always associated with ovulation

TABLE 33-4   Causes of Anovulation

WHO I	Hypogonadotropic hypogonadism	Kallmann syndrome
		Idiopathic hypogonadotropic hypogonadism
		Cranial tumors
		Radiation
		Sheehan syndrome
		Empty Sella syndrome
		Pituitary adenoma
		Lymphocytic hypophysitis (autoimmune)
		Infiltrating disease: lymphoma or histiocytosis
		Lactational amenorrhea
		Stress
		Eating disorders
		Intense exercise
		Immaturity at onset of menarche or perimenopausal decline
		Oral contraceptives
WHO II	Euestrogenic ovulatory dysfunction	Polycystic ovary syndrome
		Thyroid disorders
		Hormone producing tumors
		Chronic liver or lung disease
		Cushing's disease
		Congenital adrenal hyperplasia
		Antidepressant and antipsychotic drugs
		Corticosteroids
WHO III	Hypergonadotropic hypogonadism	Premature ovarian failure
		Turner's syndrome
		Androgen insensitivity syndrome

Adapted from Strauss JF III, Barbieri RL: *Yen & Jaffe's reproductive endocrinology: expert consult,* Philadelphia, 2009, Sanders.

- Luteal serum progesterone:
  - A level greater than 3 ng/mL is diagnostic of ovulation
  - A level greater than 10 ng/mL is always associated with a normal secretory endometrium
- LH surge (detected by laboratory values or LH detection kit):
  - Ovulation occurs 34 to 36 hours after the onset of an LH surge
  - Ten to 12 hours after the LH peak
- Ultrasound changes:
  - Follicular growth, rupture and formation of a corpus luteum
- Endometrial biopsy (EMB) that demonstrates a secretory endometrium confirms ovulation and progesterone effect
  - If anovulation is confirmed additional workup includes BMI, FSH, prolactin, TSH, androgens (if associated with hyperandrogenemia, see the discussion of PCOS)
- An EMB should be performed if a patient is anovulatory and 40 years or older or has had a long duration of exposure to unopposed estrogen regardless of age

TREATMENT

- If uterine pathology is present, treat the pathology as necessary
- Oral contraceptives are first-line therapy to regulate menses, as they are easily tolerated and protect the endometrium
- Cyclic progestins are also sufficient to protect the endometrium if OCs are not tolerated or contraception is not desired
- Occasionally bleeding is unresponsive to progesterones or combination oral contraceptives because bleeding may be secondary to a very thin or denuded endometrium rather than a thickened, unstable endometrium; in these cases, high-dose estrogen therapy can be used in both oral and intravenous forms
  - 1.25 mg conjugated estrogens or 2.0 mg micronized estradiol every 4 to 6 hours x24 hours followed by one pill a day for the next 7 to 10 days
  - 25 mg conjugated equine estrogens IV every 4 hours for 24 hours until bleeding subsides, followed by oral estrogens 7 to 10 days
- Norethindrone intrauterine device (Mirena IUD)
  - Significantly decreases menorrhagia
  - In a randomized trial comparing the Mirena IUD to endometrial resection in the treatment of menorrhagia, a significant decrease of blood loss was seen after 3 years in both groups, and two thirds of patients tolerated the Mirena IUD for the duration of the study period
- Nonsteroidal anti-inflammatory drugs (NSAIDs)
  - Decrease prostaglandin synthesis in the endometrium and can reduce blood loss by 20% to 50%
  - Should be started on the first day of menses and continued for at least five days
- Antifibrinolytic
  - More effective than NSAIDs and cyclic progestins in reducing blood flow
  - Only take 1 to 2 days before menses and for the first 2 days of the menses

- Endometrial ablation or destruction of the endometrium
  - Various techniques available
  - Amenorrhea rates 37% to 38% at 1 year for all techniques, with patient satisfaction 88% to 91% at 1 year and 87% to 93% at 2 to 5 years
  - Approximately 25% of patients will have a subsequent surgery within 5 years secondary to abnormal bleeding
  - Contraindicated if endometrial hyperplasia or cancer suspected, future fertility desired, or acute pelvic infection
- Gonadotropin-releasing hormone agonists
  - Use limited to 6 months to 1 year given risk of irreversible bone loss
- In hemodynamically unstable women, a dilation and curettage is the best option and can be followed with endometrial ablation or hysterectomy if there is no further desire for conception

FERTILITY AND ANOVULATION

- Many women can restore ovulation by normalizing BMI
- If anovulation persists, clomiphene citrate (a selective estrogen-receptor modulator) can be used for 5 days in the early follicular phase followed by timed intercourse or an intrauterine insemination
- Clomiphene citrate can only be used with an intact hypothalamic-pituitary-ovarian axis (WHO II and WHO III)
- Clomiphene citrate (CC) can be given with metformin, dexamethasone, or gonadotropins in CC-resistant patients
- Clomiphene is superior to metformin alone in achieving a live birth in infertile women with PCOS, although multiple birth is a complication (Legro et al, 2007)
- One half of PCOS women who will conceive on CC will do so at the starting dose of 50 mg; another 20% of PCOS women will conceive at the 100-mg dose
- Women with hyperandrogenemia and amenorrhea are less likely to ovulate with CC than women with normal androgen levels or oligomenorrhea
- A risk of ovarian tumors is associated with prolonged exposure to clomiphene citrate
- Current recommendation is to move to other treatments in women who do not achieve pregnancy after six cycles of clomiphene citrate

SUGGESTED READINGS

The Normal Menstrual Cycle

Rogers PA, Lederman F, Taylor N: Endometrial microvascular growth in normal and dysfunctional states, *Hum Reprod Update* 4(5):503–508, 1998.

Salamonsen LA, Woolley DE: Matrix metalloproteinases in normal menstruation, *Hum Reprod* 11(Suppl 2):124–133, 1996.

Schwab KE, Chan RW, Gargett CE: Putative stem cell activity of human endometrial epithelial and stromal cells during the menstrual cycle, *Fertil Steril* 84(Suppl 2):1124–1130, 2005.

Sehested A, Juul AA, Andersson AM, et al: Serum inhibin A and inhibin B in healthy prepubertal, pubertal, and adolescent girls and adult women: relation to age, stage of puberty, menstrual cycle, follicle-stimulating hormone, luteinizing hormone, and estradiol levels, *J Clin Endocrinol Metab* 85(4):1634–1640, 2000.

Abnormal Bleeding in Adolescents

American Academy of Pediatrics Committee on Adolescence: American College of Obstetricians and Gynecologists Committee on Adolescent Health Care, Diaz A, Laufer MR, Breech LL: Menstruation in girls and adolescents: using the menstrual cycle as a vital sign, *Pediatrics* 118(5):2245–2250, 2006.

Beasley A: Contraception for specific populations, *Semin Reprod Med* 28(2):147–155, 2010.

Biro FM, Galvez MP, Greenspan LC, et al: Pubertal assessment method and baseline characteristics in a mixed longitudinal study of girls, *Pediatrics* 126(3):e583–e590, 2010.

Cromer BA, Blair JM, Mahan JD, Zibners L, et al: A prospective comparison of bone density in adolescent girls receiving depot medroxyprogesterone acetate (Depo-Provera), levonorgestrel (Norplant), or oral contraceptives, *J Pediatr* 129(5):671–676, 1996.

Roa J, García-Galiano D, Castellano JM, et al: Metabolic control of puberty onset: new players, new mechanisms, *Mol Cell Endocrinol* 324(1-2):87–94, 2010.

Sanfilippo JS, Lara-Torre E: Adolescent gynecology, *Obstet Gynecol* 113(4):935–947, 2009.

Intermenstrual Bleeding, Fibroids, and Endometrial Polyps

American College of Obstetricians and Gynecologists: ACOG practice bulletin: alternatives to hysterectomy in the management of leiomyomas, *Obstet Gynecol* 112(2 Pt 1):387–400, 2008.

Engman M, Granberg S, Williams AR, et al: Mifepristone for the treatment of uterine leiomyomas: a prospective randomized placebo controlled trial, *Hum Reprod* 24(8):1870–1879, 2009.

Griesinger G, Felberbaum R, Diedrich K: GnRH-antagonists in reproductive medicine, *Arch Gynecol Obstet* 273(2):71–78, 2005.

Klatsky PC, Tran ND, Caughey AB, Fujimoto VY: Fibroids and reproductive outcomes: a systematic literature review from conception to delivery, *Am J Obstet Gynecol* 198(4):357–366, 2008.

van der Kooij SM, Hehenkamp WJ, Volkers NA, et al: Uterine artery embolization vs. hysterectomy in the treatment of symptomatic uterine fibroids: 5-year outcome from the randomized EMMY trial, *Am J Obstet Gynecol* 203(2):105.e1–105.e13, 2010.

Amenorrhea

Ehrmann DA, Lilijenquist DR, Kasza K, et al: Prevalence and predictors of the metabolic syndrome in women with polycystic ovary syndrome, *J Clin Endocrinology Metab* 91(1):48–53, 2006.

Gordon CM: Clinical practice: functional hypothalamic amenorrhea, *N Engl J Med* 363(4):365–371, 2010.

Kalantaridou SN, Naka KK, Papanikolaou E, et al: Impaired endothelial function in young women with premature ovarian failure: normalization with hormone therapy, *J Clin Endocrinol Metab* 89(8):3907–3913, 2004.

Meczekalski B, Podfigurna-Stopa A, Genazzani AR: Hypoestrogenism in young women and its influence on bone mass density, *Gynecol Endocrinol* 26(9):652–657, 2010.

Pleskacova J, Hersmus R, Oosterhuis JW, et al: Tumor risk in disorders of sex development, *Sex Dev* 4(4-5):259–269, 2010.

Practice Committee of the American Society for Reproductive Medicine: Current evaluation of amenorrhea, *Fertil Steril* 82(1):266–272, 2004.

Webster J, Piscitelli G, Polli A, et al: A comparison of cabergoline and bromocriptine in the treatment of hyperprolactinemic amenorrhea, *N Engl J Med* 331(14):904–909, 1994.

Welt CK, Chan J, Bullen J, Recombinant human leptin in women with hypothalamic amenorrhea, *N Engl J Med* 351(10):987–997, 2004.

Chronic Menorrhagia and Anovulation

Atsma F, Bartelink ML, Grobbee DE, van der Schouw YT: Postmenopausal status and early menopause as independent risk factors for cardiovascular disease: a meta-analysis, *Menopause* 13(2):265–279, 2006.

Chuong CJ, Brenner PF: Management of abnormal uterine bleeding, *Am J Obstet Gynecol* 175(3 Pt 2):787–792, 1996.

Nelson LM, Covington SN, Rebar RW: an update: spontaneous premature ovarian failure is not an early menopause, *Fertil Steril* 83(5):1327–1332, 2005.

Practice Committee of the American Society for Reproductive Medicine: Indications and options for endometrial ablation, *Fertil Steril* 90(Suppl 5): S236–S240: 2008.

Schlinder AE: Progestogen deficiency and endometrial cancer risk, *Maturitas* 62(4):334–337, 2009.

Strauss JF III, Barbieri RL, editors: *Yen & Jaffe's reproductive endocrinology: expert consult*, ed 6, Philadelphia, 2009, Saunders.

References

Please go to expertconsult.com to view references.

Chapter 34

Benign and Malignant Disease of the Breast

SHAGUFTA YASMEEN

KEY UPDATES

1 The incidence of benign breast disease (BBD) begins to rise during the 2nd decade of life and peaks in fourth and fifth decades. Prevalence of BBD doubled among postmenopausal women receiving hormone replacement therapy (HRT) for more than 8 years

2 Estrogens stimulate the proliferation of breast epithelial cells, and may also have direct genotoxic effects, and induce aneuploidy. Women with *BRCA1* or *BRCA2* gene mutations have a higher frequency of multiple benign and malignant breast lesions

3 Patients undergoing kidney transplantation have an increased incidence of multiple fibroadenomas. Proliferation marker Ki-67 is a helpful in differentiating phylloides tumor from fibroadenomas

4 Multiple papillomas are associated with higher risk for invasive breast cancer

5 Tamoxifen use is associated with 28% reduction in prevalence of benign breast disease

6 Breast cancer incidence has decreased by 2.2% per year from 1999 to 2005 largely due to discontinuation of HRT. Lifetime risk of developing breast cancer in the United States is estimated at 12.7% for all women. Five to 10% of women with breast cancer have an identifiable hereditary predisposition

7 Pregnancy-associated breast cancer (BC during, or within a year after a pregnancy) is expected to increase in frequency due to delay in childbearing until later in life, when the general risk of breast cancer begins to rise

Benign Breast Disease (BBD)

CLINICAL PROFILE

- Benign breast diseases frequently present with symptoms such as breast mass, thickening, nodularity, tenderness, skin changes, nipple discharge, or nipple retraction (Figures 34-1, 34-2, and 34-3)
- Breast mass that fluctuates with menstrual cycles or has been present and stable for years is more likely to be benign
- In absence of a surgical scar, a mass associated with skin dimpling is malignant until proven otherwise
- The "triple test" of a breast mass includes palpation, imaging, and core needle biopsy or fine-needle aspiration for pathologic diagnosis

UPDATE #1

There are no known modifiable risk factors for BBD. Smoking (ever, former, or current), diet (high or low fat/vitamins and fiber), and methylxanthines (caffeine, theophylline) have no substantial effect of on fibrocystic changes (FCC), fibroadenoma (FA), or across different grades of atypia. Obesity is protective for development of both fibroadenoma and fibrocystic disease; however, obesity cannot be promoted because of its other potentially deleterious effects on a woman's health (Worsham et al, 2009).

DIAGNOSIS

- Fifty percent of women with FCC present with a tender palpable breast mass or multifocal nodularities, or sudden pain, because of distension or leakage of fluid into surrounding tissue from chemical irritation
- Symptoms are usually bilateral, symmetrical, and may occur in conjunction with the menstrual cycle in the middle and late reproductive period (30 to 50 years)
- Diagnostics mammography is usually negative; ultrasound (US) is helpful differentiating simple from a complex cyst
- Breast biopsy may show adenosis, sclerosing adenosis, or microglandular adenosis

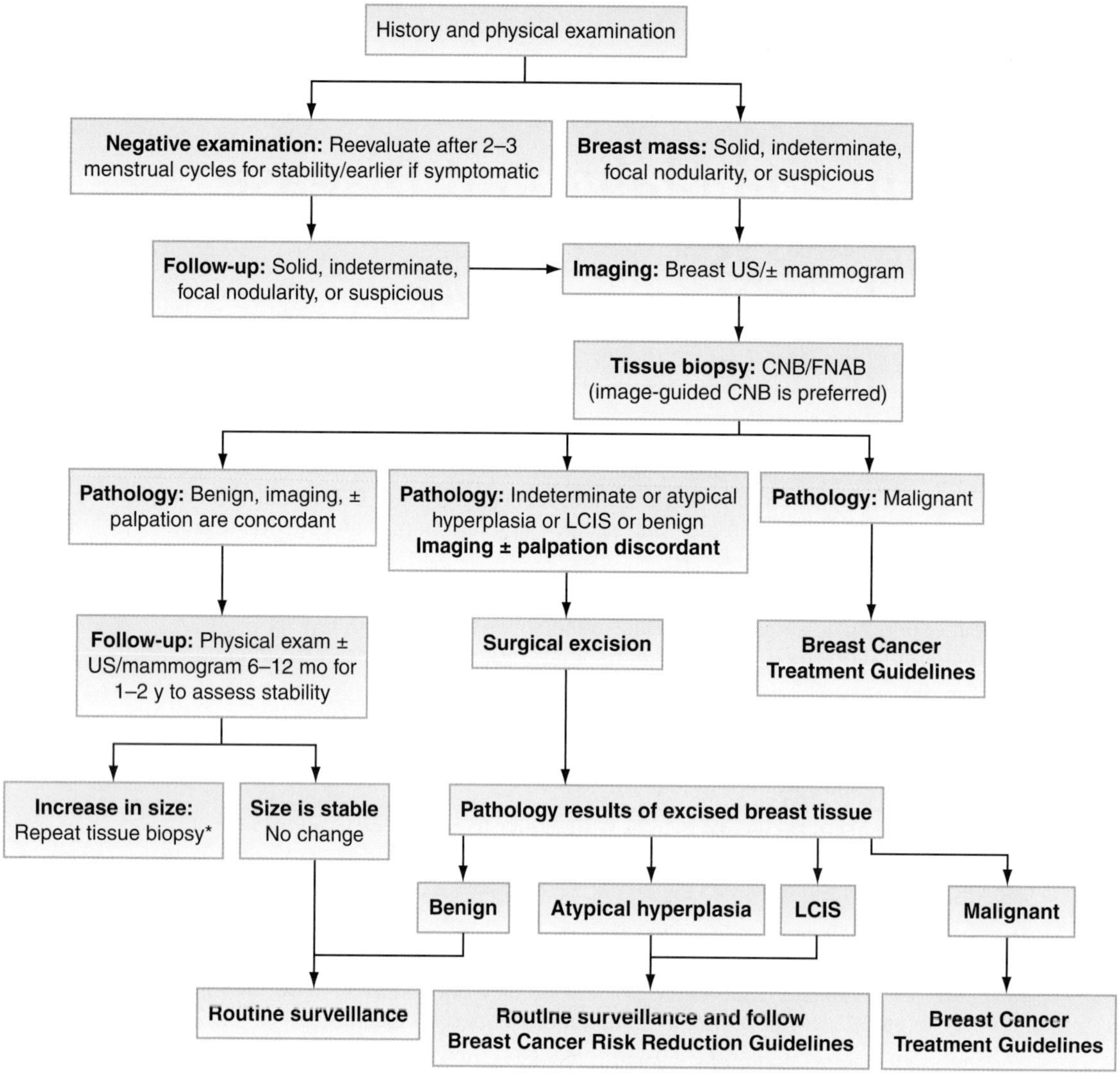

Figure 34-1. Evaluation of breast lump/mass in a woman age <30 years age.

MANAGEMENT

- Simple cysts: no increased risk for breast cancer, aspiration is indicated for symptoms (painful, tender lump)
- Complex cysts: risk of breast cancer is very low (<0.3%); US features of a complex cyst include internal echoes, septations, thickened or irregular wall, intracystic mass, absent posterior enhancement; US-guided aspiration is routinely performed to exclude malignant cells

Benign Breast Disease and Subsequent Breast Cancer Risk

CLINICAL PROFILE

- Fibrocystic changes are multifocal bilateral disorder of epithelial origin with cystic and solid lesions
- Presenting symptoms include breast tenderness, palpable breast mass, and multifocal nodularities
- Although fibrocystic breast lesions are relatively common, only a small proportion of proliferative lesions progress to invasive breast cancer
- Fibrocystic changes are present in 90% of women between ages 20 to 50 years (on incidental breast biopsies)

- Seventy percent of lesions are "nonproliferative"
- Greater than 80% of patients with a diagnosis of atypical hyperplasia (ADH) do not develop invasive breast cancer during their lifetime (Tables 34-1 and 34-2)

UPDATE #2

Benign breast diseases associated with subsequent development of invasive breast cancer include age, family history, and biopsy findings (e.g., atypical ductal hyperplasia, lobular hyperplasia, or papilloma) (Degnim et al, 2009; Hartmann et al, 2005). Estrogen and progesterone stimulate the proliferation of breast tissue and are considered mitogens for normal breast epithelium. Loss of heterozygosity is an indicator of a clonal neoplastic change and is present in some cases of atypical ductal hyperplasia (ADH), ductal carcinoma in situ (DCIS), and lobular carcinoma in situ (LCIS) (Hefler et al, 2004; Rohan et al, 2008). High levels of estrogen receptor α(ER α) and a decrease in ß (ER ß) receptor in premalignant lesions (unfolded lobules, atypical ductal hyperplasias, and ductal carcinoma in situ) are associated with a two- to threefold increased risk of developing invasive breast cancer (Hartmann et al, 2005; Visvanathan et al, 2009; Rohan et al, 2008). *BRCA1* and *BRCA2* mutations are responsible for 3% to 8% of all cases of breast cancer and 5% to

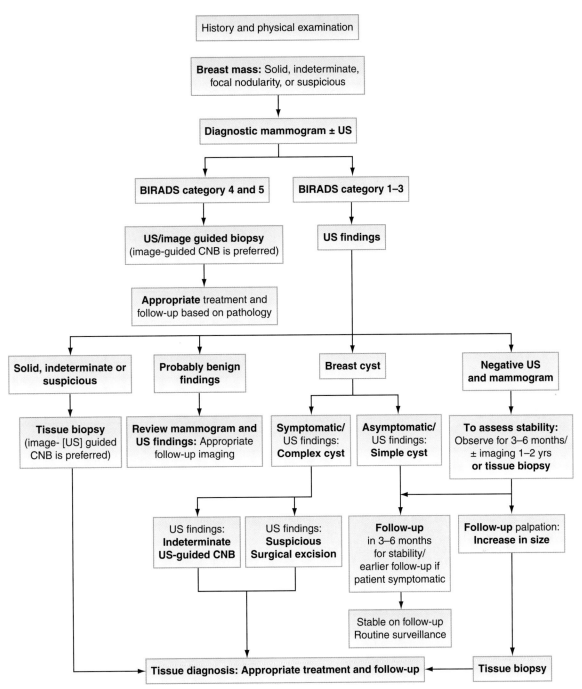

Figure 34-2. Evaluation of breast lump/mass/cyst in a woman age ≥30 years age.

10% of familial breast cancers. Women with *BRCA1* or *BRCA2* gene mutations have a higher frequency of multiple benign and malignant breast lesions. Breast magnetic resonance imaging (MRI) screening is recommended for high-risk women, including those with *BRCA1* or *BRCA2* mutations and those who have greater than a 20% lifetime risk of developing breast cancer, and women who have been treated for Hodgkin's lymphoma (see Table 34-2).

MANAGEMENT

- Surgical excision of benign breast lesions is indicated for proliferate lesions with atypia on breast biopsy, even when mammography and US are negative for abnormal findings

- Atypical ductal and lobular hyperplasia is associated with a higher relative risk of developing breast cancer in patients with no family history of breast cancer (see Table 34-2)

Fibroadenomas and Phylloides Tumor

CLINICAL PROFILE

- Fibroadenomas are common; hormonally sensitive benign breast tumor occurs in younger women (age 15 to 35 years)
- Presents as a soft rubbery, round, or lobulated well-circumscribed breast mass

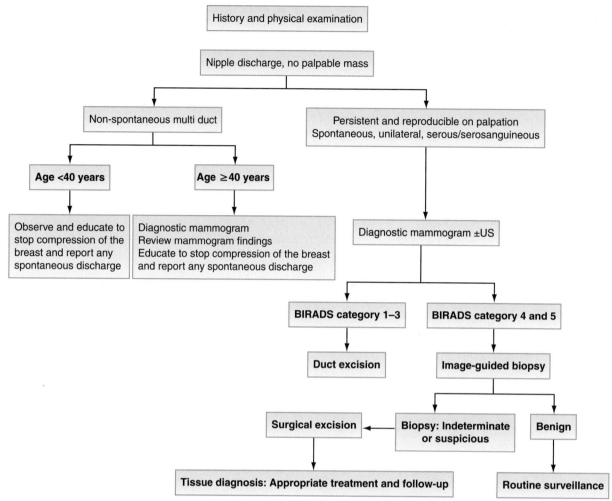

Figure 34-3. Evaluation and management of nipple discharge.

TABLE 34-1   **Histological Category of Benign Breast Lesions Associated with the Relative Risk for Breast Cancer**

Histologic Category	Relative Risk *
Nonproliferative lesions	
Cysts	1
Mild hyperplasia of the usual type	
Columnar cell change	
Proliferative lesions without atypia	
Sclerosing adenosis	1.3-1.9
Moderate or florid ductal hyperplasia of the usual type	
Radial scar	
Intraductal papilloma	
Fibroadenoma	
Atypical hyperplasia	
Atypical ductal hyperplasia	3.9-13.0
Atypical lobular hyperplasia	

*Relative risk represents the range of relative risks reported in one retrospective cohort study and three case-control studies.

- Frequently unilateral, 2 to 3 cm in size, 20% are occur bilateral, may also occur at multiple sites in the same breast
- Giant fibroadenomas are massive tumors (> 10 cm in size), more commonly observed in female adolescents
- Postmenopausal woman with a fibroadenoma shows typical stippled "popcorn" calcification on mammogram
- A phylloides tumor presents as a well-circumscribed soft to firm mass, size varies ≥10 cm, occurs at a median age of 45 years
- Phylloides tumors are classified as benign, borderline, and malignant

UPDATE #3

Chromosomal aberrations in epithelial and stromal cells of a fibroadenoma suggest neoplastic change. Complex fibroadenoma with pathologic features of sclerosing adenosis, adenosis, and epithelial hyperplasia is associated with a higher risk of breast cancer among women aged 50 years and older (Khanzada et al, 2009). The presence of fibroblast in a fibroadenoma suggests progression to phylloides tumors. Proliferation marker Ki-67 differentiates phylloides tumors from fibroadenoma. Predictors of local recurrence in phylloides tumors include cellularity, cytologic atypia, mitotic activity, positive margins, infiltrative borders, and fibroproliferative satellite nodules, and predictors for a distant metastasis include size, tumor necrosis, and stromal overgrowth (Macdonald et al, 2006).

TABLE 34-2 **Evaluation of a Patient with Benign Breast Symptoms**

History	Physical Examination
Characterize Symptoms	*1. Breast Mass*
Identify Risk Factors for Breast Cancer	
Age (current)	Palpate the four breast quadrants while patient is sitting and lying down
Age at menarche	Identify discrete lumps and examine for regional nodes
Age at first live birth	Determine whether consistency is doughy with vague nodularity → fibrocystic changes
Number of relatives with breast cancer or ovarian cancer	Look for a discrete lesion with distinct marginated borders → fibroadenoma
Age at diagnosis	Examine overlying skin, areola and axilla
Number of previous breast biopsies	Determine degree of symmetry (asymmetry suggests underlying disease)
Presence of ADH or LCIS on previous breast biopsy	Examine nipple and seek to elicit discharge
Weight gain after menopause	*2. Nipple Discharge*
Waist-to-hip ratio	Determine whether galactorrhea is present
Results of bone-density testing (if patient is postmenopausal)	Determine whether discharge is from one duct for or from multiple ducts
Age at menopause	Determine whether discharge is viscous, watery, serosanguineous, grossly bloody, clear, blue-black, or green
Duration of use of estrogen or progestin therapy	Determine whether occult blood is present
	3. Breast Pain
	Seek to elicit chest-wall pain
	Examine costochondral junctions (Tietze syndrome)
	Examine lateral chest wall while patient is lying on her side (at 90 degrees), to move breast away from chest wall
	Compare pain elicited by squeezing breast tissue with pain elicited by palpation of chest wall

MANAGEMENT

- US and core needle biopsy for tissue diagnosis in younger women (age <35 years)
- Diagnostic mammogram, US, and biopsy in women age ≥35 years
- Pathology shows proliferation of epithelial and mesenchymal elements, with densely fibrotic stroma and compressed cleftlike ducts
- Pathology review to exclude phylloides tumor and complex fibroadenomas
- Conservative approach (without surgical excision) is acceptable for women at any age if triple assessment (palpation, imaging, and biopsy) is unequivocally benign
- Surgical excision is indicated for giant and complex fibroadenomas
- US-guided cryoablation is the treatment option for simple and multiple fibroadenoma
- Pathology shows a typical leaflike pattern and a more cellular stroma than fibroadenoma
- Surgical excision with negative margins is acceptable treatment
- Recurrent phylloides tumor without metastatic disease is treated with reexcision with wide margins without axillary staging, with or without radiation
- Metastatic phylloides tumor is treated following principles of soft tissue sarcoma

Breast Papilloma, Papillomatosis/ Multiple Papillomas

CLINICAL PROFILE

- Intraductal papilloma is a benign tumor of the epithelium of mammary ducts

- Presenting symptoms are serous, serosanguineous, or bloody nipple discharge
- Juvenile papillomatosis occurs in women aged <30 years
- Solitary, central, benign duct papillomas are not associated with increased risk for subsequent invasive breast cancer
- Multiple papillomas are associated with higher risk for subsequent invasive breast cancer

UPDATE #4

Multiple papillomas, and juvenile papillomatosis present with a minimum of five clearly separate papillomas within a localized segment of breast tissue. They are usually bilateral and occur in the peripheral or subareolar location. Multiple papillomas are associated with a higher risk for subsequent invasive breast cancer (Meisner et al, 2008).

MANAGEMENT

- Bilateral diagnostic mammogram, US, and image-guided biopsy
- Excisional biopsy (duct excision) and thorough sampling of the specimen to rule out malignancy

Chemoprevention Recommendations for High-Risk Women

CLINICAL PROFILE

- Offer tamoxifen 20 mg/d for 5 years to women who are at high risk for developing breast cancer (pre and postmenopausal) (Gail score of ≥1.67 (Table 34-3)
- Raloxifene 60 mg/d for 5 years may also be considered in postmenopausal women as a chemo-preventive agent

TABLE 34-3 Risk Factors for Breast Cancer

Risk Factors	Estimated Relative Risk
Advanced age	>4
Family history	
Two or more relatives (mother, sister)	>5
One first-degree relative	>2
Family history of ovarian cancer in women <50 years	>2
Personal history	3-4
Positive *BRCA1/BRCA2* mutation	>4
Breast biopsy with atypical hyperplasia	4-5
Breast biopsy with LCIS or DCIS	8-10
Lifestyle factors	
Adult weight gain	1.5-2
Sedentary lifestyle	1.3-1.5
Alcohol consumption	1.5
Reproductive history	
Early age at menarche (<12 years)	2
Late age of first-term pregnancy (>3/nulliparity)	1.5-2
Late age of menopause	2
Use of combined estrogen/progesterone HRT	1.5-2
Current or recent use of oral contraceptives	1.25

- Hormonal exposure and risk of breast cancer: oral contraceptive pill use is associated with a modest 1.25 (relative risk [RR]) of increased breast cancer risk among current users
- Postmenopausal hormone replacement therapy (HRT) estrogen plus progestin (E&P) use is associated with a two- to threefold higher risk for developing invasive breast cancer, and the risk is directly associated with length of exposure, with the greater risk for the development of hormonally responsive lobular (RR = 2.3), mixed ductal–lobular (RR = 2.1), and tubular cancers (RR = 2.7)
- Breast cancer risk assessment models (www.cancer.gov/bcrisktool) can estimate a woman's absolute risk of developing breast cancer over time (5-year and lifetime risk)

UPDATE #5

Tamoxifen and raloxifene are equally effective in reducing risk of ER-positive breast cancer in postmenopausal women. Raloxifene is associated with lower rates of thromboembolic disease, benign uterine conditions, and cataracts compared to tamoxifen. Neither agent decreases mortality from breast cancer. Aromatase inhibitors (e.g., anastrozole, exemestane, letrozole), fenretinide, or other selective estrogen receptor modulators (SERMs) are not recommended outside of a clinical trials (Cummings et al, 2009; National Cancer Comprehensive Network [NCCN], 2011). Future breast cancer risk assessment models are being developed to assess breast cancer risk in pre and postmenopausal women; models will also incorporate other identifiable risk factors such as breast density, mammography density change across exams, hormone use, body mass index, and number of first-degree relatives with breast cancer.

Breast Cancer Screening Detection and Treatment

CLINICAL PROFILE

- An overall decrease in breast cancer mortality since 1990 (2.3% per year) has been largely attributed to mammography screening and advances in the treatment of breast cancer
- Mammography screening often reveals a lesion before it is palpable by clinical breast examination (CBE) and, on average, 1 to 2 years before it is noted by breast self-examination
- Digital mammography compared to film mammography is more accurate in women under age 50 years and premenopausal women with radiographically dense breasts; however, overall diagnostic accuracy of digital and film mammography is similar (Jemal et al, 2009)
- Human epidermal growth factor receptor-2 (HER-2) overexpression occurs in 20% to 30% of breast cancers and is associated with increased incidence of recurrence and reduced survival
- MRI screening is recommended for high-risk women including those with *BRCA1* or *BRCA2* mutations, women who have greater than 20% lifetime risk of developing breast cancer, and women who have been treated for Hodgkin's lymphoma

UPDATE #6

Specific recommendations of the U.S. Preventive Services Task Force (USPSTF) New Breast Cancer Screening Guidelines (updated November 2009) and the accompanying strength of recommendations were as follows:

- The USPSTF recommends against routine screening mammography in women age 40 to 49 years. The decision to start regular, biennial screening mammography before the age of 50 years should be an individual one and take into account patient context, including the patient's values regarding specific benefits and harms (grade C recommendation).
- Women aged 50 to 74 years should undergo biennial screening mammography (grade B recommendation).
- Current evidence is insufficient to determine additional benefits and harms of screening mammography in women 75 years or older (1 statement).
- In women 40 years or older, current evidence is insufficient to determine the additional benefits and harms of CBE beyond screening mammography (I statement).
- The USPSTF recommends against clinicians teaching women the technique of breast self-examination (BSE) (grade D recommendation).
- Current evidence is insufficient to determine additional benefits and harms of either digital mammography or MRI versus film mammography as screening modalities for breast cancer (1 statement).

Response to the USPSTF Recommendations from the American College of Obstetricians and Gynecologists (ACOG)

For the present, ACOG continues to recommend adherence to guidelines that include screening mammography every 1 to 2 years for women aged 40 to 49 years and screening mammography every year for women age 50 or older (www.acog.org/from_home/misc/uspstfresponse.cfm).

DIAGNOSIS

- Currently, most breast cancers are detected mammographically, when the mass may be quite small and nonpalpable
- Abnormal mammographic findings include asymmetry, microcalcifications, mass, or architectural distortion
- Concerning findings on CBE or BSE include breast mass, thickening, dimpling or breast pain (5%), skin thickening, swelling, redness, nipple ulceration, retraction, or spontaneous bloody discharge
- Inflammatory breast cancer is invasive breast cancer that involves the dermal lymphatic and is characterized by erythema, edema (peau d'orange) of a third or more of the breast skin, and a palpable border to the erythema
- Initial work of a suspicious breast mass includes the following:
  - Bilateral diagnostic mammogram and breast US if necessary
  - Core needle biopsy (CNB) image-guided or nonimage-guided for palpable lesions
  - Pathology review (tumor type and grade)
  - Determination of estrogen/progesterone receptor and HER-2 status
  - Genetic counseling is recommended if a patient is considered at high risk of hereditary breast cancer
- Use of MRI to evaluate women considering breast-conserving therapy is optional

MANAGEMENT

- Primary treatment of breast cancer includes surgery, radiation therapy, or both, and the treatment of systemic disease with cytotoxic chemotherapy, endocrine therapy, biologic therapy, or combinations of these. Treatment selection depends on the following:
- Tumor histology
- Clinical and pathologic characteristics of the primary tumor
- Axillary node status
- Tumor hormone receptor content
- Tumor HER-2 status
- Presence or absence of detectable metastatic disease
- Patient preferences
- Comorbid conditions
- Patient age
- Menopausal status

Treatment of Noninvasive Cancers (Stage 0)

- Lobular carcinoma in situ (LCIS): treatment options include the following:
  - Observation counseling regarding risk reduction (*tamoxifen for premenopausal women, or tamoxifen or raloxifene for postmenopausal women*)
  - Complete excision for pleomorphic LCIS
  - Bilateral mastectomy (in special cases)
- Ductal carcinoma in situ (DCIS) include the following:
  - Lumpectomy without lymph node surgery plus whole-breast radiation therapy **or**
  - Total mastectomy with or without sentinel node biopsy ± reconstruction **or**
  - Lumpectomy without lymph node surgery and without radiation therapy

Treatment of Invasive Cancer

- Stages I, II, IIIA: treatment includes breast-conserving therapy with lumpectomy, axillary dissection, and whole-breast irradiation with adjuvant systemic chemotherapy and hormonal and biologic therapy if indicated
- Preoperative chemotherapy for large clinically stage IIA and IIB tumors and T3N1M0 tumors for women who meet the criteria for breast-conserving therapy
- Chemotherapies commonly used in breast cancer treatment include anthracyclines (such as Adriamycin and epirubicin), and taxanes (paclitaxel and docetaxel)
- Side effects of chemotherapy: alopecia, nausea/vomiting, mucositis, lowering of blood counts, fatigue, and peripheral sensory neuropathy
- Long-term toxicities: cardiomyopathy, secondary leukemia, and premature menopause
- Antiestrogen therapy (tamoxifen and aromatase inhibitors) for patients with hormone-receptor (ER) or progesterone receptor (PR) positive tumors
- No survival benefits from mastectomy with axillary dissection compared to breast-conserving therapy with lumpectomy, axillary dissection, and whole-breast irradiation
- Trastuzumab (a humanized monoclonal antibody) has been shown to improve outcomes in tumors with overexpression of HER-2
- Common toxicities associated with trastuzumab include infusion reactions and cardiomyopathy
  - Lapatinib (a small molecule tyrosine kinase inhibitor) (TKI) has been shown to be useful in the management of metastatic disease
  - Toxicities associated with lapatinib include diarrhea and rash (National Cancer Comprehensive Network (NCCN), 2011)

Pregnancy-Associated Breast Cancer

CLINICAL PROFILE

- Pregnancy-associated breast cancer (breast cancer during or within a year after a pregnancy) is expected to increase in frequency because of the delay in childbearing until later in life, when the general risk of breast cancer begins to rise
- Breast cancer is the second most common malignancy in pregnancy (after cervical cancer), occurring in 1 in 5000 deliveries
- Approximately 10% of cases occur in women <40 years of age and are considered sporadic

UPDATE #7

The majority of breast cancer cases during pregnancy are considered sporadic. Mammography is safe for the evaluation of the breast in pregnant women, and the radiation dose to the properly shielded fetus is only 0.01 rad, well below the accepted 5 rad limit. Mammography is less sensitive during pregnancy because of the higher breast density. Breast US is 93% accurate for the evaluation of masses during pregnancy. The safety of breast MRI in pregnant women is not known (National Cancer Comprehensive Network (NCCN), 2011).

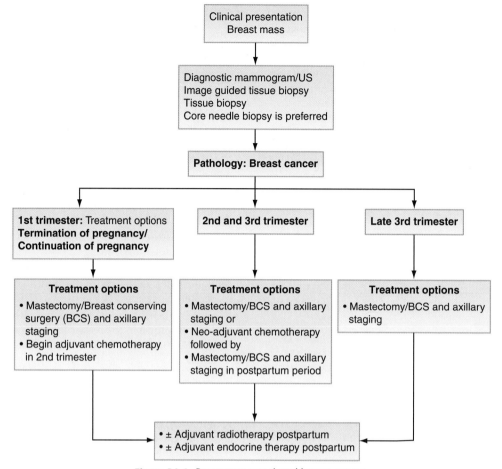

Figure 34-4. Pregnancy-associated breast cancer.

DIAGNOSIS

- Pregnancy-associated breast cancer typically presents as breast mass (Figure 34-4)
- Breast US is routinely used for initial evaluation of a breast mass
- Initial diagnostic work is the same as for any breast mass

MANAGEMENT

- First-trimester treatment options include termination of pregnancy or continuation and treatment
- Treatment includes surgery (mastectomy or breast-conserving surgery), axillary staging followed by adjuvant chemo in the second trimester, and postpartum radiotherapy
- Treatment in the second and third trimesters includes surgical (mastectomy or breast-conserving surgery), axillary staging or neoadjuvant chemotherapy followed by surgery (mastectomy or breast-conserving surgery), axillary staging, and postpartum radiotherapy (National Cancer Comprehensive Network [NCCN], 2011)

SUGGESTED READINGS

Benign Breast Disease

Degnim AC, Hartmann LC: Refining risk assessment in women with atypical hyperplasia, *Current Breast Cancer Reports* 1(3):167–174, 2009.

El Aouni N, Laurent I, Terrier P, et al: Granular cell tumor of the breast, *Diagn Cytopathol* 35(11):725–727, 2007.

Guray M, Sahin AA: Benign breast diseases: classification, diagnosis, and management, *Oncologist* 11(5):435–449, 2006.

Hartmann LC, Sellers TA, Frost MH, et al: Benign breast disease and the risk of breast cancer, *N Engl J Med* 353(3):229–237, 2005.

Hefler LA, Tempfer CB, Grimm C, et al: Estrogen-metabolizing gene polymorphisms in the assessment of breast carcinoma risk and fibroadenoma risk in Caucasian women, *Cancer* 101(2):264–269, 2004.

Khanzada TW, Samad A, Sushel C: Spectrum of benign breast diseases, *Pak J Med Sci* 25(2):265–268, 2009.

Kiluk JV, Acs G, Hoover SJ: High-risk benign breast lesions: current strategies in management, *Cancer Control* 14(4):321–329, 2007.

Macdonald OK, Lee CM, Tward JD, et al: Malignant phyllodes tumor of the female breast: association of primary therapy with cause-specific survival from the Surveillance, Epidemiology, and End Results (SEER) program, *Cancer* 107(9):2127–2133, 2006.

Meisner AL, Fekrazad MH, Royce ME: Breast disease: benign and malignant, *Med Clin North Am* 92(5):1115–1141, 2008.

Miltenburg DM, Speights VO Jr: Benign breast disease, *Obstet Gynecol Clin North Am* 35(2), 2008. 285-ix, 300.

Neal L, Tortorelli CL, Nassar A: Clinician's guide to imaging and pathologic findings in benign breast disease, *Mayo Clin Proc* 85(3):274–279, 2010.

Rohan TE, Negassa A, Chlebowski RT, et al: Conjugated equine estrogen and risk of benign proliferative breast disease: a randomized controlled trial, *J Natl Cancer Inst* 100(8):563–571, 2008.

Silvera SA, Rohan TE: Benign proliferative epithelial disorders of the breast: a review of the epidemiologic evidence, *Breast Cancer Res Treat* 110(3):397–409, 2008.

Virnig Beth A. Tuttle, Todd M. Shamliyan Tatyana, Kane Robert L: Ductal carcinoma in situ of the breast: a systematic review of incidence, treatment, and outcomes, *J Natl Cancer Inst* 102(3):170–178, 2010.

Visvanathan K, Chlebowski RT, Hurley P, et al: American society of clinical oncology clinical practice guideline update on the use of pharmacologic interventions including tamoxifen, raloxifene, and aromatase inhibition for breast cancer risk reduction, *J Clin Oncol* 27(19):3235–3258, 2009.

Worsham MJ, Raju U, Lu M, Kapke A, Cheng J, Wolman SR: Risk factors for breast cancer from benign breast disease in a diverse population, *Breast Cancer Res Treat* 118(1):1–7, 2009.

Breast Cancer

U.S. Preventive Services Task Force. Screening for Breast Cancer: *Recommendations and Rationale. Agency for Healthcare Research and Quality.* Available at http://www.ahrq.gov/clinic/3rduspstf/breastCancer/brcanrr.htm.

American Cancer Society: *Breast cancer facts & figures 2009-2010* (website). www.cancer.org/acs/groups/content/@nho/documents/document/f861009final90809pdf.pdf. Accessed August 5, 2011.

American Congress of Obstetricians and Gynecologists: *Response of the American College of Obstetricians and Gynecologists to new breast cancer screening recommendations from the U.S. Preventive Services Task Force* (website). www.acog.org/from_home/misc/uspstfresponse.cfm. Accessed August 5, 2011.

Cummings SR, Tice JA, Bauer S, et al: Prevention of breast cancer in postmenopausal women: approaches to estimating and reducing risk, *Natl Cancer Inst* 101(6):384–398, 2009.

Jemal A, Siegel R, Ward E, et al: Cancer statistics, 2009, *CA Cancer J Clin* 59(4):225–249, 2009.

National Cancer Comprehensive Network (NCCN): *Clinical practice guidelines in oncology: invasive breast cancer* (website). www.jnccn.org/content/9/2/136.full.pdf+html. Accessed August 5, 2011.

National Cancer Institute: *Breast cancer risk assessment tool* (website). www.cancer.gov/bcrisktool. Accessed August 5, 2011.

Wolff AC, Hammond ME, Schwartz JN, et al: American Society of Clinical Oncology/College of American Pathologists guideline recommendations for human epidermal growth factor receptor 2 testing in breast cancer, *J Clin Oncol* 25(1):118–145, 2007.

Chapter 35

Management of Diseases of the Vulva and Vagina

ANNE O. RODRIGUEZ • LLOYD H. SMITH

KEY UPDATES

1 Human papilloma virus (HPV) DNA is often associated with vaginal intraepithelial neoplasia (VAIN) and vaginal cancer.

2 Ultrasonic surgical aspiration is described as a treatment for VAIN.

3 Topical imiquimod 5% cream has been found to be active in the treatment of some vulvar intra-epithelial neoplasia (VIN) lesions.

4 Prophylactic HPV vaccination may affect the risk of developing vaginal cancer.

5 Primary radiotherapy treatment reports high disease-free survival rates for stage I and stage II squamous cell carcinoma of the vagina.

6 Younger HPV-positive and older HPV-negative women who develop vulvar cancer have different pathogenic mechanisms.

7 Current recommendations for early vulvar cancer include removal of the entire inguinofemoral fat pad, which may not require removal of the cribriform fascia or resection of the saphenous vein.

Vaginal Intraepithelial Neoplasia (VAIN)

CLINICAL PROFILE

- VAIN frequently discovered within 10 years following hysterectomy for cervical dysplasia
- Usually asymptomatic; abnormal pap smear may suggest VAIN in patients who have had a hysterectomy
- Upper third of the vagina is most common location
- Half to two thirds of VAIN patients have had or currently have other lower genital tract neoplasia

UPDATE #1

Multiple studies have shown that HPV DNA is often associated with VAIN and vaginal cancer. Over 90% of VAIN lesions (VAIN 2/3 or VAIN 1) harbored HPV DNA with HPV 16 found most frequently among VAIN lesions (De Vuyst et al, 2009; Smith et al, 2009). These findings suggest that women receiving multivalent HPV vaccines could experience some protection against the development of VAIN.

DIAGNOSIS

- Colposcopic findings similar to cervical intraepithelial neoplasia (CIN) lesions
- Lugol's solution may be helpful in delineating lesions
- Multifocal lesions common
- Biopsy with alligator-jaw forceps
- Women exposed to diethylstilbestrol (DES)
  - Persistent Müllerian duct epithelium within vaginal mucosa, or adenosis

- Adenosis sometimes submucosal
- Rare development of clear cell carcinoma
- Morphologic and vaginal cytologic abnormalities common
- Palpation as well as colposcopy required

MANAGEMENT

- Local excision
- CO_2 laser ablation
- Intravaginal 5-fluorouracil (5Fu)

UPDATE #2

Ultrasonic surgical aspiration has been described as a treatment for VAIN. In a study of 92 patients with VAIN treated by ultrasonic surgical aspiration and followed for a median of 4.5 years, the overall recurrence rate was 19.6%, 32.3% for VAIN 3 (Matsuo et al, 2009).

Vulvar Intraepithelial Neoplasia (VIN)

DIFFERENTIAL DIAGNOSIS

- Biopsy all vulvar lesions to establish which have neoplastic potential, Paget's disease
- Squamous cell hyperplasia
  - Associated with pruritus
  - Thickening, excoriations, hyperkeratosis
  - Treatment with topical corticosteroids
- Lichen sclerosis
  - Most patients postmenopausal, but can occur at any age
  - Pruritus, excoriation, ulceration

- Thin, crinkled epithelium ("cigarette paper")
- Atrophy of labia minora, phimosis of clitoral hood late manifestations
  - Treatment = clobetasol propionate 0.05% cream
- Other dermatoses: seborrheic dermatitis, psoriasis, tinea, lichen simplex, lichen planus

CLINICAL PROFILE

- Increasing incidence among young white women
- High risk HPV DNA in 80% to 90%
- Diagnosis: biopsy, colposcopy with 5% acetic acid helpful
- Pigmented lesions often harbor carcinoma in situ

MANAGEMENT

- Surgical excision, 5-mm disease-free margins
- Widespread carcinoma in situ: skinning vulvectomy with split-thickness skin grafting
- CO_2 laser: must rule out invasive disease, depth of destruction 3 mm in hair-bearing skin, deep burns heal slowly and may be painful
- Recurrences common: regular follow-up surveillance, biopsy of suspicious lesions

UPDATE #3

Topical imiquimod 5% cream, originally developed to treat genital condyloma, has been found to be active in the treatment of some VIN lesions. Among 52 patients with VIN lesions, imiquimod treatment was associated with a shrinkage in lesion size over 20 weeks of treatment. Nine patients had a complete response at 20 weeks and remained disease free for 12 months (van Seters et al, 2008).

Invasive Cancer of the Vagina

CLINICAL PROFILE

- Vaginal cancer only 1% to 3% of all genital cancers
- Most vaginal cancers in upper third of vagina
- Peak incidence in 1970s and 1980s
- Squamous histology 85%, adenocarcinoma 6%, melanoma 3%
- Presentation: vaginal bleeding, discharge

UPDATE #4

Among 21 patients with invasive squamous cell carcinoma of the vagina, 17 (81%) were found to be associated with HPV DNA (Ferreira et al, 2008). Other studies support these findings with 65.5% (Smith et al, 2009) and 69.9% (De Vuyst et al, 2009) of vaginal cancers harboring HPV DNA. HPV DNA 16 was the most prevalent HPV type identified in vaginal cancer, suggesting that prophylactic HPV vaccination may affect the risk of developing vaginal cancer.

- Patterns of spread: distal vaginal lesions—lymphatic spread to inguinofemoral nodes, proximal vaginal lesions—deep pelvic nodes
- International Federation of Gynecology and Obstetrics (FIGO) staging (Table 35-1)

MANAGEMENT

- Primary radiotherapy
  - Teletherapy 4000 to 5000 cGy
  - Brachytherapy 6000 to 8000 cGy
  - Interstitial implants for bulky upper vaginal lesions

TABLE 35-1   FIGO Staging of Invasive Cancer of the Vagina

Stage 0	Carcinoma in situ, intraepithelial carcinoma
Stage I	Carcinoma is limited to the vaginal wall
Stage II	Carcinoma has involved the subvaginal tissue but has not extended onto the pelvic wall
Stage III	Carcinoma has extended onto the pelvic wall
Stage IV	Carcinoma has extended beyond the true pelvis or has involved the mucosa of the bladder or rectum; bullous edema or tumor bulge into the bladder or rectum is not acceptable evidence of invasion of these organs
—Stage IVa	Spread of the growth to adjacent organs or direct extension beyond the true pelvis
—Stage IVb	Spread to distant organs

From *Staging of gynecologic malignancies handbook,* ed 3, Society of Gynecologic Oncologists, January 2010. www.sgo.org.

- Radical surgery for radiation failures
- Radical hysterectomy with upper vaginectomy may be an alternative in early-stage upper vaginal lesions in younger patients
- Five-year disease-free survival for majority of patients with FIGO stage I and II vaginal cancer

UPDATE #5

Recent retrospective reports confirm high disease-free survival rates for women with stages I and II squamous cell carcinoma of the vagina treated with primary radiotherapy (De Crevoisier et al, 2007; Frank et al, 2005; Sinha et al, 2009). Smaller studies have suggested that radiotherapy with concurrent chemotherapy may be an effective treatment for patients with advanced vaginal cancer (Dalrymple et al, 2004; Nashiro et al, 2008).

- Surgery
  - Superficially invasive squamous cell carcinoma (<2.5 mm)
  - Resection of vaginal mucosa with negative margins, primary closure
- Adenocarcinoma/clear cell carcinoma
  - Clear cell carcinoma: marked decrease in incidence since 1970s as fewer women DES exposed
  - Radical hysterectomy/upper vaginectomy with retention of ovaries in young women
- Malignant melanoma
  - Less than 1% of vaginal malignancies
  - Bleeding, vaginal discharge
  - Surgical excision treatment of choice

Invasive Cancer of the Vulva

CLINICAL PROFILE

- Five percent of all genital malignancies
- Eighty-six percent are squamous cell carcinomas

UPDATE #6

Among the same studies showing high rates of HPV DNA associated with VIN lesions, only 40% of vulvar cancers were found to harbor HPV DNA (De Vuyst et al, 2009; Smith et al, 2009).

TABLE 35-2   **FIGO Staging of Invasive Cancer of the Vulva (2010)***

Stage I: tumor confined to the vulva
— Stage IA: lesions ≦2 centimeters confined to the vulva or perineum and with stromal invasion no greater than 1.0 mm,[†] no nodal metastasis
— Stage IB: lesions >2 centimeters or with stromal invasion >1.0 mm, confined to the vulva or perineum, no nodal metastasis

Stage II: tumor of any size with extension to adjacent perineal structures (one third lower urethra, one third lower vagina, anus), no nodal metastasis

Stage III: tumor of any size with or without extension to adjacent perineal structures (one third lower urethra, one third lower vagina, anus), with positive inguinofemoral lymph nodes
— Stage IIIAi : with one lymph node metastasis (≧5 mm)
— Stage IIIAii: one to two lymph node metastases (<5 mm)
— Stage IIIBi: with two or more lymph node metastases (≧5 mm)
— Stage IIIBii: three or more lymph node metastases (<5 mm)
— Stage IIIC: with positive nodes with extracapsular spread

Stage IV: tumor invades any of the following:
— Stage IVAi: upper urethral or vaginal mucosa, bladder mucosa, rectal mucosa, or fixed to pelvic bone
— Stage IVAii: fixed or ulcerated inguinofemoral lymph nodes
— Stage IVB: any distant metastasis including pelvic lymph nodes

*Tumor, nodes, and metastases (TNM) staging differs slightly (see the American Joint Committee on Cancer [AJCC] cancer staging manual, 7th ed.)
[†]The depth of invasion is defined as the measurement of the tumor from the epithelial-stromal junction of the adjacent most superficial dermal papilla to the deepest point of invasion.
From *Staging of gynecologic malignancies handbook,* ed 3, Society of Gynecologic Oncologists, January 2010. www.sgo.org.

HPV DNA association with vulvar cancer is most prominent in younger women who also experience a lower probability of cancer-related death (Hampl et al, 2006; Launeau et al, 2009), suggesting different pathogenic mechanisms between younger HPV-positive and older HPV-negative women who develop vulvar cancer (Kumar et al, 2009).

- Chronic pruritus a common symptom
- A minority of vulvar cancers associated with HPV DNA
- Lymphatic spread: labial lesions primary to inguinofemoral nodes; midline lesions may drain to deep pelvic nodes
- Incidence of node metastases increases with lesion size and FIGO stage
  - FIGO staging (Table 35-2)

MANAGEMENT OF VULVAR CANCER

- Treatment algorithms (Figs. 35-1 through 35-3)

UPDATE #7

Controversy arose regarding the safety of "superficial" inguinal lymphadenectomy (as originally described by Di Saia et al, 1979, and Berman et al, 1989) for early vulvar cancer with the publication of the results of a prospective trial by the Gynecologic Oncology Group (protocol 74) showing an unexpected number (7.3%) of patients with isolated groin recurrences (Stehman et al, 1992). Current recommendations define the standard of care as the removal of the entire inguinofemoral fat pad, which may not require removal of the cribriform fascia or resection of the saphenous vein (Stehman et al, 2009).

Clinical trials evaluating the efficacy of sentinel lymph node biopsy (SLNB) in vulvar carcinoma are ongoing (e.g., GOG protocol 173). SLNB has proved valuable in the care of patients with early breast cancer and melanoma, and, if appropriate, it could establish which patients with vulvar cancer could avoid full inguinofemoral lymphadenectomy with all of its potential morbidity. Recent results suggest SLNB is feasible in patients

with vulvar cancer. Some studies show a low false-negative rate (2.9% groin recurrence rate among SLNB-negative patients) (Van der Zee et al, 2008); however, in others the false-negative rate was somewhat more concerning (27% false-negative SLN based on full groin dissection) (Radziszewski et al, 2010). A consensus panel of experts from the international Sentinel Node Society Meeting recommended that the best candidates for SLNB as an alternative to full groin dissection are patients with invasion >1 mm, tumors <4 cm diameter, and no obvious metastatic disease. Preoperative lymphoscintigraphy can aid identification of SLN in unexpected locations; otherwise the recommendation is for radiocolloid for SLN identification with or without blue dye. Surgeons should have a minimum of 10 consecutive successful identification procedures prior to performing SLNB without lymphadenectomy. Radiologists and pathologists experienced in SLNB should be available (Levenback et al, 2009). SLNB for vulvar cancer continues to be explored in clinical trials, and the results of GOG 173 should be helpful.

- Results
  - Complications: wound breakdown of vulvar incisions common; lower extremity edema, especially after lymphadenectomy and groin irradiation
  - Survival: 5-year disease-free survival rates
    - I: 91%
    - II: 81%
    - III: 48%
    - IV: 15%
  - Recurrent disease
    - Eighty percent of recurrences within 2 years of initial surgery; half localized near primary site; poor prognosis for groin recurrences

NONSQUAMOUS VULVAR MALIGNANCIES

- Paget's disease of vulva
  - Pruritus, burning, pain
  - Demarcated erythematous areas with excoriation, thickening

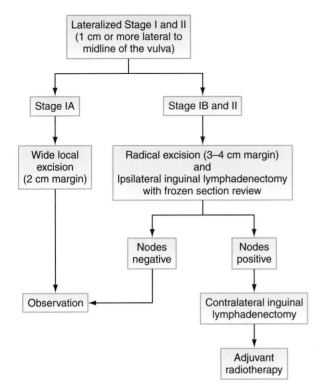

Note: Stage IA (≤2 cm diameter, ≤1 mm invasion) wide radical
      excision without lymphadenectomy if no lympho-vascular
      invasion present

Stage IB (≤2 cm diameter, invasion >1 mm) role of "superficial"
inguinofemoral lymphadenectomy controversial.

Figure 35-1. Treatment of lateralized early stage vulvar cancer.

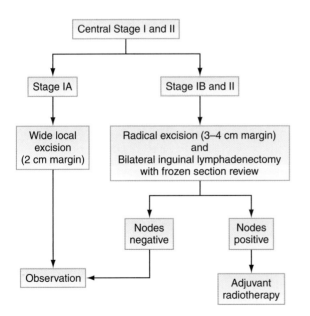

Note: Separate vulvar and inguinal incisions may limit morbidity
      from wound breakdown.

Figure 35-2. Treatment of central early stage vulvar cancer.

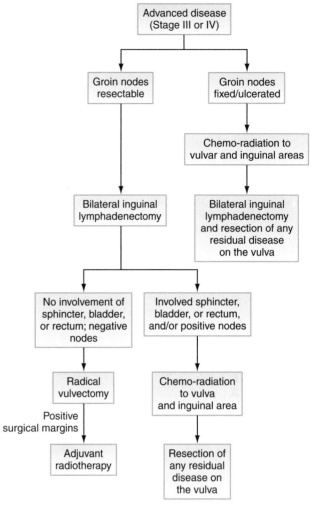

Figure 35-3. Treatment of advanced vulvar cancer.

- Biopsy, rule out underlying invasive adenocarcinoma
- Treatment: wide excision, recurrences frequent
  regardless of margin status
- Underlying invasive adenocarcinoma: treat as other
  invasive vulvar cancers
- Concurrent malignancies: breast, colon up to 25%
- Vulvar melanoma
  - Most common on labia minora and clitoris
  - Staging for depth of invasion (Clark, Breslow)
- Invasive vulvar cancer: melanoma
  - Lymph node metastases risk increases with lesion
    thickness
  - Role of lymphadenectomy for prognosis, not
    therapeutic

SUGGESTED READINGS

VAIN

De Vuyst H, Clifford GM, Nascimento MC, et al: Prevalence and type
  distribution of human papillomavirus in carcinoma and intraepithelial
  neoplasia of the vulva, vagina and anus: a meta-analysis, *Int J Cancer*
  124(7):1626–1636, 2009.
Matsuo K, Chi DS, Walker LD, et al: Ultrasonic surgical aspiration for vaginal
  intraepithelial neoplasia, *Int J Gynaecol Obstet* 105(1):71–73, 2009.
Smith JS, Backes DM, Hoots BE, et al: Human papillomavirus type-
  distribution in vulvar and vaginal cancers and their associated precursors,
  Obstet Gynecol 113(4):917–924, 2009.

VIN

van Seters M, van Beurden M, ten Kate FJW, et al: Treatment of vulvar intraepithelial neoplasia with topical imiquimod, *N Engl J Med* 358(14): 1465–1473, 2008.

Invasive Cancer of the Vagina

Dalrymple JL, Russell AH, Lee SW, et al: Chemoradiation for primary invasive squamous carcinoma of the vagina, *Int J Gynecol Cancer* 14(1):110–117, 2004.

De Crevoisier R, Sanfilippo N, Gerbaulet A, et al: Exclusive radiotherapy for primary squamous cell carcinoma of the vagina, *Radiother Oncol* 85(3):362–370, 2007.

Ferreira M, Crespo M, Martins L, Felix A: HPV DNA detection and genotyping in 21 cases of primary invasive squamous cell carcinoma of the vagina, *Mod Pathol* 21(8):968–972, 2008.

Frank SJ, Jhingran A, Levenback C, Eifel PJ: Definitive radiation therapy for squamous cell carcinoma of the vagina, *Int J Radiat Oncol Biol Phys* 62(1):138–147, 2005.

Nashiro T, Yagi C, Hirakawa M, et al: Concurrent chemoradiation for locally advanced squamous cell carcinoma of the vagina: case series and literature review, *Int J Clin Oncol* 13(4):335–339, 2008.

Sinha B, Stehman F, Schilder J, et al: Indiana University experience in the management of vaginal cancer, *Int J Gynecol Cancer* 19(4):686–693, 2009.

Smith JS, Backes DM, Hoots BE, et al: Human papillomavirus type-distribution in vulvar and vaginal cancers and their associated precursors, *Obstet Gynecol* 113(4):917–924, 2009.

Invasive Cancer of the Vulva

Berman ML, Soper JT, Creasman WT, et al: Conservative surgical management of superficially invasive stage I vulvar carcinoma, *Gynecol Oncol* 35(3):352–357, 1989.

De Vuyst H, Clifford GM, Nascimento MC, et al: Prevalence and type distribution of human papillomavirus in carcinoma and intraepithelial neoplasia of the vulva, vagina and anus: a meta-analysis, *Int J Cancer* 124(7):1626–1636, 2009.

Di Saia PJ, Creasman WT, Rich WM: An alternate approach to early cancer of the vulva, *Am J Obstet Gynecol* 133(7):825–832, 1979.

Edge SB, Byrd DR, Compton CC, et al: *AJCC [American Joint Committee on Cancer] cancer staging manual*, ed 7, New York, 2010, Springer.

Hampl M, Sarajuuri H, Wentzensen N, et al: Effect of human papillomavirus vaccines on vulvar, vaginal, and anal intraepithelial lesions and vulvar cancer, *Obstet Gynecol* 108(6):1361–1368, 2006.

Kumar S, Shah JP, Bryant CS, et al: A comparison of younger vs older women with vulvar cancer in the United States, *Am J Obstet Gynecol* 200(5):e52–e55, 2009.

Lanneau GS, Argenta PA, Lanneau MS, et al: Vulvar cancer in young women: demographic features and outcome evaluation, *Am J Obstet Gynecol* 200(6):645.e1–e5, 2009.

Levenback CF, van der Zee AGJ, Rob L, et al: Sentinel lymph node biopsy in patients with gynecologic cancers expert panel statement from the International Sentinel Node Society Meeting, February 21, 2008, *Gynecol Oncol* 114(2):151–156, 2009.

Radziszewski J, Kowalewska M, Jedrzejczak T, et al: The accuracy of the sentinel lymph node concept in early stage squamous cell vulvar carcinoma, *Gynecol Oncol* 116(3):473–477, 2010.

Smith JS, Backes DM, Hoots BE, et al: Human papillomavirus type-distribution in vulvar and vaginal cancers and their associated precursors, *Obstet Gynecol* 113(4):917–924, 2009.

Stehman FB, Ali S, Di Saia PJ: Node count and groin recurrence in early vulvar cancer: a Gynecologic Oncology Group study, *Gynecol Oncol* 113(1):52–56, 2009.

Stehman FB, Bundy BN, Dvoretsky PM, Creasman WT: Early stage I carcinoma of the vulva treated with ipsilateral superficial inguinal lymphadenectomy and modified radical hemivulvectomy: a prospective study of the Gynecologic Oncology Group, *Obstet Gynecol* 79(4):490–497, 1992.

The new FIGO staging system for cancers of the vulva, cervix, endometrium and sarcomas, *Gynecol Oncol* 115:325–328, 2009.

Van der Zee AG, Oonk MH, De Hullu JA, et al: Sentinel node dissection is safe in the treatment of early-stage vulvar cancer, *J Clin Oncol* 26(6):884–889, 2008.

Chapter 36

Management of Diseases of the Cervix

KRISHNANSU S. TEWARI • BRADLEY J. MONK

KEY UPDATES

1 Persistent oncogenic (high risk = HR) human papilloma virus (HPV) infection significantly increases the risk of high-grade cervical intraepithelial neoplasia (CIN).

2 Molecular screening with HR HPV testing is more sensitive than cytology screening (Pap). Two Food and Drug Administration (FDA)–approved HR HPV tests are available.

3 HPV genotyping is available in the triage of women with normal Paps with HR HPV.

4 Liquid cytology screening is not more sensitive than conventional cytology and does not reduce the numbers of unsatisfactory Pap tests.

5 The American Society of Colposcopy and Cervical Pathology updated its guidelines for cervical cancer screening in 2006.

6 The American College of Obstetricians and Gynecologists (ACOG) updated its guidelines for cervical cancer screening in 2009.

7 HPV vaccination prevents persistent HPV infection, CIN, vaginal intraepithelial neoplasm (VAIN), and vulvar intraepithelial neoplasm (VIN). It is indicated in young boys and girls. Two FDA-approved vaccines are available.

8 The Federation of Gynecology and Obstetrics (FIGO) staging system has been updated and IIA2 has been added as a new stage.

9 Positron emission tomography (PET) scanning is more sensitive than magnetic resonance imaging (MRI) or computed tomography (CT) in evaluating the metastatic spread of cervical cancer.

10 Fertility-sparing surgical options (cone and trachelectomy) are available for young women with adenocarcinoma in situ (AIS) and early (stage IB1) cervical cancers.

11 Minimally invasive surgery (laparoscopy and robotic) is feasible.

12 Postradical hysterectomy radiation therapy (RT) or chemo-RT is indicated for high-risk cervical factors and nodal metastases, respectively.

13 Concomitant chemotherapy and pelvic radiation (RT) (external and brachytherapy) is still the standard therapy for locally advanced cervical cancers (stage IB2-IVA).

14 Pelvic exenteration remains an option in treating isolated central recurrences in the pelvis after RT.

15 "Other platinum doublets" are not superior to cisplatin and paclitaxel in treating metastatic cervical cancer.

16 Anti-angiogenesis agents are active in treating metastatic cervical cancer and are being studied in phase III clinical trials.

Cervical Intraepithelial Neoplasia (CIN)

CLINICAL PROFILE

- In the absence of invasion, CIN is almost always asymptomatic; occasionally it is associated with postcoital bleeding
- According to a 1997-2002 Kaiser Permanente Northwest (Portland, Oregon) study, the annual incidence of CIN 1 was 1.2 per 1000 with a rate of 1.5 per 1000 for CIN 2-3; CIN 1 incidence peaked among women aged 20 to 24 years

(5.1 per 1000), with CIN 2-3 rates highest among those 25 to 29 years (8.1 per 1000)

- The evidence implicating specific human papillomavirus (HPV) types in the etiology of cervical cancer is now strong enough to establish a causative role
- Exposure to HPV is an extremely common event, especially in young sexually active women
- The top two HPV types contributing to cervical disease are CIN 1 (HPV 16/66; 15.3%), CIN 2-3 (HPV 16/31; 61.9%), and cervical cancer (HPV 16/18; 79.2%)

- The long time lag between initial HPV infection and eventual malignant conversion suggests that other events are necessary for such conversion and that spontaneous regression of many primary lesions is very common
- Potential cofactors include cigarette smoking, hormonal effects of oral contraceptives and pregnancy, dietary deficiencies, immunosuppression, and chronic inflammation

UPDATE #1
Persistent oncogenic (high risk = HR) HPV infection significantly increases the risk of high-grade cervical intraepithelial neoplasia (CIN) (Insigna et al, 2008).

DIAGNOSIS

- Biopsy of all grossly visualized lesions and colposcopically directed biopsies during evaluation of abnormal Pap or HR HPV test; biopsy with alligator-jaw forceps and endocervical curettage
- Multifocal lesions common
- Infections with multiple HPV types common

SCREENING

- In one analysis, compared with cytology, primary screening with HPV DNA testing followed by cytologic triage and repeat HPV DNA testing of HPV DNA-positive women with normal cytology appears to increase the CIN3+ sensitivity by approximately 30%, maintains a high PPV (relative PPV = 0.87), and results in a mere 12% increase in the number of screening tests
  - "Primary HPV DNA-based screening with cytology triage and repeat HPV DNA testing of cytology-negative women appears to be the most feasible cervical screening strategy"(Naucler et al, 2009)

UPDATE #2
Molecular screening with HR HPV testing is more sensitive than cytology screening (Pap). Two FDA-approved HR HPV tests are available (Naucler et al, 2009).

- HPV is a small, eight kilobases, double-stranded DNA virus and encodes a maximum of eight genes, six of which encode nonstructural or early proteins E1, E2, E4, E5, E6, and E7 and two of which encode structural or late proteins L1 and L2
  - E6 protein binds to and promotes degradation of the tumor suppressor protein, p53, whereas E7 protein complexes and inactivates the Rb protein; together, they disrupt cell cycle regulation during cervical cancer carcinogenesis; p53 and Rb are commonly mutated in other human cancers; E2 disruption caused by the integration of HR HPV into the cellular genome may induce overexpression of E6 and E7
- Digene HPV Test
  - Nucleic acid hybridization assay with signal amplification using microplate chemiluminescence
  - Types 16, 18, 31, 33, 35, 39, 45, 51, 52, 56, 58, 59, and 68
  - Indications (approvals 1999 [ASC-US]; 2003 [screening])
    - To screen patients with atypical squamous cells of undetermined significance (ASC-US) Pap smear results to determine the need for referral to colposcopy

- In women 30 years and older with Pap to adjunctively screen to assess the presence or absence of high-risk HPV types; this information—together with the physician's assessment of cytology history, other risk factors, and professional guidelines—may be used to guide patient management
- Cervista HPV HR Test
  - Signal amplification method (Invader chemistry) for detection of specific nucleic acid sequences; this method uses two types of isothermal reactions: a primary reaction that occurs on the targeted DNA sequence and a secondary reaction that produces a fluorescent signal
  - Types 16, 18, 31, 33, 35, 39, 45, 51, 52, 56, 58, 59, 66, and 68
  - Identical indication to Digene HPV test (approved 2009 [ASC-US and screening])

UPDATE #3
HPV genotyping is available in the triage of women with normal Paps with HR HPV (Smith et al, 2010).

- If positive for HPV 16 or 18 DNA when the Pap is normal, proceed to immediate colposcopy (www.asccp.org/pdfs/consensus/hpv_genotyping_20090320.pdf)

UPDATE #4
Liquid cytology screening is *not* more sensitive than conventional cytology and does not reduce the numbers of unsatisfactory Pap tests (Arbyn et al, 2008).

UPDATE #5
The American Society of Colposcopy and Cervical Pathology updated its guidelines for cervical cancer screening in 2006 (Wright et al, 2007).

- To provide revised evidence-based consensus guidelines for managing women with abnormal cervical cancer screening test results; a group of 146 experts, including representatives from 29 professional organizations, federal agencies, and national and international health organizations, met in Bethesda, Maryland, September 18-19, 2006, to develop the guidelines (www.asccp.org/consensus.shtml)

UPDATE #6
The American College of Obstetricians and Gynecologists (ACOG) updated its guidelines for cervical cancer screening in 2009 (ACOG Committee on Practice Bulletins—Gynecology, 2009).

- Both liquid-based and conventional methods of cervical cytology screening are acceptable
- The Bethesda System is the most widely used system in the United States
- Cervical cancer screening should begin at age 21 years regardless of the age of onset of sexual intercourse (level A)
- Cervical cytology screening is recommended every 2 years for women aged 21 to 29 years, with either conventional or liquid-based cytology

- "Because HPV DNA testing is more sensitive than cervical cytology in detecting CIN 2 and CIN 3, women with negative concurrent test results can be reassured that their risk of unidentified CIN 2 and CIN 3 or cervical cancer is approximately 1 in 1,000" (level A) (Naucler et al, 2009)
- Women with any of the following risk factors may require more frequent cervical cytology screening:
  - Infected with HIV
  - Immunosuppressed
  - DES in utero exposure
  - Prior CIN 2-3 or cancer
- Any attempt at setting an upper age for screening must take into consideration a woman's past screening history
  - After three consecutive negative cervical cytology screening tests in the prior decade: ACOG—age 65 to 70 (level B)
    - American Cancer Society: age 70
    - U.S. Preventive Services Task Force: age 65
- In women who have had a total hysterectomy for benign indications and have no prior history of high-grade CIN, routine cytology testing should be discontinued

VACCINATION

- GARDASIL
  - A vaccine (three doses in 6 months) indicated in girls and women 9 through 26 years of age for the prevention of cervical, vulvar, and vaginal cancers; precancerous or dysplastic lesions; and genital warts caused by human papillomavirus (HPV) types 6, 11, 16, and 18
  - Indicated in boys and men 9 through 26 years of age for the prevention of genital warts caused by HPV types 6 and 11
- CERVARIX
  - A vaccine (three doses in 6 months) indicated for the prevention of the following diseases caused by oncogenic human papillomavirus (HPV) types 16 and 18: cervical cancer, cervical intraepithelial neoplasia (CIN) grade 2 or worse and adenocarcinoma in situ, and cervical intraepithelial neoplasia (CIN) grade 1
  - Approved for use in females 10 through 25 years of age

UPDATE #7

HPV vaccination prevents persistent HPV infection, CIN, VAIN, and VIN. It is indicated in young boys and girls. Two FDA-approved vaccines are available (Advisory Committee on Immunization Practices [ACIP], 2011).

MANAGEMENT

- Local excision (large loop excision of the transformation zone [LLETZ] or cold knife cone): preferred for high-grade lesions
- Ablation (CO_2 laser or cryotherapy)
- Observation in teenagers and pregnancy is acceptable

Invasive Cervical Cancer

DIFFERENTIAL DIAGNOSIS

- Biopsy all cervical lesions to establish diagnosis
- Cell types: the majority (70%) of cervical cancers are squamous cell carcinomas, whereas the next most common type of cervical cancer is cervical adenocarcinoma (25%); adenocarcinomas consist of all epithelial types

of carcinomas with glandular differentiation, including adenosquamous tumors; HPV 18 is more common in glandular cancers (40% to 60%)

CLINICAL PROFILE OF INVASIVE CERVICAL CANCER

- Oncogenic (HR) HPV infection is a necessary cause (99.7%) of cervical cancer; worldwide, approximately 70% of all cervical cancer cases are attributable to types 16 and 18; the next two most prevalent oncogenic types are 45 and 31, which together account for an additional 10% of all cervical cancer cases
- Spreads locally into the surrounding tissues (vagina, uterine corpus, parametrium, bladder, and rectum) and metastasizes into the lymphatics (pelvic then aortic); hematogenous spread less common
- Most common symptom is bleeding although pain as well as intestinal or urinary symptoms can be associated with advanced disease
- Most lesions are exophytic; a second type of cervical carcinoma is created by an infiltrating tumor that tends to show little visible ulceration or exophytic mass but is initially seen as a stone-hard cervix; a third category of lesion is the ulcerative tumor, which usually erodes a portion of the cervix

DIAGNOSIS AND STAGING OF INVASIVE DISEASE

- Diagnosis: biopsy of all gross lesions, colposcopy with 5% acetic acid helpful

UPDATE #8

The FIGO staging system has been updated and IIA2 has been added as a new stage (FIGO Committee on Gynecologic Oncology, 2009) (Table 36-1.)

UPDATE #9

PET scanning is more sensitive than MRI or CT in evaluating the metastatic spread of cervical cancer (Choi et al, 2010).

MANAGEMENT OF INVASIVE CERVICAL CANCER

1. Minimally invasive disease (stage IA1) (Figure 36-1)

UPDATE #10

Fertility-sparing surgical options (cone and trachelectomy) are available for young women with adenocarcinoma in situ (AIS) and early (stage IB1) cervical cancers (Tewari et al, 2012).

2. Early-stage disease (stage IA2-IB1) (see Figure 36-1)

UPDATE #11

Minimally invasive surgery (laparoscopy and robotic) is feasible (Tewari et al, 2012).

UPDATE #12

Postradical hysterectomy RT or chemo-RT is indicated for high-risk cervical factors and nodal metastases, respectively (Tewari et al, 2012) (Figure 36-2).

TABLE 36-1 **International Federation of Gynecology and Obstetrics Clinical Staging System for Cervical Cancer**

Stage I	The carcinoma is strictly confined to the cervix (extension to the corpus would be disregarded)
IA	Invasive carcinoma, which can be diagnosed only by microscopy, with deepest invasion ≤ 5 mm and largest extension ≥7 mm
IA1	Measured stromal invasion of ≤ 3 mm in depth and extension of ≤ 7 mm
IA2	Measured stromal invasion of >3 mm and not >5 mm with an extension of not >7 mm
IB	Clinically visible lesions limited to the cervix uteri or preclinical cancers greater than stage IA*
IB1	Clinically visible lesion ≤ 4 cm in greatest dimension
IB2	Clinically visible lesion >4 cm in greatest dimension
Stage II	Cervical carcinoma invades beyond the uterus, but not the pelvic wall or to the lower third of the vagina
IIA	Without parametrial invasion
IIA1	Clinically visible lesion ≤ 4 cm in greatest dimension
IIA2	Clinically visible lesion >4 cm in greatest dimension
IIB	With obvious parametrial invasion
Stage III	The tumor extends to the pelvic wall or involves lower third of the vagina or causes hydronephrosis or nonfunctioning kidney†
Stage IIIA	Tumor involves lower third of the vagina, with no extension to the pelvic wall
Stage IIIB	Extension to the pelvic wall or hydronephrosis or nonfunctioning kidney
Stage IV	The carcinoma has extended beyond the true pelvis or has involved (biopsy proven) the mucosa of the bladder or rectum; a bullous edema, as such, does not permit a case to be allotted to stage IV
IVA	Spread of the growth to adjacent organs
IVB	Spread to distant organs

*All macroscopically visible lesions—even with superficial invasion—are allotted to stage IB carcinomas. Invasion is limited to a measured stromal invasion with a maximal depth of 5 mm and a horizontal extension of not >7 mm. Depth of invasion should not be >5 mm taken from the base of the epithelium of the original tissue—superficial or glandular. The depth of invasion should always be reported in mm, even in those cases with "early (minimal) stromal invasion" (~1 mm).
The involvement of vascular/lymphatic spaces should not change the stage allotment.
†On rectal examination, there is no cancer-free space between the tumor and the pelvic wall. All cases with hydronephrosis or a nonfunctioning kidney are included, unless they are known to be due to another cause.
From Current FIGO staging for cancer of the vagina, fallopian tube, ovary, and gestational trophoblastic neoplasia: FIGO Committee on Gynecologic Oncology, *Int J Gynaecol Obstet* 105(1):3-4, 2009.

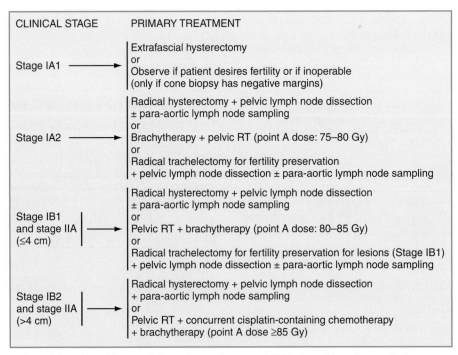

Figure 36-1. Algorithm outlining primary therapy of FIGO stage I invasive cervical cancer.

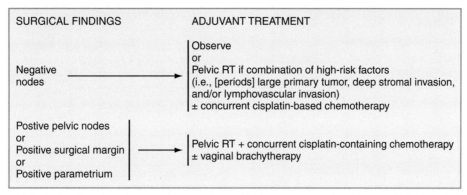

Figure 36-2. Indications for adjuvant therapy after radical hysterectomy based on pathologic risk factors.

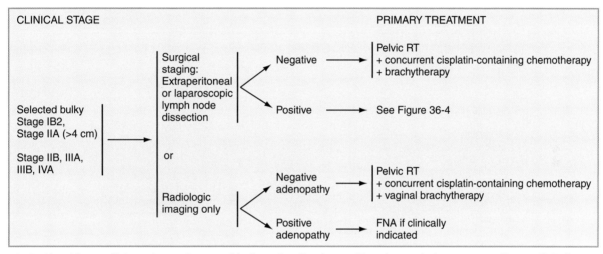

Figure 36-3. Algorithm outlining primary therapy of bulky or locally advanced invasive cervical cancer according to clinical FIGO stage.

3. Locally advanced disease (stage IB2-IVA) (Figures 36-3 and 36-4)

UPDATE #13

Concomitant chemotherapy and pelvic radiation (RT) (external and brachytherapy) is still the standard therapy for locally advanced cervical cancers (stage IB2-IVA) (Monk et al, 2007).

4. Isolated central pelvic recurrent disease after radiotherapy

UPDATE #14

Pelvic exenteration remains an option in treating isolated central recurrences in the pelvis after RT (Tewari et al, 2012).

5. Metastatic disease (stage IVB and recurrent) (Figure 36-5)
6. Metastatic disease (stage IVB and recurrent) (Figure 36-6)

UPDATE #15

"Other platinum doublets" are not superior to cisplatin and paclitaxel in treating metastatic cervical cancer (Monk et al, 2009).

UPDATE #16

Anti-angiogenesis agents are active in treating metastatic cervical cancer and are being studied in phase III clinical trials (Tewari et al, 2009).

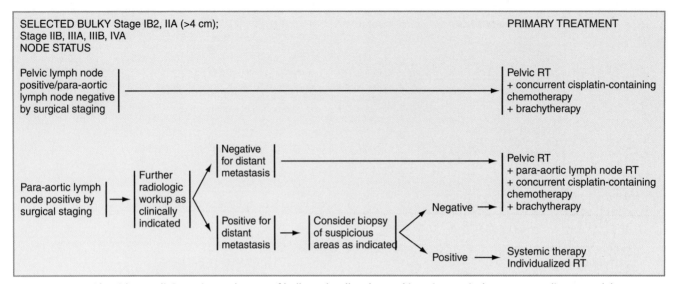

Figure 36-4. Algorithm outlining primary therapy of bulky or locally advanced invasive cervical cancer according to nodal status.

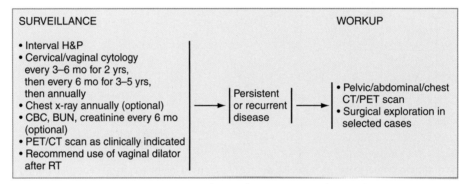

Figure 36-5. Posttreatment surveillance after treatment of cervical carcinoma.

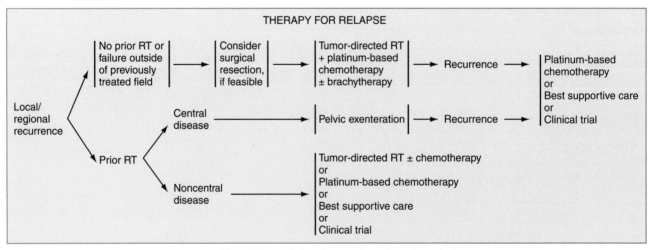

Figure 36-6. Algorithm outlining therapy for relapsed cervical cancer.

SUGGESTED READINGS

CIN

Clinical Profile

Insinga RP, Glass AG, Rush BB: Diagnoses and outcomes in cervical cancer screening: a population-based study, *Am J Obstet Gynecol* 191(1):105–113, 2004.

Insinga RP, Liaw KL, Johnson LG, Madeleine MM: A systematic review of the prevalence and attribution of human papillomavirus types among cervical, vaginal, and vulvar precancers and cancers in the United States, *Cancer Epidemiol Biomarkers Prev* 17(7):1611–1622, 2008.

Diagnosis

Driggers RW, Zahn CM: To ECC or not to ECC: the question remains, *Obstet Gynecol Clin North Am* 35(4):583–597, 2008.

Kyrgiou M, Koliopoulos G, Martin-Hirsch P, et al: Management of minor cervical cytological abnormalities: a systematic review and a meta-analysis of the literature, *Cancer Treat Rev* 33(6):514–520, 2007.

Kyrgiou M, Tsoumpou I, Vrekoussis T, et al: The up-to-date evidence on colposcopy practice and treatment of cervical intraepithelial neoplasia: the Cochrane colposcopy & cervical cytopathology collaborative group (C5 group) approach, *Cancer Treat Rev* 32(7):516–523, 2006.

Screening

American College of Obstetricians and Gynecologists: ACOG practice bulletin: clinical management guidelines for obstetrician-gynecologists no. 61, April 2005: human papillomavirus, *Obstet Gynecol* 105(4):905–918, 2005.

American College of Obstetricians and Gynecologists Committee on Practice Bulletins—Gynecology: ACOG practice bulletin no. 109: cervical cytology screening, *Obstet Gynecol* 114(6):1409–1420, 2009.

Arbyn M, Bergeron C, Klinkhamer P, et al: Liquid compared with conventional cervical cytology: a systematic review and meta-analysis, *Obstet Gynecol* 111(1):167–177, 2008.

Davey E, Barratt A, Irwig L, et al: Effect of study design and quality on unsatisfactory rates, cytology classifications, and accuracy in liquid-based versus conventional cervical cytology: a systematic review, *Lancet* 367(9505):122–132, 2006.

Hologic: *Cervista HPV* (website). www.cervistahpv.com. Accessed October 9, 2011.

Naucler P, Ryd W, Törnberg S, et al: Efficacy of HPV DNA testing with cytology triage and/or repeat HPV DNA testing in primary cervical cancer screening, *J Natl Cancer Inst* 101(2):88–99, 2009.

Naucler P, Ryd W, Törnberg S, et al: Human papillomavirus and Papanicolaou tests to screen for cervical cancer, *N Engl J Med* 357(16):1589–1597, 2007.

Qiagen: *The digene HPV test* (website). www.thehpvtest.com. Accessed October 9, 2011.

Smith RA, Cokkinides V, Brooks D, et al: Cancer screening in the United States, 2010: a review of current American Cancer Society guidelines and issues in cancer screening, *CA Cancer J Clin* 60(2):99–119, 2010.

U.S. Preventive Services Task Force: *Screening for cervical cancer* (website). www.ahrq.gov/clinic/3rduspstf/cervcan/cervcanrr.htm. Accessed October 9, 2011.

Vaccination

Advisory Committee on Immunization Practices (ACIP): *Summary report October 21-22, 2009 Atlanta, Georgia* (website). www.cdc.gov/vaccines/recs/acip/downloads/min-oct09.pdf. Accessed October 9, 2011.

Centers for Disease Control and Prevention (CDC): National vaccination coverage among adolescents aged 13-17 years—United States, 2006, *MMWR Morb Mortal Wkly Rep* 6(34):885–888, 2007.

Centers for Disease Control and Prevention (CDC): STD-prevention counseling practices and human papillomavirus opinions among clinicians with adolescent patients—United States, 2004, *MMWR Morb Mortal Wkly Rep* 55(41):1118–1120, 2006.

Centers for Disease Control and Prevention (CDC): Syncope after vaccination—United States, January 2005-July 2007, *MMWR Morb Mortal Wkly Rep* 57(17):457–460, 2008.

GlaxoSmithKline: *[Cervarix] highlights of prescribing information* (website). us.gsk.com/products/assets/us_cervarix.pdf. Accessed October 9, 2011.

Merck & Co: *Gardasil prescribing information* (website). www.gardasil.com/prescribe-gardasil/index.html. Accessed October 9, 2011.

Management

Wright TC Jr, Massad LS, Dunton CJ, et al: 2006 consensus guidelines for the management of women with abnormal cervical cancer screening tests, *Am J Obstet Gynecol* 197(4):346–355, 2007.

Wright TC Jr, Massad LS, Dunton CJ, et al: 2006 consensus guidelines for the management of women with cervical intraepithelial neoplasia or adenocarcinoma in situ, *Am J Obstet Gynecol* 197(4):340–345, 2007.

Invasive Disease

Differential Diagnosis and Clinical Profile

Tewari KS, Monk BJ: Invasive cervical cancer. In Di Saia PJ, Creasman WT, editors: *Clinical gynecologic oncology*, ed 8, Philadelphia, 2012, Mosby, pp 51–119.

Diagnosis and Staging

Choi HJ, Ju W, Myung SK, Kim Y: Diagnostic performance of computer tomography, magnetic resonance imaging, and positron emission tomography or positron emission tomography/computed tomography for detection of metastatic lymph nodes in patients with cervical cancer: meta-analysis, *Cancer Sci* 101(6):1471–1479, Jun 2010.

FIGO Committee on Gynecologic Oncology: Current FIGO staging for cancer of the vagina, fallopian tube, ovary, and gestational trophoblastic neoplasia, *Int J Gynaecol Obstet* 105(1):3–4, Apr 2009.

Management

Monk BJ, Sill MW, McMeekin DS, et al: Phase III trial of four cisplatin-containing doublet combinations in stage IVB, recurrent, or persistent cervical carcinoma: a Gynecologic Oncology Group study, *J Clin Oncol* 27(28):4649–4655, 2009.

Monk BJ, Tewari KS, Koh WJ: Multimodality therapy for locally advanced cervical carcinoma: state of the art and future directions, *J Clin Oncol* 25(20):2952–2965, 2007.

National Comprehensive Cancer Network (NCCN): *National comprehensive cancer network* (website). www.nccn.org/index.asp. Accessed October 9, 2011.

Tewari KS, Monk BJ: Recent achievements and future developments in advanced and recurrent cervical cancer: trials of the Gynecologic Oncology Group, *Semin Oncol* 36(2):170–180, 2009.

Willmott LJ, Monk BJ: Cervical cancer therapy: current, future and anti-angiogenesis targeted treatment, *Expert Rev Anticancer Ther* 9(7):895–903, 2009.

Chapter 37

Management of Diseases of the Uterus and Endometrium

KATHERINE CYNTHIA FUH • JOHN K. CHAN

KEY UPDATES

1. Novel medical and surgical therapies are under development in the treatment of symptomatic fibroids.

2. The pathologic diagnosis of atypical endometrial hyperplasia has poor reproducibility, and improved diagnostic criteria are needed.

3. Levonorgestrel containing intrauterine contraception and oral progestins therapy can be an alternative to hysterectomy to treat endometrial hyperplasia.

4. The International Federation of Obstetrics and Gynecology (FIGO) staging system of endometrial cancer was updated in 2009.

5. An increase in the number of deaths from corpus cancer over years may be associated with an increased proportion of advanced-stage cancers and high-risk histologies.

6. Uterine papillary serous and clear cell carcinomas have a worse outcome compared to endometrioid cell type.

7. A large prospective randomized trial revealed that laparoscopic surgical staging is a feasible and safe alternative to abdominal hysterectomy with fewer complications and shorter hospital stay without compromising survival.

8. Retrospective series have shown that robotic surgery is also a feasible alternative to abdominal hysterectomy.

9. Prospective trials from Europe have shown that lymphadenectomy did not improve disease-free or overall survival in early-stage endometrial cancer. However, lymphadenectomy remains the most accurate manner to identify those with nodal metastases to guide adjuvant treatment.

10. In early-stage, intermediate-risk endometrial cancer, vaginal brachytherapy is comparable to external beam pelvic radiotherapy to decrease vaginal recurrence.

11. In advanced-stage disease, chemotherapy is superior to whole abdominal irradiation.

12. In advanced cancers, the addition of paclitaxel to doxorubicin and cisplatin improved the survival compared to doxorubicin and cisplatin.

13. Treatment of advanced leiomyosarcoma with fixed-dose gemcitabine plus docetaxel yielded high response rates.

14. Carcinosarcomas are now classified as carcinomas rather than sarcomas or mixed Müllerian mesodermal tumors.

15. In those with measurable stage III or IV, persistent, or recurrent carcinosarcoma, ifosfamide plus paclitaxel improved the outcomes of those with ifosfamide alone.

16. Estrogen replacement therapy after surgery for stage I and II endometrial cancer leads to an overall low risk for recurrence (2.1%).

17. Although ovarian preservation in premenopausal, early-stage, low-grade disease was not associated with a worsened outcome in large population-based series, smaller series have shown that a significant proportion of young women with endometrial cancer have coexisting ovarian tumors.

18. In patients younger than 50 years of age with endometrial cancer, 9% were found to carry a germline Lynch syndrome–associated mutation.

Uterine Leiomyomas

CLINICAL PROFILE

- An estimated 70% of Caucasian and 80% of African American women have leiomyomas
- Most patients present with increased uterine bleeding, pelvic pressure and pain, or reproductive dysfunction
- Good maternal and neonatal outcomes are expected in pregnancies with uterine fibroids (Klatsky et al, 2008[*])
  - Submucosal fibroids associated with lower pregnancy rates primarily are the result of decreased implantation
  - Intramural fibroids are associated with more miscarriages (20.4% versus 2.9%) and slightly lower cumulative pregnancy rates (36.9% versus 41.1%)
  - Leiomyomas during pregnancy increase the risk of malpresentation, cesarean delivery, and preterm delivery (Table 37-1)

DIAGNOSIS

- Most patients have a physical finding of an enlarged, mobile uterus
- Routine radiologic assessment is not required and does not improve outcome but confirms the presence of a leiomyoma versus an adnexal mass
- Transvaginal ultrasound has a high sensitivity and specificity (99% and 91%) of detecting leiomyomas in uteri less than 10 weeks in size (Dueholm et al, 2002)
- Magnetic resonance imaging (MRI) also has a high sensitivity and specificity (99% and 86%) of detecting leiomyomas; MRI is better at detecting multiple and larger leiomyomas (Dueholm et al, 2002)

MANAGEMENT

UPDATE #1

Novel medical and surgical therapies are under development in the treatment of symptomatic fibroids (American College of Obstetricians and Gynecologists [ACOG], Practice Bulletin No. 96, 2008; Fiscella et al, 2006; Goodwin et al, 2008; Hindley et al, 2004).

- Two most common symptoms for which women seek treatment for leiomyomas are abnormal uterine bleeding (usually heavy or prolonged menstrual bleeding leading to iron deficiency anemia) and pelvic pressure (American College of Obstetricians and Gynecologists, Practice Bulletin No. 96, 2008[*])
- Medical treatment (American College of Obstetricians and Gynecologists, Practice Bulletin No. 96, 2008)
  - Contraceptive steroids (estrogen and progestin or progestin alone) are often first-line therapy and used to achieve short-term relief; crossover rate to surgical therapies is high
  - Gonadotropin releasing hormone (GnRH) agonists can decrease volume of leiomyomas by 35% to 65% within 3 months of treatment but will recur within several months after cessation of treatment; if treatment is continued for more than 6 months, add-back therapy should be considered to minimize bone loss and vasomotor symptoms (Olive, 2004)

- Sequential regimen gives maximal results: GnRH agonist is first used to achieve down-regulation, then add contraceptive steroids after 1 to 3 months of therapy
  - Low-dose preparations (equivalent to menopausal hormonal therapy) have been studied as add-back therapy during GnRH therapy
  - However, the addition of progestin add-back therapy resulted in an increase in mean uterine volume up to 95% of baseline within 24 months (Friedman et al, 1993)
- Aromatase inhibitors block ovarian and peripheral estrogen production and decrease estradiol after 1 day of treatment; small studies have shown a reduction in leiomyoma size and symptoms, although not approved by the Food and Drug Administration (FDA) (Attilakos et al, 2005; Shozu et al, 2003; Varelas et al, 2007)
- Progesterone modulators act at the level of the progesterone receptors found in high concentration in leiomyomatous uteri
  - Mifepristone is the most extensively studied (Fiscella et al, 2006[*])
    - Recent randomized controlled trial with mifepristone 5 mg daily for 26 weeks versus placebo showed an improvement in quality of life and activities, energy and fatigue, and sexual functioning
    - Anemia was decreased after 6 months of treatment in the treatment group by 9% versus 60% of controls
    - Reduction of uterine size by 47% in the treatment group
    - Amenorrhea is 41% in treated women by the sixth month
- Uterine artery embolization (UAE)
  - Embolization occurs via transcutaneous femoral artery approach resulting in leiomyoma devascularization and involution; uterine arteries are embolized using polyvinyl alcohol particles of trisacryl gelatin microspheres
- Uterine Artery Embolization in the Treatment of Symptomatic Uterine Fibroid Tumors (EMMY) randomized trial compared UAE to total abdominal hysterectomy (TAH) (Hehenkamp et al, 2005, 2006)
  - UAE: less pain during the first 24 hours postoperatively and returned to work sooner; overall complication rate of 5%
  - TAH: fewer minor complications such as vaginal discharge, leiomyoma expulsion, and hematoma; lower readmission rate (0% versus 11%); overall complication rate of 2.7%
  - Fibroid Registry for Outcomes Data (FIBROID) assessed the long-term outcomes of UAE with similar results as the EMMY trial (Goodwin et al, 2008[*])
  - Of 1278 women with follow-up, further surgical care was required: 2.82% for myomectomy, 9.79% for hysterectomy, 1.83% for repeat UAE
  - Symptoms of heavy bleeding, use of prior medication, and leiomyoma size and morphology normalized 3 years after the procedure
  - Symptoms of bulk and pain did not change from baseline to after treatment

---

[*]Denotes a maintenance of certification (MOC) article.

TABLE 37-1   Cumulative Obstetric Outcomes Associated with Fibroid Uterus

	Fibroids	No Fibroids	*P* value	Unadjusted OR (95% CI)
Cesarean	48.8%	13.3%	<0.001	3.7 (3.5-3.9)
Malpresentation	13.0%	4.5%	<0.001	2.9 (2.6-3.2)
Labor dystocia	7.5%	3.1%	<0.001	2.4 (2.1-2.7)
Postpartum hemorrhage	2.5%	1.4%	<0.001	1.8 (1.4-2.2)
Peripartum hysterectomy	3.3%	0.2%	<0.001	13.4 (9.3-19.3)
Retained placenta	1.4%	0.6%	0.001	2.3 (1.3-3.7)
Chorio or endometritis	8.7%	8.2%	0.63	1.06 (0.8-1.3)
IUGR	11.2%	8.6%	<0.001	1.4 (1.1-1.7)
Preterm labor	16.1%	8.7%	<0.001	1.9 (1.5-2.3)
Preterm delivery	16.0%	10.8%	<0.001	1.5 (1.3-1.7)
Placenta previa	1.4%	0.6%	<0.001	2.3 (1.7-3.1)
First-trimester bleeding	4.7%	7.6%	<0.001	0.6 (0.5-0.7)
Abruption	3.0%	0.9%	<0.001	3.2 (2.6-4.0)
PPROM	9.9%	13.0%	0.003	0.8 (0.6-0.9)
PPROM or PROM	6.2%	12.2%	<0.001	0.5 (0.4-0.6)

CI, confidence interval; IUGR, intrauterine growth rate; OR, odds ratio; PPROM, preterm premature rupture of membranes; PROM, premature rupture of membranes.
Modified from Klatsky, Tran, Caughey, et al. Fibroids and reproductive outcomes: a systematic literature review from conception to delivery. *Am J Ob Gyn* 198:357-366, 2008.)

- Factors associated with failure of UAE examined in a retrospective Canadian study (Huang et al, 2006*)
  - Total of 233 patients, 211 became asymptomatic after UAE; 22 others required surgical reintervention; overall failure rate of UAE is 9.4%, mainly due to persistent menorrhagia and abdominal pain
  - Concomitant findings of adenomyosis in 25% of hysterectomy specimens
- Magnetic resonance imaging-guided focused ultrasound surgery (American College of Obstetricians and Gynecologists, Practice Bulletin No. 96, 2008*)
  - In 2004, the FDA approved the use of MRI-guided system for localization and treatment with focused ultrasound therapy
  - Ultrasound energy penetrates soft tissue and produces well-defined regions of protein denaturation, irreversible cell damage, and coagulative necrosis
  - Outcomes of 109 patients undergoing MRI-guided focused ultrasound surgery were reported at 6 months and 12 months; modest reductions of uterine volume noted at 13.5% at 6 months and 9.4% at 12 months; 71% and 51% reported a reduction of symptoms at 6 months and 12 months, respectively (Hindley et al, 2004; Stewart et al, 2006)
  - Adverse events included heavy menses, requiring transfusion, persistent pain and bleeding, hospitalization for nausea, and leg, and buttock pain caused by sonification of the sciatic nerve, which eventually resolved (Fraser et al, 2007)

Endometrial Hyperplasia

CLINICAL PROFILE

- Peaks in the early 50s without atypia versus in the early 60s with atypia
- Diagnosis should be suspected with heavy, prolonged, frequent (less than 21 days), or irregular uterine bleeding, particularly in patients >35 years

DIAGNOSIS

- Endometrial biopsy
  - A meta-analysis of 39 studies including 7914 women assessed the accuracy of endometrial sampling devices in the detection of endometrial carcinoma and atypical hyperplasia; the results of endometrial sampling with findings at dilation and curettage (D&C), hysteroscopy, and hysterectomy were compared; the Pipelle was found to have detection rates for endometrial carcinoma of 99.6% and 91% for premenopausal and postmenopausal women, respectively; for detection of atypical hyperplasia, the Pipelle was the most sensitive technique at 81% (Dijkhuizen et al, 2000)
- Dilation and curettage
- Saline-infusion sonography endometrial sampling
  - In one retrospective study, saline-infusion sonography was found to be superior to endometrial biopsy in obtaining tissue for diagnosis in 89% of cases versus 52% of cases by endometrial biopsy; the positive predictive value of endometrial biopsy was 61% and the negative predictive value was 75%; for saline-infusion sonography, the positive predictive value was 80% and the negative predictive value was 74% (Moschos et al, 2009*)
  - Progression to endometrial cancer is 1% for simple hyperplasia without atypia, 3% for complex hyperplasia without atypia, 8% for simple hyperplasia with atypia, and 29% for complex hyperplasia with atypia (Kurman et al, 1985)

UPDATE #2

The pathologic diagnosis of atypical endometrial hyperplasia has poor reproducibility, and improved diagnostic criteria are needed (Trimble et al, 2006; Zaino et al, 2006).

- In Gynecologic Oncology Group (GOG) 167, only 38% of the diagnosis of atypical endometrial hyperplasia (AEH) from the referring institution was supported by the panel of GOG gynecologic pathologists (Zaino et al, 2006)
  - The prevalence of endometrial carcinoma in patients with a biopsy diagnosis of AEH was as high as 42.6% (Trimble et al, 2006)

MANAGEMENT

- Treatment depends more on the presence of atypia and menopausal status; simple or complex hyperplasia does not determine treatment as much as atypia

UPDATE #3

Levonorgestrel containing intrauterine contraception and oral progestins therapy can be an alternative to hysterectomy to treat endometrial hyperplasia (Ushijima et al, 2007; Wildemeersch et al, 2007).

- Progestins reverse endometrial hyperplasia by activation of progesterone receptors, which results in stromal decidualization and subsequent thinning of the endometrium; progestins also decreases estrogen and progesterone receptors and activate hydroxylase enzymes to convert estradiol to its less active metabolite estrone
- Response rate is highest in women without atypia and with therapy of 12 to 14 days per month
- In premenopausal patients without atypia: medroxyprogesterone acetate (MPA) at 10 mg daily for 12 to 14 days each month × 3 to 6 months; regression has been seen in 80% of treated patients; levonorgestrel containing intrauterine contraception (IUC) is also effective (Wildemeersch et al, 2007)
- In premenopausal patients with atypia: if atypia is found on initial endometrial biopsy, further evaluation with a dilation and curettage may be indicated given the high concurrent risk of carcinoma; if maintaining fertility is desired, use medroxyprogesterone acetate (Ushijima et al, 2007) or megestrol acetate at 80 mg twice daily; levonorgestrel containing IUC is also an effective option for treating hyperplasia in premenopausal women (Wildemeersch et al, 2007)
- In postmenopausal women without atypia: medroxy progesterone acetate at 10 mg daily for 3 months with follow-up endometrial biopsy after cessation of drug therapy
- In postmenopausal women with atypia: if hysterectomy is not an option, continuous oral megestrol acetate at 80 mg twice daily or levonorgestrel IUC (Wildmeersch et al, 2007)

Staging of Endometrial Cancer

UPDATE #4

The International Federation of Obstetrics and Gynecology (FIGO) staging system of endometrial cancer was updated in 2009.

MERGING OF STAGES IA AND IB

- Because of the overall favorable prognosis, tumor confined to the endometrium cannot be reliably distinguished from tumors invading the superficial endometrium

TABLE 37-2 2009 FIGO Staging for Carcinoma of the Endometrium

Stage I*	Tumor confined to the corpus uteri
IA*	No or less than half myometrial invasion
IB*	Invasion equal to or more than half of the myometrium
Stage II†	Tumor invades cervical stroma, but does not extend beyond the uterus
Stage III*	Local or regional spread of the tumor
IIIA*	Tumor invades the serosa of the corpus uteri or adnexae
IIIB*	Vaginal or parametrial involvement#
IIIC*	Metastases to pelvic or para-aortic lymph nodes#
IIIC1*	Positive pelvic nodes
IIIC2*	Positive para-aortic lymph nodes with or without positive pelvic lymph nodes
Stage IV*	Tumor invades bladder or bowel mucosa, or distant metastases
IVA*	Tumor invasion of bladder or bowel mucosa
IVB*	Distant metastases, including intra-abdominal metastases or inguinal lymph nodes

*Either G1, G2, or G3.
†Endocervical glandular involvement only should be considered as stage I, not stage II.
#Positive cytology has to be reported separately without changing the stage.
From FIGO Committee on Gynecologic Oncology: Revised FIGO staging for carcinoma of the vulva, cervix, and endometrium. *Int J Gynecol Obstet* 105:103-104, 2009.

- Merging of stage IIA with stage I disease
- Because the prognostic significance of cervical mucosa is not well defined, endocervical glandular involvement should be considered as stage I.

ELIMINATION OF POSITIVE CYTOLOGY FROM STAGING CRITERIA

- Because of the uncertain prognostic importance of isolated positive peritoneal cytology, positive cytology should be reported separately without influencing the stage
- There is a significant heterogeneity of prior International Federation of Gynecology and Obstetrics (FIGO) 2003 stage IIIA, which included peritoneal cytology with serosal or adnexal invasion that resulted in a range of overall survival (Slomovitz et al, 2005*)
- In fact, the 5-year overall survival for those with endometrioid histology with positive cytology, endometrioid with adnexal or serosal spread, nonendometrioid with positive cytology, and nonendometrioid with adnexal spread was 79%, 65%, 64%, and 13%, respectively

SUBDIVIDING STAGE IIIC INTO TWO DIFFERENT RISK CATEGORIES BASED ON THE LOCATION OF METASTATIC DISEASE

- Para-aortic lymph node metastasis is recognized as a predictor of poor outcome; in fact, the 5-year survival for those with pelvic node metastasis is significantly better (70% to 80%) than it is for those with positive para-aortic nodes (30% to 40%)

Trends in Uterine Cancer

UPDATE #5

The increase in the number of deaths from corpus cancer over years may be associated with an increased proportion of advanced-stage cancers and high-risk histologies (Ueda et al, 2008).

- From 1988 to 2001, there was an increase in grade 3 disease, serous histology, and sarcomas; these trends may partially explain the increase in the number of deaths from corpus cancer over years

Endometrial Cancer

CLINICAL PROFILE

- The most common presentation of endometrial cancer is abnormal uterine bleeding

UPDATE #6

Uterine papillary serous carcinoma (UPSC) and clear cell cancer of the uterus (CC) have a worse survival compared to grade 3 endometrioid uterine cancer (G3EC) (Hamilton et al, 2006).

- UPSC, CC, and G3EC patients represent 10%, 3%, and 15% of endometrial cancers; however, the 5-year disease-specific survival was 55%, 68%, and 77% of cancer deaths, respectively (Hamilton et al, 2006[*])
- To identify patients at risk for extrauterine recurrence, a retrospective study showed that depth of myometrial invasion predicted the risk of hematogenous recurrence; positive lymph nodes and cervical stromal invasion predicted the risk for lymphatic recurrence; stage IV disease or a combination of nonendometrioid histology, cervical stromal invasion, positive lymph nodes, and positive peritoneal cytology was predictive for peritoneal recurrence
- Using the preceding criteria, 35% of patients were predicted to have a risk for recurrence in one or more of the three sites; 46% of the patients predicted to have a risk for recurrence subsequently had recurrence in one or more of the three sites compared with 2% of patients not at risk for relapse (Mariani et al, 2004[*])

DIAGNOSIS

- Endometrial biopsy with Pipelle or dilation and curettage in women older than 35 years of age with anovulatory uterine bleeding to rule out endometrial hyperplasia or cancer based on ACOG guidelines

TREATMENT

- Surgical management of endometrial cancer

UPDATE #7

A large prospective randomized trial revealed that laparoscopic surgical staging is a feasible and safe alternative to abdominal hysterectomy with fewer complications and shorter hospital stay without compromising survival (Walker et al, 2009).

- Stage I to IIA uterine cancer assigned to laparoscopy (n = 1696) or open laparotomy (n = 920)
  - Main study end points were 6-week morbidity and mortality, hospital length of stay, and patient-reported quality of life outcomes
  - Laparoscopy had fewer moderate to severe postoperative adverse events than laparotomy (14% versus 21%, respectively, with longer operative time [204 versus 130 minutes])
  - Pelvic and para-aortic nodes were not removed in 8% of laparoscopy and 4% of laparotomy patients; no difference in overall detection of advanced stage disease (Walker et al, 2009)

UPDATE #8

Retrospective series have shown that robotic surgery is a feasible alternative to abdominal hysterectomy (Veljovich et al, 2008).

- Robotic surgery is feasible in gynecologic oncology with the advantage of three-dimensional high-definition optics, greater range of motion, and ergonomics over laparoscopic surgery
- In a retrospective series compared with open surgery, robotic surgery was longer (283 versus 139 minutes), had less blood loss (66.6 versus 197.6 ml), and had a shorter length of stay (40.3 versus 127 hours) with comparable number of nodes removed (17.5 versus 13.1) (Veljovich et al, 2008)
- In another retrospective study of 455 patients, the mean operative time was 170.5 minutes with a mean lymph node count of 15.5, and mean hospital stay was 1.8 days; intraoperative complications occurred in 6.7% and postoperative complications were reported in 14.6% with a 2% rate of conversion; fewer than 10 cases were required to achieve proficiency of the procedure (Lowe et al, 2009)

UPDATE #9

Prospective trials from Europe have shown that lymphadenectomy did not improve disease-free or overall survival in early-stage endometrial cancer. However, lymphadenectomy can accurately identify those with nodal metastases to guide adjuvant treatment (A Study in the Treatment of Endometrial Cancer trial [ASTEC], 2009; Benedetti Panici et al, 2008).

- Prior retrospective studies have demonstrated the survival advantage associated with lymphadenectomy in early-stage endometrial cancer (Chan et al, 2006; Cragun et al, 2005)
- Others showed that lymphadenectomy does not benefit patients with grades 1 and 2 endometrioid lesions with myometrial invasion ≤50% and primary tumor diameter ≤2 cm; nevertheless, 67% of patients with lymphatic dissemination had para-aortic metastases; in fact, some patients with intermediate or high-risk histologies have a significant rate of lymphatic metastasis above the inferior mesenteric artery (Mariani et al, 2008)
- Recently the results of the British randomized clinical trial (A Study in the Treatment of Endometrial Cancer trial [ASTEC]) and Italian CONSORT randomized clinical trial provided significant information on the role of therapeutic lymphadenectomy and adjuvant therapy

TABLE 37-3   Role of Lymphadenectomy with Intermediate-Risk or High-Risk Early-Stage Endometrial Cancer in Recurrence and Survival

Study	Study Arms	Percentage of Patients with Positive Lymph Nodes Detected with LN	Percentage of Patients with Positive Lymph Nodes without LN	Rate of Overall Recurrence	Five-Year DFS and Overall Survival
CONSORT Benedetti et al.	264 patients with LN 250 pts without LN	13.3%	3.2%	12.9% with LN 13.2% without LN	5-year DFS: 81% with LN 81.7% without LN Overall survival: 85.9% with LN 90% without LN
ASTEC Kitchner et al.	684 patients with LN 685 patients with standard surgery (without LN)	9%	1%	14% with LN 11% with standard surgery (without LN)	5-year DFS: 73% with LN 79% without LN Overall survival: 81% with LN 80% without LN

DFS, Disease-free survival; LN, lymphadenectomy.

- In the British ASTEC study of 1408 early-stage endometrial cancer patients, pelvic lymphadenectomy did not confer an overall or recurrence-free survival benefit; the 5-year recurrence-free survival was 79% in the standard surgery group versus 73% in the lymphadenectomy group; likewise, the 5-year overall survival was 81% in the standard surgery group and 80% in the lymphadenectomy group (ASTEC, 2009[*])

- However, the limitation of this randomized trial includes a significant number of patients with low-risk disease and thus may not have sufficient statistical power to discern the true therapeutic role of lymphadenectomy in those with high-risk disease; in addition, a systematic lymph node dissection inclusive of para-aortic nodes was not performed, making it difficult to determine the therapeutic role of a lymphadenectomy; one of the most important roles of surgical staging with lymphadenectomy is to guide postoperative treatment; however, the radiation component of the ASTEC trial did not enable the investigators to evaluate the effect of adjuvant therapy guided by staging surgery

- In the Italian CONSORT study of 514 women with early-stage endometrial cancer, these investigators showed that systematic pelvic lymphadenectomy improved surgical staging but did not improve disease-free or overall survival in early-stage endometrial cancer (Benedetti Panici et al, 2008); more specifically, pelvic lymphadenectomy improved surgical staging by identifying those with lymph node metastases compared to those without the lymphadenectomy arm (13.3% versus 3.2%); however, the 5-year disease-free and overall survival rates in an intention-to-treat analysis were similar between arms (81% and 85.9% in the lymphadenectomy arm and 81.7% and 90% in the no-lymphadenectomy arm, respectively)

- Some of the limitations of the trial include the extent of lymphadenectomy, which did not systematically include para-aortic lymph nodes, as only 26% of patients in the lymphadenectomy arm underwent an aortic lymphadenectomy; some studies have shown that the expected rate of para-aortic involvement can be as high as 30% to 50%; moreover, there was a lack of strict criteria for adjuvant therapies

- These prospective randomized trials have shown that pelvic lymphadenectomy did not provide any therapeutic benefit in early-stage endometrial cancer; nevertheless, these studies consistently demonstrate that lymphadenectomy provides significant prognostic information and can direct adjuvant therapies individualized to each patient; clearly, future investigations are needed to enrich the population of endometrial cancer patients to identify the subgroup of women with high-risk disease who are more likely to benefit from a systematic lymphadenectomy to direct postoperative treatment (Table 37-3)

- Others have also investigated the cost-effectiveness of surgical staging to estimate the costs and outcomes of various treatment strategies used for grade 1 endometrial cancer and showed that surgical staging of all patients with grade 1 endometrial cancer is the most cost-effective strategy and decreases the use of radiation therapy without negatively impacting survival (Cohn et al, 2007[*])

- This study presented a model assuming that all patients were "treated" by each of the three management strategies: (1) surgical staging in all patients (including hysterectomy and lymphadenectomy), (2) frozen section at the time of hysterectomy with surgical staging based on the results of tumor grade and depth of myometrial invasion, and (3) hysterectomy without surgical staging; adjuvant treatment was further stratified by clinical stage of disease including intermediate-risk stage I and stage II disease receiving whole pelvic radiation therapy

- The cost-effectiveness model showed total costs for the three strategies were $240.4 million (surgical staging), $252.4 million (frozen section), and $255.8 million (no staging); the 5-year disease-free survival was 87.9% for surgical staging, 87.3% frozen section, and 86.7% for no staging

TABLE 37-4   **Role of Radiation Therapy in Early-Stage, Intermediate, and High-Risk Endometrial Cancer in Recurrence and Survival**

Study	Study Arms	Local Recurrence Rate	Distal Recurrence Rate	Survival
GOG 99 Keys et al.	202 patients with NAT 190 patients with external beam whole pelvic radiation (RT)	7% with NAT 2% with RT	8% with NAT 5% with RT	4-year overall survival: 86% with NAT 92% with RT
PORTEC I Creutzberg et al.	354 patients with external beam whole pelvic radiation (RT) 360 patients with no further treatment	14% with no further treatment 4% with RT	7% with no further treatment 8% with RT	5-year overall survival: 85% with no further treatment 81% with RT
PORTEC II Nout et al.	214 patients with pelvic EBRT 213 patients with VBT	2.1% with EBRT 5.1% with VBT	5.7% with EBRT 8.3% with VBT	DFS: 78.1% EBRT 82.7% VBT Overall survival: 79.6% EBRT 84.8% VBT
ASTEC/EN.5	453 patients to observation 452 patients to EBRT		88.5% with EBRT 89.9% with observation	83.5% with EBRT 83.9% with observation

DFS, Disease free survival; EBRT, external beam radiation; NAT, no adjuvant treatment; VBT, vaginal brachytherapy.

- Adjuvant treatment of endometrial cancer
  - Several prospective randomized trials have shown that pelvic radiation can decrease locoregional recurrence but does not improve survival
    - The Post Operative Radiation Therapy in Endometrial Carcinoma (PORTEC)-1 trial was made up of patients with stage 1 endometrial carcinoma grade 1 with deep myometrial invasion, grade 2 with any invasion, grade 3 with superficial invasion; the results showed that postoperative radiotherapy reduces locoregional recurrence but has no impact on overall survival (Creutzberg et al, 2000)
    - The 5-year locoregional recurrence rates were 4% in the radiotherapy group and 14% in the control group; the 5-year overall survival rates were similar in the two groups (81% in the radiotherapy and 85% in the control group)
      - The GOG 99 trial enrolled patients with early-stage intermediate-risk disease and showed that adjuvant radiation therapy decreases the risk of recurrence from 12% in those with no additional treatment (NAT) to 3% in patients who underwent pelvic radiation; however, there was a difference in 4-year survival: 86% in NAT and 92% in radiation therapy (RT); more specifically, in those with high intermediate risk—which included those with (1) moderate to poorly differentiated tumor, presence of lymphovascular invasion, and outer third myometrial invasion; (2) age 50 or greater with any two risk factors listed above; or (3) age of at least 70 with any risk factor listed previously—the 2-year recurrence in the NAT versus RT group was 26% versus 6%; however, the survival was not significantly different: 86% in the NAT arm and 92% for the RT arm (Keys et al, 2004)
  - Recent results from the ASTEC trial also showed that adjuvant external beam radiation did not improve the survival of those with intermediate risk or high risk

TABLE 37-5   **Risk of Distant Recurrence in Intermediate High Risk, Early-Stage Endometrial Cancer**

Study	Distant Recurrence
GOG 99	6.4% overall 19% for high intermediate risk early stage
PORTEC	7%
PORTEC 2	6.3%
ASTEC/EN.5	7%

early stage with 5-year overall survival of 84% in both groups; the local recurrence rate in the external beam radiotherapy was 3% versus 6.1% in the observation group (Blake et al, 2009) (Table 37-4)

- In summary, these trials showed that pelvic radiation reduces the recurrence in the pelvis but does not improve survival

UPDATE #10

In early intermediate risk endometrial cancer, vaginal brachytherapy is just as effective as external beam pelvic radiotherapy (EBRT) for decreasing the risk of vaginal recurrence (Nout et al, 2010).

- Recently, investigators from the PORTEC II trial, a prospective randomized trial of stage I, IIA high intermediate risk disease, demonstrated that vaginal brachytherapy (VBT) is just as effective as external beam pelvic radiotherapy (EBRT) for decreasing the rates of locoregional relapse (5.1% for VBT versus 2.1% for EBRT) and isolated pelvic recurrence (1.5% versus 0.5%) and distant metastases (8.3% versus 5.7%) (Table 37-5)

TABLE 37-6   Hormonal Treatment as Adjuvant Therapy in Endometrial Cancer

Study	Study Arms	Recurrence	Overall Survival
Vergote, 1989	531 patients with observation 553 patients with progesterone caproate	14% with observation 12% with progesterone caproate	22 months with observation 30 months with progesterone caproate
GOG 121 Lentz et al, 1996	58 patients with high-dose MA 800 mg/day	24%	7.6 months
GOG 81 Thigpen et al, 1999	154 patients with MPA 200 mg/day 145 patients with MPA 1000 mg/day	15% with 200 mg/day dose 25% with 1000 mg/day dose	11.1 months with 200 mg/day 7 months with 1000 mg/day
GOG B1F Thigpen et al, 2001	68 patients with tamoxifen 20 mg bid	10%	8.8 months
GOG 119 Whitney et al, 2004	58 patients with daily tamoxifen 20 mg bid + MPA 100 mg bid	33%	12.8 months

MA, Megestrol acetate; MPA, medroxyprogesterone acetate.

- There was no difference in overall survival (84.8% versus 79.6%) (Nout et al, 2010); moreover, vaginal brachytherapy provides a better quality of life (QOL) and should be the preferred treatment from a QOL perspective; patients who received EBRT had significantly higher levels of bowel symptoms, limiting their daily activities (Nout et al, 2010)
- In those with early-stage, high intermediate risk disease, the risk of distant failure ranges from 10% to 30%; as such, current clinical trials are investigating the role of systemic chemotherapy with and without pelvic radiation to improve survival
  - In another prospective trial by the Japanese GOG on women with endometrioid adenocarcinoma with deeper than 50% myometrial invasion, investigators showed no significant differences in overall survival comparing adjuvant pelvic radiation therapy (RT) versus cyclophosphamide-doxorubicin-cisplatin (CAP) chemotherapy in the overall study group at 85.3% RT and 86.7% CAP groups, respectively; however, in the high- to intermediate-risk group defined as (1) stage IC in patients over 70 years old or with G3 endometrioid adenocarcinoma or (2) stage II or IIIA (positive cytology), the CAP group had a significantly higher progression-free survival (PFS) rate (83.8% versus 66.2%) and a higher overall survival (OS) rate (89.7% versus 73.6%) (Susumu et al, 2008)
- In the ongoing GOG 249, investigators are comparing the effect of pelvic radiotherapy versus vaginal cuff brachytherapy combined with intravenous carboplatinum and paclitaxel × three cycles in the treatment of high intermediate risk disease

UPDATE #11

In advanced stage disease, chemotherapy is superior to whole abdominal irradiation (Randall et al, 2006).

- In the GOG 122 study of stage III/IV endometrial cancer with a maximum of 2 cm of postoperative residual disease, doxorubicin + cisplatin (AP) improved progression-free survival (PFS) and overall survival (OS) over whole abdominal irradiation (WAI); at 60 months, overall survival was 55% for patients who received AP compared to 42% for patients who received whole abdominal irradiation (GOG 122;[*] Randall et al, 2006)

UPDATE #12

In advanced cancers, the addition of paclitaxel to doxorubicin and cisplatin improved the survival compared to doxorubicin and cisplatin (Fleming et al, 2004).

- In this randomized clinical trial composed of women with advanced or recurrent endometrial carcinoma, the combination of cisplatin, doxorubicin, and paclitaxel (TAP) significantly improved the response rate and progression-free survival compared to cisplatin and doxorubicin (AP) (Fleming et al, 2004[*])
- Seventeen randomized controlled trails (RCTs) compared regimens involving chemotherapy or hormonal therapies; the addition of cisplatin to doxorubicin in two RCTs significantly improved response rates (1.7- to 2.5-fold higher) but did not impact survival; two other RCTs using cisplatin and doxorubicin as standard therapy and the addition of paclitaxel improved response rates (57% versus 34%) and median survival (15.3 versus 12.3 months) when combined with cisplatin and doxorubicin but not doxorubicin only (Carey et al, 2006[*])
- In the ongoing trial of GOG 258 composed of stage III/IVΛ, patients are randomized to cisplatin + tumor volume irradiation followed by paclitaxel and carboplatin × four cycles compared to paclitaxel and carboplatin × six cycles

HORMONAL TREATMENT IN ADVANCED AND RECURRENT ENDOMETRIAL CANCER

- Hormone receptor assessments should be performed in all patients entered on clinical trial and may aid clinical treatment; in previously untreated patients with grade 1 or 2 tumors, the response rate for progestogens ranged from 11% to 56% (Decruze et al, 2007) (Table 37-6)

NOVEL TARGETED THERAPIES FOR RECURRENT DISEASE

- An ongoing trial of GOG 86p involves a three-arm randomized study of paclitaxel/carboplatin/bevacizumab versus paclitaxel/carboplatin/temsirolimus versus ixabepilone/

carboplatin/bevacizumab as initial therapy for measurable stage III or IVA, stage IVB, or recurrent endometrial cancer
- Another ongoing prospective trial investigates the molecular staging of endometrial cancer (GOG 210); this is a 10-year project collecting endometrial tumors with extensive follow-up; investigators use high-throughput methodologies (e.g., genomics and proteomics) and more traditional techniques (e.g., immunoassays) to examine cellular and extracellular factors, including chromosomes, DNA, RNA, proteins, lipids, and carbohydrates

Leiomyosarcoma (LMS)

CLINICAL PROFILE

- There are 0.55 cases per 100,000 women, which accounts for 1.3% of all uterine cancers
- Fifty percent of patients with disease limited to the uterus have recurrence within 2 years and 5-year survival rates of less than 50%
- FIGO staging for leiomyosarcomas (Table 37-7)

DIAGNOSIS

- Usually diagnosed after a myomectomy or hysterectomy for fibroids
- The incidence of sarcoma is 1% to 2% in women with new or enlarging pelvic mass, abnormal uterine bleeding, and pelvic pain
- Rapidly growing fibroids is not a risk factor for leiomyosarcoma
- Twenty-seven percent of hysterectomies performed for rapidly growing fibroids are found to be leiomyosarcoma

MANAGEMENT

- In unsuspected LMS, reoperation for staging is case dependent
  - In a small series, up to 15% who underwent staging procedures were upstaged (Einstein et al, 2008)

TABLE 37-7   **FIGO Staging for Uterine Leiomyosarcoma and Endometrial Stromal Sarcoma**

Stage I	Tumor limited to uterus
Stage IA	Tumor ≤5cm
Stage IB	Tumor >5cm
Stage II	Tumor extends to the pelvis
Stage IIA	Adnexal involvement
Stage IIB	Tumor extends to extrauterine pelvic tissue
Stage III	Tumor invades abdominal tissues (not just protruding into the abdomen)
Stage IIIA	One site
Stage IIIB	> One site
Stage IIIC	Metastasis to pelvic or para-aortic lymph nodes
Stage IV	
Stage IVA	Tumor invades bladder or rectum
Stage IVB	Distant metastasis

From FIGO Committee of Gynecologic Oncology: Revised FIGO staging for carcinoma of the vulva, cervix, and endometrium. *Int J Gynecol Obstet* 104:179, 2009.

- There is also a low risk of pelvic lymph node metastasis at 6.6% to 8% (Giuntoli et al, 2003; Kapp et al, 2008; Leitao et al, 2003)
- The risk of ovarian metastasis is approximately 2.3% (Giuntoli et al, 2003; Leitao et al, 2003; Major et al, 1993; Wu et al, 2006); however, premenopausal ovaries can still secrete estrogen and have the potential to stimulate tumor growth

UPDATE #13

Treatment of advanced leiomyosarcoma has a higher response rate with fixed-dose gemcitabine plus docetaxel (38%) than the first-line therapy with doxorubicin (25%) (Hensley et al, 2008*).

Carcinosarcoma

CLINICAL PROFILE

- Presents with vaginal bleeding, abdominal distension, and symptoms related to distant metastases (pulmonary)

UPDATE #14

Carcinosarcomas are now classified as carcinomas rather than sarcomas or mixed Müllerian mesodermal tumors. These tumors originate from monoclonal carcinoma cells that display sarcomatous metaplasia (McCluggage et al, 2002).

DIAGNOSIS

- Diagnosis is based on histology and sometimes only made after the hysterectomy
- Extrauterine disease is found in 30% of women at the time of diagnosis

MANAGEMENT

- Approach to management has shifted from chemotherapy used for high-grade sarcomas to that used for high-grade endometrial carcinomas
  - A prospective randomized study showed that pelvic radiation decreased local relapse without a significant improvement in survival (Reed et al, 2008)
  - In a prospective randomized trial of GOG 150 comparing whole abdominal irradiation (WAI) versus cisplatin, ifosfamide, and mesna (CIM), the estimated crude probability of recurrence within 5 years was 58% (WAI) and 52% (CIM); adjusting for stage and age, the estimated death rate was 29% lower among the CIM group (Wolfson et al, 2007)

UPDATE #15

In those with measurable stage III or IV, persistent, or recurrent carcinosarcoma, ifosfamide plus paclitaxel improved the outcomes of those with ifosfamide alone. Of these patients, ifosfamide plus paclitaxel improved the median PFS and OS from 3.6 versus 5.8 months and 8.4 versus 13.5 months over ifosfamide alone, respectively (Homesley et al, 2007).

UPDATE #16

Estrogen replacement therapy after surgery for stages I and II endometrial cancer has a low risk for disease recurrence (Barakat et al, 2006).

- GOG 137 studied patients with stage IA to IIB grade 1 to 3 histologic endometrial cancers to determine the effect of estrogen replacement therapy on the recurrence rate for women who have undergone surgery for stage I or II endometrial cancer; the planned duration of treatment was 3 years with 2 years of additional follow-up; there were 1236 eligible patients, with 618 assigned to estrogen replacement therapy; 41% were compliant (251 patients) for the entire treatment period; disease recurrence was found in 14 patients (2.3%); eight patients (1.3%) developed a new malignancy; there were five deaths (0.8%) as a result of endometrial cancer; although this incomplete study did not conclusively refute or support the safety of exogenous estrogen use with respect to the risk of endometrial recurrence, it is noteworthy that the absolute recurrence rate (2.1%) and the incidence of new malignancy were low (Barakat et al, 2006)

Young Women and Endometrial Cancer

UPDATE #17

Although ovarian preservation in premenopausal, early-stage, low-grade disease was not associated with a worsened outcome in large population-based series, smaller series have shown that a significant proportion of young women with endometrial cancer have coexisting ovarian tumors. Among 102 women who had hysterectomy for endometrial cancer, 26 (25%) had coexisting ovarian malignancies (Walsh et al, 2005*). The ovarian cancer histology was endometrioid in 92% of cases.

UPDATE #18

In patients younger than 50 years of age with endometrial cancer, 9% were found to carry a germline Lynch syndrome–associated mutation (Lu et al, 2007).

- In a prospective study, investigators determined the prevalence of Lynch syndrome in young women (<50 years) with endometrial cancer and found that 9% were found to carry germline Lynch syndrome–associated mutations; in addition to young age of onset, family history, body mass index (BMI), and molecular tumor studies can improve the likelihood of identifying a Lynch syndrome–associated germline mutation MLH1, MSH2, and MSH6 (Lu et al, 2007*)

- In half of the women, the gynecologic cancer preceded the development of colon cancer by an average of 5.5 years (ovarian cancer presenting first) or 11 years (endometrial cancer presenting first)
- Median age for germline Lynch syndrome mutations was 44 years
- Women with a first-degree relative with a Lynch syndrome–associated cancer had a 43% chance of having a germline Lynch mutation compared with women without an affected first-degree relative

SUGGESTED READINGS

Uterine Leiomyomas

American College of Obstetricians and Gynecologists: ACOG practice bulletin no. 96: alternatives to hysterectomy in the management of leiomyomas, *Obstet Gynecol* 112(2 Pt 1):387–400, 2008.

Goodwin SC, Spies JB, Worthington-Kirsch R, et al: Uterine artery embolization for treatment of leiomyomata: long-term outcomes from the FIBROID registry, *Obstet Gynecol* 111(1):22–33, 2008.

Klatsky PC, Tran ND, Caughey AB, Fujimoto VY: Fibroids and reproductive outcomes: a systematic literature review from conception to delivery, *Am J Obstet Gynecol* 198(4):357–366, 2008.

Endometrial Cancer

ASTEC/EN.5 Study Group, Blake P, et al: Adjuvant external beam radiotherapy in the treatment of endometrial cancer (MRC ASTEC and NCIC CTG EN.5 randomised trials): pooled trial results, systematic review, and meta-analysis, *Lancet* 373(9658):137–146, 2009.

Panici PB, Basile S, Maneschi F, et al: Systematic pelvic lymphadenectomy vs no lymphadenectomy in early-stage endometrial carcinoma: randomized clinical trial, *J Natl Cancer Inst* 100(23):1707–1716, 2008.

Carey M, Gawlik C, Fung MF, et al: Systematic review of systemic therapy for advanced or recurrent endometrial cancer, *Gynecol Oncol* 101(1):158–167, 2006.

Lu KH, Schorge JO, Rodabaugh KJ, et al: Prospective determination of prevalence of lynch syndrome in young women with endometrial cancer, *J Clin Oncol* 25(33):5158–5164, 2007.

Reed NS, Mangioni C, Malmstrom H, et al: Phase III randomized study to evaluate the role of adjuvant pelvic radiotherapy in the treatment of uterine sarcomas stages I and II: an European Organisation for Research and Treatment of Cancer Gynaecological Cancer Group Study (protocol 55874), *Eur J Cancer* 44(6):808–818, 2008.

Sutton G, Kauderer J, Carson LF, et al: Adjuvant ifosfamide and cisplatin in patients with completely resected stage I or II carcinosarcomas (mixed mesodermal tumors) of the uterus: a Gynecologic Oncology Group study, *Gynecol Oncol* 96(3):630–634, 2005.

Visco AG, Advincula AP: Robotic gynecologic surgery, *Obstet Gynecol* 112(6):1369–1384, 2008.

References

Please go to expertconsult.com to view references.

Chapter 38

Carcinoma of the Ovary and Fallopian Tube

NICOLE D. FLEMING • ROBIN FARIAS-EISNER

KEY UPDATES

1 Risk reducing salpingo-oophorectomy (RRSO) was associated with a statistically significant reduction in both breast and ovarian/fallopian tube cancer in *BRCA1* or 2 mutation carriers.

2 The positive predictive value for routine screening for ovarian cancer was 3.7% for an abnormal CA-125, 1% for an abnormal transvaginal ultrasound (TVUS), and 23.5% if both tests were abnormal.

3 Maximal cytoreduction is one of the most powerful determinants of survival in patients with stage III or IV ovarian cancer.

4 Complete resection of all macroscopic disease at primary cytoreduction or interval cytoreduction following neoadjuvant chemotherapy is the strongest independent variable predicting overall survival.

5 Intravenous paclitaxel plus intraperitoneal cisplatin and paclitaxel improves survival compared to intravenous paclitaxel plus cisplatin.

6 Intravenous dose-dense paclitaxel (80 mg/m^2 weekly for 3 weeks) plus carboplatin (AUC 6 every 3 weeks) improved survival compared to conventional paclitaxel (175 mg/m^2) plus carboplatin (AUC 6) every 3 weeks.

7 Immediate treatment of recurrence based on CA-125 elevation (doubling from baseline) alone may have similar overall survival with that of the delayed treatment arm (await clinical symptoms).

8 Targeted agents including vascular endothelial growth factor (VEGF) inhibitors and poly (ADP-ribose) polymerase (PARP) inhibitors may have response in ovarian cancer.

9 PARP is a key enzyme involved in repair of DNA single-strand breaks using the base excision repair pathway. PARP inhibition results in the accumulation of DNA double-strand breaks that are repaired by homologous recombination, which requires functional *BRCA1* or *BRCA2* activity. Thus the use of PARP inhibitors in *BRCA1* or *BRCA2* mutation carriers results in synthetic lethality, inducing selective tumor cytotoxicity and sparing normal cells.

Clinical Profile: Ovarian Cancer

INCIDENCE

- Second most common gynecologic malignancy (following uterine cancer)
- Fifth leading cause of death in females in the United States
- Lifetime risk is about 1 in 70 (1.4%)
- Peak incidence in 60s and 70s
- Overall 5-year survival is 46%

RISK FACTORS

- Nulliparous, early menarche, late menopause, infertility
- Incessant ovulation hypothesis
- Ovulatory trauma to surface epithelium of the ovary may predispose to malignant transformation
- White (14.2 per 100,000) more than black (9.3 per 100,000) women
- European Jewish descent
- *BRCA1* and *BRCA2* mutation carriers

FAMILIAL SYNDROMES

- *BRCA* mutation carriers
  - One in 800 mutation carriers in general population
  - One in 40 mutation carriers in Ashkenazi Jewish population
  - *BRCA1* risk of ovarian cancer 36% to 46%
  - *BRCA2* risk of ovarian cancer 10% to 27%

- Three founder mutations account for 90% cases of hereditary breast-ovarian cancer
  - 185delAG and 5382insC (*BRCA1*)
  - 6174delT (*BRCA2*)
- Hereditary nonpolyposis colorectal cancer (HNPCC)/Lynch II syndrome
  - Two percent of familial ovarian cancer
  - Mutations in DNA mismatch repair genes (*MSH2, MLH1, MSH6, PMS2, PMS1*)
  - Synchronous or metachronous colon, endometrial, ovarian, gastric, biliary tract, urinary tract carcinomas

SCREENING

- Third-generation family history should be assessed
- Genetic testing for *BRCA* mutations
  - Personal or family history of breast cancer before age 50
  - Ovarian cancer diagnosed at any age
  - *BRCA* carrier in first-degree relative
  - Family history of two or more cases of ovarian cancer
  - Personal or family history of bilateral breast cancer
  - Family history of male breast cancer
  - Ashkenazi Jewish ancestry with personal or family history of breast or ovarian cancer
- Genetic testing for HNPCC mutations
  - Family history of at least two successive generations affected by colorectal cancer
  - Family history of colon cancer diagnosed before age 50
  - Colon cancer diagnosed in at least three relatives
  - Increased incidence of other cancers (ovarian, endometrial, gastric, urinary tract, biliary)

PREVENTION

- Oral contraceptive use for at least 5 years confers a 30% to 50% risk reduction of ovarian cancer
- Annual or semiannual transvaginal ultrasound (TVUS) and CA-125 starting at age 25 to 35 in known *BRCA* mutation carriers
- Tubal ligation +/− oral contraceptives decreased risk of ovarian cancer in *BRCA1* mutation carriers only

UPDATE #1

Risk reducing salpingo-oophorectomy (RRSO) was associated with a statistically significant reduction in both breast and ovarian/fallopian tube cancer in *BRCA1* or *BRCA2* mutation carriers. RRSO decreased the risk of ovarian/fallopian tube cancer by 80% to 90% and the risk of breast cancer by 50% in *BRCA* mutation carriers (Rebbeck et al, 2009).

UPDATE #2

The positive predictive value for routine screening for ovarian cancer was 3.7% for an abnormal CA-125, 1% for an abnormal TVUS, and 23.5% if both tests were abnormal. If surgery was done to evaluate an abnormal CA-125, 1 neoplasm was identified per 3.9 surgeries, 1 neoplasm per 24 surgeries based on an abnormal TVUS, and 1 neoplasm per 3 surgeries if both TVUS and CA-125 were abnormal (Buys et al, 2005).

PRESENTATION/PATTERNS OF SPREAD

- Symptoms of increasing abdominal girth, abdominopelvic pain, weight loss, decreased appetite, early satiety, nausea/vomiting, changes in bowel/bladder habits
- Spread by peritoneal dissemination, direct extension, lymphatic or hematogenous spread

INTERNATIONAL FEDERATION OF GYNECOLOGY AND OBSTETRICS (FIGO) STAGING (Table 38-1)
HISTOLOGY

- Epithelial (86%)
  - Serous, borderline, mucinous, endometrioid, clear cell, transitional cell, squamous
- Sex cord-stromal tumors (4%)
  - Granulosa cell, theca-fibroma, Sertoli-Leydig, sex cord tumors with annular tubules, gynandroblastoma
- Germ cell tumors (6%)
  - Dysgerminoma, endodermal sinus tumor, embryonal, choriocarcinoma, teratomas (immature, mature, struma ovarii, carcinoid)
- Gonadoblastoma
- Other (small cell carcinoma, lymphoma/leukemias, metastatic tumors)

Clinical Profile: Fallopian Tube Carcinoma
INCIDENCE

- <1% lifetime risk
- Most common carcinoma of the fallopian tube is metastatic from another site

HISTOLOGY AND PATHOLOGIC DIAGNOSIS

- Most frequent site of origin is ampulla

TABLE 38-1 FIGO Staging of Ovarian Cancer

Stage I	
Stage IA	Growth limited to one ovary, capsule intact, no ascites
Stage IB	Growth limited to both ovaries, capsule intact, no ascites
Stage IC	Stage IA or IB, tumor on surface, ruptured capsule, ascites, or positive washings
Stage II	
Stage IIA	Extension or mets to uterus or tubes
Stage IIB	Extension to other pelvic tissues
Stage IIC	Stage IIA or IIB, tumor on surface, ruptured capsule, ascites, or positive washings
Stage III	
Stage IIIA	Tumor grossly limited to pelvis, negative nodes, microscopic seeding of abdominal peritoneal surfaces
Stage IIIB	Abdominal peritoneal implants less than or equal to 2 cm, negative nodes
Stage IIIC	Abdominal peritoneal implants greater than 2 cm or positive nodes
Stage IV	Distant metastasis (parenchymal liver or lung mets, positive cytology in pleural effusion)

Adapted from 1985 FIGO staging criteria. Petterson F, Kelstad P, Ludwig H, Ulfelder H: *Annual report on the results of treatment in Gynecologic cancer*, Stockholm, Sweden, 1985, International Federation of Gynecology and Obstetrics; p 19.

- Bilateral involvement in 5% to 30% cases
- Occult invasive or in situ carcinomas of the fallopian tube in BRCA mutation carriers undergoing risk-reducing salpingo-oophorectomy (RRSO)
  - Entire fallopian tube should be serially sectioned and examined microscopically
- Histologic subtypes: serous (90%), mucinous, endometrioid, clear cell, transitional, squamous, glassy cell, mixed
- Criteria for pathologic diagnosis
  - Main tumor in the tube and arises from endosalpinx
  - Histologically reproduces the epithelium of mucosa
  - Transition from benign to malignant epithelium
  - Ovaries and endometrium normal or contain less tumor than tube
- Exfoliative spread of tubal carcinoma occurs frequently
  - Recommend cytologic examination of peritoneal washings
- Depth of invasion into tubal mucosa is an important prognostic factor

FIGO STAGING (Table 38-2)

Primary Management

SURGERY

- Surgical staging (salpingo-oophorectomy +/− hysterectomy, pelvic and periaortic lymphadenectomy, infracolic omentectomy, peritoneal biopsies, washings)
- Primary cytoreductive surgery
  - Reduce number of cancer cells for chemotherapy to act on

TABLE 38-2 FIGO Staging of Fallopian Tube Carcinoma

Stage I	
Stage IA	Growth limited to one tube, no extension to serosa, no ascites
Stage IB	Growth limited to both tubes, no extension to serosa, no ascites
Stage IC	Stage IA or IB, extension to serosa, ascites, or positive washings
Stage II	
Stage IIA	Extension or mets to uterus or ovaries
Stage IIB	Extension to other pelvic tissues
Stage IIC	Stage IIA or IIB, ascites, or positive washings
Stage III	
Stage IIIA	Tumor grossly limited to pelvis, negative nodes, microscopic seeding of abdominal peritoneal surfaces
Stage IIIB	Abdominal peritoneal implants less than or equal to 2 cm, negative nodes
Stage IIIC	Abdominal peritoneal implants greater than 2 cm or positive nodes
Stage IV	Distant metastasis (parenchymal liver or lung mets, positive cytology in pleural effusion)

Adapted from 1991 FIGO staging criteria. Petterson F: Staging rules for gestational trophoblastic tumors and fallopian tube cancer, *Acta Obstet Gynecol Scan* 71:224-225, 1992.

- Less chemotherapy-resistant cells (Goldie-Coldman model)
- Large bulky tumor is hypoperfused with suboptimal chemotherapy concentrations
- Majority of large tumor cells are in the G0 phase of cell cycle
- Chemotherapy works on cells in active cell cycle
- Goal is no gross residual disease

UPDATE #3

- Maximal cytoreduction is one of the most powerful determinants of survival in patients with stage III or IV ovarian cancer.
- Improved progression-free survival for microscopic (22 months) versus 0.1 to 1 cm (12 months) residual tumor.
- Improved median overall survival for microscopic (76 months), compared to 0.1 to 1 cm (32 months) versus greater than 1 cm (19 months) residual tumor (Eisenkop et al, 2003).

- Interval cytoreductive surgery
  - Performed after short course of chemotherapy
  - Need initial pathologic confirmation of ovarian cancer
  - Candidates include those who underwent initial suboptimal cytoreduction, medical comorbidities precluding initial surgery, or extent/distribution of disease

UPDATE #4

A retrospective review of the literature showed survival rates as follows: neoadjuvant chemotherapy and interval cytoreduction (26 months), suboptimal cytoreduction (20 months), and optimal primary cytoreduction (51 months) (Holschneider et al, 2006). However, a recent randomized controlled trial showed neoadjuvant chemotherapy followed by interval cytoreduction was not inferior to primary cytoreduction in stage IIIC or IV ovarian cancer in survival outcomes. Complete resection of all macroscopic disease at primary or interval cytoreduction is the strongest independent variable predicting overall survival (Vergote et al, 2010).

CHEMOTHERAPY

- Standard first-line treatment for advanced epithelial ovarian cancer: platinum compound combined with a taxane every 3 weeks for six cycles

UPDATE #5

Intravenous paclitaxel plus intraperitoneal cisplatin and paclitaxel improves survival compared to intravenous paclitaxel plus cisplatin. Median progression-free survival in the intravenous and intraperitoneal groups was 18.3 and 23.8 months, respectively ($p = 0.05$). Median overall survival in the intravenous and intraperitoneal groups was 49.7 and 65.6 months, respectively ($p = 0.03$) (Armstrong et al, 2006).

UPDATE #6

Intravenous dose-dense paclitaxel (80 mg/m^2 weekly for 3 weeks) plus carboplatin (AUC 6 every 3 weeks) improved survival compared to conventional paclitaxel (175 mg/m^2) plus carboplatin (AUC 6) every 3 weeks. Median progression-free survival was longer in the dose-dense group (28 versus 17.2 months, $p = 0.03$) than in the conventional group. Median overall survival at 3 years was higher in the dose-dense group (72% versus 65%, p = 0.03) than in the conventional group. The most common adverse event in the dose-dense group was neutropenia (92% versus 88%, p = NS). The frequency of grade 3 to 4 anemia was higher in the dose-dense group (69% vs. 44%, p < 0.0001) (Katsumata et al, 2009).

Management of Recurrence

SURVEILLANCE

- Serial serum CA-125 levels and radiographic imaging

UPDATE #7

Recent results from a randomized controlled trial revealed that immediate treatment based on CA-125 elevation (doubling from baseline) alone had similar overall survival with that of the delayed treatment arm (await clinical symptoms). Furthermore, the patients in the immediate treatment arm reported worse quality of life compared to those in the delayed treatment arm (Rustin et al, 2010). Rates of optimal versus suboptimal secondary cytoreduction were not addressed, and patients in both arms did not receive the same treatment after recurrence.

SECONDARY CYTOREDUCTION

- Candidates generally have a 12-month disease-free interval and are platinum sensitive
- Poor clinical indicators include the presence of ascites, carcinomatosis, and greater than three sites of recurrence

SECOND-LINE CHEMOTHERAPY

- Platinum and taxane-based chemotherapy typically used for platinum-sensitive recurrence
- Common second-line agents in platinum-resistant disease include liposomal doxorubicin, gemcitabine, topotecan, cyclophosphamide, etoposide
- Targeted agents currently being studied:
  - Anti-angiogenesis/VEGF inhibitors

UPDATE #8

Angiogenesis is a complex and highly regulated process by which tumors develop new vasculature, a feature essential for growth of tumors beyond 1 mm in size. VEGF signaling is one of the most promising angiogenic targets because of its central role in tumor growth. Bevacizumab (Avastin, Genentech), a humanized monoclonal antibody that targets VEGF, has been evaluated in combination with standard chemotherapy in patients with advanced colorectal cancer, breast cancer, and non-small-cell lung cancer, and it has demonstrated improved progression-free and overall survival. Several retrospective studies in persistent or recurrent ovarian cancer have shown response rates up to 35%. The first prospective phase II trial of single-agent bevacizumab in persistent or recurrent ovarian cancer, Gynecologic Oncology Group (GOG) 170-D, showed 21% relative risk (RR) with 40% patients showing no signs of progression at 6 months. We are awaiting results from recent phase III trials in the front-line adjuvant setting: for example, GOG 218, a three-arm, placebo-controlled, randomized clinical trial comparing carboplatin and paclitaxel with or without bevacizumab followed by placebo or bevacizumab maintenance therapy, and ICON-7, an open-label, randomized Gynecologic Cancer InterGroup trial comparing carboplatin, paclitaxel, and bevacizumab with or without bevacizumab maintenance therapy. In addition, GOG 213 will

evaluate the use of bevacizumab in platinum-sensitive recurrent disease in the presence or absence of secondary surgical cytoreduction (Spannuth et al, 2008).

- Epidermal growth factor receptor inhibitors
- Tyrosine kinase and multikinase inhibitors
- Poly (ADP-ribose) ribose polymerase (PARP) inhibitors

UPDATE #9

PARP is a key enzyme involved in repair of DNA single-strand breaks using the base excision repair pathway. PARP inhibition results in the accumulation of DNA double-strand breaks that are repaired by homologous recombination, which requires functional BRCA1 or BRCA2 activity. Thus, the use of PARP inhibitors in BRCA1 or BRCA2 mutation carriers results in synthetic lethality, inducing selective tumor cytotoxicity and sparing normal cells. In vitro, BRCA1 or BRCA2 deficient cells were up to 1000-fold more sensitive to PARP inhibitors than wild-type cells. A phase I trial of an orally active PARP inhibitor, olaparib, was studied in patients with advanced solid tumors, including ovarian, breast, and colorectal cancers. Durable objective antitumor activity was observed only in confirmed carriers of a BRCA1 or BRCA2 mutation; 63% of BRCA carriers had a clinical benefit from treatment with olaparib, with radiologic or tumor-marker responses. No objective antitumor responses were observed in patients without BRCA mutations (Fong et al, 2009).

SUGGESTED READINGS

Hereditary Ovarian Cancer

Rebbeck TR, Kauff ND, Domchek SM: Meta-analysis of risk reduction estimates associated with risk-reducing salpingoophorectomy in BRCA1 or BRCA2 mutation carriers, *J Natl Cancer Inst* 101(2):80–87, 2009.

Ovarian Cancer Screening

Buys SS, Partridge E, Greene MH, et al: Ovarian cancer screening in the prostate, lung, colorectal and ovarian (PLCO) cancer screening trial: findings from the initial screen of a randomized trial, *Am J Ob Gyn* 193(5):1630–1639, 2005.

Cytoreductive Surgery in Ovarian Cancer

Eisnenkop SM, Spirtos NM, Friedman RL, et al: Relative influences of tumor volume before surgery and the cytoreductive outcome on survival for patients with advanced ovarian cancer: a prospective study, *Gynecol Oncol* 90(2):390–396, 2003.

Holschneider CH, Berek JS: Cytoreductive surgery: principles and rationale. In Bristow RE, Karlan BY, editors: *Surgery for ovarian cancer*, Abingdon, Oxon (UK), 2006, Taylor & Francis, pp 87–125.

Vergote I, Trope CG, Amant F, et al. Neoadjuvant chemotherapy or primary surgery in stage IIIC or IV ovarian cancer. *N Engl J Med* 363(10):943-953, 2010.

Primary Chemotherapy in Ovarian Cancer

Armstrong DK, Bundy B, Wenzel L, et al: Intraperitoneal cisplatin and paclitaxel in ovarian cancer, *N Engl J Med* 354(1):34–43, 2006.

Katsumata N, Yasuda M, Takahashi F, et al: Dose-dense paclitaxel once a week in combination with carboplatin every 3 weeks for advanced ovarian cancer: a phase 3, open-label, randomized controlled trial, *Lancet* 374(9698):1331–1338, 2009.

Surveillance for Recurrent Ovarian Cancer

Rustin GJ, Van der Burg ME, Griffin CL, et al: Early versus delayed treatment of relapsed ovarian cancer (MRC OV05/EORTC 55955): a randomised trial, *Lancet* 376(9747):1155–1163, 2010.

Targeted Therapies in Ovarian Cancer

Fong PC, Boss DS, Yap TA, et al: Inhibition of poly(ADP-Ribose) polymerase in tumors from BRCA mutation carriers, *N Engl J Med* 361(2):123–134, 2009.

Spannuth WA, Sood AK, Coleman RL: Angiogenesis as a strategic target for ovarian cancer therapy, *Nat Clin Pract Oncol* 5(4):194–204, 2008.

Chapter 39

Pelvic Floor Disorders

FELICIA L. LANE • JENNIFER K. LEE

KEY UPDATES

1. The 2010 Joint Report on the Terminology for Female Pelvic Floor Dysfunction.
2. Weight loss reduces the risk of urinary incontinence.
3. Tension-free vaginal tape (TVT) and Burch colposuspension have similar efficacy at 5 years.
4. Autologous fascial sling is more effective than Burch colposuspension but has greater morbidity (SISTEr Trial).
5. Sacral nerve stimulation (InterStim) demonstrates long-term efficacy for urge incontinence, urgency-frequency, and urinary retention.
6. Botulinum toxin A is an effective treatment alternative for refractory overactive bladder.
7. International Continence Society adopts pelvic organ (POP-Q) prolapse quantification (POP-Q) system.
8. Burch colposuspension reduces postoperative symptoms of stress incontinence in stress-continent women undergoing abdominal sacrocolpopexy.
9. Abdominal sacrocolpopexy is associated with a lower rate of recurrent vault prolapse and dyspareunia than vaginal sacrospinous colpopexy.
10. McCall culdoplasty found to be a superior method to prevent enterocele at time of vaginal hysterectomy.
11. Society of Gynecologic Surgeons publishes clinical practice guidelines for use of transvaginal mesh.
12. Food and Drug Administration (FDA) issues updated safety communication on use of transvaginally placed mesh for prolapse or stress urinary incontinence.
13. Sacral nerve stimulation for fecal incontinence.

Urinary Incontinence

CLINICAL PROFILE

- The observation of involuntary loss of urine on examination: this may be urethral or extraurethral
- The National Health Survey concluded that between 25% to 75% of women have urinary incontinence, and the prevalence increases with age
- Projections for 2050 are that 41.3 million women will have urinary incontinence
- Total cost related to urinary incontinence in the United States in 2000 was nearly $20 billion
- Stress incontinence is most prevalent, followed by mixed incontinence and urge incontinence; proportions change as women age with urge incontinence becoming more common; extraurethral incontinence is a rare occurrence in developed countries

UPDATE #1

In 2010, the International Urogynecological Association (IUGA) and International Continence Society (ICS) published a joint report on female pelvic floor dysfunction. The new terminology is included throughout this chapter. Patients report symptoms, physicians identify signs, and these lead to the common diagnoses discussed here (Haylen et al, 2010).

DIFFERENTIAL DIAGNOSIS

- Stress urinary incontinence (SUI)
  - Symptom: involuntary loss of urine on effort or physical exertion
  - Sign: observation of involuntary leakage from the urethra
  - Urodynamic stress incontinence (USI): symptoms and signs noted previously, plus involuntary leakage during filling cystometry in the absence of a detrusor contraction

- Female continence is complex; any deficit in urethral support, coaptation, sphincter mechanism, or neurovascular supply can result in incontinence
- Urgency (urge) urinary incontinence
  - Symptom: complaint of involuntary loss of urine associated with urgency
  - Sign: observation of leakage from the urethra synchronous with the sudden desire to void
  - Overactive bladder syndrome: urinary urgency, accompanied by frequency and nocturia
- Mixed urinary incontinence
  - Symptom: complaint of involuntary loss of urine associated with urgency and also with effort or physical exertion or sneezing or coughing
- Extraurethral incontinence
  - Symptom: complaint of continuous involuntary loss of urine
  - Sign: observation of urine leakage through channels other than the urethral meatus— for example, fistula
- Stress incontinence on prolapse reduction (NEW)
  - Sign: stress incontinence only observed after the reduction of coexistent prolapse

RISK FACTORS

- Childbearing
- Obesity
- Mobility impairment
- Advancing age/menopause
- Unclear if race is a factor

DIAGNOSIS

- History of symptoms alone can be misleading
  - Correlation of symptoms with identification of urine loss (signs) is necessary prior to intervention
- Identify reversible causes of incontinence, determine severity, contributing factors, and impact on quality of life (Table 39-1)
- A 24-hour voiding diary to measure fluid intake and output and leakage episodes
- Neurologic examination including mental status, gait, coordination, motor strength, and reflexes
- Asymmetric strength or hyperreflexia can be indicative of upper motor nerve lesions; patients with these findings need further neurologic assessment for conditions such as multiple sclerosis, stroke, and Parkinson's disease
  - Atrophy of the vaginal and urethral tissue should be corrected

TABLE 39-1 **Reversible Causes of Urinary Incontinence**

Delirium
Infection
Atrophic vaginitis
Pharmacologic
Psychological
Endocrine
Restricted mobility
Stool impaction

- Inspect for urethral cysts and diverticulum
- Speculum examination to exclude mass lesion and neoplasm
- Vaginal pool of urine suggests vesicovaginal or ureterovaginal fistula
- Pelvic organ prolapse quantification system (POP-Q) to measure support
- Pelvic floor muscles are assessed for strength and tenderness
- Q-tip testing
  - Introduced by Crystle et al. in 1971 as a nonradiographic measurement of urethral mobility
  - The urethra is prepped and anesthetic jelly applied; a sterile Q-tip is advanced past the urethrovesical junction and drawn back until slight resistance is noted; this ensures that the tip is at the bladder neck; hypermobility by convention is defined as a straining angle of 30 degrees from the horizontal, but there is no clear cutoff between normal and abnormal; Q-tip testing does not diagnose SUI; however, women with a fixed or nonmobile urethra have higher surgical failure rates and may be better candidates for transurethral bulking agents
- Postvoid residual
  - Obtain prior to initiating medical and surgical therapy; this assessment should take place immediately after the patient voids by either clean catheterization or bladder scanner; volumes less than 50 cc are normal, and volumes greater than 200 cc are abnormal; values in between should be confirmed on several separate occasions
- Urinalysis to rule out reversible causes of incontinence such as infection
- A cough stress test may be performed to demonstrate stress incontinence
- In complicated cases or after treatment failures, urodynamic testing is recommended
  - A filling cystometrogram can assess detrusor overactivity, bladder sensation, and compliance
  - Uroflowmetry and pressure voiding studies are necessary in patients with voiding dysfunction
- Cystoscopy is indicated with hematuria, recurrent cystitis, and when extraurethral urinary incontinence is suspected
- Prolapse beyond the hymen
  - Anatomic changes associated with advanced prolapse may mask stress incontinence; therefore, patients should undergo prolapse reduction at the time of stress testing or urodynamics

MANAGEMENT OF SUI

- Conservative
  - Pelvic floor exercises
  - Pessary (Figure 39-1)
- Weight loss

UPDATE #2

Weight loss can reduce urinary incontinence in overweight and obese women. A randomized trial of 338 women with a mean weight loss of 8% of baseline body weight experienced a 47.4% decrease in the total number of weekly incontinence episodes (Subak et al, 2009).

- Vaginal estrogen replacement
- Urethral bulking agents; transurethral or periurethral injection techniques include the following:
  - Collagen (Contigen: Bard Urological Products); need sensitivity skin test, may need to be repeated in 9 to 12 months; manufacturing to cease in 2011
  - Calcium hydroxyapatite (Coaptite; Bioform Medical); no skin test required; may need to be repeated in 12 months
  - Carbon bead particles (Durasphere: Carbon Medical Technologies); no skin test required, nonbiodegradable bulking agent; slower degradation than Contigen and Coaptite
  - Polydimethylsiloxane (Macroplastique: Uroplasty Inc.); permanent material, yields excellent efficacy at 12 months; current U.S. studies on its long-term efficacy in progress
  - Hyaluronic acid/dextranomer (Deflux: Oceana Therapeutics Inc.); nonimmunogenic, microspheres last 4 years; FDA approval pending
  - Success rates 63% to 65%
- Surgical treatments
  - Retropubic urethropexy (Burch)
    - Tanagho (1976) described the modified Burch colposuspension performed today; an open or laparoscopic incision is used to access the space of Retzius, and two nonabsorbable sutures are placed 2 cm lateral to the urethrovesical junction and two additional sutures are placed 2 cm lateral to the proximal third of the urethra; these sutures are then passed through pectineal (Cooper's) ligament; a suture bridge is common to avoid overcorrecting the urethral angle, which should remain −10 to +10 degrees relative to the horizontal; studies with 10-year follow-up report success rates ranging from 63% to 81%
  - Midurethral sling (retropubic and transobturator)
    - The tension-free vaginal tape (TVT) was the first synthetic sling and was described by Petros and Ulmsten in 1995
    - The synthetic material is made of macroporous polypropylene
    - Approximately 1 cm wide and 40 cm long
    - Two stainless-steel needles are passed through the retropubic space; this can be done by either a bottom-up or top-down approach; the vascular retropubic space can be bypassed via the transobturator approach (TOT) (Figures 39-2, 39-3, and 39-4)
    - Randomized data suggest the TVT approach is more effective than TOT for severe incontinence complicated by intrinsic sphincter deficiency

UPDATE #3

TVT and Burch colposuspension have similar efficacy at 5 years; 404 women with urodynamic stress incontinence randomized to TVT versus Burch. The primary outcome measure was a negative 1-hour pad test (81% versus 90%, $P = 0.21$). The authors noted more vault and posterior vaginal wall prolapse in the Burch group and tape erosion in the TVT group (Ward et al, 2007). The midurethral sling has widely replaced Burch because of its ease of placement and similar efficacy.

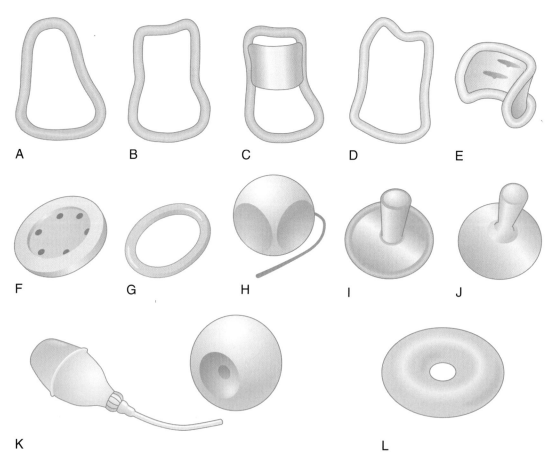

Figure 39-1. Incontinence and support pessaries. (From Foster DC, Duecy E: Gynecologic disorders. In Duthie EH, Katz PR, Malone ML: *Practice of geriatrics,* ed 4, Philadelphia, 2007, Saunders.)

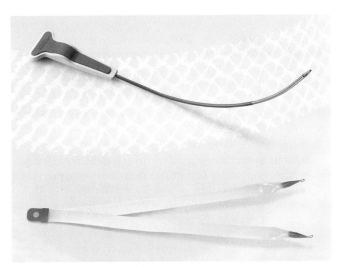

Figure 39-2. Lynx retropubic midurethral system; includes macro-porous polypropylene mesh sling and 3-mm trocars. (Courtesy of Boston Scientific.)

- Pubovaginal sling
  - First described in 1907 and again by Aldridge in 1942; a strip of autologous fascia or donor material is placed transvaginally at the level of the proximal urethra and bladder base; the fascial strip is then anchored to the rectus fascia with permanent sutures. Success rates range from 70% to 85%

UPDATE #4

Pubovaginal sling with autologous fascia results in higher rates of successful treatment of stress incontinence than Burch (66% versus 49%, $P < 0.001$) and greater patient satisfaction. However, the sling group had higher rates of urinary tract infections, urge incontinence, voiding dysfunction, and the need for surgical revision (Albo et al, 2007). Despite these recent data, most providers are using minimally invasive procedures such as midurethral slings.

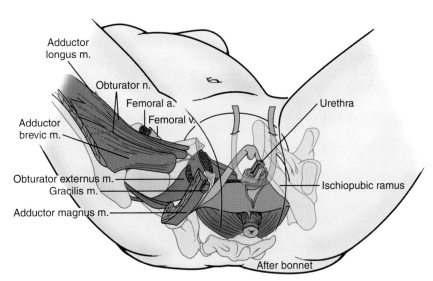

Figure 39-3. Anatomic illustration of retropubic midurethral sling in situ. (From Dmochowski R, Scarpero H, Starkman J. Tension-free vaginal tape procedures. In Wein AJ, Kavoussi LR, Novick Andrew C, et al: *Campbell-Walsh urology,* ed 9, Philadelphia, 2007, Saunders, pp 2251-2271.)

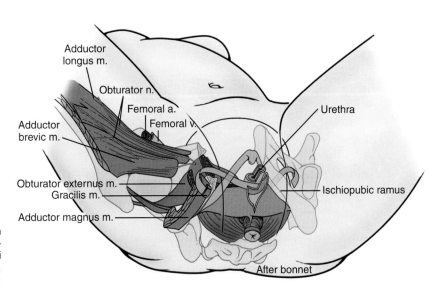

Figure 39-4. Transobturator sling. (From Dmochowski R, Scarpero H, Starkman J. Tension-free vaginal tape procedures. In Wein AJ, Kavoussi LR, Novick Andrew C, et al: *Campbell-Walsh urology,* ed 9, Philadelphia, 2007, Saunders, pp 2251-2271.)

MANAGEMENT OF URGE URINARY INCONTINENCE AND OVERACTIVE BLADDER

- Pelvic floor exercises, timed voiding, fluid management and bladder retraining
- Weight loss
- Anticholinergics
  - Oxybutynin
  - Tolterodine
  - Darifenacin
  - Solifenacin
  - Trospium chloride
  - Imipramine
  - Pharmacologic therapy still considered first line; potential side effects include dry mouth, constipation, dry eyes, and confusion; contraindicated in patients with narrow-angle glaucoma; side effect profile leads to high discontinuation rates (>50%) irrespective of medication
- Neuromuscular electrical stimulation (E-Stim)
  - Utilizes electrical current to the pelvic floor to help patients gain awareness and control
- Neuromodulation
  - Urgent PC (tibial nerve stimulation)
    - This is an office-based procedure; an acupuncture needle is placed at the level of the posterior tibial nerve and stimulation administered; sessions are 30 minutes weekly for 12 weeks; maintenance therapy is necessary; success rates of 37% to 92%
  - InterStim (sacral nerve stimulation)
    - System includes a lead wire and implantable pulse generator similar to a pacemaker; the lead wire is placed adjacent to the S3 nerve root; the therapy is trialled prior to implantation of the programmable system; improvement of greater than 50% meets criteria for implant; FDA approved for urge incontinence, urinary frequency/urgency, and retention (Figure 39-5)

UPDATE #5

Sacral nerve stimulation (InterStim; Medtronic, Minneapolis, Minnesota) has been FDA approved since 1997. A prospective worldwide trial including 17 sites yielded 152 subjects; data on 105 participants were available at 5 years. InterStim demonstrates long-term efficacy for treatment of urge incontinence (68%), urgency-frequency (56%), and nonobstructive urinary retention (71%). No irreversible adverse effects were reported; however, minor surgical procedures were required for pain at the implantation site or device exchange (van Kerrebroeck et al, 2007).

- Intravesical botulinum toxin type A (Botox)
  - Inhibits the presynaptic release of acetylcholine causing localized reduction in detrusor muscle activity; this is an office-based procedure; through a cystoscope, 10 to 30 sites are injected with avoidance of the trigone

UPDATE #6

A randomized, double-blind placebo trial was conducted by the Pelvic Floor Disorders Network. Women who failed medical management of urge incontinence were enrolled. Twenty-three received 200 U of Botox, 15 received placebos. Sixty percent of subjects in the Botox arm had a significant improvement, with the median response of 373 days. However, the study was halted due to elevated postvoid residuals and the need for intermittent self-catheterization in 12 (43%) patients (Brubaker et al, 2008). These data suggest efficacy, and current National Institutes of Health trials are under way to determine efficacy, dosing, and safety. Patients should be made aware that Botox is still experimental and not yet approved by the FDA.

MANAGEMENT OF EXTRAURETHRAL INCONTINENCE

- Vesicovaginal
- Urethrovaginal
- Ureterovaginal
- Vesicouterine
- In developed countries, fistulas occur as a result of gynecologic surgery, neoplasm, or radiation; in developing countries, they are associated with childbirth
- Vaginal exam may reveal a fistula tract or just granulation tissue
- Cystoscopy with methylene blue dye (Moir test) can confirm the presence of a vesicovaginal fistula; if negative, oral Pyridium test is used to identify ureterovaginal fistula; cyclic blood in the urine is suggestive of a vesicouterine fistula
- A simple post hysterectomy fistula can often be treated immediately postoperatively with simple bladder drainage; a simple fistula with mature tracts can be approached vaginally with a Latzko procedure; distal and complex fistula may require Martius flap interposition or an abdominal approach; success rates vary based on the complexity of the fistula from 74% to 100%

Pelvic Organ Prolapse

CLINICAL PROFILE

- The descent of one or more of the anterior vaginal wall, posterior vaginal wall, uterus, or the apex of the vagina from normally supported locations
- Estimated that 200,000 surgeries are performed annually for treatment of prolapse

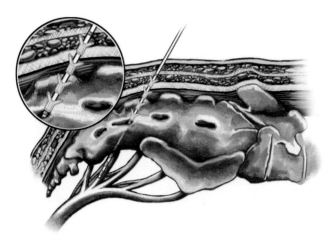

Figure 39-5. Sacral nerve stimulation-lead wire placed in S3 foramen. (Courtesy of Medtronic.)

- Eleven percent lifetime risk of prolapse surgery, with approximately one third requiring repeat surgery for recurrence
- Risk factors
  - Vaginal birth/operative vaginal delivery
  - Obesity
  - Advancing age/ menopause/ estrogen deficiency
  - State of chronic increased intra-abdominal pressure (chronic obstructive pulmonary disease [COPD], chronic cough, occupational lifting)
  - Connective tissue/neuromuscular disorders
  - Genetic predisposition
- Anatomy of pelvic support
  - The pelvic organs are supported by a complex interplay between the uterosacral/cardinal ligament complex, levator ani muscles, and endopelvic fascia; these structures form the pelvic girdle and attach to the bony pelvis; the urethra, vagina, and anus collectively open to the perineum/vulva through the genital hiatus; damage to supportive ligaments results in protrusion of pelvic organs through the urogenital hiatus
  - Delancey's levels of support (Figure 39-6)
    - Level I: attachment of the vaginal apex/cervix to the cardinal/uterosacral ligaments
      - Defect results in vault/uterine prolapse
    - Level II: attachment of the midvagina to levator muscles via the arcus tendineus fascia pelvis
      - Defect results in lateral cystocele/anterior wall defect
    - Level III: support of distal vagina via pubourethral ligaments and perineal body
      - Defect results in perineocele, posterior wall defect

DIAGNOSIS

- Symptoms
  - Vaginal bulge
  - Pelvic pressure
  - Bleeding/discharge
  - Low backache
  - Splinting/digitation to facilitate voiding or defecation
  - Outlet constipation
- Evaluation
  - Examine in both recumbent and upright positions to maximize prolapse descent
  - May apply traction to maximize descent
  - Complete a site-specific split speculum examination to evaluate anterior, posterior, and apical compartments with valsalva
  - Verify extent of prolapse with patient
  - Evaluate postvoid residual (severe prolapse can cause urethral kinking and urinary retention)
  - Evaluate occult stress incontinence by prolapse-reduced stress testing
- Classification and staging systems
  - Baden-Walker Halfway classification
    - 1st degree: Prolapse descent halfway to hymen
    - 2nd degree: Prolapse descent to hymen
    - 3rd degree: Prolapse halfway beyond hymen
    - 4th degree: Total prolapse

UPDATE #7

The International Continence Society adopts the pelvic organ prolapse quantification (POP-Q) system (Bump et al, 1996).

- POP-Q classification system
  - Developed in 1995 by the International Continence Society
  - Includes six site-specific measurements corresponding to segments of the lower reproductive tract (replaces cystocele, rectocele, enterocele)
  - Hymen is a fixed reference point (assigned to be 0)
  - Proximal points to hymen assigned negative values (in cm)

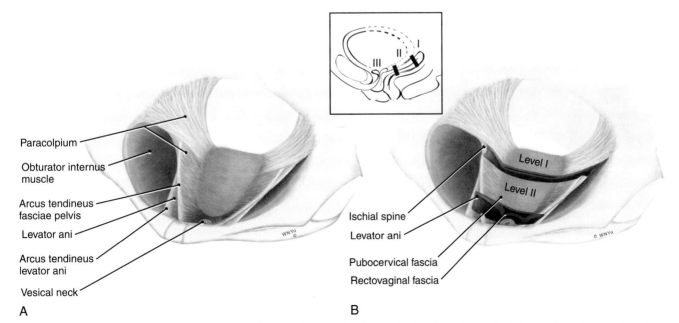

Figure 39-6. Delancey's levels of support. **A,** In level III, the distal vagina is attached to the pubourethral ligaments and perineal body. **B,** Defects in level III support can lead to perineoceles, rectoceles, and urethral hypermobility. (From Delancey JO: Anatomic aspects of vaginal eversion after hysterectomy, *Am J Obstet Gynecol* 166:1717-1728, 1992.)

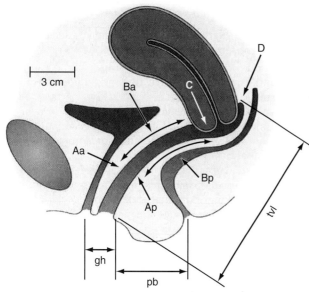

Figure 39-7. POP-Q site-specific points. (From Bump RC, Mattiasson A, Bø K, et al: The standardization of terminology of female pelvic organ prolapse and pelvic floor dysfunction. *Am J Obstet Gynecol* 175:10, 1996. Copyright ©1996 Mosby, Inc.)

- Distal points assigned positive values (Figure 39-7)
  - Anterior sites
    - Point Aa: located 3 cm proximal to external urethral meatus on anterior vaginal wall, corresponds to urethrovesical crease
    - Range: −3 to +3
    - Point Ba: represents the most distal position of any part for upper anterior vaginal wall, up to the vaginal cuff/anterior vaginal fornix
    - Range: −3 to +total vaginal length (TVL)
  - Apical sites
    - Point C: represents most distal edge of cervix or leading edge of vaginal cuff after total hysterectomy
    - Range: −TVL to +TVL
    - Point D: represents posterior fornix in women with cervix present; omitted if no cervix present; represents level of uterosacral attachment to cervix, and can help distinguish between cervical elongation and a level I defect
    - Range: −TVL to +TVL
  - Posterior sites
    - Point Ap: located midline of posterior vaginal wall, 3 cm proximal to hymen
    - Range: −3 to +3
    - Point Bp: point of most distal (most dependent) aspect of upper posterior wall proximal to point Ap
    - Range: −3 to + TVL
  - TVL: greatest depth of vagina when cervix/vaginal vault fully reduced (no range)
  - Genital hiatus (GH): measured from midportion of external urethral meatus to the posterior hymen
  - Perineal body (PB): measured from posterior hymen to midanus (Table 39-2)
- Stages of pelvic organ prolapse by POP-Q system
  - Stage 0: No prolapse is demonstrated; points Aa, Ap, Ba, and Bp are all at −3 cm, and either point C or D is between −TVL (total vaginal length) cm and −(TVL-2) cm

TABLE 39-2 Pelvic Organ Prolapse Quantification Exam Grid

Anterior wall Aa	Anterior wall Ba	Cervix or cuff C
Genital hiatus GH	Perineal body Pb	Total vaginal length tvl
Posterior wall Ap	Posterior wall Bp	Posterior fornix D

(quantitation value for point Aa, Ap, Ba, Bp = −3, and value for point C or D is ≤−[TVL-2] cm)
- Stage I: the criteria for stage 0 are not met, most distal portion of the prolapse is >1 cm above the level of the hymen (value is <−1 cm)
- Stage II: the most distal portion of the prolapse is ≤1 cm proximal to or distal to the plane of the hymen (value is ≥−1 cm but ≤+1 cm)
- Stage III: the most distal portion of the prolapse is >1 cm below the plane of the hymen but protrudes no further than 2 cm less than the total vaginal length in centimeters (value >+1 cm but <+[TVL-2] cm)
- Stage IV: complete eversion of the total length of the lower genital tract is demonstrated; the distal portion of the prolapse protrudes to at least (TVL-2) cm (value is ≥+[TVL-2] cm)

MANAGEMENT
Conservative Management of Pelvic Organ Prolapse

- Expectant management
  - Regression of prolapse may occur in postmenopausal women with prolapse proximal to hymen
  - Regression with higher stage prolapse is less likely
- Pessary
  - Success rate approximately 62%
  - Candidates
    - Preference for nonsurgical approach
    - Poor surgical candidates
    - Desire for future childbearing
  - Contraindications
    - Mesh erosion
    - Severe vaginal erosion
  - Risk factors for failure
    - Short vaginal length (≤ 6 cm)
    - Widened genital hiatus/introitus (≥4 fingerbreadths in width)
  - Types
    - Support pessaries (two dimensional): fill the vertical axis of vagina
      Examples: Ring, Shaatz, dish
    - Space occupying (three dimensional): best for severe prolapse
      Examples: Gellhorn, cube, donut, inflatoball
  - Risks
    - Vaginal erosion/bleeding
      - Can be mitigated with concomitant local estrogen therapy
      - May require pessary-free interval for healing
    - Vaginal infections
    - Urinary tract infections

Surgical Management

- Anterior compartment
  - Standard anterior colporrhaphy with midline plication
    - Success rates range from 42% to 100% in published literature
  - Augmentation with graft material for anterior wall defects:
    - Several small studies show improved success compared to anterior colporrhaphy
  - Addition of polyglactin mesh versus no mesh
    - 25% versus 45% recurrence (beyond midvaginal plane) at 1 year p = 0.02
    - Findings confirmed in Cochrane database meta-analysis: higher recurrence of traditional anterior colporrhaphy compared to polyglactin inlay (relative risk [RR] 1.39)
  - Addition of porcine collagen implant (Pelvicol) versus standard anterior repair
    - 7% versus 19% recurrence (Ba>−1) p = 0.019
  - Addition of nonabsorbable mesh (polypropylene) versus standard anterior repair (two trials)
    - No recurrence with mesh versus 33% with standard anterior repair, 25% mesh erosion
    - 7% versus 38% recurrence, 17% mesh erosion
- Abdominal paravaginal repair (Richardson)
  - Success rate 75% to 97% (case series)
  - Abdominal procedure in retropubic space
  - Corrects lateral defect by reattaching paravaginal fascia to arcus tendineus fascia pelvis (ATFP)
  - Obturator nerve is susceptible to injury, lies lateral to ATFP
- Vaginal paravaginal repair (Shull)
  - Success rate 67% to 100% (case series)
  - Usually graft augmented with concomitant bilateral sacrospinous vault suspension
  - Corrects lateral defect and suspends apex
  - Involves dissection of vaginal epithelium off anterior wall and attaching trapezoidal graft to ATFP and sacrospinous ligament
  - Pudendal neurovascular bundle susceptible to injury during sacrospinous suturing; therefore, sutures are placed medial to ischial spine

Apical Compartment

- Colpocleisis
  - Obliterative procedure for nonsexually active women
  - Involves removal of vaginal epithelium and imbrication of vaginal muscularis, partial colpocleisis leaves lateral tunnels to allow for drainage
  - Success rates 90% to 100%
  - Regret 0% to 13%
  - Low morbidity
  - No evidence that concomitant hysterectomy improves success
  - Ninety percent resolution of preoperative urinary retention
- Abdominal sacral colpopexy (ASCP)
  - Abdominal procedure that involves synthetic mesh attachment to anterior and posterior aspects of vagina distally and to anterior longitudinal ligament of sacrum proximally

- Considered most durable procedure for apical prolapse
- Success rates 76% to 100%
- Risks
  - Presacral hemorrhage from presacral plexus and middle sacral artery (bone tacks, bone wax, indirect coagulation, thrombin)
  - Mesh erosion (3%)

UPDATE #8

Burch colposuspension reduces postoperative symptoms of stress incontinence in stress-continent women undergoing abdominal sacrocolpopexy (Brubaker et al, 2006).

Results from the Colpopexy and Urinary Reduction Efforts (CARE) trial demonstrated reduction of bothersome stress incontinence symptoms (6% versus 25%) and stress incontinence prevalence at 3 months (24% versus 44%) with performing a concomitant Burch procedure with sacrocolpopexy in stress continent women. Based on results of this study, women should be offered Burch colposuspension at time of sacrocolpopexy irrespective of urodynamic testing results for stress incontinence. No large published randomized trials exist for concomitant transvaginal midurethral sling procedures in stress continent women, but such procedures may present a viable option. In addition, although data is limited, practitioners may consider offering stress continent patients with prolapse undergoing vaginal reconstructive procedures a concomitant anti-incontinence procedure if they have occult stress incontinence. Another approach would be undergoing a staged procedure for symptomatic stress urinary incontinence post-operatively.

- Sacrospinous ligament vault suspension
  - Vaginal procedure for vault prolapse, which may be performed unilaterally or bilaterally
  - Requires opening pararectal space and isolation of sacrospinous ligament
  - Approximates vaginal apex to sacrospinous ligament
  - Success rates: 63% to 97%
  - Pudendal neurovascular bundle susceptible to injury
  - Sacral root/sciatic nerve injury: can result in entrapment syndrome with severe buttock pain radiating down posterior leg, requires immediate suture removal
- Uterosacral vault suspension
  - Vaginal procedure, which enters peritoneal cavity
  - Three permanent sutures placed on each uterosacral ligament
  - Sutures are placed through anterior and posterior endopelvic fascia
  - Success rates 85% to 89%
  - Ureters susceptible to injury, lie approximately 1.5 cm lateral to sutures
  - Cystoscopy performed with sutures on tension to evaluate for ureteral obstruction
  - Sacral nerves also susceptible if suture placement laterally (presents with sensory neuropathy); therefore, place sutures medial and posterior to ischial spine

UPDATE #9

Abdominal sacrocolpopexy is associated with a lower rate of recurrent vault prolapse and dyspareunia than vaginal sacrospinous colpopexy (Benson et al, 1996; Maher et al, 2004, 2008).

- Summary of findings
  - Surgical effectiveness (asymptomatic, <50% vault inversion/supported above levator place, no prolapse beyond hymen) 58% versus 29% abdominal versus vaginal (Benson et al, 1996)
  - Reoperation 16% versus 33%
  - Recurrent incontinence 2% versus 12%
  - Subjective success (not symptomatic) 94% versus 91% abdominal versus vaginal p = 0.19 (Maher et al, 2004)
  - Objective success (no prolapse beyond halfway point of vagina): 76% versus 61% p = 0.48
  - Operating time: 106 versus 76 (min) p < 0.01
  - Return to activities of daily living: 34 versus 25 days p < 0.01
  - Average cost: $6450 versus $4575 p < 0.01

A 2007 Cochrane database review combined these studies and confirmed lower rates of recurrent vault prolapse, postoperative dyspareunia, and postoperative stress incontinence, as well as longer operating time, longer time to recover, and greater cost with abdominal surgery. Subjective success and reoperation rates were not statistically different. Benefits of abdominal surgery need to be balanced with the risks of longer operating time, cost, and recovery. These factors should be discussed with patients to meet their individual goals and expectations.

- Uterine prolapse
  - Usually managed in combination with approach for vault prolapse
  - Abdominal sacrohysteropexy associated with a greater reoperation rate for recurrent uterine prolapse

UPDATE #10

McCall culdoplasty is recommended at time of vaginal hysterectomy for prevention of enterocele formation (Cruikshank et al, 1998).

McCall-type culdoplasty is superior to prevent subsequent enterocele versus simple peritoneal closure or Moschcowitz-type procedure at time of vaginal hysterectomy. Two-year data showed 6% stage I or greater prolapse with McCall culdoplasty versus 17% with Moschcowitz and 65% with simple peritoneal closure.

- Robotic surgery
- Advantages of robotic versus traditional laparoscopy
  - Intuitive movements: "wristed instruments" with increased degrees of freedom
  - Enhanced 12× magnification
  - Three-dimensional depth perception
  - Tremor filtration
  - Enhanced surgeon comfort/ergonomics
- Disadvantages
  - Steep learning curve
  - Cost
  - Prolonged operating time
  - Absence of haptic/tactile feedback

Robotic-assisted laparoscopic hysterectomy not found to be superior to laparoscopic hysterectomy.

Several case series demonstrated that robotic-assisted sacrocolpopexy is feasible with no significantly increased adverse events. A case-control study by Geller et al. compared robotic sacrocolpopexy to conventional sacrocolpopexy. The authors demonstrated a statistically significant lower blood loss, shorter length of stay, and improvement in point C by the POP-Q staging system, but also a statistically significant increase in operative time and higher incidence of postoperative fever.

There have been no published prospective randomized trials comparing either laparoscopic or robotic ASCP to conventional ASCP.

- Posterior compartment
  - Standard posterior colporrhaphy
    - A Cochrane review concluded that the vaginal approach to rectocele or enterocele repair was associated with lower recurrence than transanal approach (RR 0.24, 95% confidence interval [CI] 0.09 to 0.64); recurrence rate 15%
  - Site-specific defect repair
    - Defect approach requires identification of discrete tears in the rectovaginal septum (apical, central, lateral, or distal), and then one or more discrete sites are repaired, thus avoiding a mass closure
    - Recurrence rate 18%
  - Graft augmentation
    - To date, no randomized trials support the use of graft augmentation for rectocele repair; current evidence supports suture only repair over augmentation with porcine small intestines
  - Prolapse repair kits
    - Commercially marketed to duplicate the success of midurethral slings; safety and outcome data lacking; these procedures remain without enough data to merit recommendation.

UPDATE #11

The Society for Gynecologic Surgeons publishes clinical practice guidelines on the use of vaginal mesh (Murphy et al, 2008).

RECOMMENDATIONS

- Native tissue repair is appropriate compared to biologic or absorbable synthetic mesh in the anterior compartment (weak)
- Nonabsorbable synthetic mesh may improve outcomes in the anterior compartment, with significant trade-offs with adverse events (weak)
- Native tissue repair is recommended in the posterior compartment compared to biologic, absorbable synthetic, or nonabsorbable synthetic graft (weak)

TYPES OF RECONSTRUCTIVE MATERIALS

- Synthetic mesh: includes absorbable and nonabsorbable options; risk of infection decreased with large pore size, loose weave, low mesh density, and monofilament structure
- Autografts: harvested from patient at time of surgery (fascia lata, rectus fascia)
- Allografts: harvested from human cadaver
- Xenografts: nonhuman source (bovine, porcine), theoretic risks of infectious transmission

Due to additional 2500+ reported complications since 2008, FDA states that complications are "not rare" and include:

- Mesh erosion
- Infection
- Dyspareunia/pain due to mesh contracture
- Injury to bowel/bladder/vessels/nerves from minimally invasive placement kits
- Repeat surgery necessary to manage above complications
- Abdominally placed mesh for prolapse has lower risks than vaginal mesh
- FDA to present further recommendations on transvaginal mesh (sling procedures) for stress incontinence

RECOMMENDATIONS

- Use mesh with caution and in carefully selected patients
- Consider nonmesh repairs
- Obtain specialized training in placement/use of mesh kits
- Provide patient with product labeling information
- Inform patient of potential serious, irreversible complications that may require further surgery

Anal Incontinence (AI)

CLINICAL PROFILE

- Complaint of involuntary loss of feces or flatus
- Prevalence 9%
- Continence requires normal stool consistency, intact neurovascular supply, anorectal sensation plus a coordinated rectum, puborectalis, and anal sphincter
- Risk factors
  - Age
  - Childbirth (forceps, macrosomia, and episiotomy increase risk)
    - Thirty-five percent of primiparous and 45% of multiparous women have ultrasound-proven sphincter defects after vaginal delivery; only a third of these women are symptomatic (Sultan et al, 1993)
  - Diarrheal states
  - Fecal impaction and overflow
  - Fistula
    - Occur following obstetric trauma, pressure necrosis, unsuccessful primary repair of third- and fourth-degree laceration, postsurgical, neoplastic, radiation, diverticulitis, and inflammatory bowel disease
  - Hemorrhoids
  - Inflammatory bowel diseases
  - Neurologic diseases
  - Rectal neoplasia
  - Rectal prolapse
  - Trauma (nonobstetric)
  - Urinary incontinence

DIAGNOSIS

- Differentiate flatal, liquid, or solid incontinence
- Obstetric history, mode of delivery, episiotomy, birth weight
- Neurologic history and screening neurologic exam
- Digital rectal exam, exclude mass, hemorrhoids, rectal mucosal prolapse, and assess resting and squeeze tone
- Inspection for fistula
  - Anovaginal fistula within the first 3 cm of anal orifice below dentate line; fistulas above dentate line are rectovaginal; tender tract from anus to skin is a fistula-in-ano and is commonly inflammatory; simple and pinpoint fistulas can be difficult to isolate; colposcopy, transrectal methylene blue enema, endoanal sonography with peroxide solution, and examination under anesthesia with sigmoid scope and air insufflation can improve detection; high vaginal fistula or size greater than 2.5 cm are considered complex
- Endoanal ultrasound to detect internal and external sphincter lacerations
- Neurophysiologic (electromyography and manometry) testing may aid in counseling

MANAGEMENT

- Most modifiable factor is stool consistency
  - High fiber to bulk stool
  - Reduction of motility with medications, loperamide hydrochloride (Imodium), and diphenoxylate hydrochloride (Lomotil)
- Pelvic floor exercises, biofeedback, and electrical stimulation
  - Anal sphincter strengthening
  - Coordination of distension and contraction (rectoanal coordination)
  - Rectal sensory perception
  - Improvement with biofeedback reported between 63% to 90%
- Anal sphincteroplasty
  - Overlapping
  - End to end
    - Three randomized studies show similar success between overlapping and end to end; despite either repair, 25% to 59% of patients have persistent symptoms; long-term outcomes for sphincteroplasty are discouraging with 0% to 28% continence at 10 years; research using myoblast transplantation and stem cell therapeutics holds future promise
- Repair of fistula
  - Active infection completely treated prior to closure
  - Preoperative broad-spectrum antibiotics
  - Sphincter imaging preoperatively
  - Mobilization with wide dissection
  - Excision of fistula tract
  - Multiple layer closure without overlapping suture lines
  - Tension-free repair
  - Vascularized tissue or martius flap if deficient
  - Rectal mucosa advancement flap can be done concurrently
  - Diversion/colostomy in recurrent and complex cases
  - Postoperative management includes maintenance of loose stools with fiber and softeners to eliminate straining; no consensus exists on type or duration of postoperative antibiotics

- Repair of rectal prolapse
- Sacral nerve stimulation

UPDATE #13

Sacral nerve stimulation is a safe and effective treatment for patients with AI. It has been approved in Europe since 1994. A multicenter prospective study of 120 patients included a mean follow-up at 28 months. Patients were excluded if the anal sphincter defect was over 60 degrees. Therapeutic success was 85% at 2 years, and incontinence episodes reduced from 9.4 to 2.9 per week. No adverse device effects were reported. Sacral nerve modulation was FDA approved for AI in the United States in 2011 (Wexner et al, 2010).

- Artificial anal sphincter
- Colostomy

SUGGESTED READINGS

Urinary Incontinence

Albo ME, Richter HE, Brubaker L, et al: Burch colposuspension versus fascial sling to reduce urinary stress incontinence, *N Engl J Med* 356(21):2143–2155, 2007.

Aldridge AH: Transplantation of fascia for relief of urinary stress incontinence, *Am J Obstet Gynecol* 44:398–411, 1943.

Brubaker L, Richter HE, Visco A, et al: Refractory idiopathic urge incontinence and botulinum A injection, *J Urol* 180(1):217–222, 2008.

Crystle CD, Charme LS, Copeland WE: Q-tip test in stress urinary incontiennce, *Obstet Gynecol* 38:313–315, 1971.

Haylen BT, Ridder DD, Freeman RM, et al: An International Urogynecological Association (IUGA)/International Continence Society (ICS) joint report on the terminology for female pelvic floor dysfunction, *Neurourol Urodyn* 29(1):4–20, 2010.

Nygard I, Barber MD, Burgio KL, et al: Prevalence of symptomatic pelvic floor disorders in US women, *JAMA* 300(11):1311–1316, 2008.

Schierlitz L, Dwyer PL, Rosamilia A, et al: Effectiveness of tension-free vaginal tape compared with transobturator tape in women with stress urinary incontinence and intrinsic sphincter deficiency: a randomized controlled trial, *Obstet Gynecol* 112(6):1253–1261, 2008.

Subak LL, Wing R, Smith West D, et al: Weight loss to treat urinary incontinence in overweight and obese women, *N Engl J Med* 360(5):481–490, 2009.

Tanagho EA: Colpocystourethropexy: the way we do it, *J Urol* 116:751–753, 1976.

Ulmsten UI, Petros P: Intravaginal slingplasty (IVS): an ambulatory surgical procedure for treatment of female urinary incontinence, *Scand J Urol Nephrol* 29(1):75–82, 1995.

van Kerrebroeck PE, van Voskuilen AC, Heesakkers JP, et al: Results of sacral neuromodulation therapy for urinary voiding dysfunction: outcomes of a prospective, worldwide clinical study, *J Urol* 178(5):2020–2034, 2007.

Ward KL, Hilton P, UK and Ireland TVT Trial Group. Tension-free vaginal tape versus colposuspension for primary urodynamic stress incontinence: 5 year follow up, *BJOG* 115(2):226–233, 2007.

Pelvic Organ Prolapse

Benson JT, Lucente V, McClellan E: Vaginal versus abdominal reconstructive surgery for the treatment of pelvic support defects: a prospective randomized study with long term outcome evaluation, *Am J Obstet Gynecol* 175(6):1418–1422, 1996.

Brubaker L, Cundiff GW, Fine P, et al: Abdominal sacrocolpopexy with Burch colposuspension to reduce urinary stress incontinence, *N Engl J Med* 354(15):1557–1566, 2006.

Bump RC, Mattiasson A, Bø K, et al: The standardization of terminology of female pelvic organ prolapse and pelvic floor dysfunction, *Am J Obstet Gynecol* 175(1):10–17, 1996.

Cruikshank S, Kovac SR: Randomized comparison of three surgical methods used at the time of vaginal hysterectomy to prevent posterior enterocele, *Am J Obstet Gynecol* 180(4):859–865, 1999.

Maher C, Baessler K, Glazener C, et al: Surgical management of pelvic organ prolapse in women: a short version Cochrane review, *Neurourol Urodyn* 27(1):3–12, 2008.

Maher CF, Qatawneh AM, Dwyer PL, et al: Abdominal sacral colpopexy or vaginal sacrospinous colpopexy for vaginal vault prolapse: a prospective randomized study, *Am J Obstet Gynecol* 190(1):20–26, 2004.

Murphy M, Society of Gynecologic Surgeons Systematic Review Group. Clinical practice guidelines on vaginal graft use from the society of gynecologic surgeons, *Obstet Gynecol* 112(5):1123–1130, 2008.

U.S. Department of Health and Human Services, U.S. Food and Drug Administration: *FDA Safety Communication: UPDATE on Serious Complications Associated with Transvaginal Placement of Surgical Mesh for Pelvic Organ Prolapse* (website). http://www.fda.gov/MedicalDevices/Safety/AlertsandNotices//UCM262435.htm. July 2011.

Weber AM, Walters MD, Piedmonte MR, Ballard LA: Anterior colporrhaphy: a randomized trial of three surgical techniques, *Am J Obstet Gynecol* 185(6):1299–1306, 2001.

Anal Incontinence

Lorenzi B, Pessina F, Lorenzoni P, et al: Treatment of experimental injury of anal sphincters with primary surgical repair and injection of bone marrow-derived mesenchymal stem cells, *Dis Colon Rectum* 51(4):411–420, 2008.

Sultan AH, Kamm MA, Hudson CN, et al: Anal sphincter disruption during vaginal delivery, *New Engl J Med* 329:1905–1911, 1993.

Wexner SD, Coller JA, Devroede G, et al: Sacral nerve stimulation for fecal incontinence, *Ann Surg* 251(3):441–449, 2010.

Chapter 40

Perioperative Care

STEVEN A. VASILEV

KEY UPDATES

1 Pneumatic compression devices should be activated before induction of anesthesia to achieve maximum thromboprophylactic effect.

2 Patients undergoing laparoscopy should be categorized according to risk of thromboembolic complications and provided thromboprophylaxis similar to patients undergoing laparotomy with the same risk factor category.

3 Very high risk patients should be considered for dual modality thromboprophylaxis.

4 Single-dose antibiotic prophylaxis for hysterectomy, regardless of route of surgery, should be administered within 1 hour of incision.

5 Assess for presence of chronic obstructive pulmonary disease, age greater than 60 years, American Society of Anesthesiologists (ASA) class of II or greater, functional dependency, and congestive heart failure as indications for perioperative risk reducing interventions.

6 Most routine medications patients take can be continued and administered up to the morning of surgery (major exceptions are specifically noted).

7 Primary prevention of coronary ischemia with beta-blockers should be considered in high-risk patients who have more than one risk factor.

8 Plavix (clopidogrel) effectiveness can be reduced by the Prilosec (omeprazole) stomach acid reducing agent.

9 Up to 70% of preoperative patients do not disclose herbal and supplement use unless asked specifically, and many of these substances can adversely affect perioperative outcomes.

The following guidelines and recommendations regarding perioperative care are focused on gynecologic surgery, but in some areas the data are drawn from surgical patients in general who undergo abdominal and pelvic surgery. If nongynecologic components are to be performed during a gynecologic surgery, such as vascular or urologic surgery, specific guidelines should be reviewed for additional details.

Venous Thromboembolism Prophylaxis

Recommendations for thromboprophylaxis are based on type of surgery and additional well-defined risk factors:

- Low risk: surgery time less than 30 minutes in length, in patients younger than 40 years with no additional risk factors
- Moderate risk: surgery time less than 30 minutes in patients with additional risk factors; surgery time less than 30 minutes in patients age 40 to 60 years with no additional risk factors; major surgery in patients younger than 40 years with no additional risk factors
- High risk: surgery time less than 30 minutes in patients older than 60 years or with additional risk factors; major

surgery in patients older than 40 years or with additional risk factors
- Highest risk: major surgery in patients older than 60 years plus prior venous thromboembolism, cancer, or hypercoagulable state

VENOUS THROMBOEMBOLISM RISK FACTORS

- Surgery
- Trauma (major or lower extremity)
- Immobility, paresis
- Obesity
- Malignancy
- Cancer therapy (hormonal, chemotherapy, or radiotherapy)
- Acute medical illness
- Previous venous thromboembolism
- Increasing age
- Pregnancy and the postpartum period
- Estrogen-containing oral contraception or hormone therapy

- Selective estrogen receptor modulators
- Heart or respiratory failure
- Inflammatory bowel disease
- Myeloproliferative disorders
- Paroxysmal nocturnal hemoglobinuria
- Nephrotic syndrome
- Smoking
- Varicose veins
- Central venous catheterization
- Inherited or acquired thrombophilia

The following recommendations are based on good and consistent scientific evidence:

- Thromboprophylaxis for moderate-risk patients undergoing gynecologic surgery includes the following options:
  - Graduated compression stockings placed before initiation of surgery and continued until the patient is fully ambulatory
  - Pneumatic compression devices ideally placed and activated prior to induction of anesthesia and continued until the patient is fully ambulatory
  - Unfractionated heparin (5000 units) administered subcutaneously 2 hours before surgery and every 12 hours after surgery until discharge
  - Low-molecular-weight heparin administered subcutaneously, 12 hours before surgery and once a day postoperatively until discharge

UPDATE #1

Pneumatic compression devices should be activated before induction of anesthesia to achieve maximum thromboprophylactic effect (Caprini, 2010; Geerts et al, 2004).

- Thromboprophylaxis for high-risk patients undergoing gynecologic surgery, especially for malignancy, includes the following options:
  - Pneumatic compression devices placed before surgery and continued until hospital discharge
  - Unfractionated heparin (5000 units) administered subcutaneously 2 hours before surgery and every 8 hours postoperatively and continued until discharge
  - Low-molecular weight-heparin administered subcutaneously, 12 hours before surgery and once daily postoperatively until discharge

The following recommendations are based on limited scientific evidence:

- Thromboprophylaxis for highest-risk patients includes the following options:
  - Combination prophylaxis (such as the combination of pneumatic compression device and either low-dose unfractionated heparin or low-molecular-weight heparin)
  - Consideration of continuing low-molecular-weight heparin prophylaxis as an outpatient for up to 28 days postoperatively
- If administration of low-molecular-weight heparin 12 hours before surgery is impractical, initial dose should be given 6 to 12 hours postoperatively
- Low-risk patients who are undergoing gynecologic surgery do not require specific prophylaxis other than early

ambulation; this includes short minor vaginal procedures; however, observational studies suggest that the incidence of thromboembolic complications after sling procedures for incontinence is approximately 1%; when concomitant prolapse surgery is performed, the odds ratio almost triples, suggesting the need for thromboprophylaxis with complex vaginal surgery

- Patients undergoing laparoscopic surgery should be categorized by risk (and provided thromboprophylaxis) similar to patients undergoing the same surgery by laparotomy route

UPDATE #2

Patients undergoing laparoscopy should be categorized according to risk of thromboembolic complications and provided thromboprophylaxis similar to patients undergoing laparotomy with the same risk factor category (Kakkos et al, 2008).

SPECIFIC INTERVENTION BENEFITS

- *Graduated compression stockings.* These stockings prevent blood pooling in the calves; low cost and ease of use are the main advantages of using graduated compression stockings; knee-length stockings are just as effective as thigh-length stockings.
- *Pneumatic compression.* Intermittent pneumatic compression devices reduce stasis by regularly compressing the calves. When used during and after major gynecologic surgery, the devices are just as effective as low-dose heparin and low-molecular-weight heparin in reducing venous thrombosis.
- *Low-dose unfractionated heparin.* Two large meta-analyses of randomized clinical trials of patients who had undergone general surgery showed a two-thirds reduction in fatal pulmonary embolism with the use of low-dose unfractionated heparin every 8 hours compared with placebo or no prophylaxis. Advantages of low-dose unfractionated heparin include well-studied efficacy and low cost.
- *Low-molecular-weight heparin.* Advantages of low-molecular-weight heparin include greater bioavailability and a once-daily dosage, although the drug itself is more expensive. These benefits result from a longer half-life, more predictable pharmacokinetics, and equivalent efficacy when compared with prophylactic use of low-dose unfractionated heparin. Low-molecular-weight heparin has more antifactor-Xa and less antithrombin activity than low-dose unfractionated heparin, which may decrease medical bleeding and wound hematoma formation. Heparin-induced thrombocytopenia is rarely observed with short-term use of low-molecular-weight heparin, and screening for this is not required.
- *Combined modality prophylaxis.* Although data from randomized trials in gynecology patients are lacking, a combined approach using stockings/devices and heparin seems appropriate in the highest-risk patients, and the Seventh American College of Chest Physicians Consensus Conference recommends this practice. To support this approach, the Cochrane group reviewed 11 studies, 6 of which were randomized controlled trials. The trials included 7431 patients in total. Compared with compression alone, the use of combined modalities

reduced significantly the incidence of both symptomatic pulmonary embolism (PE) (from about 3% to 1%; odds ratio [OR] 0.39, 95% confidence interval [CI] 0.25 to 0.63) and deep vein thrombosis (DVT) (from about 4% to 1%; OR 0.43, 95% CI 0.24 to 0.76). Compared with pharmacologic prophylaxis alone, the use of combined modalities significantly reduced the incidence of DVT (from 4.21% to 0.65%; OR 0.16, 95% CI 0.07 to 0.34), but the included studies were underpowered with regard to PE. The comparison of compression plus pharmacologic prophylaxis versus compression plus aspirin showed a nonsignificant reduction in PE and DVT in favor of the former group. Compared with compression alone, combined prophylaxis significantly decreased the incidence of venous thromboembolism.

UPDATE #3
Very high risk patients should be considered for dual modality thromboprophylaxis (Kakkos et al, 2008).

SPECIFIC INTERVENTION RISKS
- Improperly fitted stockings may act as a tourniquet at the knee or mid-thigh, causing an increase in venous stasis
- Blood loss during surgery does not seem to be increased by the preoperative use of low-dose unfractionated heparin administration
- An increase in *post*operative bleeding has been noted, specifically in wound hematoma formation.
- Use of heparin for more than 4 days warrants monitoring of platelet counts because 6% of patients will experience heparin-induced thrombocytopenia

Antibiotic Prophylaxis

The following recommendations and conclusions are based on good and consistent scientific evidence:
- Patients undergoing hysterectomy, regardless of route, should receive single-dose antimicrobial prophylaxis preoperatively
- Antibiotic prophylaxis is indicated for elective suction curettage abortion
- Antibiotic prophylaxis is not recommended in patients undergoing *diagnostic* laparoscopy

UPDATE #4
Single-dose antibiotic prophylaxis for hysterectomy, regardless of route of surgery, should be administered within 1 hour of incision (American College of Obstetricians and Gynecologists, ACOG Committee on Practice Bulletins—Gynecology, Practice Bulletin No. 104, 2009).

The following recommendations and conclusions are based on limited or inconsistent scientific evidence:
- In patients with no history of pelvic infection, hysterosalpingography (HSG) can be performed without prophylactic antibiotics. If HSG demonstrates dilated fallopian tubes, antibiotic prophylaxis should be given to reduce the incidence of post-HSG pelvic inflammatory disease (PID).

- Routine antibiotic prophylaxis is not recommended for the general patient population undergoing hysteroscopic surgery.
- Cephalosporin prophylaxis is acceptable in those patients with a history of penicillin allergy not felt to be immunoglobulin E mediated (immediate hypersensitivity).
- Patients found to have preoperative bacterial vaginosis should be treated before hysterectomy.
- Randomized controlled data involving antibiotics for vaginal surgery other than hysterectomy, hysteroscopic surgery, and suction curettage are limited. However, based on available data, the American Urological Association (AUA) guidelines recommend antibiotic prophylaxis for urology-related vaginal procedures, on the strength of evidence for vaginal hysterectomy, which is considered to have a similar infection risk profile. Parenthetically, the AUA guidelines do not recommend antibiotic prophylaxis for uncomplicated cystourethroscopy with negative urine cultures.

The following recommendations and conclusions are based primarily on consensus and expert opinion:
- Antibiotic prophylaxis is not recommended in patients undergoing exploratory laparotomy.
- For transcervical procedures such as HSG, chromotubation, and hysteroscopy, prophylaxis may be considered in those patients with a history of PID or tubal damage noted at the time of the procedure.
- Patients with a history of an immediate hypersensitivity reaction to penicillin should not receive cephalosporin antibiotics.

Pulmonary Assessment

Perioperative recommendations regarding pulmonary risk assessment and resulting risk-reducing strategies are limited by a lack of randomized controlled data. However, the following are prudent measures recommended by the American College of Physicians.
- All patients undergoing noncardiothoracic surgery should be evaluated for the presence of the following significant risk factors for postoperative pulmonary complications in order to receive pre- and postoperative interventions to reduce pulmonary risk: chronic obstructive pulmonary disease, age older than 60 years, American Society of Anesthesiologists (ASA) class of II or greater, functional dependency, and congestive heart failure.
- Obesity and mild or moderate asthma are *not* significant risk factors for postoperative pulmonary complications.

UPDATE #5
Assess for the presence of chronic obstructive pulmonary disease, age greater than 60 years, American Society of Anesthesiologists (ASA) class of II or greater, functional dependency, and congestive heart failure as indications for perioperative risk-reducing interventions (Qaseem et al, 2006).

- Patients undergoing the following procedures are at higher risk for postoperative pulmonary complications and should be evaluated for other concomitant risk factors and receive pre- and postoperative interventions to reduce pulmonary complications: prolonged surgery (>3 hours), abdominal surgery, emergency surgery, and general anesthesia.

- A low serum albumin level (<3.5 g/dL) is a powerful marker of increased risk for postoperative pulmonary complications and should be measured in all patients who are clinically suspected of having hypoalbuminemia; measurement should be considered in patients with one or more risk factors for perioperative pulmonary complications.

- All patients who after preoperative evaluation are found to be at higher risk for postoperative pulmonary complications should receive the following postoperative procedures to reduce postoperative pulmonary complications: (1) deep breathing exercises or incentive spirometry and (2) highly limited use of a nasogastric (NG) tube (as needed for overt postoperative nausea or vomiting, inability to tolerate oral intake, or symptomatic abdominal distention; the tube should be removed as soon as possible, as the presence of an NG tube can paradoxically increase the risk of aspiration).

- Preoperative spirometry and chest radiography should *not* be used routinely for predicting risk for postoperative pulmonary complications.

- Preoperative pulmonary function testing or chest radiography may be appropriate in patients with a previous diagnosis of chronic obstructive pulmonary disease or asthma.

The following procedures should not be used solely for reducing postoperative pulmonary complication risk: (1) right-heart catheterization and (2) total parenteral nutrition or total enteral nutrition (for patients who are malnourished or have low serum albumin levels).

Cardiovascular Assessment

Myocardial hypoxia remains the major cardiac risk in gynecologic surgery. The reported incidence rate of perioperative infarction is approximately 0.15% to 2%. However, patients with a history of previous myocardial infarction have a 6.6% chance of having a second postoperative infarction.

If surgery is performed within 6 months of an infarction, these patients are at significant risk for reinfarction. In such cases, postponing elective surgery for at least 6 months is advisable. Likewise, unstable angina of less than 3 months' duration is an absolute contraindication to noncardiac surgery except in the emergency setting.

- Active cardiac conditions for which the patient should undergo evaluation and treatment before noncardiac surgery condition
  - Unstable coronary syndromes (e.g., unstable or severe angina, recent myocardial infarction [MI] <30 days)
  - Decompensated heart failure (HF) (New York Heart Association [NYHA] functional class IV; worsening or new-onset HF)
  - Significant arrhythmias (e.g., high-grade atrioventricular block, Mobitz II atrioventricular block, third-degree atrioventricular heart block, symptomatic ventricular arrhythmias, supraventricular arrhythmias [including atrial fibrillation] with uncontrolled ventricular rate [heart rate {HR} greater than 100 beats per minute at rest], symptomatic bradycardia, newly recognized ventricular tachycardia)
  - Severe valvular disease (e.g., severe aortic stenosis [mean pressure gradient greater than 40 mmHg], aortic valve area less than 1.0 cm², or symptomatic), symptomatic mitral stenosis (progressive dyspnea on exertion, exertional presyncope, or HF)

Perioperative Medication Management

Routine medications that patients take may interact with drugs used during surgery. This is a much broader topic than others reviewed in this chapter, and strict recommendations are more limited due to the complex effects of many drugs, dosing, absorption differences, and duration of therapy. The following represent major areas of concern that are based on best available evidence.

UPDATE #6

Most routine medications patients take can be continued and administered up to the morning of surgery (major exceptions are specifically noted) (Fleisher et al, 2007).

Many routine medications can and should be continued through the perioperative period, with the last dose being possible within 2 hours of a procedure. Liquids are cleared from the stomach within 2 hours, and there are no stomach fluid volume or pH differences between patients who stop taking clear fluids 9 hours before surgery (i.e., approaching the traditional nothing by mouth (NPO) after midnight recommendation).

CARDIOVASCULAR SYSTEM

Beta-Blockers

Ischemia frequently presents atypically, with chest pain occurring only 50% of the time. Beta-blockers provide the single best therapy for prevention of ischemia during the perioperative period. Recommendations are now stratified based on primary or secondary prevention, and extreme caution should be applied in patients with decompensated heart failure, nonischemic cardiomyopathy, or severe valvular heart disease in the absence of coronary heart disease.

When used for primary prevention, a beta-blockade should ideally be initiated several weeks before surgery and titrated to a resting heart rate of 60 beats per minute. The last dose can be taken with sips of water on the morning of surgery.

Beta-blockers should be continued in patients undergoing surgery who are already receiving them to treat angina, symptomatic arrhythmias, hypertension, or other cardiac disease.

UPDATE #7

Primary prevention of coronary ischemia with beta-blockers should be considered in high-risk patients who have more than one risk factor (Fleisher et al, 2007).

Beta-blockers are probably recommended for patients in whom preoperative assessment identifies coronary heart disease or high cardiac risk, as defined by the presence of more than one clinical risk factor.

Hypertension

Patients with elevated blood pressure are more likely to experience significant fluctuations in intraoperative blood pressure and associated MI. Adequate blood pressure control is essential prior to elective surgeries because this reduces perioperative ischemia and subsequent cardiac morbidity.

Antihypertensive medications should be continued throughout the perioperative period, with a change of formulation or substitution if needed. Abrupt withdrawal of beta-blocking agents may adversely affect the heart rate and blood pressure and may precipitate MI.

Antihypertensive medications, except diuretics, should be continued until the last dose on the morning of surgery (with a sip of water). Diuretics should not be administered on the day of surgery because of the potential adverse interaction of diuretic-induced volume depletion and hypokalemia and the use of anesthetic agents. Similarly, potassium supplementation should be stopped the day before surgery and the potassium level checked.

Surgeons can reduce postoperative blood pressure elevations by appropriate management of pain, anxiety, hypoxia, and hypothermia with rewarming.

Congestive Heart Failure

Patients with congestive heart failure (CHF) need stabilization with diuretics, digoxin, angiotensin-converting enzyme (ACE) inhibitors, and nitroglycerides prior to surgery. Preoperative CHF is the strongest predictor of postoperative pulmonary edema.

Although postoperative CHF occurs in only approximately 1% to 6% of patients, the associated mortality rate is 15% to 20%.

Following surgery, most sequestered fluid is mobilized within the first 48 hours, placing an increased load on the heart. This is also a period of greatly increased metabolic and neurohumoral stress. Most postoperative CHF occurs within 1 hour following surgery, and, in 50% of these cases, inappropriate fluid administration is a major factor.

Anti-Platelet Therapy

After percutaneous coronary intervention or stent placement, patients are routinely managed with aspirin and clopidogrel (Plavix) to reduce reocclusion. After balloon angioplasty or bare metal stent placement, elective noncardiac surgery should be postponed 4 to 6 weeks. If a drug-eluting stent is placed, elective surgery is not recommended for 12 months. Plavix effectiveness can be reduced by the Prilosec (omeprazole) stomach acid reducing agent.

Additional discussion about aspirin is presented later, in the Perioperative Nonsteroidal Anti-inflammatory Drugs section.

UPDATE #8

Plavix (clopidogrel) effectiveness can be reduced by the Prilosec (omeprazole) stomach acid reducing agent (Fleisher et al, 2007).

Heart Valve Prostheses

For patients with heart valve prostheses, anticoagulant management is an important component of perioperative care.

For major surgeries, substituting warfarin with heparin is recommended to maintain anticoagulation until the time of surgery. The short half-life of heparin allows the patient to safely undergo surgery within a few hours after discontinuation. Heparin should be discontinued 6 hours prior to surgery and then restarted 12 to 24 hours after surgery, when postoperative hemorrhage is no longer a threat. Activated partial thromboplastin time (aPTT) should be titrated to 1.5 to 2 times normal. For patients on warfarin, checking the prothrombin time 1 day prior to the day of the operation and administering vitamin K (1 to 3 mg is generally sufficient), if necessary, is recommended.

Therapeutic anticoagulation is typically not reestablished for several days after warfarin is reinitiated. Therefore, the patient should receive heparin in the postoperative period until oral anticoagulation is fully therapeutic. Warfarin should be started and adjusted to an international normalized ratio (INR) based on the underlying reason for the long-term anticoagulation.

Arrhythmias

- *Digoxin.* For control of atrial fibrillation and supraventricular tachycardia in the perioperative period, digoxin should be continued. Bioavailabilities differ with oral and parenteral preparations, which needs to be considered in dosing. Because a risk of digitalis toxicity and perioperative arrhythmia exists, some clinicians prefer to withhold the medication 12 hours before surgery.

- *Quinidine.* Patients should receive their last preoperative dose on the night before surgery. Intravenous lidocaine may be used for ventricular arrhythmia, and intravenous propranolol or verapamil can be used for supraventricular arrhythmias. Quinidine is restarted as soon as the patient is tolerating liquids.

- *Procainamide.* Patients should receive their last preoperative dose on the night before surgery. To control arrhythmia in the intraoperative period, intravenous procainamide or lidocaine may be used. Poorly tolerated supraventricular arrhythmia may be treated with propranolol and verapamil.

- *Disopyramide.* This drug has a negative inotropic effect with adverse anticholinergic effects of urinary retention and constipation. For this reason, it should be discontinued on the night prior to surgery and substituted with intravenous lidocaine in the perioperative period.

- *Tocainide.* This oral agent is similar to lidocaine and may be used to treat ventricular arrhythmia. The last preoperative dose should be administered the night before surgery. Intravenous lidocaine is then used until the patient resumes oral tocainide.

- *Amiodarone.* This drug is usually used to manage life-threatening arrhythmias, and should be discontinued on the night before surgery. It has a long half-life (30 to 60 d). Therefore, it can be restarted safely after the patient has resumed a diet. If arrhythmia develops in the perioperative period, there is an intravenous preparation. Rarely patients on amiodarone can experience acute respiratory distress syndrome, the etiology of which is unclear.

- *Verapamil.* The last dose can be given with a sip of water on the morning of surgery, and an intravenous formulation can be used to cover the perioperative period.

In summary, those patients on long-term therapy for supraventricular tachycardia should receive their usual medication in the perioperative period. Supplemental rate control can be achieved with calcium channel blockers, beta-blockers, or the cautious use of digoxin. Treatment of sustained ventricular arrhythmia with oral medication should continue until the day of surgery, when intravenous procainamide or lidocaine can be substituted.

Respiratory System

Beta-agonists and bronchodilators should not be discontinued in patients with asthma, and beta-agonists and atropine analogs should not be discontinued in patients with chronic obstructive pulmonary disease. The patient should take the usual inhaled medication or tablet until the day of surgery and also on the morning of the operation.

- In patients who have a forced vital capacity of less than 1 L or a forced expiratory volume in 1 second of less than 500 cm^3, consider preoperative bronchodilator therapy.
- In the case of productive cough, reschedule elective surgery and treat the patient with a course of antibiotics to reduce the risk of bronchospasm.
- For patients on long-term steroid therapy, some degree of hypothalamic-pituitary-adrenal axis suppression can be assumed. Increase the dose on the day of surgery (hydrocortisone 100 mg q8h for 24 h), then decrease the dose by 50% every day until back to the usual dose (N.B. Keep in mind that prednisone is four times stronger than hydrocortisone.)

ENDOCRINE SYSTEM

Diabetes

Diabetics are at an increased risk of perioperative complications, including up to a fivefold increase of infection. This increased infection rate may be due to delayed wound healing or an alteration in leukocyte function in patients with poorly controlled diabetes.

Good control prior to an elective surgery may help reduce the risks. The blood glucose level on the morning of surgery ideally should be lower than 200 mg. If glucose levels are greater than 300 mg, elective surgery should be postponed.

The primary perioperative goal is to avoid ketosis and to maintain glucose levels in the range of 100 to 200 mg/dL.

Type 1 diabetics always require insulin perioperatively, even if the addition of glucose is required to minimize hypoglycemia. Type 2 diabetics require insulin perioperatively, especially if their diabetes is usually controlled with insulin and they are undergoing major surgery. Administer insulin either subcutaneously at approximately 50% of the patient's usual morning human insulin isophane suspension dose on the morning of surgery or by an intravenous infusion at approximately 1 U/h. To avoid hypoglycemia, dextrose must be given along with insulin while the patient is NPO. Restart the patient's usual regimen when a diet is resumed.

Monitor serum glucose levels every 2 to 4 hours during surgery and every 4 to 6 hours while NPO postoperatively; then administer supplemental short-acting insulin as dictated by the blood sugar level.

In diabetics controlled by oral agents, discontinue hypoglycemic agents 1 day before surgery. Biguanides (metformin) may increase the risk of developing lactic acidosis because of possible alterations in perioperative renal function. Sulfonylureas are routinely continued on the day before surgery and withheld on the operative day.

Glucose levels should be measured every 6 hours while the patient is NPO. Regular insulin can be administered as needed to patients with glucose levels greater than 250 mg/dL. Resume their routine oral agent when the baseline diet is resumed.

Thyroid Dysfunction

Hypothyroid patients may take their thyroxine replacement until the night before or the day of surgery. One can withhold this medication for as long as a week because of its long half-life of 7 days. However, it should be restarted as soon as the patient is tolerating a diet. Monitor for hypothermia, hypoventilation, hyponatremia, and hypoglycemia.

Urgent surgery should not be deferred in a newly diagnosed patient with hypothyroidism. In patients with severe hypothyroidism, intravenous L-thyroxine, with an initial dose of 500 mcg, followed by 50 to 100 mcg/d, may be given. Elective surgery should be delayed in patients with symptomatic hypothyroidism.

In newly diagnosed patients, possible pituitary-adrenal hypofunction should be assessed and the patient treated with steroids if necessary. Patients with hypothyroidism or thyrotoxicosis should be under good control prior to surgery. In a case of nonthyroid surgery in the presence of hyperthyroidism, patients should receive their antithyroid drug with propranolol on the day of surgery with a sip of water.

Oral Contraceptives and Hormone Replacement

Patients taking oral contraceptives have an increased risk of postoperative venous thromboembolism because of the combined effects of hormones and the hypercoagulable state, which accompanies surgical stress and postoperative immobility. Controversy exists regarding whether or not combined oral contraceptive pills (OCPs) should be stopped preoperatively, and when. Best evidence suggests that if OCPs are to be discontinued, this should occur 4 to 6 weeks prior to surgery and alternative contraception initiated.

Hormone replacement therapy (HRT) in postmenopausal women may also increase the risk of postoperative venous thromboembolism. Because of the limited data, controversy exists in this area as well. However, in this group additional risk factors for thromboembolism exist because of age.

Thromboprophylaxis should be employed in patients on OCPs or on HRT, but the decision regarding interruption is situation specific.

Perioperative Steroids

Several studies have shown that a stress dose is needed only when the hypothalamic-pituitary-adrenal axis (HPAA) is suppressed. However, the corticosteroid dose below which HPAA suppression is unlikely is difficult to predict.

The time to recovery of normal adrenal function after discontinuation of corticosteroids varies from a few days to several months. It is prudent to assume that patients receiving a course of corticosteroid therapy within 3 months of surgery have some degree of HPAA suppression, and perioperative supplementation should be considered.

When using perioperative corticosteroid supplementation, doses should parallel the physiologic response of the normal adrenal gland to surgical stress, providing only very short-term supplementation.

In the case of a minor surgery, in a patient on more than 10 mg/d of prednisone (or the equivalent), 25 to 100 mg of hydrocortisone at induction is sufficient. Postoperatively, patients resume the usual dose of corticosteroid the next day.

Remember that when calculating the hydrocortisone dose, prednisone is four times stronger.

CENTRAL NERVOUS SYSTEM

Seizures

Grand mal seizures substantially increase the risks of surgery. Considerable morbidity may follow grand mal seizures in the perioperative period (e.g., pulmonary aspiration and wound dehiscence, or other physical seizures). Identifying patients with preexisting seizure disorders assures that their anticonvulsant medications can be continued.

Neither absence nor focal seizures appreciably increase the risk of surgery and anesthesia.

In general, if control of epilepsy has been adequate during the year before surgery, measuring blood levels of antiepileptic medications or repeating an electroencephalogram evaluation is not required.

Phenytoin and phenobarbital should be continued in the perioperative period with parenteral formulations, if needed. However, carbamazepine and valproic acid are not available in parenteral form. If patients are on these medications, they should be loaded with phenytoin or phenobarbital, which are effective for all types of seizures.

Parkinson Disease

Patients with Parkinson disease who take dopamine (combination of L-dopa and carbidopa) should stay on their usual medication schedule as much as possible perioperatively because no parenteral form of Sinemet is available and withholding the drug can cause a parkinsonian crisis. Anticholinergics, such as benztropine mesylate in a dose of 0.5 to 1 mg twice daily, may be given intramuscularly during the perioperative period without serious cardiovascular risk. L-dopa should be resumed postoperatively as soon as possible, and the patient should be carefully monitored for hypotension.

Psychotropic Agents

Perioperative exacerbation of psychoses can lead to increased morbidity. However, psychotropic agents can exert complex effects on cardiovascular and autonomic nervous system function.

Patients treated with psychotropic drugs may have altered responses to other medications commonly used in the perioperative period. However, with proper precautions and careful monitoring, psychotropic drugs can be managed safely in surgical patients.

Most antidepressants, anxiolytics, and neuroleptics can be given perioperatively with the following cautionary notes:

- Tricyclic antidepressants (TCAs) are related to a number of important drug interactions. With caution TCAs may be administered until just before surgery and restarted when the patient resumes a diet. If they are interrupted, tapering should occur over several weeks in order to minimize sleep disorders.
- Use of meperidine in patients taking monoamine oxidase inhibitors (MAOIs) is contraindicated because of a possible life-threatening reaction similar to neuroleptic malignant syndrome (characterized by fever, hallucinations, and rigidity).
- Lithium may potentiate the effect of depolarizing and competitive neuromuscular blocking agents. The clearance

of lithium can be reduced and its toxicity increased by factors that cause negative fluid balance, negative sodium balance, and decreased glomerular filtration rate. It should be discontinued 2 to 3 days before major surgery and resumed when renal function and electrolyte levels are stable.

- Patients who have been on benzodiazepines (BZs) for a long time develop tolerance and have an increased risk of serious withdrawal symptoms. Maintaining these patients on BZs in adequate doses and appropriate formulations at timely intervals is indicated to avert withdrawal in the perioperative period.
- The use of phenothiazines, butyrophenones, and BZs can lead to problems with hypotension and myocardial depression in the perioperative period in patients with heart disease. The recommendation is to discontinue tranquilizing agents several days before surgery and resume as needed on the second or third postoperative day.

PERIOPERATIVE NONSTEROIDAL ANTI-INFLAMMATORY DRUGS (NSAIDS)

NSAIDs are often prescribed for patients with rheumatic diseases. The majority of NSAIDs inhibit platelet cyclooxygenase-1 (COX-1), which blocks the formation of thromboxane A2. This impairs thromboxane-dependent platelet aggregation and variably prolongs the bleeding time, depending on the half-life.

Conflicting data exist regarding the use of NSAIDs and perioperative bleeding. However, the general consensus is to withhold aspirin and platelet active–nonaspirin NSAIDs before surgery. The inhibitory effect of aspirin on platelet aggregation may persist for 7 to 10 days, and in nonaspirin NSAIDs it is variable. Discontinuing aspirin and other NSAIDs at least 1 week before surgery is prudent.

In situations where angioplasty or cardiac stenting has been previously performed, the risk and benefit of ischemic heart disease exacerbation versus bleeding should be considered. In general, aspirin increases the frequency of procedural bleeding (relative risk 1.5) but not the severity of bleeding complications or postoperative mortality.

Patients with inflammatory arthritis may be highly dependent on their NSAID therapy for control of their symptoms. Alternative therapy, such as analgesics or low-dose corticosteroids, should be considered.

RHEUMATIC DISEASE

Whether or not perioperative methotrexate increases the risk of postoperative complications (e.g., infections, poor wound healing) is unclear. Because the drug is predominantly cleared from the body by the kidneys, withholding it 48 hours before surgery, which may be associated with transient renal insufficiency, is prudent. Some surgeons also prefer to withhold the drug for 2 weeks postoperatively to ensure appropriate wound healing.

Similarly, withholding cyclophosphamide (also excreted renally) a few days prior to surgery is recommended. Other antirheumatic drugs (e.g., hydroxychloroquine, colchicine, gold, sulfasalazine, azathioprine) should be discontinued prior to surgery, although little data exist regarding their use in the perioperative period.

Depending on the severity of the rheumatologic condition, methotrexate should be started as soon as possible after surgery to avoid a rebound flare in arthritis.

GASTROINTESTINAL SYSTEM

Patients with a history of peptic ulcer disease, gastrointestinal bleeding, or active symptoms of dyspepsia should receive prophylactic histamine-2 receptor blocker therapy throughout the perioperative period. Patients may also require motility-enhancing agents (e.g., metoclopramide), especially in the presence of nausea and gastric atony. If patients are on proton pump inhibitors, these can be continued in the perioperative period.

Perioperative Herbs and Supplements Management

As many as 70% of preoperative patients do not disclose their use of herbal or supplement products unless asked specifically. Numerous potential drug-herb/supplement interactions are possible. Some are theoretic, and many are well documented clinically. The following summary focuses on those herbs and supplements that are most likely to be problematic, but it should not be regarded as a complete list. In most cases, it is prudent to stop herb and supplement use at least 7 to 10 days before surgery.

UPDATE #9

Up to 70% of preoperative patients do not disclose herbal and supplement use unless asked specifically, and many of these substances can adversely affect perioperative outcomes (Ang-Lee et al, 2001).

Herbs and supplements that may affect platelet aggregation and bleeding risk:

- Andrographis
- Black and green tea
- Chondroitin
- Danshen
- Dong quai
- Fenugreek
- Garlic
- Ginger
- Ginkgo
- Glucosamine
- Guarana
- Horse chestnut
- Policosanol
- Resveratrol
- Saw palmetto
- Vitamin E

Herbs and supplements that might cause central nervous system depression and potentiate anesthetic drugs:

- German chamomile
- Kava
- L-tryptophan
- Lavender
- Lemon balm
- Melatonin
- Passion flower
- Valerian

Herbs and supplements that might cause hypoglycemia:

- Alpha-lipoic acid
- American ginseng
- Banaba
- Bitter lemon
- Fenugreek
- Glucomannan
- Gymnema
- Panax ginseng
- Prickly pear cactus
- Vanadium

Herbs and supplements that might affect blood pressure:

- Andrographis (hypo)
- Coenzyme-Q (hypo)
- Epimedium (hypo)
- L-arginine (hypo)
- Licorice (hyper)
- Theanine (hypo)

Herbs and supplements that may exert stimulant effects, with potential for stroke, MI, and arrhythmias:

- Ephedra
- Bitter orange
- Green tea extracts
- Mate
- Guarana
- Cola nut

The preceding combinations are often present in popular "energy drinks," and Ephedra, although banned in the United States, is still available on the Internet.

Herbs and supplements that may affect serotonin levels, which may impact vascular activity and blood pressure to the point of vascular collapse:

- St. John's wort
- 5-HTP
- SAMe
- L-tryptophan

SUGGESTED READINGS

Thromboprophylaxis

Anger J, Weinberg A, Gore J, et al: Thromboembolic complications of sling surgery for stress urinary incontinence among female Medicare beneficiaries, *Urology* 74(6):1223–1226, 2009.

Caprini JA: Venous thromboembolism in surgery: a preventable complication. Introduction, *Am J Surg* 199(Suppl 1):S1–S2, 2010.

Committee on Practice Bulletins—Gynecology, et al: ACOG practice bulletin no. 84: prevention of deep vein thrombosis and pulmonary embolism, *Obstet Gynecol* 110(2 Pt 1):420–429, 2007.

Geerts WH, Pineo GF, Heit JA, et al: Prevention of venous thromboembolism: the Seventh ACCP Conference on Antithrombotic and Thrombolytic Therapy, *Chest* 126(Suppl):338S–400S, 2004.

Kakkos SK, Caprini JA, Geroulakos G, et al: Combined intermittent pneumatic leg compression and pharmacological prophylaxis for prevention of venous thromboembolism in high-risk patients, *Cochrane Database Syst Rev* (4):CD005258, 2008.

Infection Prophylaxis

American College of Obstetricians and Gynecologists Committee on Practice Bulletins—Gynecology: ACOG practice bulletin no. 104: antibiotic prophylaxis for gynecologic procedures, *Obstet Gyencol* 113(5):1180–1189, 2009.

Wolf JS Jr, Bennett CJ, Dimochowski RR, et al: Best practice policy statement on urologic surgery antimicrobial prophylaxis, *J Urol* 179(4):1379–1390, 2008.

Pulmonary Assessment and Prophylaxis

Qaseem A, Snow V, Fitterman N, et al: Risk assessment for and strategies to reduce perioperative pulmonary complications for patients undergoing noncardiothoracic surgery: a guideline from the American College of Physicians, *Ann Intern Med* 144(8):575–580, 2006.

Cardiovascular Assessment and Prophylaxis

Fleisher LA, Beckman JA, Brown KA, et al: ACC/AHA 2007 guidelines on perioperative cardiovascular evaluation and care for noncardiac surgery, *J Am Coll Cardiol* 50(17):e159–e241, 2007.

Perioperative Medications

Fleisher LA, Beckman JA, Brown KA, et al: ACC/AHA 2007 guidelines on perioperative cardiovascular evaluation and care for noncardiac surgery, *J Am Coll Cardiol* 50(17):e159–e241, 2007.

Perioperative Herbs and Supplements

Ang-Lee MK, Moss J, Yuan CS: Herbal medicines and perioperative care, *JAMA* 286(2):208–216, 2001.

Therapeutic Research Faculty: *Natural medicines comprehensive database.* www.naturaldatabase.com. Accessed May 31, 2011.

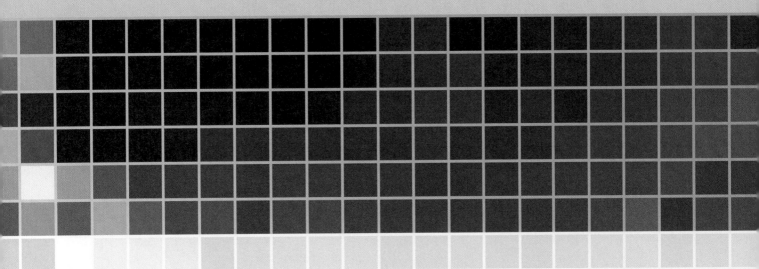

SECTION 9

Gynecologic Health: The Peri- and Postmenopausal Woman

Chapter 41

Lower Genital Tract Infections

KAREN SMITH-MCCUNE

KEY UPDATES

1 Human papillomavirus (HPV)–naïve women can be protected against cervical precancer by vaccination with the bivalent or quadrivalent HPV vaccine.

2 The quadrivalent HPV vaccine protects against external genital warts.

3 In women with preexisting infection with HPV 16 or 18, HPV vaccination does not accelerate HPV clearance.

4 Genetic host factors that regulate immune activity such as polymorphisms in the tumor necrosis factor (TNF) promoter can affect the risk of preterm labor associated with bacterial vaginosis.

5 Prophylactic long-term treatment with oral fluconazole is effective in reducing the recurrence rate of symptoms in women with recurrent vulvovaginal candidiasis. Two effective regimens are available.

6 Women with metronidazole sensitivity can be effectively treated for *Trichomonas vaginalis* using either oral or intravenous metronidazole desensitization regimens.

7 Chronic vaginitis is commonly associated with noninfectious diagnoses including vulvar vestibulitis syndrome, contact dermatitis, atrophic dermatitis, and desquamative inflammatory vaginitis.

Human Papillomavirus (HPV)

CLINICAL PROFILE

- HPV is a DNA virus that infects skin surfaces; genital HPV infection is acquired through sexual contact
- There are more than 100 HPV types, of which approximately 30 are tropic for genital skin
- Genital HPV infection is usually subclinical and resolves spontaneously, but it can also result in a range of clinical manifestations including genital warts and abnormal Pap tests
- Women are most likely to be exposed to HPV infection at the time of onset of sexual activity; prevalence of HPV infection is highest in women in their 20s and declines thereafter
- Some genital HPV types are associated with cancer of the cervix, anus, vagina, and vulva, called high-risk or oncogenic HPV types; the most common high-risk HPV types are HPV 16, 18, 31, 33, 35, 39, 45, 51, 52, 56, 58, 59, and 68; other genital HPV types that are not associated with cancer are termed low-risk or nononcogenic; the most common low-risk HPV types are HPV 6 and 11
- HPV 16 and 18 are the most common high-risk HPV types associated with cervical cancer, accounting for approximately two thirds of cervical cancer cases globally

DIAGNOSIS

- Two tests are available that have been approved by the Food and Drug Administration (FDA) and can detect one or more of the oncogenic HPV types: these tests can be used for triage of minimally abnormal Pap tests or as co-tests with the Pap in cervical cancer screening
- There is no clinical indication for testing for low-risk HPV types
- HPV changes in cell growth can also be detected on the Pap test as atypia, warts, precancer, or cancer
- Genital warts are papular, flat, or pedunculated lesions on the genital mucosa; biopsy is not necessary for diagnosis unless the diagnosis is uncertain, the lesion does not respond to standard therapy or progresses during therapy, or the lesion is fixed or indurated or ulcerated

TREATMENT

- There are no known therapies for eradication of HPV infection per se
- Numerous therapies are available for treatment of external genital warts, both provider- or patient-administered

Provider-Administered Therapies for Treatment of External Genital Warts

- Cryotherapy with liquid nitrogen or a cryoprobe: application may need to be repeated in 1 to 2 weeks
- Topical application of 80% to 90% bi- or trichloroacetic acid (chemical desiccation): avoid application to adjacent normal skin to enhance patient comfort; application may need to be repeated weekly for several weeks to completely eradicate the warts
- Topical application of 10% to 25% podophyllin resin in a compound tincture of benzoin (contains antimitotic

activity): do not apply to open skin and wash off after 1 to 4 hours to avoid systemic toxicity; application may need to be repeated; not recommended during pregnancy

- Surgical removal (excision, electrosurgery, shave biopsy): requires local or general anesthesia
- Laser ablation: requires local or general anesthesia

Patient-Applied Therapies for Treatment of External Genital Warts

- A treatment of 0.5% podofilox gel or solution applied to the warts twice daily for 3 days then 4 days off, repeated for a total of 4 weeks; total volume of podofilox should not exceed 0.5 mL per day
- A treatment of 5% imiquimod cream applied to the warts three times a week at bedtime for up to 16 weeks. Skin should be washed 6 to 10 hours later
- A treatment of 15% sinecatechin ointment applied to the warts three times daily for up to 16 weeks
- Patient-applied topical therapies for external genital warts are not recommended for use in pregnant women due to an unknown safety profile
- Two FDA-approved HPV vaccines have been designed to prevent infection with HPV; the HPV vaccine consists of virus-like particles composed of the L1 coat proteins in combination with immune adjuvant; the vaccine does not contain the viral genome nor any other viral proteins, and hence it is nonreplicative and noninfectious
- The bivalent vaccine contains L1 proteins from HPV 16 and 18 (the HPV types most commonly associated with cervical cancer), whereas the quadrivalent vaccine contains L1 proteins from HPV 16 and 18 as well as HPV 6 and 11 (the HPV types most commonly associated with genital warts)

UPDATE #1

Recent results from large randomized trials of the bivalent and quadrivalent vaccines indicate that inoculation of HPV-naïve females with either the bivalent or quadrivalent HPV vaccine significantly decreases the incidence of cervical precancers. End-of-study results from the quadrivalent HPV vaccine clinical trial indicate that women naïve to 12 oncogenic HPV types had a 43% reduction in CIN 3 lesions after vaccination compared to the placebo group (Muñoz et al, 2010). Event-driven final analysis from the bivalent HPV vaccine trial indicates that women naïve to 14 oncogenic HPV types had an 87% reduction of cervical intraepithelial neoplasia (CIN) 3 lesions (Pavenon et al, 2009). Population-based vaccination of girls and adolescents before the onset of sexual activity is expected to decrease the risk of cervical cancer.

- Because the vaccines target only two of the oncogenic HPV types, vaccinated women should continue to get cervical cancer screening at recommended intervals

UPDATE #2

The quadrivalent HPV vaccine protects against external genital warts. End-of-study data indicate that women naïve to HPV 6 and 11 who received the vaccine had an 83% reduction in genital warts compared to the placebo group after an average follow-up of 3.6 years (Muñoz et al, 2010).

UPDATE #3

In a large randomized trial, the rates of clearance of HPV infection were unchanged in the group of women who received vaccination with the bivalent HPV vaccine (HPV 16 and 18) compared to the placebo control group. At 12 months, clearance rates of HPV 16/18 were 48.8% in the vaccinated groups and 49.8% in the control group. Therefore, HPV vaccination does not accelerate clearance of infection in women who are already infected with the vaccine HPV types, nor is it indicated for treatment in women with HPV-associated changes (Hildesheim et al, 2007).

Bacterial Vaginosis (BV)

CLINICAL PROFILE

- One of the commonest causes of vaginitis
- Clinical signs and symptoms include vaginal discharge, irritation, and odor
- BV is associated with an alteration in the vaginal microflora with decreased amounts of lactobacillus and increased presence of other bacteria including *Gardnerella vaginalis*, *Atopobium vaginae*, *Megasphera-a*, *Prevotella* and *Mobiluncus* species
- BV is associated with increased susceptibility to some sexually transmitted infections, to HIV, to ascending infections including pelvic inflammatory disease, postabortion and postpartum endometritis, and to adverse pregnancy outcomes (preterm birth, delivery of low-birth-weight infants)

UPDATE #4

Genetic polymorphisms may explain why only a minority of pregnant women with BV experience adverse pregnancy outcomes. Women with the tumor necrosis factor (TNF)-2 allele of the TNF gene promoter had a significantly increased risk of preterm delivery (odds ratio [OR] 2.7, 95% confidence interval [CI] 1.7 to 4.5). In women with both the TNF-2 allele and BV, the OR of preterm delivery was increased to 6.1 (95% CI 1.9 to 21.0) (Macones et al, 2004). Therefore, the interaction of both genetic and infectious factors can contribute to the risk of preterm labor.

DIAGNOSIS

- For diagnosis of BV, ≥3 of the following must be present (Amsel criteria):
  - Homogeneous, thin, white discharge that coats the vaginal walls
  - Clue cells on saline wet mount
  - pH of vaginal fluid >4.5
  - Positive whiff test: a fishy odor of vaginal discharge before or after the addition of 10% potassium hydroxide (KOH)
- BV can also be diagnosed by assessment of bacterial populations on Gram stain (Nugent score), but this technique is used primarily in research protocols

TREATMENT OF NONPREGNANT WOMEN

- Table 41-1 lists Centers for Disease Control and Prevention (CDC) regimens for treatment of BV
- Benefits of therapy in nonpregnant women include alleviation of symptoms, reduction of risk for sexually transmitted infections and HIV, and reduced

TABLE 41-1 CDC Recommended Regimens for Treatment of BV in Nonpregnant Women

Metronidazole 500 mg orally twice a day for 7 days
OR
Metronidazole gel, 0.75%, one full applicator (5 g) intravaginally, once a day for 5 days
OR
Clindamycin cream, 2%, one full applicator (5 g) intravaginally at bedtime for 7 days

CDC Alternative Regimens for Treatment of BV
Clindamycin 300 mg orally twice a day for 7 days
OR
Clindamycin ovules 100 mg intravaginally once at bedtime for 3 days

From Centers for Disease Control and Prevention: Sexually transmitted diseases treatment guidelines, 2006, *MMWR* 55(RR-11), 2006.

TABLE 41-2 CDC Recommended Regimens for Treatment of BV in Pregnant Women

Metronidazole 500 mg orally twice a day for 7 days
OR
Metronidazole 250 mg orally three times a day for 7 days
OR
Clindamycin 300 mg orally twice a day for 7 days

From Centers for Disease Control and Prevention: Sexually transmitted diseases treatment guidelines, 2006, *MMWR* 55(RR-11), 2006.

postprocedure complications after abortion, hysterectomy, and other invasive procedures
- BV is not a conventional sexually transmitted infection but can be considered a *sexually enhanced disease* (Verstraelen et al, 2010); treatment of sex partners of women with BV is not indicated, as it does not alter the woman's response or recurrence rates
- Recurrence rates of BV (diagnosed primarily on Gram stain) are high after standard oral treatment with metronidazole: 58% of women after 6 months and 69% after 1 year had abnormal vaginal flora (Bradshaw et al, 2006)
- Follow-up for test of cure in asymptomatic women is unnecessary

PREGNANT WOMEN
- Detection and treatment of BV is important for reduction of adverse pregnancy outcomes, including premature preterm rupture of the membranes, preterm labor, preterm birth, intra-amniotic infection, and postpartum endometritis
- Table 41-2 lists CDC regimens for treatment of BV
- Topical clindamycin preparations should not be used in the second half of pregnancy

Vulvovaginal Candidiasis

CLINICAL PROFILE
- Approximately 75% of women will have at least one episode of vulvovaginal candidiasis during their lifetime
- Clinical signs and symptoms can be pruritus, vaginal soreness, dyspareunia, dysuria, vulvar pain, abnormal

TABLE 41-3 CDC Recommendations for Treatment of Uncomplicated Vulvovaginal Candidiasis

Intravaginal Butoconazole 2% cream 5 g intravaginally for 3 days
OR
Intravaginal Butoconazole-sustained release 2% cream 5 g single intravaginal application
OR
Intravaginal Clotrimazole 1% cream 5 g intravaginally for 7 to 14 days
OR
Intravaginal Clotrimazole 100 mg vaginal tablet for 7 days
OR
Intravaginal Clotrimazole 100 mg vaginal tablet, two tablets for 3 days
OR
Miconazole 2% cream 5 g intravaginally for 7 days

From Centers for Disease Control and Prevention: Sexually transmitted diseases treatment guidelines, 2006, *MMWR* 55(RR-11), 2006.

vaginal discharge, vulvar swelling, vulvar erythema, and vulvar fissures
- Diagnosis is made with a wet mount (saline or 10% KOH) of vaginal discharge
- In women with symptoms but negative wet mount, culture should be considered
- The usual etiology is *Candida albicans*, but other species such as *Candida glabrata* can be found
- Candida species can colonize the vagina; therefore, a positive culture result or detection on a cytology sample in an asymptomatic woman is not an indication for treatment
- Vaginal pH is usually <4.5 in women with Candida infection

TREATMENT
- Eighty percent to 90% of patients with uncomplicated vulvovaginal candidiasis will respond to topical (intravaginal) azole therapy for 1 to 3 days
- Table 41-3 lists CDC recommendations for treatment of uncomplicated vulvovaginal candidiasis

RECURRENT VULVOVAGINAL CANDIDIASIS (RVC)
- Defined as ≥ four documented attacks per year
- Occurs in <5% of women
- Non–*C. albicans* species such as *C. glabrata* are more common in women with RVC

UPDATE #5
After induction of remission with three sequential oral fluconazole doses (150 mg) every 72 hours for three doses, women with RVC were randomized to weekly fluconazole (150 mg) versus placebo for 6 months. Women in the treatment group had a 91% cure rate at 6 months versus 36% in the placebo group (p < 0.001); 6 months later, after ending prophylactic therapy, 43% of women in the treatment groups versus 28% in the placebo group remained symptom free (p < 0.001) (Sobel et al, 2004). Treatment of RVC with an induction dose of 600 mg of oral fluconazole in the first week followed by an individualized, digressive prophylactic regimen lasting

1 year resulted in 90% of women being disease-free at 6 months and 77% after 1 year (Donders et al, 2008). Both prophylactic regimens were considered safe.

SPECIAL POPULATIONS

- Women receiving immunosuppressive therapy for autoimmune disease or organ transplant are less likely to respond to short-term topical therapy; treatment for 7 to 14 days is recommended
- In diabetic women, control of blood sugar is an important component of management/treatment of RVC
- Pregnant women should be treated with topical (not oral) therapies, and treatment should be for 7 days

Trichomoniasis

CLINICAL PROFILE

- Caused by the protozoan *Trichomonas vaginalis*
- Symptoms include yellow-green thin vaginal discharge, odor, and vulvar irritation
- Organisms can also be detected in women with minimal or no symptoms
- Organisms reside in the vagina, cervix, urethra, bladder, and Bartholin's and Skene's glands; therefore, systemic therapy rather than topical therapy is essential

DIAGNOSIS

- Usual method is detection of organisms on wet mount
- Requires immediate microscopic assessment after preparation of the wet mount while the protozoans are still motile
- Wet mount has low sensitivity (60% to 70%)
- FDA-approved point-of-care tests are also available, which provide improved sensitivity but higher false-positive rates in populations with low prevalence
- Optimal test in women with symptoms but negative wet mount is to perform culture for *T. vaginalis* on a sample of vaginal discharge

TREATMENT

- Trichomoniasis is effectively treated with nitroimidazoles, typically metronidazole 2 g orally in a single dose
- Trichomoniasis is a sexually transmitted infection, so sex partners should also be offered treatment
- Patients who recur despite treatment of the partner can be offered treatment with metronidazole 500 mg orally twice daily for 7 days or tinidazole 2 g orally in a single dose
- Consumption of alcohol should be avoided for 24 hours after treatment with metronidazole and 72 hours after tinidazole
- Topical therapy with metronidazole gel or other intravaginal products is significantly less effective than oral treatment
- Women with metronidazole hypersensitivity (flushing, urticaria, fever, angioedema, and anaphylactic shock) are also likely to react to tinidazole, given their similar chemical structures

TABLE 41-4   CDC Recommended Regimens for Initial First Clinical Episodes

Acyclovir 400 mg orally three times a day for 7 to 10 days
OR
Acyclovir 200 mg orally five times a day for 7 to 10 day
OR
Famciclovir 250 mg orally three times a day for 7 to 10 days
OR
Valacyclovir 1 g orally twice a day for 7 to 10 days

From Centers for Disease Control and Prevention: Sexually transmitted diseases treatment guidelines, 2006, *MMWR* 55(RR-11), 2006.

UPDATE #6

Women with metronidazole hypersensitivity can be desensitized by either oral or intravenous administration of increasing doses of metronidazole resulting in successful treatment of trichomoniasis with a 100% cure and minimal side effects (n = 15) (Helms et al, 2008).

- Follow-up for test-of-cure after oral treatment of trichomoniasis is not necessary unless the woman has symptoms

Herpes Simplex Virus (HSV)

CLINICAL PROFILE

- Clinical symptoms of primary infection can range from no symptoms, to multiple painful genital vesicles or ulcers, to fever, and flulike symptoms in severe cases
- Two types of HSV can infect the lower genital tract: HSV-1 and HSV-2; both types can cause genital outbreaks, although HSV-2 is a more common cause of recurrent genital herpes
- Most HSV infections are clinically asymptomatic but can result in intermittent genital HSV shedding

DIAGNOSIS

- HSV-1 and HSV-2 can be diagnosed by virologic testing (culture or polymerase chain reaction [PCR]) of material collected from genital lesions
- Serologic detection of antibodies to HSV-1 and HSV-2 indicates prior infection

TREATMENT

- Systemic antiviral therapy can reduce the symptoms associated with HSV either during acute outbreaks or as suppressive therapy
- Acyclovir, valacyclovir, and famciclovir are effective oral agents
- Table 41-4 lists CDC-recommended regimens for initial first clinical episodes

ESTABLISHED HSV-2 INFECTION

- For women with recurrent genital herpes, therapy can ameliorate or shorten the duration of symptoms, reduce the frequency of recurrences, and reduce HSV shedding; therapy can be either episodic (initiated immediately upon onset of symptoms) or continuous (for HSV suppression)

TABLE 41-5 CDC Recommended Regimens for HSV Suppression

Acyclovir 400 mg orally twice a day
OR
Famciclovir 250 mg orally twice a day
OR
Valacyclovir 500 mg orally once a day
OR
Valacyclovir 1.0 g orally once a day

From Centers for Disease Control and Prevention: Sexually transmitted diseases treatment guidelines, 2006, *MMWR* 55(RR-11), 2006.

- Table 41-5 lists CDC-recommended regimens for HSV suppression
- Daily treatment with valacyclovir 500 mg daily may decrease the rate of transmission in discordant heterosexual couples and in persons with multiple sex partners

Chronic Vaginitis

CLINICAL PROFILE

- Characterized by persistent or recurrent vaginal discharge or odor
- Vulvar itching or irritation may also be present
- Can result in significant morbidities including discomfort, pain, decreased productivity, dyspareunia, alterations in sexual interest, depression, and other psychiatric sequelae
- Although the usual etiology of vaginitis is infectious (candida, bacterial vaginosis, or trichomoniasis), in women with chronic vaginitis the diagnosis more commonly includes noninfectious etiologies

UPDATE #7

Among 200 women referred to a tertiary center for chronic vaginitis, the most common diagnoses were contact dermatitis (21%), recurrent vulvovaginal candidiasis (20.5%), atrophic vaginitis (14.5%), vulvar vestibulitis syndrome (12.5%), lichen simplex or sclerosus (11%), physiologic leukorrhea (9%), desquamative inflammatory vaginitis (8%), and bacterial vaginosis (6.5%) (Nyirjesy et al, 2006).

DIAGNOSIS

- Physical exam: assess vulva for signs of inflammation, abnormal pigmentation, or leukoplakia; perform biopsy if indicated
- Physical exam: assess vestibule for point tenderness to cotton-tipped application
- Speculum exam: assess cervix for signs of inflammation (cervicitis): perform cultures for gonococcus or chlamydia if indicated
- Speculum exam: collect vaginal discharge for wet mounts (saline and 10% KOH)
- Collect vaginal discharge for yeast culture and trichomonas culture if indicated
- Perform amine test of vaginal discharge (fishy odor when added to 10% KOH)
- Perform pH measurement of vaginal discharge (normal is pH is <4.5)

- Perform microscopic assessment of vaginal discharge to determine the presence and relative proportions of leukocytes, clue cells, hyphae, trichomonads, epithelial cells, lactobacilli, and coccobacilli

MANAGEMENT

- The key to successful management is accurate diagnosis
- In women with recurrent or chronic symptoms, do not automatically assume an infectious etiology
- Culturing for candida and trichomonas is useful in women with recurrent symptoms
- Desquamative inflammatory vaginitis can be treated with intravaginal steroids and clindamycin (which has anti-inflammatory properties)
- Psychological support is an important component of treatment

SUGGESTED READINGS

HPV

Hildesheim A, Herrero R, Wacholder S, et al: Effect of human papillomavirus 16/18 L1 viruslike particle vaccine among young women with preexisting infection: a randomized trial, *JAMA* 298(7):743–753, 2007.

Muñoz N, Kjaer SK, Sigurdsson K, et al: Impact of human papillomavirus (HPV)-6/11/16/18 vaccine on all HPV-associated genital diseases in young women, *J Natl Cancer Inst* 102(5):325–339, 2010.

Paavonen J, Naud P, Salmeron J, et al: Efficacy of human papillomavirus (HPV)-16/18 AS04-adjuvanted vaccine against cervical infection and precancer caused by oncogenic HPV types (PATRICIA): final analysis of a double-blind, randomised study in young women, *Lancet* 374(9686): 301–314, 2009.

BV

Bradshaw CS, Morton AN, Hocking J, et al: High recurrence rates of bacterial vaginosis over the course of 12 months after oral metronidazole therapy and factors associated with recurrence, *J Infect Dis* 193(11):1478–1486, 2006.

Macones GA, Parry S, Elkousy M, et al: A polymorphism in the promoter region of TNF and bacterial vaginosis: preliminary evidence of gene-environment interaction in the etiology of spontaneous preterm birth, *Am J Obstet Gynecol* 190(6):504–508, 2004. discussion 3A.

Marrazzo JM: A persistent(ly) enigmatic ecological mystery: bacterial vaginosis, *J Infect Dis* 193(11):1475–1477, 2006.

Romero R, Chaiworapongsa T, Kuivaniemi H, Tromp G: Bacterial vaginosis, the inflammatory response and the risk of preterm birth: a role for genetic epidemiology in the prevention of preterm birth, *Am J Obstet Gynecol* 190(6):1509–1519, 2004.

Verstraelen H, Verhelst R, Vaneechoutte M, Temmerman M: The epidemiology of bacterial vaginosis in relation to sexual behavior, *BMC Infect Dis* 10:81, 2010.

Vulvovaginal Candidiasis

Donders G, Bellen G, Byttebier G, et al: Individualized decreasing-dose maintenance fluconazole regimen for recurrent vulvovaginal candidiasis (ReCiDiF trial), *Am J Obstet Gynecol* 199(6):613.e1–e9, 2008.

Sobel JD, Wiesenfeld HC, Martens M, et al: Maintenance fluconazole therapy for recurrent vulvovaginal candidiasis, *N Engl J Med* 351(9):876–883, 2004.

Trichomoniasis

Helms DJ, Mosure DJ, Secor WE, Workowski KA: Management of trichomonas vaginalis in women with suspected metronidazole hypersensitivity, *Am J Obstet Gynecol* 198(4):370.e1–e7, 2008.

Chronic Vaginitis

Nyirjesy P, Peyton C, Weitz MV, et al: Causes of chronic vaginitis: analysis of a prospective database of affected women, *Obstet Gynecol* 108(5): 1185–1191, 2006.

Chapter 42

Upper Genital Tract Infections

CRAIG R. COHEN

KEY UPDATES

1 Because of risks and costs associated with invasive diagnostic procedures and the potential for tubal scarring in women with apparent "mild" and "subclinical" disease, a low threshold should be used to make the diagnosis of pelvic inflammatory disease (PID).

2 Anaerobic bacteria and facultative bacteria are frequently isolated from women with PID. Using molecular techniques, novel bacteria including *Mycoplasma genitalium*, *Leptotrichia spp.*, and *Atopobium vaginae* have been isolated from the upper genital tract of women with PID.

3 Most laboratory test and imaging studies are nonspecific for the diagnosis of PID.

4 Broad-spectrum antibiotics are required to treat PID.

5 Human immunodeficiency virus (HIV)-1 testing and counseling should be performed after informing the woman.

6 Primary measures to identify and treat asymptomatic genital tract infections such as chlamydia and gonorrhea have proved useful to decrease the risk of PID.

Pelvic Inflammatory Disease

CLINICAL PROFILE

- Pelvic inflammatory disease (PID) is a general term that refers to infection of the uterus, fallopian tubes, and ovaries; it is the most common serious infection acquired by sexually active females and one of the most common causes of tubal factor infertility
- In the United States, from 750,000 to 1 million women develop PID annually, with a 1.5% annual incidence among adolescents and higher rates among non-white populations
  - Since the early 1990s, the number of hospitalizations and initial visits to outpatient facilities, including physicians' offices, has steadily declined
- Circumstantial evidence suggests that a large percentage of PID goes unrecognized, undiagnosed, and, therefore, untreated
- For this reason, clinicians should have a low threshold to make a diagnosis of PID, and women at risk of a sexually transmitted disease (STD) should be educated to recognize the symptoms of PID and to seek immediate care
- Although most women with PID recover completely from acute infection, serious irreversible reproductive organ damage can occur; scarring can cause fallopian tube obstruction and pelvic adhesions that lead to sequelae such as tubal factor infertility, ectopic pregnancy, and chronic pelvic pain

- Following PID, infertility occurs in 11% of women, the risk of ectopic pregnancy increases 7- to 10-fold, and approximately 20% of women develop chronic pelvic pain
- Alternative diagnosis of PID includes other gynecologic, urologic, and gastrointestinal disorders (Table 42-1)

UPDATE #1

Because of the risks and costs associated with invasive diagnostic procedures and the potential for tubal scarring in women with apparent "mild" and "subclinical" disease, a low threshold should be used to make the diagnosis of PID (Centers for Disease Control and Prevention, 2010). In sexually active young women and other women at risk for sexually transmitted diseases, PID should be diagnosed and treated if the patient presents with acute (usually defined as ≤ 30 days), low abdominal or pelvic pain with uterine/adnexal (i.e., ovaries and fallopian tubes) or cervical motion tenderness present, and no other cause(s) for the illness can be identified. The criteria found in Table 42-2 may be used to enhance the diagnostic potential of these minimum criteria.

Early diagnosis of PID is important for effective treatment and prevention of sequelae. However, because of the complexity and lack of objective clinical criteria to diagnose PID, women with mild PID may go undiagnosed, and those with severe disease may be misdiagnosed with gastrointestinal or noninfectious gynecologic conditions. No set of signs and symptoms are sufficiently sensitive and specific to diagnose PID. In comparison to laparoscopy (i.e., direct visualization of the ovaries and exterior of the fallopian tubes and uterus through a surgical instrument inserted through a small incision), the clinical diagnosis of PID correctly identifies women with confirmed disease in 65% to 90% of cases (Bukusi et al, 1999; Ness et al, 2002). Although

TABLE 42-1   Differential Diagnosis

Ectopic pregnancy

Septic abortion

Rupture, torsion, hemorrhage of an ovarian cyst

Endometriosis

Acute appendicitis

Inflammatory bowel disease

Urinary tract infection

Kidney stone

TABLE 42-2   Centers for Disease Control Criteria for the Clinical Diagnosis of PID

Minimal Criteria*	Additional Criteria†
Acute low abdominal/ pelvic pain *and* at least one of the following on examination: uterine, adnexal, or cervical motion tenderness	Oral temperature ≥ 38.3⁰ C
	Abnormal cervical or vaginal mucopurulent discharge
	White blood cells on saline microscopy of vaginal secretions (≥ 1 per 400×)
	Elevated C-reactive protein
	Elevated sedimentation rate
	Cervical gonorrhea or chlamydia infection

*Empiric treatment should be started in women with a mild to moderately severe clinical presentation, if they meet the minimal criteria, are at risk for a sexually transmitted infection, and have no other cause for illness identified.

†Additional criteria can be used to more accurately diagnose PID and should be reserved for women with severe presentations to help rule out other serious diagnoses. Further evaluation of women with uncertain diagnoses can be made by laparoscopy and ultrasound.

Adapted from Centers for Disease Control and Prevention: *Sexually transmitted diseases treatment guidelines, 2010: pelvic inflammatory disease* (website). www.cdc.gov/std/treatment/2010/pid.htm. Accessed June 16, 2010.

laparoscopy and biopsy of the uterus provide objective criteria for the diagnosis of PID, the risk of these procedures, potential delay in treatment, and underdiagnosis of PID in comparison to the risk of overtreatment weigh in favor of relying on sensitive clinical criteria in most cases.

ETIOLOGY

- Gonorrhea and chlamydia historically are the most common causes of PID and account for 5% to 80% and 5% to 50% of cases, respectively
- Half to two thirds of women with proved PID are not infected with gonorrhea or chlamydia
- Anaerobic bacteria and facultative bacteria have frequently been isolated from women with PID
  - Many of the anaerobic bacteria isolated from the upper genital tract are commonly found in low concentrations in normal vaginal flora and at far greater concentrations among women with bacterial vaginosis

- *Prevotella bivius, Bacteroides spp., Peptostreptococcus spp.,* staphylococci, group B-D streptococci, *Gardnerella vaginalis,* and *Escherichia coli* can be isolated from the upper genital tract of women with PID
- Because of the empiric data just cited, anaerobic coverage is included in all the inpatient treatment regimens and as an option for outpatient treatment recommended for the treatment of PID by the U.S. Centers for Disease Control

UPDATE #2

Novel bacteria including *Mycoplasma genitalium, Leptotrichia spp.,* and *Atopobium vaginae,* among others, have more recently been isolated from the upper genital tract of women with PID using molecular diagnostic techniques (Cohen et al, 2002, 2005; Haggerty, 2008; Hebb et al, 2004).

LABORATORY DIAGNOSTICS AND DIAGNOSTIC IMAGING STUDIES

- Most laboratory tests are nonspecific in the diagnosis of PID
- Any woman of reproductive age presenting with acute abdominal/pelvic pain should have a urine human pregnancy test performed to rule out an ectopic pregnancy
- An elevated white blood cell count (≥10,000 cells/mm³) has a relatively poor positive and negative predictive value but may be useful to rule out other causes of acute abdominal/pelvic pain, such as appendicitis
- Although the minority of PID is caused by gonorrhea and chlamydia, a positive test for either is highly indicative of a diagnosis of PID, may influence the treatment of sexual contacts, and may help to target prevention messages to reduce the risk of recurrent infection
- Ultrasound provides a noninvasive test to help diagnose PID
- Ultrasound may be used to follow the course of patients with a tubo-ovarian abscess, or pyosalpinx (pus-filled fallopian tube), and help rule out other causes of acute pelvic pain

UPDATE #3

The presence of vaginal polymorphonuclear leukocytes (PMN) (≥1 per 400× field) has a high sensitivity and negative predictive value for the diagnosis of upper genital tract infection (Yudin et al, 2003) and thus can be used to help rule out PID if PMNs are not present.

The sensitivity of pelvic ultrasonography is approximately 94% for severe PID, 80% for moderate PID, and 64% for mild PID. Transvaginal ultrasonography appears to improve the sensitivity for ultrasonographically diagnosing mild PID. In general, thickening or dilation of the fallopian tubes, fluid in the cul-de-sac, multicystic ovary, and tubo-ovarian abscess can be used to help confirm the clinical diagnosis of PID. Furthermore, pelvic ultrasound is available in most clinical settings and is a useful tool for determining other causes of acute pelvic pain. However, because of its low sensitivity in cases of mild PID, the routine use of transvaginal ultrasonography to confirm the diagnosis of mild-to-moderately severe PID has limited clinical utility (Boardman et al, 1997).

TREATMENT

- Broad-spectrum antibiotics are required to treat the infections present in PID
- Early antibiotic therapy, within the first 3 days after the onset of symptoms, has been associated with a reduced risk of sequelae and therefore is highly recommended
- Although single-agent treatment regimens have been used successfully to treat PID, two- and three-drug regimens that cover gonorrhea, chlamydia, and common aerobic and anaerobic isolates are recommended
- Treatment should be empiric and not based on lower genital tract tests, which are costly, may delay the onset of treatment, and often do not predict pathogens in the upper genital tract
- Surgical drainage of pelvic abscesses is reserved for ruptured pelvic abscesses, masses that persists after antibiotic treatment, abscesses ≥ 4 to 6 cm as observed by ultrasound, and fluctuant pelvic masses attached to the cul-de-sac that can easily be drained through the vagina
  - Transabdominal drainage under laparoscopic guidance is used for persistent pelvic abscesses that are not suitable for colpotomy drainage; ultrasound-guided placement of percutaneous catheters is also possible

---

UPDATE #4

A multicenter randomized controlled trial of treatment of women with clinical signs and symptoms of mild-to-moderate PID, comparing inpatient intravenous cefoxitin and doxycycline treatment versus outpatient treatment consisting of a single intramuscular injection of cefoxitin and oral doxycycline, demonstrated that short-term clinical and microbiologic improvement were similar between the two groups, and pregnancy rates (42% in both arms), time to pregnancy, proportion of women with PID recurrence, chronic pelvic pain, or ectopic pregnancy were equivalent (Ness et al, 2002). Therefore, inpatient treatment and hospitalization should be reserved for patients with an unclear diagnosis (particularly if a serious surgical diagnosis cannot be excluded), patients with abscesses, and those who have failed oral antibiotic therapy or are unable to tolerate oral medication. HIV-1 infection, unless associated with severe immunodeficiency (CD4 T-cell count <200/mm³), is not an absolute indication for hospitalization (Bukusi et al, 1999). Table 42-4 lists parenteral treatments for PID and Table 42-4 for oral treatments.

COUNSELING

- Most PID is sexually transmitted; therefore, counseling efforts should focus on decreasing one's sexual exposure (reduction of number of partners, increased condom use, etc.)
- Often a women's risk of exposure to sexually transmitted infections is related to the promiscuity of her male sexual partner; therefore, in addition to counseling the patient, clinicians need to direct sexually transmitted disease prevention messages toward the patient's male partner
- Although the sexual behaviors of homosexual women are associated with a reduced risk of most sexually transmitted infections, female partners of women with PID should also receive appropriate treatment and counseling

---

TABLE 42-3   Parenteral Treatment for PID

Recommended Parenteral Treatment

Parenteral Regimen A

Cefotetan 2 g IV every 12 hours

OR

Cefoxitin 2 g IV every 6 hours

PLUS

Doxycycline 100 mg orally or IV every 12 hours

Parenteral Regimen B

Clindamycin 900 mg IV every 8 hours

PLUS

Gentamicin loading dose IV or IM (2 mg/kg of body weight) followed by a maintenance dose (1.5 mg/kg) every 8 hours; single daily dosing may be substituted

Alternative Parenteral Regimens

Ampicillin/Sulbactam 3 g IV every 6 hours

PLUS

Doxycycline 100 mg orally or IV every 12 hours

Adapted from Centers for Disease Control and Prevention: *Sexually transmitted diseases treatment guidelines, 2010: pelvic inflammatory disease* (website). www.cdc.gov/std/treatment/2010/pid.htm. Accessed June 16, 2010.

- To provide incentive for women to reduce their sexual exposure, counseling may also include messages concerning the increased risk of infertility and other sequelae associated with subsequent episodes of PID (infertility risk: 12% after one episode, 21% after two episodes, and 40% after three or more episodes)

UPDATE #5

Among hospitalized patients with PID, the risk of HIV-1 infection has been demonstrated to be two to seven times greater than in similarly aged women receiving prenatal care in the same community (Centers for Disease Control and Prevention, 2010). Thus, HIV-1 testing and counseling should be performed after informing the woman, unless she decides to opt out of testing.

PREVENTION

- Sexually active women ≤25 years old should be screened annually for chlamydia, as well as for gonorrhea depending on their risk factors and the prevalence of gonorrhea in the community
- Older women should be screened for chlamydia and gonorrhea based on their risk factors (e.g., new or multiple sex partners)
- Secondary measures to prevent the sequelae of PID include early identification and treatment of upper genital tract infection; not surprisingly, antibiotic treatment helps prevent tubal damage

---

UPDATE #6

Screening and identification of women for asymptomatic chlamydia infection has proven useful to decrease the risk of PID (Scholes et al, 1996). However, a recent study suggests that the effectiveness of a single chlamydia test in preventing PID over 12 months may have been overestimated (Oakeshott et al, 2010).

TABLE 42-4   Oral Treatment for PID

Recommended Oral Regimens

Ceftriaxone 250 mg IM in a single dose

PLUS

Doxycycline 100 mg orally twice a day for 14 days

WITH or WITHOUT

Metronidazole 500 mg orally twice a day for 14 days

Cefoxitin 2 g IM in a single dose and **Probenecid**, 1 g orally administered concurrently in a single dose

OR

Other parenteral third-generation **cephalosporin** (e.g., **ceftizoxime** or **cefotaxime**)

PLUS

Doxycycline 100 mg orally twice a day for 14 days

WITH or WITHOUT

Metronidazole 500 mg orally twice a day for 14 days

Other parenteral third-generation **cephalosporin** (e.g., **ceftizoxime** or **cefotaxime**)

PLUS

Doxycycline 100 mg orally twice a day for 14 days

WITH or WITHOUT

Metronidazole 500 mg orally twice a day for 14 days

Alternative Oral Regimens

If parenteral cephalosporin therapy is not feasible, use of fluoroquinolones (levofloxacin 500 mg orally once daily or ofloxacin 400 mg twice daily for 14 days), with or without metronidazole (500 mg orally twice daily for 14 days), may be considered if the community prevalence and individual risk for gonococcal infection are low. However, quinolone resistance of gonorrhea has increased in up to >10% of isolates in some regions. Therefore, tests for gonorrhea must be performed prior to instituting therapy with fluoroquinolones and the patient managed as follows if the test is positive: if the nucleic acid amplification test (NAAT) test is positive, parenteral cephalosporin is recommended; if culture for gonorrhea is positive, treatment should be based on results of antimicrobial susceptibility. If the isolate is quinolone resistant or antimicrobial susceptibility cannot be assessed, a parenteral cephalosporin is recommended (Centers for Disease Control and Prevention: Updated recommended treatment regimens for gonococcal infections and associated conditions, 2007).

Although information regarding other outpatient regimens is limited, amoxicillin/clavulanic acid and doxycycline or azithromycin with metronidazole has demonstrated short-term clinical cure. No data have been published regarding the use of oral cephalosporins for the treatment of PID. A recent publication compared ceftriaxone 250 mg plus azithromycin 1 gram per week for 2 weeks or doxycycline 200 mg/day for 2 weeks to treat mild PID; the regimen containing azithromycin was equivalent in regard to clinical cure at 2 weeks (Savaris et al, 2007). Azithromycin may have other advantages over doxycycline, including its easier dosing and improved coverage of *M. genitalium* infection (Haggerty et al, 2008).

Adapted from Centers for Disease Control and Prevention: *Sexually transmitted diseases treatment guidelines, 2010: pelvic inflammatory disease* (website). www.cdc.gov/std/treatment/2010/pid.htm. Accessed June 16, 2010.

SUGGESTED READINGS

Clinical Profile

Centers for Disease Control and Prevention: *Pelvic inflammatory disease (PID): CDC fact sheet* (website). www.cdc.gov/std/PID/STDFact-PID.htm. Accessed June 20, 2011.

Centers for Disease Control and Prevention: *Sexually transmitted diseases treatment guidelines 2010: pelvic inflammatory disease* (website). www.cdc.gov/std/treatment/5-2010TG.htm#PelvicInflammatoryDisease. Accessed June 20, 2011.

Etiology

Cohen CR, Manhart LE, Bukusi EA, et al: Association between *Mycoplasma genitalium* and acute endometritis, *Lancet* 359(9308):765–766, 2002.

Cohen CR, Mugo NR, Astete SG, et al: Detection of *Mycoplasma genitalium* in women with laparoscopically diagnosed acute salpingitis, *Sex Transm Infect* 81(6):463–466, 2005.

Haggerty CL: Evidence for a role of *Mycoplasma genitalium* in pelvic inflammatory disease, *Curr Opin Infect Dis* 21(1):65–69, 2008.

Hebb JK, Cohen CR, Astete SG, et al: Detection of novel organisms associated with salpingitis, by use of 16S rDNA polymerase chain reaction, *J Infect Dis* 190:2109–2120, 2004.

Laboratory Diagnostics and Diagnostic Imaging Studies

Boardman LA, Peipert JF, Brody JM, et al: Endovaginal sonography for the diagnosis of upper genital tract infection, *Obstet Gynecol* 90(1):54–57, 1997.

Yudin MH, Hillier SL, Wiesenfeld HC, et al: Vaginal polymorphonuclear leukocytes and bacterial vaginosis as markers for histologic endometritis among women without symptoms of pelvic inflammatory disease, *Am J Obstet Gynecol* 188(2):318–323, 2003.

Treatment

Bukusi EA, Cohen CR, Stevens CE, et al: Effects of human immunodeficiency virus 1 infection on microbial origins of pelvic inflammatory disease and on efficacy of ambulatory oral therapy, *Am J Obstet Gynecol* 181(6):1374–1381, 1999.

Centers for Disease Control and Prevention (CDC): *Updated recommended treatment regimens for gonococcal infections and associated conditions: United States, April 2007* (website). www.cdc.gov/std/treatment/2006/updated-regimens.htm. Accessed June 20, 2011.

Centers for Disease Control and Prevention (CDC): Update to CDC's sexually transmitted diseases treatment guidelines, 2006: fluoroquinolones no longer recommended for treatment of gonococcal infections, *MMWR Morb Mortal Wkly Rep* 56(14):332–336, 2007.

Haggerty CL, Totten PA, Astete SG, et al: Failure of cefoxitin and doxycycline to eradicate endometrial *Mycoplasma genitalium* and the consequence for clinical cure of pelvic inflammatory disease, *Sex Transm Infect* 84(5): 338–342, 2008.

Ness RB, Soper DE, Holley RL, et al: Effectiveness of inpatient and outpatient treatment strategies for women with pelvic inflammatory disease: results from the Pelvic Inflammatory Disease Evaluation and Clinical Health (PEACH) Randomized Trial, *Am J Obstet Gynecol* 186(5):929–937, 2002.

Savaris RF, Teixeira LM, Torres TG, et al: Comparing ceftriaxone plus azithromycin or doxycycline for pelvic inflammatory disease: a randomized controlled trial, *Obstet Gynecol* 110(1):53–60, 2007.

Prevention

Oakeshott P, Kerry S, Aghaizu A, et al: Randomised controlled trial of screening for Chlamydia trachomatis to prevent pelvic inflammatory disease: the POPI (prevention of pelvic infection) trial, *BMJ* 340:c1642, 2010.

Scholes D, Stergachis A, Heidrich FE, et al: Prevention of pelvic inflammatory disease by screening for cervical chlamydial infection, *N Engl J Med* 334(21):1362–1366, 1996.

Chapter 43

Human Immunodeficiency Virus Infection in Women

KHADY DIOUF • DEBORAH COHAN

KEY UPDATES

1   Women represent a growing proportion of adults infected with the human immunodeficiency virus (HIV).

2   The most common route of HIV acquisition for women is heterosexual.

3   Women are more vulnerable to HIV than men because of both biologic and socioeconomic factors.

4   Male circumcision protects men from HIV acquisition. Antiretrovirals for preexposure prophylaxis are currently being investigated. A tenofovir-based gel used as a vaginal microbicide was recently shown to decrease HIV acquisition in women by 39%.

5   A package of interventions during pregnancy—including antenatal HIV testing, use of highly active antiretroviral therapy (HAART), and rapid HIV testing in labor and delivery—has led to a decline of the perinatal transmission of HIV to less than 2% in the United States.

6   There are safe reproductive options for couples affected by HIV.

7   The IUD and Depo Provera are safe contraceptive options for HIV-positive women. Other forms of hormonal contraception are also safe, though there are potential drug-drug interactions with antiretrovirals.

8   Women with HIV are at higher risk of developing preinvasive cervical lesions and cervical cancer. Cervical cancer is considered an acquired immune deficiency syndrome (AIDS)–defining condition in HIV-infected women. The impact of HAART on the natural history of human papilloma virus (HPV) is unclear, though effective and adherent HAART may improve HPV-related outcomes. For all HIV-infected women, Pap smears should be done twice in the first year after diagnosis, and if normal, then yearly thereafter. Studies are needed to investigate the efficacy and safety of the HPV vaccine in HIV-infected women and adolescents.

Epidemiology

• Globally, HIV/AIDS is the leading cause of death and disease among women of reproductive age

• Women represent the fastest growing portion in the epidemic: 50% of infections globally, 60% of infections in sub-Saharan Africa, and 30% of infections in the United States; in the United States, minority women are disproportionately affected by HIV/AIDS

UPDATE #1

Two recent reports indicate that HIV is affecting women at a large scale both in the United States and globally (Centers for Disease Control and Prevention, 2011; World Health Organization, 2011). Of the 33.4 million current HIV cases in the world, half represent women (47% prevalence, 48% incidence). In sub-Saharan Africa, HIV disproportionately affects women, who represent 60% of infections. In the United States, the proportion of women with HIV/AIDS increased from 7% in 1985 to 28% in 2009. HIV is a growing epidemic among minority women in the United States. African Americans and Latinas represent 80% of the new infections. HIV/AIDS is the leading cause of death among African American women age 25 to 34.

How Do Women Acquire HIV?

• Most common route of HIV transmission for women: heterosexual route, followed by injection drug use (IDU); in 2002, a significant proportion of women (48%) were not aware of their risk factor for HIV acquisition

The Women Interagency HIV Study (WIHS) cohort surveyed its participants regarding route of HIV transmission at two time points (1994-1995 cohort versus 2001-2002 cohort). The most common routes of transmission in the initial cohort were heterosexual (42%), IDU (34%), and blood transfusion (4%). The more recently recruited cohort (2001-2002) showed similar trends, with heterosexual transmission as the most common route (40%) followed by IDU (10%), with almost half of women not aware of their route of transmission (Barkan et al, 1998; Statepi et al, 2011).

Women Are More Vulnerable to HIV

- Women are particularly vulnerable to HIV because of a combination of biologic and socioeconomic factors

BIOLOGIC VULNERABILITY

- Women are twice as likely as men to acquire HIV from heterosexual intercourse
- The presence of a sexually transmitted disease (STD) increases the risk of HIV transmission
- The presence of an STD increases the risk of HIV acquisition
- Although the data are conflicting, hormonal contraception use, particularly depo-medroxyprogesterone acetate, may be associated with increased acquisition of HIV

SOCIOECONOMIC VULNERABILITY

- Linked to gender inequalities including lack of information/knowledge about HIV and inability to negotiate safer sex
- Most-at-risk groups are the following:
  - Ethnic minorities (African American women and Latinas represent 80% of the new infections in the United States)
  - Younger women
  - Incarcerated women

A systematic review of 43 publications among 25 different study populations showed that per coital risk of HIV transmission was 0.08% for male-to-female and 0.04% for female-to-male in high-income countries. Estimates were higher and more heterogenous in low-income countries (Boily et al, 2009). Both viral load and type of sexual act affect risk of transmission.

HIV acquisition and transmission can also be enhanced by the presence of other sexually transmitted diseases (Fleming et al, 1999). Both ulcerative diseases (syphilis, chancroid, and herpes) and nonulcerative diseases (gonorrhea, chlamydia, trichomoniasis, bacterial vaginosis) increase the risk of acquiring HIV, as individuals with other STDs are more likely to recruit HIV target cells to the endocervix. HIV-infected individuals with other STDs also have higher levels of viral shedding in the genital tract and are more likely to transmit the virus.

Additionally, socioeconomic factors are important in explaining vulnerability to HIV in women. Because of sexual inequalities, women are often unable to negotiate safe sex for fear of rejection or violence from their partners. Younger women are also a high-risk group; in a Centers for Disease Control and Prevention (CDC) study of urban high schools, more than one third of black and Hispanic women had their first sexual encounter with a male who was older (3 or more years) (Centers for Disease Control and Prevention, 2011).

Updates in HIV Prevention for Women

CIRCUMCISION OF MALE PARTNERS

- Though male circumcision significantly decreases risk of HIV acquisition by men, there is no evidence that circumcision of HIV-positive men decreases risk of HIV transmission to their female partners

PREEXPOSURE PROPHYLAXIS

- In preexposure prophylaxis (PrEP), an HIV-uninfected individual starts antiretroviral medications prior to exposure to HIV and continues throughout periods of risk
- The rationale behind preexposure prophylaxis for women:
  - More female-controlled prevention methods are needed to combat the HIV epidemic
  - Animal studies show that using the antiretroviral tenofovir in macaques inoculated with simian immunodeficiency virus (SIV/SHIV) confers protection against viral infection
  - Compared to other antiretroviral agents, tenofovir has a long intracellular half-life and is present in higher levels in the male and female genital tracts

PrEP is currently being investigated in multiple trials as one of several new prevention approaches (Figure 43-1).

Male Circumcision

Results from three randomized trials conducted in Africa have shown strong evidence that male circumcision decreases the risk of HIV acquisition from heterosexual sex by up to 60% for men (Siegfried et al, 2009). However, data from two randomized controlled trials assessing the effect of circumcision on male-to-female transmission show no protection for women. One randomized trial showed no benefit of circumcision for female protection after 2 years of follow-up (Wawer et al, 2009) and even increased risk of HIV acquisition if sexual activity resumed before healing of the circumcised penis; another trial showed no increased risk but potentially a decreased risk from circumcision on male-to-female transmission of HIV (Baeten et al, 2010).

Microbicides

Large randomized trials have looked at four different HIV nonspecific microbicides and found no benefit in HIV protection for women (Skoler-Karpoff et al, 2008; Van Damme et al, 2000, 2008). One of these products (nonoxynol-9) may even lead to increased HIV transmission (Van Damme et al, 2000). Most recently, a large clinical trial of PRO-2000, involving more than 9000 women, showed no protection against HIV infection (Roehr, 2009). In contrast, new-generation microbicides are giving promising results. In July 2010, the Centre for the Aids Programme of Research in South Africa (CAPRISA) trial conducted in South Africa, which enrolled more than 800 sexually active women and provided a vaginal gel containing an antiretroviral (tenofovir), showed a 39% reduction in HIV acquisition among women who received the gel compared to the placebo (Abdool Karim, 2011).

- *Tenofovir-containing pills.* The recently completed Chemoprophylaxis for HIV Prevention in Men (iPrEx) study in men who have sex with men and transgender women showed a 44% decrease in HIV acquisition among those who took oral tenofovir/emtricitabine compared to those who took placebo (Grant et al, 2010); PrEP trials involving women are ongoing.
- *Vaccines.* So far, vaccines have shown minimal to no efficacy against HIV acquisition.

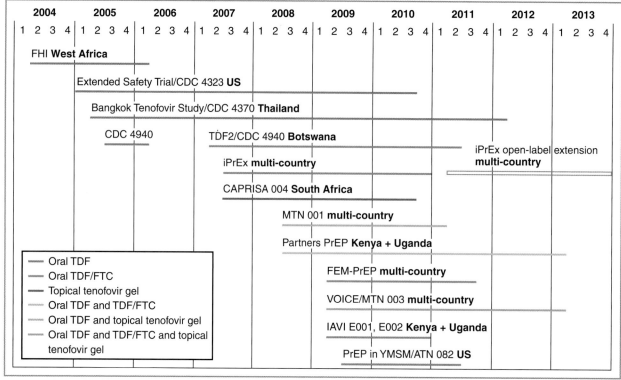

May 2011   *The trial end-dates listed in this table are estimates. Due to the nature of clinical trials the actual dates may change. AVAC will continue to monitor trial progress and will update the timeline accordingly. To view or download an updated timeline visit *www.avac.org/prep.*

Figure 43-1. **Oral and Topical PrEp Trials timeline.** (Adapted from AVAC. For an updated timeline, visit www.avac.org/trials/prep/ongoing.)

Interventions Performed in the United States to Decrease HIV Transmission during Pregnancy

UPDATE #5

Perinatal transmission of HIV in the United States and Europe is less than 2% with a combination of universal testing of pregnant women, HAART during pregnancy and labor, cesarean delivery for viral load >1000, infant zidovudine prophylaxis, and avoidance of breast-feeding (Cooper et al, 2002; Townsend et al, 2008).

- In the United States, all HIV-infected women should be on highly active antiretroviral therapy while pregnant, regardless of CD4 count or viral load; for women needing treatment for their disease (CD4 count <500), antiretrovirals should be continued throughout pregnancy and beyond; for women whose indication is prevention of perinatal HIV transmission, antiretrovirals are typically initiated between 12 to 14 weeks (Department of Health and Human Services, perinatal guidelines, 2011); the decision to continue versus stop HAART postpartum for women at high CD4 cells is complex and evolving; the PROmoting Maternal Infant Survival Everywhere (PROMISE) randomized controlled trial is currently under way to address this issue
- Antiretroviral safety during pregnancy
  - Most antiretroviral medications are thought to be safe for both the woman and the exposed fetus

- Efavirenz should be avoided in the first trimester of pregnancy because of the potential association with neural tube defects in exposed fetuses; efavirenz appears safe in the second and third trimesters
- Nevirapine should be avoided for women with CD4 counts above 250 cells/mm3 because of the increased risk of severe hepatotoxicity; single-dose nevirapine, sometimes given in labor to previously untreated women, can be given, regardless of CD4 count
- Stavudine and didanosine should be avoided, if possible, during pregnancy because of the increased risk of lactic acidosis
- Protease inhibitors have been associated with hyperglycemia; some experts recommend an early glucose loading test in women on protease inhibitors; protease inhibitors also have been associated with a slight increased risk of preterm birth
- HIV screening during pregnancy
  - All women should be screened for HIV at their first prenatal visit
  - A third-trimester screening test is recommended for at-risk women and those living in certain states and clinical facilities with high HIV prevalence and incidence (a compendium of all state testing laws is available at www.nccc.ucsf.edu/StateLaws/Index.html)
  - Rapid testing on labor and delivery for women without documented HIV status or at risk for HIV acquisition during pregnancy is also recommended; the Mother Infant Rapid Intervention At Delivery (MIRIAD) study proved that rapid testing is feasible, acceptable, and effective (Bulterys et al, 2004)

REPRODUCTIVE OPTIONS FOR COUPLES AFFECTED BY HIV

- Many couples affected by HIV have the desire to have children
- Options for safe conception are available for both seroconcordant couples (both partners are HIV infected) and serodiscordant ones (one partner is HIV infected) (Thornton et al, 2004)

SERODISCORDANT COUPLES

- Main concerns are the risk of transmission between partners and the risk of transmission to the child; the risk of transmission is increased with higher plasma HIV ribonucleic acid (RNA) levels in the HIV-infected partner and the presence of sexually transmitted diseases in either partner (Donnell et al, 2010; Lee et al, 1996)
- Options for reproduction are as follows:
  - When only the man is HIV infected: artificial insemination via intrauterine insemination (IUI) *or* in vitro fertilization (IVF), after sperm washing *or* self-insemination with washed sperm
  - Timed intercourse if HIV-infected partner is on HAART, has an undetectable viral load, and has no other STDs has been suggested (Vernazza et al, 2011); studies suggest a minimal risk of transmission from an HIV-infected partner on HAART with an undetectable viral load (Attia et al, 2009; Donnell et al, 2010)
- Another potential option currently under investigation is preexposure prophylaxis (PrEP) (see update #6)

SEROCONCORDANT COUPLES (BOTH HIV INFECTED)

- Superinfection, or transmission of different strains of HIV, is extremely rare, though it has been documented
- Counseling and testing each partner for sexually transmitted infections (STIs), which may increase risk of transmission, and encouraging medication adherence to keep the viral load undetectable for each partner will decrease the risk of transmission to the infant once conception occurs

UPDATE #6

In a small study presented at the 2007 International AIDS Society annual meeting, HIV-discordant couples wanting to conceive received risk reduction counseling, urine luteinizing hormone (LH) peak measurements, and tenofovir at 36 hours and 12 hours before intercourse. All male partners were on HAART with HIV RNA <50 copies/mL for more than 3 months. HIV RNA was tested and found to be undetectable in the semen of HIV-infected men at baseline. All female partners tested HIV negative 3 months after last unprotected intercourse (Vernazza et al, 2011). Though these results are promising, larger trials are needed. In a recent randomized controlled trial, early initiation of antiretroviral therapy (ART) in serodiscordant couples decreased risk of HIV transmission to uninfected partners by 96% compared to delayed initiation of ART (Cohen MS, Chen YQ, McCaughley M, et al, 2011)

Contraception Counseling for HIV-Positive Women

- According to the World Health Organization's Medical Eligibility Criteria for Contraceptive Use, most contraceptive methods are considered to be safe and effective for HIV-infected women, both with asymptomatic HIV and AIDS
- Hormonal contraceptives in general do not appear to affect antiretroviral drug effectiveness, but certain antiretrovirals (including protease inhibitors and efavirenz) do affect hormonal levels; the clinical significance of these interactions is unclear
- Long-acting reversible contraceptives (such as the intrauterine device [IUD]) are effective and safe in HIV-infected women who are on antiretrovirals
- Condoms represent the only contraceptive method effective in decreasing the sexual transmission of HIV
- Though hormonal contraception has been effectively used by HIV positive women, there is some evidence that HIV transmission in the absence of antiretroviral therapy may be increased with hormonal contraception, especially injectable methods.

UPDATE #7

In a recent observational study of serodiscordant couples, HIV negative women who were using hormonal contraception were almost twice as likely to acquire HIV from their male HIV positive partners not receiving antiretroviral therapy than those who did not. In this same study, HIV positive women not receiving antiretroviral therapy who used hormonal contraception were more likely to transmit HIV to their partners than those women who did not. This was a secondary analysis of a prospective study; results need to be confirmed with a randomized controlled trial.

HPV and Cervical Dysplasia in HIV-Infected Women

- HIV-infected women have a higher prevalence of HPV infection, as well as vulvovaginal and cervical dysplasia
- The risk of cervical cancer is five- to eightfold higher in HIV-infected women
- It is unclear if treatment with HAART affects the progression of cervical dysplasia; however, prior studies might have overlooked the importance of adherence to HAART and effectiveness of the treatment regimen

UPDATE #8

Two hundred and eighty-six women who initiated HAART during follow-up in a prospective cohort were assessed semiannually for HPV infection and squamous intraepithelial lesions (SILs). Adherence to HAART and effectiveness of the regimen were also assessed. The prevalence, incident detection, and clearance of HPV infection or SILs before versus after HAART initiation were compared (using women as their own comparison group). HAART initiation among adherent women was associated with a significant reduction in prevalence, incident detection of oncogenic HPV infection, and decreased prevalence and more rapid clearance of oncogenic HPV-positive SILs. Effects were smaller among nonadherent women (Minkoff et al, 2010).

SUGGESTED READINGS

Epidemiology of HIV in Women

Barkan S, Melnick SL, Preston-Martin S, et al: The Women's Interagency HIV Study: WIHS Collaborative Study Group, *Epidemiology* 9(2):117–125, 1998.

Boily MC, Baggaley RF, Wang L, et al: Heterosexual risk of HIV-1 infection per sexual act: systematic review and meta-analysis of observational studies, *Lancet Infect Dis* 9(2):118–129, 2009.

Centers for Disease Control and Prevention: *Cases of HIV infection and AIDS in the United States and dependent areas, 2007: Table 6a* (website). www.cdc.gov/hiv/topics/surveillance/resources/reports/2007report/table6a.htm. Accessed August 6, 2011.

Centers for Disease Control and Prevention: *HIV/AIDS and women* (website). www.cdc.gov/hiv/topics/women/index.htm. Accessed August 6, 2011.

Fleming DT, Wasserheit JN: From epidemiological synergy to public health policy and practice: the contribution of other sexually transmitted diseases to sexual transmission of HIV infection, *Sex Transm Infect* 75(1):3–17, 1999.

http://statepiaps.jhsph.edu/wihs. Accessed August 6, 2011.

World Health Organization: *Women and health: today's evidence tomorrow's agenda* (website). www.who.int/gender/documents/9789241563857/en/index.html. Accessed August 6, 2011.

Male Circumcision

Baeten JM, Donnell D, Kapiga SH, et al: Male circumcision and risk of male-to-female HIV-1 transmission: a multinational prospective study in African HIV-1 serodiscordant couples, *AIDS* 24(5):737–744, 2010.

Siegfried N, Muller M, Deeks JJ, Volmink J: Male circumcision for prevention of heterosexual acquisition of HIV in men, *Cochrane Database Syst Rev*(2): CD003362, 2009.

Wawer MJ, Makumbi F, Kigozi G, et al: Circumcision in HIV-infected men and its effect on HIV transmission to female partners in Rakai, Uganda: a randomised controlled trial, *Lancet* 374(9685):229–237, 2009.

Microbicides

Roehr B: Microbicide offers no protection against HIV infection, *BMJ* 339:b5538, 2009.

Skoler-Karpoff S, Ramjee G, Ahmed K, et al: Efficacy of Carraguard for prevention of HIV infection in women in South Africa: a randomised, double-blind, placebo-controlled trial, *Lancet* 372(9654):1977–1987, 2008.

Van Damme L, Chandeying V, Ramjee G, et al: Safety of multiple daily applications of COL-1492, a nonoxynol-9 vaginal gel, among female sex workers: COL-1492 phase 2 study group, *AIDS* 14(1):85–88, 2000.

Van Damme L, Govinden R, Mirembe FM, et al: Lack of effectiveness of cellulose sulfate gel for the prevention of vaginal HIV transmission, *N Engl J Med* 359(5):463–472, 2008.

Preexposure Prophylaxis

Abdool Karim Q: *Safety and effectiveness of 1% tenofovir vaginal microbicide gel in South African women: results of the CAPRISA 004 Trial*, Vienna, Austria, 2010, Oral presentation, XVIII International AIDS Conference. (website) globalhealth.kff.org/AIDS2010/July-20/Safety-and-Effectiveness.aspx. Accessed August 6, 2011.

AVAC: *Pre-Exposure Prophylaxis (PrEP)* (website). www.prepwatch.org Accessed March 15, 2010.

Cohen MS, Chen YQ, McCaughley M, et al: Prevention of HIV-1 infection with Early Antiretroviral Therapy, *NEJM* 365:493–505, 2011.

Grant RM, Lama JR, Anderson PL, et al: Preexposure chemoprophylaxis for HIV prevention in men who have sex with men, *N Engl J Med* 363(27):2587–2599, 2010.

Vernazza PL, Graf I, Sonnenberg-Schwan U, et al: *Pre-exposure prophylaxis and timed intercourse for HIV-discordant couples willing to conceive a child*. *AIDS* 25:2005–2008, 2011.

HIV in Pregnancy

Bulterys M, Jamieson DJ, O'Sullivan MJ, et al: Rapid HIV-1 testing during labor, *JAMA* 292(2):219–223, 2004.

Cooper ER, Charurat M, Mofenson LM, et al: Combination antiretroviral strategies for the treatment of pregnant HIV-1 infected women and prevention of perinatal HIV-1 transmission, *J Acquir Immune Defic Syndr Hum Retrovirol* 29(5):484–494, 2002.

Panel on Treatment of HIV-Infected Pregnant Women and Prevention of Perinatal Transmission: *Recommendations for use of antiretroviral drugs in pregnant HIV-1-infected women for maternal health and interventions to reduce perinatal HIV transmission in the United States*, May 24, 2010; pp 1-117 (website). aidsinfo.nih.gov/ContentFiles/PerinatalGL.pdf. Accessed January 19, 2011.

Townsend CL, Cortina-Borja M, Peckham CS, Tooke PA: Trends in management and outcome of pregnancies in HIV-infected women in the UK and Ireland, 1990-2006, *BJOG* 115(9):1078–1086, 2008.

Conception in HIV-Infected Couples

Attia S, Egger M, Müller M, et al: Sexual transmission of HIV according to viral load and antiretroviral therapy: systematic review and meta-analysis, *AIDS* 23(11):1397–1404, 2009.

Donnell D, Baeten JM, Kiarie J, et al: Heterosexual HIV-1 transmission after initiation of antiretroviral therapy: a prospective cohort analysis, *Lancet* 375(9731):2092–2098, 2010.

Lee TH, Sakahara N, Fiebig E, et al: Correlation of HIV-1 RNA levels in plasma and heterosexual transmission of HIV-1 from infected transfusion recipients, *J Acquir Immune Defic Syndr Human Retrovirol* 12(4):427–428, 1996.

Thornton AC, Romanelli F, Collins JD: Reproduction decision making for couples affected by HIV: a review of the literature, *Top HIV Med* 12(2):61–67, 2004.

Contraception in HIV-Infected Women

Cohn SE, Park JG, Watts DH, et al: Depot-medroxyprogesterone in women on antiretroviral therapy: effective contraception and lack of clinically significant interactions, *Clin Pharmacol Ther* 81(2):222–227, 2007.

Heffron R, Donnell D, Rees H, et al: Use of hormonal contraceptives and risk of HIV-1 transmission: a prospective cohort study, *The Lancet Infectious Diseases* doi:10.1016, 70247(11):S1473–3099, 2011. .

Heikinhimo O, Lahteenmaki P: Contraception and HIV infection in women, *Hum Reprod Update* 15(2):165–176, 2009.

Heikinheimo O, Lehtovirta P, Suni J, Paavonen J: The levonorgestrel-releasing intrauterine system (LNG-IUS) in HIV-infected women: effects on bleeding patterns, ovarian function and genital shedding of HIV, *Hum Reprod* 21(11):2857–2861, 2006.

Kapiga SH, Lyamuya EF, Lwihula GK, Hunter DJ: The incidence of HIV infection among women using family planning methods in Dar es Salaam, Tanzania, *AIDS* 12(1):75–84, 1998.

Martin HL Jr, Nyange PM, Richardson BA, et al: Hormonal contraception, sexually transmitted diseases, and risk of heterosexual transmission of human immunodeficiency virus type 1, *J Infect Dis* 178(4):1053–1059, 1998.

HPV and Cervical Dysplasia in HIV-Infected Women

American College of Obstetricians and Gynecologists Committee on Practice Bulletins—Gynecology: ACOG practice bulletin no. 109: cervical cytology screening, *Obstet Gynecol* 114(6):1409–1420, 2009.

Conley LJ, Ellenbrock TV, Bush TJ, et al: HIV-1 infection and risk of vulvovaginal and perianal condylomata acuminata and intraepithelial neoplasia: a prospective cohort study, *Lancet* 359(9301):108–113, 2002.

Delmas MC, Larsen C, van Benthem B, et al: Cervical squamous intraepithelial lesions in HIV-infected women: prevalence, incidence and regression, *AIDS* 14(12):1775–1784, 2000.

Minkoff H, Zhong Y, Burk RD, et al: Influence of adherent and effective antiretroviral therapy use on human papillomavirus infection and squamous intraepithelial lesions in human immunodeficiency virus-positive women, *J Infect Dis* 201(5):681–690, 2010.

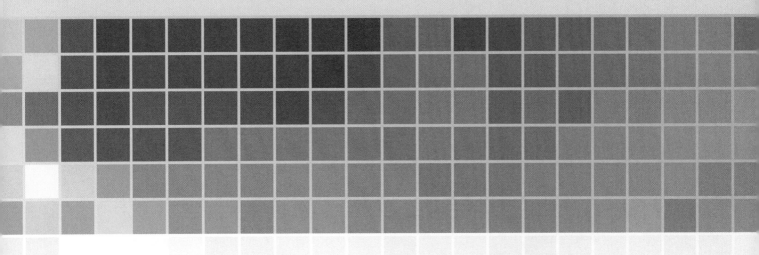

Sexuality and Women's Health Psychology

Chapter 44

Chronic Pelvic Pain

ANDREA J. RAPKIN • WENDY SATMARY

KEY UPDATES

1 Chronic pelvic pain (CPP) accounts for 10% of referrals to obstetrician-gynecologists and is a primary indication for at least 40% of laparoscopies performed by gynecologists and 20% of hysterectomies performed annually in the United States.

2 CPP is a multifactorial process. The differential diagnosis includes both gynecologic and nongynecologic disorders, often involving more than one visceral or somatic structure or a neuropathic etiology.

3 Hormonal treatment—including hormonal contraceptives, progestins, danazol, and gonadotropin-releasing hormone agonists—has been studied extensively for chronic pelvic pain of gynecologic origin and should be considered first line for women with dysmenorrhea, suspected endometriosis, or cyclic pelvic pain.

4 Myofascial pain arising from the anterior abdominal wall and pelvic floor muscles is prevalent and is a frequently overlooked cause of chronic pelvic pain.

5 Women with CPP often have higher levels of depression, anxiety, and sexual dysfunction as well as a greater incidence of past emotional, physical, or sexual trauma. Referral to psychologists, psychiatrists, social workers, marriage counselors, or sex therapists is often indicated.

6 Endometriosis is increasingly diagnosed in the adolescent population. Adolescent patients typically present with progressive and severe dysmenorrhea interfering with school, physical, or social activities. Because endometriosis is thought to be progressive and estrogen dependent, medical treatment for adolescents is particularly important and may prevent the disease from progressing and preserve future fertility.

7 Vulvar pain disorders, including generalized vulvodynia or localized vulvodynia, provoked, unprovoked, or mixed, present a significant health problem for women. It is estimated that up to 15% of women have vulvodynia. Response rates of at least 50% have been reported for the treatment of localized provoked vestibulodynia (formerly vulvar vestibulitis syndrome) with any of the following modalities: physical therapy, cognitive behavioral therapy, tricyclic antidepressants, local anesthetics applied topically or injected, or vestibulectomy.

8 Gastrointestinal and genitourinary pathologies are common among women with CPP. As many as 60% of patients referred to gynecologists for CPP are thought to have irritable bowel syndrome (IBS) and 30% to 40% have interstitial cystitis/bladder pain syndrome (IC/BPS).

9 IBS affects up to 10% of the general population and affects women two times more frequently than men.

10 Neuropathic pain caused by nerve entrapment from scar formation or injury is a commonly overlooked cause of lower quadrant pain. Ilioinguinal and iliohypogastric nerve injuries, which occur in about 3.7% of gynecologic surgeries, are more common with Pfannenstiel incisions but can also occur with trocar incisions.

11 The diagnosis and treatment of CPP can be challenging, particularly when traditional approaches fail to relieve pain. Treatment should involve a multidisciplinary, multiplatform approach.

Chronic Pelvic Pain (CPP): Overview

CLINICAL PROFILE

- CPP is characterized as the presence of pelvic pain of at least 6 months duration that is severe enough to warrant medical attention or cause functional impairment
- CPP can emanate from the pelvic visceral or somatic structures or altered central nervous system (CNS) neural processing
- CPP is defined anatomically as pain in the region delineated by the anterior superior iliac spine and umbilicus superiorly to the pubis inferiorly, including the pelvic floor, lower back, buttocks, vagina, and vulva

UPDATE #1

CPP accounts for 10% of referrals to obstetrician-gynecologists and is a primary indication for at least 40% of laparoscopies performed by gynecologists and 20% of hysterectomies performed annually in the United States (Howard, 2003).

- The prevalence of CPP in the United States is difficult to accurately establish because of differing definitions, study design, and measurements used
- Estimates of the prevalence range from 3.8% to over 15% in large-scale population-based studies
- CPP is an important cause of morbidity and suffering in women and a significant health care cost burden, with estimated annual direct costs of $880 million in the United States and billions in indirect costs

UPDATE #2

CPP is a multifactorial process, and the differential diagnosis includes both gynecologic and nongynecologic diagnoses, often involving more than one visceral, somatic or neuropathic etiology (Rapkin et al, 2011).

- The most common and often overlapping diagnoses include endometriosis, interstitial cystitis/bladder pain syndrome (IC/BPS), irritable bowel syndrome (IBS), myofascial pain, neuropathy, depression, and anxiety; central nervous system "up-regulation" and altered descending inhibition of impulses can account for the observation that the pain is generally out of proportion to visualized pathology
- Myofascial pain from the anterior abdominal wall and pelvic floor muscles is prevalent and an often overlooked source of CPP

Common Gynecologic Causes of CPP

- The most common gynecologic diagnosis is endometriosis
- There may not be a cause-and-effect relationship for many of the disorders in Table 44-1 but rather an association; in clinical practice, treatment must be individualized; excessive surgery that may result in further tissue damage or loss of reproductive and hormonal function should be avoided

TABLE 44-1   Differential Diagnosis of CPP

Gynecologic

Primary or secondary dysmenorrhea

Endometriosis

Adenomyosis

Leiomyomata

Ovarian neoplasm, recurrent functional ovarian cysts, ovarian remnant syndrome, residual ovary syndrome

Pelvic inflammatory disease

Pelvic congestion syndrome

Pelvic relaxation

Pelvic adhesions

Gastrointestinal

Irritable bowel syndrome (IBS)

Functional abdominal pain and bloating syndrome

Inflammatory bowel disease

Colorectal cancer and other gastrointestinal tumors

Celiac sprue

Genitourinary

Interstitial cystitis/ bladder pain syndrome

Recurrent urinary tract infections/urethritis

Benign or malignant tumors, hydronephrosis, calculosis

Musculoskeletal

Myofascial pain: abdominal wall, pelvic floor, lower back

Fibromyalgia

Lumbar radiculopathy

Sacroiliac joint dysfunction/sacroiliitis

Pyriformis syndrome

Neuropathic

Neuropathy or entrapment of nerve or branches of nerves:

—Iliohypogastric or ilioinguinal nerves (L1, L2)

—Sciatic nerve (L4,5; S2-4)

—Pudendal nerve (S2-4)

—Genitofemoral nerve (L2)

Multiple sclerosis

- There is consistent scientific evidence of a causal relationship to CPP in the following:
  - Endometriosis, gynecologic neoplasms, pelvic inflammatory disease (PID), ovarian remnant syndrome
- There are fewer or limited data for a causal relationship with the following:
  - Adhesions, fibroids, adenomyosis, small adnexal cysts, pelvic organ prolapse
  - Endometriosis in women who do not respond to usually effective medical or surgical therapy
- Determine if the pain is cyclic or noncyclic, as there are implications for treatment
  - Nongynecologic causes of CPP are more often noncyclic, but pain from these disorders can also be exacerbated in the premenstrual or menstrual phases; explanations for this phenomenon include hormonal modulation, neuropeptide or neurotransmitter alterations, and shared neural substrates for the pelvic viscera and somatic tissues (muscles, fascia, and nerves)

- Subtypes of CPP have been proposed, although none are universally accepted
  - In a study aimed at categorizing subtypes of CPP in patients who presented to a tertiary referral-based center, the most common categories were as follows:
    - Diffuse abdominal/pelvic pain (42.2%), vulvovaginal pain (20.4%), cyclic pain (10.0%), neuropathic pain (9%), nonlocalizable pain with inability to reproduce or localize the pain on exam (6.6%), myofascial pain with trigger points (5.9%) and fibroids (5.9%)
  - Endometriosis was common in both cyclic and diffuse abdominal/pelvic pain subtypes
  - Women with diffuse abdominal/pelvic pain had more trauma and worse mental and physical health status as compared to women with vulvovaginal or cyclic pain

Common Nongynecologic Causes of CPP

- Musculoskeletal: myofascial pain involving abdominal wall or pelvic floor muscle pain or trigger points, lumbar radiculopathy, sacroiliac joint dysfunction, pyriformis syndrome, hip disorders
- Gastrointestinal: IBS/functional bowel syndromes, carcinoma
- Genitourinary: IC/BPS, recurrent urinary tract infections, carcinoma
- Neurologic: neuropathy, nerve entrapment, neuroma formation

MUSCLES OF THE PELVIC FLOOR

- Levator ani, composed of the following:
  - Pubococcygeus–anterior and main part of levator ani
  - Iliococcygeus–posterior part of levator ani
  - Puborectalis–inferior to the pubococcygeus
- Coccygeus–reinforces pelvic floor posteriorly
- Obturator internus and pyriformis line lateral walls of the pelvis anteriorly and posteriorly, respectively

Mechanisms Underlying Pain

- Biologic mechanisms underlying pain include nociceptive, inflammatory, and neuropathic

- **Nociceptive** pain is a response to noxious stimuli, such as ischemia, spasm, distention, or injury
- Nociceptive pain may be of somatic or visceral origin
- **Inflammatory** pain is due to a response of tissue injury and the inflammatory response, and it may also lead to a chronic pain state through a pathologic pain mechanism
- **Neuropathic** pain is caused by nerve dysfunction or damage or up-regulation in the central or peripheral nervous systems (central and peripheral sensitization)

Complexity of Pelvic Neuroanatomy

- Afferent stimuli from a visceral source can affect somatic structures through visceral-somatic reflexes
- Nerve cell bodies in the dorsal horn of the spinal cord and other CNS regions receive convergent input from both somatic and visceral structures
- Afferent signals converge, leading to aberrant interactions that can result in a painful sensation from organs that are not directly inflamed or stimulated (cross-talk) and from nearby somatic structures (cross-sensitization)
- The concept of viscerovisceral and viscerosomatic convergence helps explain why there is so much overlap in the prevalence of conditions such as endometriosis, IC/BPS, IBS, and vulvodynia
- Endometriosis may generate pain through inflammatory, neuropathic mechanisms, and nociceptive mechanisms
  - This can explain the common finding of recurrent or persistent pain in women who have been adequately treated medically or surgically for endometriosis
  - This may underlie the fact that the extent of disease does not correlate with the severity of pain
- Both central and peripheral sensitization or amplification can occur with neuropathic pain
- In central sensitization, there is amplification of the CNS response; although this is initially adaptive, it may lead to pathologic allodynia (pain with usually nonpainful stimulation), hyperalgesia (increased pain with a potentially painful stimulus), or enlargement of the receptive field (pain spreading beyond the site of injury)
- Central sensitization is a proposed mechanism for endometriosis-related pain syndrome; women with symptomatic endometriosis were shown to manifest both central sensitization and inhibition in a case-controlled study in which women with laparoscopically diagnosed endometriosis and controls were injected with saline into a distal muscle; compared to control subjects, patients with endometriosis had increased pain intensity and larger painful areas
- Physiologic, environmental, and psychological stress can alter release of neuropeptides, neurotransmitters, and cytokines, which play roles in neuromodulation and pain perception
  - Pain sensitivity has been shown to increase by 40% in the premenstrual and menstrual phases in normal women

Pain History

- Obtaining a thorough pain history is critical; allow 5 minutes or so for the patient to give her pain "narrative"

- A useful sample previsit history questionnaire is available at the International Pelvic Pain Society website (www.pelvicpain.org)
- History should include the following:
  - Nature of the pain: character, intensity, location and radiation, aggravating and alleviating factors, effect of menses, activity, intercourse
  - Severity of pain on a 0-to-10 on verbal or visual analog pain scale
  - Chronology of the pain: In what context does the pain arise? Was there an inciting event? Has the pain changed over time? What does the patient think is causing the pain?
  - Associated symptoms, specifically related to the following:
    - *Genital:* abnormal vaginal bleeding, discharge, dysmenorrhea, dyspareunia, infertility
    - *Gastrointestinal:* constipation, diarrhea, flatulence, tenesmus, alteration in pain before and after bowel movement, blood, changes in color or caliber of stool
    - *Musculoskeletal:* pain distribution, radiation, association with injury, exercise, fatigue, postural changes, exercise, and lifting
    - *Urinary tract:* dysuria, hematuria, urgency, frequency, nocturia, suprapubic pain
    - *Neurologic:* burning, lancinating pain, allodynia, or numbness in distribution of a particular peripheral nerve or scar or tight muscle
  - Documentation of prior evaluation or treatment of pain including operative and pathology reports as well as doses, side effects, and success or failure of prior pharmacologic treatments
  - Impact of pain on family, occupation, and daily activities: Is the degree of pain such that the pain prevents the patient from usual activities and responsibilities? Is litigation or workers' compensation an issue? What is the attitude of the patient and family toward the pain and resultant behavior?
  - Past medical, surgical, gynecologic, obstetric history, allergies, and current medications; document history of sexually transmitted infections, obstetric trauma, and so on
  - Current and past psychological history; include history of past or current physical, sexual, or emotional abuse, history of hospitalization, suicide attempts, and drug or ethanol use or dependence
  - Sexual history
  - Social and family history

UPDATE #5

Many studies suggest that women with CPP have higher levels of depression, anxiety, and sexual dysfunction and a greater incidence of past emotional, physical, or sexual trauma. Referral to psychologists, psychiatrists, social workers, marriage counselors, or sex therapists is often indicated (Fricchione, 2004; Latthe et al, 2006; Meltzer-Brody et al, 2007; Weijenborg et al, 2009).

- Screen for depression, anxiety, stress, quality of relationships, and intimacy
- Take a sexual history include libido, arousal, orgasm, pain/primary or secondary
  - Screening tools for anxiety, depression, and sexual functioning are useful

- A screening tool for trauma and posttraumatic stress disorder (PTSD) in women with CPP has also been described; as many as 25% of individuals with a history of trauma will develop PTSD, and it is more common in women; one third of patients with CPP had a positive PTSD screen; stress response, particularly when associated with childhood trauma, may cause CNS dysregulation and contribute to CPP
- Depression is a risk factor for narcotic addiction and poor treatment outcome; referral for psychiatric or psychological services should be considered on an individual basis

Physical Exam for CPP

- Physical exam should be thorough and gentle
- Ask patient to localize her pain
- Localize the pain by careful palpation to a particular tissue or innervation, in an effort to reproduce the pain
- Educate the patient regarding anatomy, adaptive sexual functioning, and the broad range of normalcy
- Assess basic muscle strength and range of motion
- Perform a basic neurologic exam of the perineum and lower extremities for sensation and weakness
- Evaluate abdominal muscles in tender areas for trigger points using one-finger palpation in both the relaxed state and with the muscles tensed and include the inguinal areas; the hip, sacroiliac areas, and buttocks (gluteus) can also be palpated for trigger points
- In the supine position, localize the most tender point(s), mark with a pen, then ask the patient to raise both straightened legs (Carnett's test) or to perform an abdominal crunch by lifting her head and shoulders off the table ("sit-up"); again, palpate the tender areas of the abdominal wall origin and if they are still tender, pain is suggested; this maneuver will help to differentiate abdominal wall (myofascial/neuropathic/hernia) from visceral pain
- Pelvic exam should include a thorough inspection of the vulva and perineum, including skin changes, scars, sign of trauma, and the presence of any lesions that may indicate an underlying infectious or inflammatory process (i.e., herpes, dermatoses, lichen planus, dermatitis); the vulva is composed of five parts: clitoris, vestibule, hymen, labia minora, and labia majora
- A "cotton swab" test can be performed to assess for vestibular allodynia (detailed instruction follows)
- A speculum exam should be done to inspect the vagina and cervix, again noting any lesions, abnormalities, or displacement of the cervix, as seen with endometriosis
- The vaginal exam should include vaginal pH, microscopy, and assessment of estrogen status
- Examine the muscles of the vagina and introitus both at rest and during the process of squeezing and releasing; patients with hypertonic disorders may be unable to tighten because of a high basal resting tone
- Using a single finger, palpate the anterior vagina, urethra, bladder base, and vaginal side walls; tenderness or induration in these areas may suggest chronic urethritis, urethral diverticulum, IC/BPS, or vaginal wall cyst

- Palpate the cervix, paracervical areas, vaginal fornices, uterosacral ligaments, and coccyx, again noting any tenderness or nodularity, which may indicate endometriosis or infection
- Using a single finger, apply gentle pressure downward against the levator ani, obturator internus, and pyriformis; note areas of exquisite tenderness, trigger points, and reproduction of the patient's pain
- The pyriformis may be difficult to palpate; rectal exam may be easier to palpate both the coccyx and pyriformis; in the lithotomy position, palpate the ipsilateral pyriformis just superior to the ischial spine as the patient is asked to abduct her thigh against resistance; exquisite tenderness may indicate pyriformis syndrome or the presence of trigger points
- Palpate the pudendal nerve in Alcock's canal, assessing for increased pain with palpation
- Trigger point injections or nerve blocks can be both diagnostic and therapeutic; if pain reduction occurs for the next 1 to 2 weeks, then a significant myofascial or neuropathic component is present and injections should be repeated
  - Trigger point injections or nerve blocks can be done a variety of ways, commonly using a 22- to 25-guage needle to inject 1 to 3 cc of local anesthetic into the trigger point or around the tender area; once the needle penetrates the trigger point and elicits pain response, inject and then back out the needle to redirect and inject parallel planes 1 to 3 mm away in surrounding muscle; if performing a nerve block, do not inject directly into the nerve but instead redirect the needle if there is an electrical sensation with injection
  - Some authors recommend addition of corticosteroid to the local anesthetic when pain is associated with prior surgery
  - Bimanual exam should be performed to palpate the uterus and adnexa, noting any enlargement, masses, tenderness, and abnormalities in position or shape, including pelvic relaxation or prolapse; uterine tenderness may be indicative of adenomyosis, pelvic congestion syndrome, or infection; lateral cervical displacement or a fixed, immobile, or retroflexed uterus may indicate endometriosis or adhesions
  - Rectovaginal exam should be performed, noting uterosacral nodularity, tenderness, rectal disease, or occult blood

Special Circumstances

- Virginity or atrophic postmenopausal vagina
  - A bimanual exam may not always be necessary in the virginal girl with CPP
  - Consider one-finger bimanual or rectal-abdominal exam in the dorsal lithotomy position with a very narrow introitus; abdominal ultrasound is usually adequate
- Vaginismus
  - Vaginismus refers to involuntary contraction of the perineal and muscles of the pelvic floor prior to or during vaginal penetration

Additional Tests

- Diagnostic studies should be individualized and based on history and physical exam

- Complete blood count, urinalysis, and pelvic ultrasound are indicated; perform pregnancy test if indicated; transvaginal ultrasound is the imaging study of choice in evaluation for endometriosis; additional imaging such as computed tomography (CT) or magnetic resonance imaging (MRI) with and without contrast of pelvis or lumbar sacral area should be ordered based on individual symptoms and clinical judgment
- The use of laparoscopy in women with CPP should be individualized, as histologic confirmation of endometriosis is not needed before starting medical therapy; disadvantages include the cost, operative complications, and nondiagnosis, in that a negative laparoscopy may often miss occult, microscopic implants or retroperitoneal; potential major complications include vascular, visceral, or nerve injury; major complication rates vary from 0.1% to 2.3%; minor complication rates range from 5% to 11%
- The literature does not find benefit for conscious laparoscopic pain mapping, that is, laparoscopy under sedation with probing of tissues, lesions or organs for pain response, and targeted excision of painful regions
- Colonoscopy and cystoscopy may be indicated

Management of Common Gynecologic Disorders

ENDOMETRIOSIS
Background and Diagnosis

- Endometriosis affects 1% to 10% of the general population and is the most common gynecologic cause of CPP
- Endometriosis is defined by the presence of endometrial tissue (glands and stroma) outside the uterine cavity, most commonly the peritoneum or ovaries
- Different theories include retrograde menstruation, lymphatic spread, and coelomic metaplasia, which may explain the existence of endometriosis before puberty
- Most common presenting symptoms include the following:
  - Dysmenorrhea: affects up to 90% of premenopausal menstruating women; it is often described as cramping pain in the lower abdomen before and during menstrual flow; pain related to endometriosis is considered secondary dysmenorrhea
    - Primary dysmenorrhea is defined as pain without underlying pathology and is the most common gynecologic complaint among adolescent females and young women; it usually begins with the onset of ovulatory menstrual cycles and tends to decrease after childbirth
    - The etiology of primary dysmenorrhea is not fully understood; one classic theory is related to an overproduction of prostaglandins
    - Secondary dysmenorrhea is defined as pain caused by underlying pathology: endometriosis, adenomyosis, fibroids, and uterine polyps or anomalies, the latter of which should be considered in the adolescents
    - Atypical dysmenorrhea is common in endometriosis and consists of pain/pressure symptoms starting 7 or more days prior to menses not just localized to the uterus, but also the lower abdomen, back, or rectum

- Deep dyspareunia: pelvic not introital
  - Subfertility
  - In women undergoing laparoscopy for CPP, endometriosis is found in approximately in 30% to 80%
  - Other symptoms may include heavy or break-through bleeding, dyschezia, hematochezia, urinary urgency, frequency, bladder pain, or hematuria

UPDATE #6

Endometriosis is diagnosed with increasing frequency in the adolescent population. Adolescent patients typically present with progressive and severe dysmenorrhea, and often pain interferes with school, physical, or social activities. Because endometriosis is thought to be progressive and estrogen dependent, medical treatment for adolescents is important and may prevent disease progression and preserve future fertility (American College of Obstetricians and Gynecologists, Committee Opinion No. 310, 2005).

- The typical presentation of endometriosis in adolescence may differ from that in the adult
- Progressive dysmenorrhea, dyspareunia, gastrointestinal complaints, and both cyclic and acyclic pain are common
- In the adult, classic findings on exam may include uterosacral nodularity, focal tenderness, adnexal masses, and a fixed or retroverted uterus; in the adolescent, these findings are commonly absent
- Transvaginal ultrasound or other imaging study may be helpful but not specific for diagnosing endometriosis; transvaginal ultrasound is more accurate for detecting severe endometriosis, such as disease involving the bowel or bladder
- Lab studies, including CA 125 and C reactive protein are also nonspecific

Treatment

- Laparoscopy is the gold standard in diagnosis and treatment of endometriosis, but it is not necessary in order to initiate medical treatment
- Combined or progestin-only cyclic or continuous hormonal contraceptives and depo progestins are safe and effective even in the adolescent population, but there are no studies of the long-term effect of gonadotropin-releasing hormone (GnRH) agonist therapy in the adolescent population
- GnRH agonist therapy should be considered with add-back therapy with a progestin, with or without a low-dose estrogen, for patients who do not respond to continuous hormonal contraceptives
- The goal of medical treatment is hormonal suppression to reduce cyclic hormonal stimulation and lead to atrophy or dedidualization of lesions
- There are no published clinical trials comparing medical and surgical therapy in the treatment of CPP and endometriosis
- An approach based on expert panel consensus is the following:
  - Initial trial of medical therapy (first and second line) unless laparoscopy is indicated

- First-line medical therapy: nonsteroidal anti-inflammatory medications (NSAIDs), hormonal combined estrogen/progestin contraceptives, or both; OCPs or vaginal ring or transdermal patches can be used in cyclic or continuous fashion
- Second-line therapies include danazol, GnRH agonists, GnRH agonists with aromatase inhibitors, and progestins, including the levonorgestrel-releasing intrauterine system (LNG-IUS); the LNG-IUS or depo progestins can also be first line
- Laparoscopy is indicated if an adnexal mass or infertility is present
- Other factors to consider with regard to choosing laparoscopy or medical management include surgical risks, contraindications to hormonal management cost, desire for immediate conception, and patient preference
  - OCPs may be useful by inhibiting ovulation and decreasing menstrual flow
  - Second-line agents:
- Danazol, an androgenic and antiestrogenic agent, is very effective in treating symptomatic endometriosis in adults at doses ranging 400 to 800 mg, divided into twice daily doses; androgenic side effects are common
- Danazol acts primarily by inhibiting the luteinizing hormone (LH) surge and steroidogenesis and by increasing free testosterone levels
- Progestins, including medroxyprogesterone acetate, norethindrone acetate, and LNG-IUS, have also been found to be more effective than placebo in randomized controlled trials (RCTs)
- GnRH agonists via binding to GnRH receptors cause down-regulation or gonadotropins and hypoestrogenism
  - Add-back therapy should be considered for vasomotor symptoms and if therapy extends beyond 6 months because of bone loss; add-back therapy, commonly norethindrone or norethindrone acetate alone or combined with low-dose conjugated equine estrogens, may alleviate vasomotor symptoms associated with therapy as well as extend pain relief and bone mineral density preservation after completion of therapy for 12 months
  - RCTs of GnRH agonist therapy in laparoscopically confirmed endometriosis showed reduction in pain and decrease in size of lesions; a recent RCT (Petta CA et al, 2005) compared LNG-IUS with GnRH agonist for the treatment of CPP-associated endometriosis and found that both were effective treatments and one was not better than the other; the LNG-IUS has the advantage of not causing hypoestrogenism
  - GnRH agonist relieves CPP in 50% of patients
  - Aromatase inhibitors, such as letrozole, have been described in case reports to reduce pain in postmenopausal women with endometriosis-associated pain and can be added to hormonal or GnRH agonist therapy for premenopausal women in selected cases
  - Aromatase is the rate-limiting enzyme for estrogen synthesis from androgens, and side effects (joint pain, myalgia) are common; data on the effectiveness of aromatase inhibitors in treating endometriosis are limited, and further studies are needed

- Surgical and nonsurgical treatments for CPP are associated with improvement in pain, and there are no published clinical trials comparing medical and surgical therapy in the treatment of CPP and endometriosis
- Surgical treatment can be "conservative" (i.e., removing endometriosis lesions) or "definitive," with removal of the uterus and ovaries
- Bilateral salpingo-oophorectomy (BSO) with hysterectomy has been shown to reduce CPP from endometriosis and should be considered for some women; issues to consider include completion of childbearing and impact on general health including menopause and osteoporosis
- Hysterectomy alone has limited value in surgical management of women with endometriosis-associated CPP
- When a surgical approach is planned, it is well established that laparoscopic approaches are associated with reduced morbidity and decreased postoperative morbidity as compared to laparotomy
- If endometriosis is suspected at the time of diagnostic laparoscopy, biopsy, and pathology confirmation should be performed, because early lesions may be missed; clearly document the extent of disease; conservative surgical treatment with excision or ablation or both should be considered; surgeon skill may be an important limiting factor, however, because extensive disease may involve deeply infiltrating lesions—for example, into the bowel
- In comparison to expectant management, there is significant pain relief at 6 months after laparoscopic surgery for endometriosis
- No randomized controlled trials have compared surgical excision to energy-based techniques (vaporization, fulguration, coagulation); improved pain scores in general have been reported 6 and 12 months postoperatively, and improved surgical outcomes have also been reported with GnRH agonist and surgery as compared to surgery alone
- A trial evaluating use of OCPs postsurgery for resection of endometriomas showed no long-term benefit for reducing their recurrence
- Presacral neurectomy (PSN) and laparoscopic uterine nerve ablation (LUNA) involve transection of the superior hypogastric plexus at the level of the sacrum and uterosacral nerve transaction/ablation, respectively
- A 2005 Cochrane database meta-analysis of eight RCTs concluded that adding LUNA with conservative surgical management of endometriosis implants did not improve results; no pain relief differences were seen between LUNA or PSN; however, long-term PSN was shown to be significantly more effective than LUNA with regard to long-term pain relief at both 6 (87.3% versus 60.3%) and 12 months (85.7% versus 57.1%)
- Alternative treatments
  - Acupuncture
    - A small cohort study in men with chronic pelvic pain syndrome underwent treatment with acupuncture for 6 weeks; short-term (24-week) follow-up showed a significant reduction in pain scores with more than a 50% decrease from baseline
    - Acupuncture has also been described in the treatment of primary dysmenorrhea, but data to support its efficacy are limited efficacy are limited.

- Transcutaneous electrical nerve stimulation (TENS)
  - A meta-analysis of nine RCTs found TENS effective in the treatment of dysmenorrhea
- Complementary herbal medicine
  - Although data are limited, two trials included in the Cochrane review of Chinese herbal medicine for endometriosis suggest Chinese herbal medicine may be as useful as conventional treatment and associated with fewer side effects in relief of endometriosis pain; better studies are needed in the future to investigate the role of other potential alternative therapies in the treatment of endometriosis

OTHER GYNECOLOGIC DISORDERS AND MANAGEMENT

- History, physical exam, laboratory or imaging data will frequently lead to the diagnosis of *other* common gynecologic conditions that may be associated with signs and symptoms other than those related to chronic pelvic pain (i.e., bleeding)
- Management of neoplasia, fibroids, adenomyosis, prolapse, and adnexal pathology should be individualized
- Pelvic congestion syndrome is a vague disorder infrequently described in the U.S. gynecologic literature
  - Associated with ovarian or uterine vein incompetence and with symptoms often described as a "heaviness," dysmenorrhea, postcoital pain, and pain that is worse with prolonged activity or standing
  - Common after pregnancy and disappears after menopause
  - Dilatated tortuous veins may be seen on pelvic ultrasound or MRI or venography
  - Proposed treatments but may include high-dose progestins, danazol, and GnRH agonists, psychological therapy, NSAIDs, vein embolization, and hysterectomy and oophorectomy
- Adhesions
  - A causal relationship between adhesions and CPP is controversial
  - There is no evidence that adhesions cause CPP or that lysis of adhesions is more effective than placebo (laparoscopy without adhesiolysis)
- Ovarian remnant syndrome can result from ovarian tissue left in situ after difficult salpingo-oophorectomy, such as in the setting of severe endometriosis or PID; treatment consists of hormonal suppression or excision
- Residual ovary syndrome refers to recurrent, large painful functional ovarian cysts occurring in a patient posthysterectomy; treatment is with hormonal suppression; if this is effective but the patient prefers not to continue hormonal therapy, then surgery would be warranted

UPDATE #7

Vulvar pain disorders, including generalized vulvodynia or localized vulvodynia, provoked, unprovoked or mixed, present a significant health problem for women. It is estimated that up to 15% of women have vulvodynia. Response rates of at least 50% have been reported for the treatment of localized provoked vestibulodynia (formerly vulvar vestibulitis syndrome) with any of the following modalities: physical therapy, cognitive behavioral therapy, tricyclic antidepressants, local anesthetics applied topically or injected, or vestibulectomy.

VULVODYNIA

Diagnosis

- Vulvodynia is most commonly described as chronic and persistent vulvar burning, pain, stinging, or itching in the absence of any visible findings or identifiable disorder
- The differential includes infection (i.e., candida, herpes, trichomonas), inflammation (i.e., lichen planus, lichen sclerosis, lichen simplex chronicus, psoriasis), neoplasia (Paget's disease, vulvar intraepithelial neoplasia, squamous cell cancer), neurologic disorders (i.e., herpes, pudendal or sciatic neuropathy), and hypoestrogenization (menopause or long-term, low-dose [20 mcg ethinyl estradiol or less] hormonal contraception)
- In 30% of women evaluated for chronic "vaginitis" with standard evaluation, no diagnosis is found
- A prospective cohort study of patients referred for evaluation of chronic vulvovaginal symptoms found the most common diagnoses were contact dermatitis (21%), recurrent vulvovaginal candida (20.5%), atrophic vaginitis (14.5%), desquamative inflammatory vaginitis (8.0%), and bacterial vaginosis (6.5%)
- Vulvodynia is a complex disorder often requiring multidisciplinary, multiplatform approach
- Etiology is unknown and likely multifactorial; several causes have been proposed
  - These include embryologic abnormalities, allergic, infectious, genetic, hormonal, and neuropathic factors
  - The allodynia, hyperalgesia, and burning quality of pain are most consistent with neuropathic pain; potential triggers (in particular infection, tissue damage possibly, low-dose hormonal contraceptives) lead to tissue changes and nerve fiber proliferation or damage and pain feedback loop via central sensitization
- Vulvar pain disorders can be further subdivided as follows: generalized vulvar pain (vulvodynia) or localized pain to one region of the vulva and as provoked (with contact) or unprovoked vulvodynia or mixed
- In 2003 the International Society for the Study of Vulvovaginal Disease (ISSVD) suggested Friedrich's term "vulvar vestibulitis" be replaced with "provoked vestibulodynia" (PVD)
- Exam should include a thorough inspection of the vulva and perineum, including skin changes, muscle tone of the perineum and pelvic floor, presence of scars, lesions, and trigger points
- "Cotton swab" test of the vestibule is still the gold standard for assessing vulvodynia
  - Using a cotton swab, the examiner touches the vestibule to test for pain with gentle pressure (allodynia)
- The vestibule is bordered by the clitoris, the fourchette, and Hart's line; the hymen separates the vestibule from the vagina
  - The Bartholin's glands, Skene's glands, and urethral meatus all empty onto the vestibule
  - The vestibule is covered by nonkeratinized squamous epithelium rich in nerve endings

Treatment

- Many treatment options have been proposed including basic vulvar care measures, topical, oral or injected medication, cognitive behavioral therapy, biofeedback, physical therapy, dietary modifications, sexual counseling, and vestibulectomy for vestibulodynia
- Basic vulvar care measures to minimize vulvar irritation include the following:
  - Wearing 100% cotton underwear and using 100% cotton menstrual pads, avoid daily pad use, avoid soap on the vulva, and apply a preservative-free emollient such as plain petrolatum; avoid irritants such as perfumes, dyes, detergents, body wash, shampoo, douching, and fabric softeners
  - Topical nightly application of 5% lidocaine has been shown to reduce symptoms; after a mean of 7 weeks, 76% of patients were able to have intercourse as compared with 36% at baseline; lidocaine can also be applied just prior to intercourse
  - Oral tricyclic antidepressants (TCAs) (nortriptyline, amitriptyline, and desipramine) have shown up to a 60% response rate in various chronic pain conditions; however, few randomized controlled studies have looked specifically at vulvodynia
  - TCAs should be started at a low dose of 10 mg and gradually titrated up to 50 to 100 mg until therapeutic benefit is seen; it may take up to 3 weeks to see results; tolerance to common side effects (sedation, dry mouth, dizziness) also develops over time; medications should not be discontinued abruptly; needs to be tapered off slowly as well
  - However, a recent placebo-controlled, double-blinded RCT looking at women with vulvodynia treated with oral desipramine and topical lidocaine, both alone or in combination, showed *no* difference in any of the treatment groups as compared to placebo in reducing vulvodynia pain
  - Therefore, discussion with patients regarding treatment options, including discussion of risks, benefits, and efficacy, should include oral and topical medications, physical therapy, surgery, and alternative therapies
  - A multidisciplinary-type approach incorporating pelvic floor physical therapy, as well as psychological services including sex therapy, couples counseling, or individual psychotherapy has shown efficacy
  - Pelvic floor physical therapy is considered standard treatment for vulvodynia and is especially important in treatment if vaginismus or trigger points are present; physical therapy of pelvic floor muscles has been associated with a 50% improvement in women with vestibulodynia
  - Alternative therapies may include the following:
    - Anticonvulsants such as oral gabapentin have been used in a similar fashion as TCAs or as a 6% compounded topical cream; however, more research is needed
    - Topical steroids are generally of no benefit, although two uncontrolled studies have shown local injections with a combination of steroid and local anesthetic were successful
    - Local anesthetic nerve blockade incorporating caudal epidural, pudendal, and vestibular local anesthesia blockade showed a 50% response rate in an uncontrolled study for the treatment of vestibulodynia (78% were provoked and 22% mixed)

- Botulinum toxin type A was helpful in vulvodynia and pelvic floor muscle spasm in several small case reports
- Surgical management should be considered after conservative treatments fail; success rates of vestibulectomy vary, depending on the definition of "success," and have been reported to be as high as 80% to 90% but are generally accepted to be around 50%
- Potential complications after vestibulectomy include bleeding, wound complications, Bartholin's duct cyst formation, and continued or increased pain
- Cognitive behavioral therapy (CBT) has been shown to be an effective treatment for chronic pain syndromes including vulvodynia; the goal of CBT is for patients to develop self-management skills and a perspective on personal control of their condition

Special Categories

- Women who have undergone pelvic surgery for gynecologic cancer have a higher risk of dyspareunia and sexual dysfunction
- More than half of postmenopausal women have signs or symptoms resulting from atrophic changes with symptoms of dryness, soreness, irritation, discharge, or dyspareunia
  - Findings on exam include loss of rugae, paleness on the vaginal epithelium, increased pH, increased parabasal (immature) cells on saline prep microscopy
  - Local vaginal estrogen treatment is very effective at relieving symptoms of atrophic vaginitis
- Vaginal estradiol tablets, estrogen creams, and rings are effective treatments
- Systemic absorption is not substantial and the use of a progestin with local, low-dose estrogen is not needed
- Desquamative inflammatory vaginitis (DIV) and atrophic vaginitis can look similar on inspection of the vaginal epithelium and saline wet mount; both are more common after menopause and can cause dyspareunia; DIV may represent early form of lichen planus (biopsy will confirm)
  - With DIV there is purulent discharge, copious leukocytes on wet prep, and a "strawberry appearance" of the cervix may be present; vaginal pH is elevated, amine test and trichomonas cultures are negative, and wet prep shows increased parabasal and intermediate cells
  - Treatment is with intravaginal antibiotics that have an anti-inflammatory effect (clindamycin suppository or cream) and corticosteroid suppositories or cream
- Lichen planus manifests with erosions, ulcerations, and vaginal adhesions; usually also involves the vulva and oral cavity; and is treated with hydrocortisone vaginal suppositories or topical high potency corticosteroid cream
- Lichen sclerosis can cause vulvar itching, burning, irritation, and dyspareunia; biopsy confirms the diagnosis
- Vaginismus can be associated with vulvodynia or can present as a solitary finding; it can cause dyspareunia and vice versa
  - Patient education about anatomy, often with the use of a hand held mirror, as well as discussions of female sexual response are important

- Physical therapy and sexual cognitive-behavioral therapy has been found to be effective treatments for vaginismus; a stepwise use of vaginal dilators is often employed
- Botulinum toxin type A has also been found to be useful but is still in experimental stages

UPDATE #8

Gastrointestinal and genitourinary pathologies are extremely common among women with CPP. As many as 60% of patients referred to gynecologists for CPP are thought to have irritable bowel syndrome (IBS), and 30% to 40% have interstitial cystitis/bladder pain syndrome (IC/BPS) (Williams et al, 2005; Zondervan et al, 2001).

Nongynecologic Causes of CPP and Their Management

UROLOGIC CAUSES OF CPP

- CPP with urinary urgency, frequency, and nocturia in the absence of an identifiable disease or infection are suggestive of painful bladder syndrome/interstitial cystitis
- IC/BPS is a chronic, neuropathic, and inflammatory condition of the bladder
- IC/BPS seems more prevalent in women with prior surgeries for CPP than in controls
- Diagnostic criteria for IC/BPS vary, but currently it is generally accepted that the diagnosis can be made on the basis of the symptoms of suprapubic, vaginal and or vulvar/urethral pain, urinary frequency, urgency and nocturia in the absence of infectious, neoplastic, or other inflammation such as radiation
  - Classic appearance of glomerulations can be found on cystoscopy, but cystoscopy is not necessary for the diagnosis
  - Positive Potassium Sensitivity test (PST) suggests for abnormal bladder permeability, but false positives occur; women with healthy, normal bladders do not usually have pain after the instillation of intravesical potassium chloride solution
    - Seventy percent to 90% of patients with IC/BPS have a positive test
    - Up to 85% of women presenting to gynecologists with pelvic pain have a positive test
- The Interstitial Cystitis Symptom Index, described by O'Leary in 1997, can also be used as a screening tool to diagnose IC/BPS; 72% of women with a score of 5 or more on the index were shown to have cytoscopically confirmed IC/BPS; this may be a useful screening tool to determine which patients should be referred for urologic consultation
- Hydrodistension of the bladder or intravesical therapy with lidocaine, heparin, pentosan polysulfate, or dimethylsulfoxide are a mainstay of treatment
  - Goal of treatment is symptom control and prolonged remission, not cure; multidisciplinary therapy is often needed
- Sodium pentosan polysulfate (Elmiron) is an oral treatment approved by the Food and Drug Administration for IC
  - About one third of patients will respond, it is well tolerated, and it should be tried for at least 6 months

- Various other medications have been used with some success (antihistamines, antidepressants, and cyclosporine)
- Bladder training, dietary restrictions (avoiding acidic and spicy foods, alcohol, carbonated beverages, and artificial sweeteners), physical therapy, and relaxation therapy are very helpful but not well studied

GASTROINTESTINAL CAUSES OF CPP

UPDATE #9

IBS affects up to 10% of the general population and affects women two times more often than men (Boyce et al, 2000; Choung et al, 2010; Williams et al, 2004); IBS seen in up to 60% of patients presenting with CPP (Williams et al, 2005; Zondervan et al, 2001).

- Patients with IBS have increased rates of depression, somatization, abuse, sexual dysfunction, and utilization of the health care system
- Women with IBS have more severe dysmenorrhea, possibly because of shared neural pathways between the uterus and lower gastrointestinal (GI) tract
- The location of referred pain from the gastrointestinal tract overlaps with that of the reproductive organs
- IBS is characterized by abdominal pain, bloating, and is temporarily associated with alterations in form or consistency or frequency of stool (diarrhea or constipation)
- Diagnosis of IBS based on the Rome criteria
  - Pain is associated with altered form or frequency of stool
  - Pain is relieved by a bowel movement
  - Pain is increased by eating and stress
  - Associated symptoms include presence of mucous in stool, straining, urgency, incomplete evacuation, abdominal distention, nausea, fecal soiling
  - Anxiety, depression, and somatization, posttraumatic stress disorder (PTSD), fibromyalgia, temporal-mandibular joint syndrome, migraines, and IC/BPS are present more often in women with IBS
  - Treatment of IBS is multimodal and may include antispasmodic/anticholinergic, serotonergic medications, fiber, laxative or stool softeners, antidepressants, cognitive behavioral and relaxation therapy, meditation, hypnosis, or yoga; based on consensus opinion, treatment involves oral medications as well as dietary modifications
  - Subclassification of women into abdominal pain/bloating dominant, constipation or diarrhea dominant, may help guide therapy with antispasmodics or increased fiber, stool softeners, or antimotility agents
- Red flags for malignancy include older age of onset, GI bleeding, positive family history of GI malignancy, anorexia, and weight loss; for infection they include persistent watery stools and dietary, antibiotic (*C. difficile*), or travel history; rule out infectious and iatrogenic causes of GI symptoms with a dietary, travel, and medication history
- Crohn's and ulcerative colitis are inflammatory bowel diseases associated with crampy abdominal pain, weight loss, diarrhea and rectal bleeding (with ulcerative colitis), and not necessarily seen more frequently in the CPP population

MUSCULOSKELETAL CAUSES OF CPP

- Myofascial pain from the anterior abdominal wall and pelvic floor muscles is prevalent and frequently overlooked as a source of chronic pelvic pain
- Myofascial pain syndrome is a chronic form of widespread muscle pain
- Pain emanates from sensitive points in muscles called trigger points; the pain may spread throughout the affected muscle
- Trigger points are hypersensitive regions within a taut band of skeletal muscle compressing blood vessels and nerves; this should be distinguished from fibromyalgia, which involves multiple areas of tenderness throughout the body that are diffuse and in general not associated with trigger points
- Pain symptoms are frequently vague, not well localized, and described as "achy" or "throbbing"; pain may worsen with activities and radiate to the back or hip
- Hypertonic pelvic floor muscle conditions may be the primary source of pain or a component of another chronic pain syndrome, such as endometriosis, IC/BPS, IBS, or vulvodynia; if not identified and treated, symptoms will often persist or recur (Tu et al, 2008)
- Anatomic changes in pregnant women result in an increased rate of sacroiliac joint (SIJ) pain or posterior pelvic pain; increased muscle tension may lead to more muscle recruitment, thus exacerbating the problem and further increasing posterior pelvic pain and low back pain; physiologic changes of pregnancy, recognition, and treatment of common musculoskeletal disorders in pregnancy are beyond the scope of this chapter

UPDATE #10

Neuropathic pain resulting from nerve entrapment from scar formation or injury is a commonly overlooked cause of lower quadrant pain; ilioinguinal and iliohypogastric nerve injuries, which occur in about 3.7% of gynecologic surgeries, are more common with Pfannenstiel incisions, but they can also occur with trocar incisions (Rahn et al, 2010)

- Care should be taken to avoid extending the Pfannenstiel incision beyond the lateral edges of the rectus sheath; in laparoscopic procedures, to avoid these nerves place lateral trocars superior to the anterior superior iliac spine (ASIS) and >8 cm from midline to minimize vessel injury; other causes of injury to these nerves include exercise, lifting, or physical trauma

NEUROPATHIC CAUSES OF CPP

- Neuropathy involving any peripheral nerves with origins T10-L4 or S2-4 may present as CPP
- Nerve injury may be due to trauma, laceration, entrapment, or neuroma formation
- Most neuropathies associated with pelvic surgery resolve spontaneously
- Iatrogenic nerve injuries recognized at the time of surgery should be repaired immediately usually with removal of the suture that is entrapping the nerve

- Local anesthetic nerve blocks and physical therapy should be started immediately
- Surgical release or nerve resection may be helpful in some patients but long-term studies are lacking
- Lumbar radiculopathy may lead to an increase in the resting state of pelvic floor musculature, presenting as pelvic pain; patients with lumbar radiculopathy or pelvic floor pain reproduced with hip maneuvers may benefit from epidural or nerve root injections, which can be both diagnostic and therapeutic
- Pudendal nerve injury or entrapment can lead to deep pelvic pain, vulvar pain, and urinary symptoms
  - Pudendal nerve supplies motor fibers to the urinary and external anal sphincter, pelvic floor muscles, as well as sensation to the vagina and external genitalia; the pudendal nerves are prone to injury from childbirth, chronic constipation, or pelvic reconstructive surgery using mesh; symptoms are classically unilateral but can be bilateral; burning type perineal pain either located in the vulva/vagina or the anorectal region; the pain is worse in the sitting position and may be relieved upon standing; on physical exam, pain may be reproduced with unilateral vaginal palpation; relief of pain with pudendal nerve block is diagnostic; treatment consists of one or a combination of the following modalities: physical therapy, nerve blocks (pudendal or regional caudal epidural), anticonvulsants, antidepressants, sacral nerve stimulation, and, if indicated for pudendal nerve entrapment, surgical release

Treatment for Musculoskeletal and Neuropathic Causes of CPP

PHYSICAL THERAPY

- Principles of physical therapy treatment include the following:
  - Manual techniques such as myofascial release, acupressure, joint mobilization, massage, teaching relaxation, biofeedback, strain-counterstrain, transcutaneous electrical nerve stimulation, use of ice or heat
  - Prescribed home exercise program
  - Facilitation of "restorative sleep," lifestyle modifications and exercise

MEDICATIONS FOR CPP

- Nonsteroidal anti-inflammatory agents (NSAIDs)
- Antidepressants, anticonvulsants, and local anesthetics (injected or topically) are also first-line treatments, used for "off-label" indications in the treatment of CPP with a neuropathic component; common drugs include the following:
- Tricyclic antidepressants: the anticholinergic and antihistaminergic side effects can be beneficial for urinary frequency/urgency or insomnia but can lead to drowsiness, constipation, and dry mouth
  - Dosage usually begins 10 to 25 mg at bedtime, increasing slowly weekly or biweekly until effective dose is reached; 25 to 100 mg at bedtime
  - Nortriptyline and desipramine are less sedating and can be prescribed with similar dosing schedules

- Serotonin-norepinephrine reuptake inhibitors (SNRIs), such as venlafaxine and duloxetine, have also been studied and used for neuropathic and myofascial pain; venlafaxine helps alleviate neuropathic pain and also has anxiolytic and antidepressant side effects; duloxetine 20 to 60 mg daily is approved for depression and is helpful for neuropathic pain
- Anticonvulsants such as gabapentin and pregabalin are used off-label in the management of neuropathic pain and can be combined with TCAs or SNRIs
  - Gabapentin is usually started at 100 to 300 mg at bedtime and is increased by 300 mg every 4 to 7 days up to 1800 to 3600 mg/daily
  - Pregabalin is usually started at 50 mg q 12 hours and is increased weekly to a dosage ranging up to 450 to 600 mg per day
  - Side effects include sedation, dizziness, confusion, constipation, and weight gain
- Topical analgesics have been studied for neuropathic conditions, such as postherpetic neuralgia and vestibulodynia; lidocaine cream 5%, lidocaine patches 5%, or eutectic mixture of local anesthetics lidocaine 2.5% and prilocaine 2.5% cream have been used successfully
- Muscle relaxants: cyclobenzaprine is a centrally acting myorelaxant that has not been studied with regard to CPP, per se, but its use for myofascial pain is established
- Opioid agonists are controversial in the management of nonmalignant pain; however, they are to be considered based on individual risk assessment and availability of practitioners who are aware of management guidelines and of risks associated with opioid abuse, addiction, and diversion
- Tramadol has become useful in the treatment of neuropathic pain and is a weak tricyclic and u-opioid agonist; it has sedating side effects, and maximal dosage is 300 to 400 mg per day
- Injections of local anesthetics are a mainstay for down-regulation of nerve pain and myofascial trigger points
- A stepwise pharmacologic approach in the management of neuropathic pain was proposed in the Canadian Pain Society Consensus statement
  - *First-line* treatments include analgesics, TCAs, anticonvulsants (gabapentin and pregabalin)
  - *Second-line* treatments include SNRIs and topical lidocaine
  - *Third-line* treatments include tramadol and opioids
  - *Fourth-line* agents include cannabinoids, methadone, and anticonvulsants of lesser efficacy, such as valproic acid

SPECIAL CATEGORIES OF TREATMENT

- Sacral nerve stimulation is a relatively new treatment modality for refractory CPP in the S2-S4 nerve distribution and for pelvic floor dysfunction; early reports suggest up to 50% to 85% resolution of pain and urinary urgency in the setting of IC/BPS
- A group of neurolytic therapies that transect, excise, or destroy neural tissue via heat, cold, or laser has been described involving paracervical ganglion, presacral nerve, or hypogastric plexus

CPP without Obvious Pathology

The International Association for the Study of Pain (IASP) classification includes a category titled chronic pelvic pain without obvious pathology. This may account for up to 30% of CPP in which pain is out of proportion with pathology, particularly with some cases of endometriosis (endometriosis related pain syndrome), IC/BPS, IBS, vulvodynia, and myofascial pain. The etiology of the pain likely involves central nervous system sensitization and neural up-regulation and neuroplasticity. Stress, anxiety, and depression are common in these patients. This diagnosis should not imply that the pain is psychogenic. The management of pain must be a multidisciplinary approach, including pharmacologic and psychological interventions.

Psychological Factors in CPP

- There is a consistent association of CPP with psychological morbidity and with a history of emotional, physical, or sexual trauma
- Anxiety and depressive disorders are common among women with chronic pain in general and CPP specifically
- A history of sexual and physical abuse is an independent risk factor for CPP
- Recognition and treatment of these common psychological disorders is paramount, and related anxiety and fear, depression (hopelessness), and loss of control (helplessness) can lead to persistent pain
- Cognitive behavioral therapy and relaxation therapy focus on teaching self-efficacy, learning, pain-coping strategies, reducing stress, and increasing readiness to change; these approaches are a mainstay of multidisciplinary management and can help prevent or break the cycle of chronic pain
- Psychological screening of women with CPP should be routine
- The physician should be prepared to discuss these issues and, when appropriate, make referrals to psychologists, psychiatrists, social workers, marriage counselors, or sex therapists

UPDATE #11

Both the diagnosis and treatment of patients can be quite challenging. Treatment should involve a multidisciplinary, multiplatform approach, particularly when traditional approaches fail to relieve pain. Basic components of a multidisciplinary effort include a physician, physical therapist, and psychologist or psychiatrist. Multidisciplinary treatment of CPP has been shown to be more effective than traditional gynecologic medical or surgical approaches (Peters et al, 1991).

SUGGESTED READINGS

CPP

American College of Obstetricians and Gynecologists Committee on Practice Bulletins—Gynecology: ACOG practice bulletin no. 51: chronic pelvic pain, *Obstet Gynecol* 103(3):589–605, 2004.

Howard FM: Chronic pelvic pain, *Obstet Gynecol* 101(3):594–611, 2003.

Jarrell JF, Vilos GA: Consensus guidelines for the management of chronic pelvic pain, *JOCG* 64(2):869–887, 2005.

Jarrell JF, Vilos GA, Allaire C, et al: Consensus guidelines for the management of chronic pelvic pain, *J Obstet Gynaecol Can*, 27(9):869–910;2005 Sep.

Latthe P, Mignini L, Gray R, et al: Factors predisposing women to chronic pelvic pain: systematic review, *BMJ* 332(7544):749–755, 2006.

Peters AA, van Dorst E, Jellis AB, et al: A randomized clinical trial to compare two different approaches in women with chronic pelvic pain, *Obstet Gynecol* 77(5):740–744, 1991.

Rapkin AJ, Hartshorn TG, Partownavid P: Pain management, *Clinical Updates in Women's Health Care* 10(5):1–158, 2011.

Tu FF, Holt J, Gonzales J, Fitzgerald CM: Physical therapy evaluation of patients with chronic pelvic pain: a controlled study, *Am J Obstet Gynecol* 198(3):272.e1–.e7, 2008.

Endometriosis

American College of Obstetricians and Gynecologists: ACOG committee opinion no. 310, April 2005: endometriosis in adolescents, *Obstet Gynecol* 105(4):921–927, 2005.

American College of Obstetricians and Gynecologists: Practice bulletin no. 114: management of endometriosis, *Obstet Gynecol* 116(1):223–236, 2010.

Bajaj P, Bajaj P, Madsen H, Arendt-Nielsen L: Endometriosis is associated with central sensitization: a psychophysical controlled study, *J Pain* 4(47):372–380, 2003.

Davis LJ, Kennedy SS, Moore J, Prentice A: Oral contraceptives for pain associated with endometriosis, *Cochrane Database Syst Rev*(3)CD001019, 2007.

Gambone JC, Mittman BS, Munro MG, et al: Consensus statement for the management of chronic pelvic pain and endometriosis: proceedings of an expert-panel consensus process, *Fertil Steril* 78(5):961–972, 2002.

Giudice LC: Clinical practice: endometriosis, *N Engl J Med* 362(25):2389–2398, 2010.

Howard FM: Endometriosis and mechanisms of pelvic pain, *J Minim Invasive Gynecol* 16(5):540–550, 2009.

Vulvodynia

American College of Obstetricians and Gynecologists Committee on Gynecologic Practice: ACOG committee opinion no. 345, October 2006: vulvodynia, *Obstet Gynecol* 108(4):1049–1052, 2006.

Anderson MR, Klink K, Cohrssen A: Evaluation of vaginal complaints, *JAMA* 291(11):1368–1379, 2004.

Bergeron S, Khalife S, Glazer I, Binik YM: Surgical and behavioral treatments for vestibulodynia: two-and-one-half year follow-up and predictors of outcome, *Obstet Gynecol* 111(1):159–166, 2008.

Bohm-Starke N, Rylander E: Surgery for localized, provoked vestibulodynia: a long-term follow-up study, *J Repro Med* 53(2):83–89, 2008.

Foster DC, Kotok MB, Huang LS, et al: Oral desipramine and topical lidocaine for vulvodynia: a randomized controlled trial, *Obstet Gynecol* 116(3):583–593, 2010.

Harlow BL, Wise LA, Stewart EG: Prevalence and predictors of chronic lower genital tract discomfort, *Am J Obstet Gynecol* 185(3):545–550, 2001.

Rapkin AJ, McDonald JS, Morgan M: Multilevel local anesthetic nerve blockade for the treatment of vulvar vestibulitis syndrome, *Am J Obstet Gynecol* 198(1):41.e1–41.e5, 2008.

Genitourinary Causes of CPP

Clemons JL, Arya LA, Myers DL: Diagnosing interstitial cystitis in women with chronic pelvic pain, *Obstet Gynecol* 100(2):337–341, 2002.

Langenberg PW, Wallach EE, Clauw DJ, et al: Pelvic pain and surgeries in women before interstitial cystitis/painful bladder syndrome, *Am J Obstet Gynecol* 202(3):286.e1–e6, 2010.

Zondervan KT, Yudkin PL, Vessey MP, et al: Chronic pelvic pain in the community: symptoms, investigations, and diagnoses, *Am J Obstet Gynecol* 184(6):1149–1155, 2001.

Gastrointestinal Causes of CPP

Boyce PM, Koloski NA, Talley NJ: Irritable bowel syndrome according to varying diagnostic criteria: are the new Rome II criteria unnecessarily restrictive for research and practice? *Am J Gastroenterol* 95(11):3176–3183, 2000.

Choung RS, Herrick LM, Locle DR 3rd, et al: Irritable bowel syndrome and chronic pelvic pain: a population-based study, *J Clin Gastroenterol* 44(10):696–701, 2010.

Mayer EA: Clinical practice: irritable bowel syndrome, *N England J Med* 358(16):1692–1699, 2008.

Williams RE, Hartmann KE, Sandler RS, et al: Prevalence and characteristics of irritable bowel syndrome among women with chronic pelvic pain, *Obstet Gynecol* 104(3):452–458, 2004.

Williams RE, Hartmann KE, Sandler RS, et al: Recognition and treatment of irritable bowel syndrome among women with chronic pelvic pain, *Am J Obstet Gynecol* 192(3):761–767, 2005.

Musculoskeletal Causes of CPP

Butrick CW: Pathophysiology of pelvic floor hypertonic disorders, *Obstet Gynecol Clin North Am* 36(3):699–705, 2009.

Carter JE: Abdominal wall and pelvic myofascial trigger points. In Howard FM, Perry CP, Carter JE, El-Minawi AM, editors: *Pelvic pain: diagnosis and management*, Philadelphia, 2000, Lippincott, Williams & Wilkins, pp 314–358.

Neuropathic Causes of CPP

Cardosi RJ, Cox CS, Hoffman MS: Postoperative neuropathies after major pelvic surgery, *Obstet Gynecol* 100(2):240–244, 2002.

Moulin DE, Clark AJ, Gilron I, et al: Pharmacologic management of chronic neuropathic pain: consensus statement and guidelines from the Canadian Pain Society, *Pain Res Manag* 12(1):13–21, 2007.

Rahn DD, Phelan JN, Roshanravan SM, et al: Anterior abdominal wall nerve and vessel anatomy: clinical implications for gynecologic surgery, *Am J Obstet Gynecol* 202(3), 234.e.1–e5, 2010.

Psychologic/Psychiatric Associations

Aerts L, Enzlin P, Verhaeghe J, et al: Sexual and psychological functioning in women after pelvic surgery for gynaecological cancer, *Eur J Gynaecol Oncol* 30(6):652–656, 2009.

Fricchione G: Clinical practice: generalized anxiety disorder, *N Engl J Med* 351(7):675–682, 2004.

Lorencatto C, Petta CA, Navarro MJ, et al: Depression in women with endometriosis with and without chronic pelvic pain, *Acta Obstet Gynecol Scand* 85(1):88–92, 2006.

Meltzer-Brody S, Leserman J, Zolnoun D, et al: Trauma and posttraumatic stress disorder in women with chronic pelvic pain, *Obstet Gynecol* 109(4):902–908, 2007.

Weijenborg PT, Ter Kuile MM, Stones W: A cognitive behavioral based assessment of women with chronic pelvic pain, *J Psychosom Obstet Gynaecol* 30(4):262–268, 2009.

Chapter 45

Sexual Abuse and Sexual Assault

KATHRYN P. HIRST

KEY UPDATES

1   Women with a history of childhood sexual abuse (CSA) are at increased risk for developing borderline personality disorder.

2   CSA is not associated with increased risk for sexual pain disorders.

3   Women with CSA have increased risk for developing posttraumatic stress disorder following childbirth.

4   Women seeking care within 72 hours of nonoccupational exposure to body fluids from an individual with known HIV should receive a 28-day course of highly active antiretroviral treatment.

5   Two percent to 3% of drug-facilitated sexual assault involves covert administration of medication.

Childhood Sexual Abuse

BACKGROUND

- Childhood sexual abuse (CSA) can cause a wide array of symptoms that impact psychological and physical health
- Obstetricians and gynecologists commonly encounter women with a history of CSA, and knowledge of a woman's history can provide insight into a woman's current health issues

DEFINITION

- The Child Abuse Prevention and Treatment Act defines child sexual abuse as follows:
  - The employment, use, persuasion, inducement, enticement, or coercion of any child to engage in, or assist any other person to engage in, any sexually explicit conduct or simulation of such conduct for the purpose of producing a visual depiction of such conduct; or
  - The rape, and in cases of caretaker or inter-familial relationships, statutory rape, molestation, prostitution, or other form of sexual exploitation of children, or incest with children (U.S. Department of Health and Human Services, 2011)
- CSA can involve any exposure to sexual acts for a child who lacks the emotional, maturational, and cognitive development to understand or consent to such acts
- Exposure does not need to involve intercourse or sexual acts, but it can include exposure to sexual acts or posing in child pornography
- Motivation for the perpetrator can be sexual gratification for the perpetrator or demonstration of power to coerce

PREVALENCE

- Estimates vary widely of prevalence of CSA
- Studies show a range from 25% to 40% of U.S. women have experienced some form of CSA (Felitti et al, 1998; Bolen et al, 1999)
- Ethnicity is not independently associated with CSA (Finkelhor et al, 1993)
- Exposure to CSA is often accompanied by other adverse childhood experiences, including physical abuse and neglect, violence against the mother, or exposure to household members who were substance abusers (Felitti et al, 1998)
- Underreporting is common, and the majority of CSA victims do not report the abuse until adulthood
- The 1998 National Violence Against Women Survey found that 9% of all women surveyed had been raped before age 18 years
- Of women who have been raped in their lifetime, more than 50% were under 17 years old
- The most common perpetrators of child and adolescent sexual abuse and rapes are relatives and acquaintances (Tjaden et al, 2000)

GENERAL SEQUELAE

- Sequelae of CSA are common and pervasive for many survivors
- CSA has been linked to poorer general physical health extending past age 60 (Draper et al, 2008)
- Both psychological and physical sequelae often represent conscious or unconscious coping strategies in response to abnormal and traumatic events (Table 45-1)
- Obstetricians and gynecologists can play a significant role in preventing the misdiagnosis of symptoms that are evaluated outside of their original context

TABLE 45-1 Common Symptoms in Adult Survivors of Childhood Sexual Abuse

Physical Presentations
Chronic pelvic pain
Gastrointestinal symptoms/distress
Musculoskeletal symptoms
Obesity, eating disorders
Insomnia, sleep disorders
Pseudocyesis
Sexual dysfunction
Asthma, respiratory ailments
Addiction
Chronic headache
Chronic back pain

Psychologic and Behavioral Presentations
Depression and anxiety
Posttraumatic stress disorder symptoms
Dissociative states
Repeated self-injury
Suicide attempts
Lying, stealing, truancy, running away
Poor contraceptive practices
Compulsive sexual behaviors
Sexual dysfunction
Somatizing disorders
Eating disorders
Poor adherence to medical recommendations
Intolerance of or constant search for intimacy
Expectation of early death

From American College of Obstetricians and Gynecologists: ACOG educational bulletin: adult manifestation of childhood sexual abuse, no. 259, July 2000: clinical management guidelines for obstetrician-gynecologists, *Int J Gynaecol Obstet* 74(3):311-320, 2001.

TABLE 45-2 Common Life Event Symptom Triggers for Childhood Sexual Abuse Survivors

Pregnancy or birth of a child
Illness or death of parent or perpetrator
Divorce of parents
Age of survivor's child the same as onset of abuse
Key "anniversary" dates or holidays
Family reunions
Illness or injury of a child
Hospitalization or medical workup
Workplace situation that mirrors a relationship with abuser
Home relocation, especially to geographic area where abuse occurred
Viewing movies or television shows with abuse content

From American College of Obstetricians and Gynecologists: ACOG educational bulletin: adult manifestation of childhood sexual abuse, no. 259, July 2000: clinical management guidelines for obstetrician-gynecologists, *Int J Gynaecol Obstet* 74(3):311-320, 2001.

- The National Comorbidity Survey-Replication showed the following adjusted odds ratio for women with CSA:
  - Posttraumatic stress disorder: 2.41
  - Panic disorder with or without agoraphobia: 1.93
  - Social anxiety disorder: 1.65 (Cougle et al, 2010)
- Posttraumatic stress disorder (PTSD)
  - Posttraumatic stress disorder involves reexperiencing of trauma (by nightmare or flashback), avoidance or denial of memories or experiences associated with the trauma, and a heightened sense of physical arousal
  - Studies show that a high proportion of women with CSA meet criteria for posttraumatic stress disorder at some point in their lifetime and that symptoms are similar to those who have war-related trauma (McNew et al, 1995)
  - Duration and severity of CSA is associated with more severe PTSD (Rowan et al, 1994)
- Eating disorders
  - The link between CSA and eating disorders, including bulimia nervosa and anorexia nervosa, is controversial
  - Case-control and retrospective studies have found inconsistent results
  - The largest prospective, longitudinal study showed a 5.7-fold increase in risk for bulimia nervosa with two or more discrete episodes of CSA
  - There was no increase in risk for anorexia nervosa with CSA (Sanci et al, 2008)
- Substance use disorders
  - Women with CSA have consistently been shown to have elevated rates and risk for substance use disorders (Simpson et al, 2002)
- Self-perception and borderline personality disorder
  - Development of a positive self-perception is thought to be one of the most important tasks of early relationships in childhood
  - Borderline personality disorder is a pattern of behavior that starts in childhood and extends through adulthood, involving negative self-perception, poor personal boundaries, impulsive behavior, and difficulty controlling emotions (American Psychiatric Association, 2000)

MENTAL HEALTH SEQUELAE
- More extreme symptoms are associated with more severe abuse, earlier onset of CSA, incest by a parent, or use of force (Hanson et al, 2001; Molnar et al, 2001)
- Emotional responses to CSA can be mitigated by resiliency and supportive responses by individuals who are important to the victim (Lam et al, 1997)
- Some survivors may outwardly appear to be unharmed, but most have persistent negative consequences (Table 45-2)
- Severity of symptoms can vary with time, and fluctuation of severity is normal
- Major depressive disorder
  - Childhood physical abuse and neglect have been shown to increase the risk of lifetime and current major depressive disorder (Widom et al, 2007)
  - However, the effect of CSA on major depressive disorder remains somewhat controversial, with studies showing both an increased risk and lack of effect (Molnar et al, 2001; Widom et al, 2007)
- Anxiety disorders
  - CSA is uniquely associated with a higher risk for a variety of anxiety disorders, even after controlling for comorbid depression and a history of physical abuse

UPDATE #1

Women with a history of childhood trauma, including sexual abuse, are at increased risk for developing borderline personality disorder (Ball et al, 2009). Women with borderline personality disorder are at increased risk of inappropriate and strong emotional reactions to perceived stress, such as that associated with childbearing, medical complications, and limit setting by providers in the prescribing of controlled substances. These patients may benefit significantly from ongoing psychotherapy.

- Sexual abuse can interfere with this development, and the development of a positive sense of self can be negatively affected by CSA in the following manners:
  - Traumatic sexualization by premature or coerced sexual involvement with an adult
  - Creation of a sense of powerlessness when a child is exploited by those in authority
  - Betrayal of trust in an early relationship, especially when a parent commits the abuse
  - Shame over victimization and belief that the individual is fundamentally defective because of the abuse
- Negative self-perception can lead to the view that the victim deserved the abuse, and survivors may maintain the image of abuser as good
- This negative self-perception can lead to risky and self-destructive behaviors, including sexual promiscuity and substance abuse, as well as involvement in abusive relationships
- CSA by a parent can be the most destructive form of CSA because of the disruption of trust
- As a result, the child can lose the ability to trust and may learn to view the world as unsafe
- This will disrupt the ability to cope with stressful events and will lead to overreaction to stressful and emotionally or physically painful events
- The disruption of the parental relationship by sexual abuse can also lead to disruption of the sense of personal boundaries, which is important for psychological stability
- Difficulty with establishing personal boundaries can be manifested in clinical practice as a patient who is inappropriately demanding of time and resources and has emotional reactions that are abnormal for the level of perceived stress
- Dissociation
  - Dissociation is a lack of the normal integration of thoughts, feelings, and experiences into the stream of consciousness and memory (Bernstein et al, 1986); this can lead to a dreamlike state and may be accompanied by poor memory of surrounding events
  - In many cases, this is a subconscious action to protect a woman with CSA from allowing stressful events to affect her
  - Use of dissociation to cope with stress in the obstetric or gynecologic setting may increase a woman's risk for posttraumatic stress disorder or negative reaction to perceived stress

PHYSICAL HEALTH SEQUELAE

- Women with CSA are at higher risk of a variety of chronic pain conditions that are not associated with pathophysiologic changes, such as chronic pelvic pain and irritable bowel syndrome (Table 45-3)

TABLE 45-3 Examples of Chronic and Diffuse Pain in Sexual Abuse Survivors*

Headaches
Migraine
Temporomandibular joint syndrome
Muscle tension

Genitourinary Symptoms
Chronic pain
Rectal discomfort
Hemorrhoids
Constipation
Diarrhea
Irritable bowel syndrome
Spastic colon

Gastrointestinal Problems
Gagging
Nausea, vomiting
Choking

Conversion Symptoms
Fainting
Vertigo
Seizures
Muscle tension/spasms
Joint pain
Tinnitus
Respiratory problems
—Asthma
—Shortness of breath

*May be suggestive of the abuse or somatic signs of depression.
From American College of Obstetricians and Gynecologists: ACOG educational bulletin: adult manifestation of childhood sexual abuse, no. 259, July 2000: clinical management guidelines for obstetrician-gynecologists, *Int J Gynaecol Obstet* 74(3):311-320, 2001.

- This may represent dysregulation of pain perception, which has been hypothesized to represent mediation of both pain perception and emotional stress through shared limbic pathways (Fenton, 2007)
- Pain is commonly present in areas that were sexually traumatized
- Bowel symptoms
  - Irritable bowel syndrome (IBS) is a classic example of symptoms occurring in the absence of demonstrable physical pathology
  - Women with IBS have significantly higher rates of CSA compared to women with inflammatory bowel disease (IBD) (Ross, 2005)
- Interstitial cystitis and painful bladder syndrome (IC/PBS)
  - Women with IC/PBS may have higher rates of CSA than the general population (Goldstein et al, 2008)
  - Women with a history of CSA have been shown to have more severe pain manifestations and fewer irritative voiding complaints, compared to women without a history of CSA (Mayson et al, 2009)
- Gynecologic syndromes
  - Dyspareunia, vulvodynia, and provoked vestibulodynia

UPDATE #2
There is no consistent evidence showing an association between childhood sexual abuse and sexual pain disorders (Plant et al, 2008).

- Chronic pelvic pain
- Studies have found between 58% to 82% of women with chronic pelvic pain to have a history of CSA (Randolph et al, 2006)
- Increased severity of abuse is correlated with increased severity of pelvic pain (Randolph et al, 2006)
- Forms of physiotherapy, cognitive therapy, and somatocognitive therapy have been shown superior to standard care for patients without treatable biologic causes of chronic pelvic pain (Albert, 1999; Haugstad et al, 2008)

SEXUAL HEALTH

- Disturbances in sexual functioning, health, and identity are common among survivors
- Differences in severity of sexual abuse can lead to different effects on sexual functioning and attitudes toward sexual behavior
- Women with greater coercion in sexual abuse and women who have been raped are more likely to engage in risky sexual behavior (Campbell et al, 2004; Gore-Felton et al, 2002)
- Women with less severe sexual abuse (e.g., inappropriate touching of a breast) may have increased rates of anxiety about sexual experience and, therefore, increased sexual aversion (Noll et al, 2003)
- Role of negative self-perception: as CSA can lead to negative self-perception, women may develop a sexual identity that involves self-worth based on sexuality
- This can lead to high numbers of sexual partners and the resulting increased risk for sexually transmitted infections and unintended pregnancies
- Women may also confuse sexuality with nurturing behavior
- For women who report sexual problems in adulthood, the most commonly reported problems are as follows:
  - Fear of intimate relationships
  - Feelings of repulsion or lack of enjoyment
  - Flashbacks during sexual activity
  - Dysfunctions of desire and arousal, including lubrication difficulties
  - Primary or secondary anorgasmia

EFFECTS ON INTERPERSONAL RELATIONSHIPS

- CSA can profoundly damage the ability to have healthy relationships in adulthood, because of effects on trust, personal boundaries, and self-perception
- Women are more likely to maintain the role of victim and enter into abusive relationships
- Difficulty with personal boundaries can lead to unstable relationships with extreme dependence on others, overcompliance, learned helplessness, and nonassertion
- Women may create a pattern of volatile relationships, in which there is excessive dependence or involvement, withdrawal, and then hostility

EFFECTS ON REPRODUCTIVE HEALTH

- Adolescents and women with CSA have higher rates of the following:
  - Prostitution
  - Sexually transmitted infections
  - Unintended pregnancy
  - Human immunodeficiency virus (HIV)–risk behavior
- They have lower rates of contraceptive use and earlier onset of consensual sexual activity (Loeb et al, 2002)
- Survivors may also be less likely to have regular Pap tests (Farley et al, 2002)
- The vaginal examination can be a source of significant fear and pain for CSA survivors

EFFECTS ON PREGNANCY, CHILDBIRTH, AND THE POSTPARTUM PERIOD

- Feelings of vulnerability during pelvic examinations, prenatal care, and labor can lead to the reexperiencing of feelings of terror, powerlessness, and violation, though scientific data reporting the prevalence of such experiences are lacking
- Physical pain and lack of control during labor and delivery can also trigger memories of past abuse
- Women with CSA have more complications of pregnancy compared to those without CSA:
  - Increased discomfort and health complaints (Grimstad et al, 1999)
  - More abuse experiences during pregnancy
  - More nonscheduled contacts with antenatal care providers (Grimstad et al, 1999)
  - Higher number of ultrasounds during first pregnancies (Leeners et al, 2006)
  - Higher risk for nonoptimal weight gain; one study reported women with CSA were threefold more likely to have inadequate weight gain and 2.4-fold more likely to have excessive weight gain (Johnson et al, 2002)
  - Higher risk for alcohol use, illicit substance use, and smoking (Grimstad et al, 1999; Hans, 1999; Leonardson et al, 2003)
  - No difference in mode of delivery or use of forceps or vacuum extraction has been found for women with CSA (Leeners et al, 2006)
- Women with CSA tend to feel higher levels of pain and anxiety during labor (Leeners et al, 2006)
- Perineal scars from past abuse may be specifically associated with increased pain for some women (Grant, 1991)
- CSA has not been shown to impact birth weight, gestational age at delivery, or neonatal jaundice (Grimstad et al, 1999)
- Women with CSA have higher rates of postpartum depression than those without, though this may be related to a higher baseline rate of past depressive histories than with abuse, per se (Grimstad et al, 1999; LaCoursiere et al, 2009)
- CSA has been associated with more severe depression and longer length of stay for inpatient mental health hospitalization (Lev-Wiesel et al, 2009)
- Women with CSA have higher rates of using dissociation to cope with the pain and emotional stress of labor, which can increase their risk for birth-related posttraumatic stress disorder

UPDATE #3

Women with childhood sexual abuse have increased risk for birth-related posttraumatic stress disorder (Lev-Wiesel et al, 2009).

SCREENING

- There is no consistent screening method for CSA recommended by any major medical organization
- The American College of Obstetricians and Gynecologists Committee on Genetics (ACOG) recommends conducting psychosocial screening, which includes screening for current and past abuse, at least once each trimester of pregnancy
- Patients are often reluctant to initiate a conversation about sexual abuse but generally prefer a universal screening approach
- Screening can be done via standardized form, along with other psychosocial screening questions, or by personal interview
- Having a list of follow-up resources that are available to the woman if she desires additional help is an important component of successful screening

INTERVENTION

- Traumatized patients generally benefit from a counseling referral but have low compliance rates with mental health referrals in general
- Ideally, referral to a counselor should be made after discussion with the patient

AVOIDING RETRAUMATIZATION

- The nature of obstetrics and gynecology means an increased risk of triggering negative memories with routine care among women with a history childhood sexual abuse
- Explanation of all touches and procedures is important for avoiding retraumatization
- Whenever possible, the patient should be allowed to suggest ways in which the procedure can be done to lessen her fear
- It is important to ask permission to touch the patient, especially during particularly invasive examinations and procedures, such as pelvic, rectal, and vaginal ultrasound and breast examinations

Sexual Assault

DEFINITION

- Sexual assault is also called "sexual violence," which is defined as any sexual act that is perpetrated against someone's will
- According to the Centers for Disease Control and Prevention (CDC), sexual violence encompasses a range of offenses, including the following:
  - A completed nonconsensual sex act (i.e., rape)
  - An attempted nonconsensual sex act, abusive sexual contact (i.e., unwanted touching)
  - Noncontact sexual abuse (e.g., threatened sexual violence, exhibitionism, verbal sexual harassment)

- All sexual violence involves victims who do not consent or who are unable to consent or refuse to allow the act (Centers for Disease Control and Prevention, 2010)
- Criminal sexual assault is also called rape and is further characterized to include acquaintance rape, date rape, "statutory rape," child sexual abuse, and incest
- These terms relate to the age of the victim and her relationship to the abuser
- Acquaintance and date rape refer to sexual assaults committed by someone who is known to the victim
- "Statutory rape" refers to consensual sexual intercourse with female younger than a specified age; the age of consent varies by state
- In California, adolescents are able to consent to sexual intercourse at 16 years old, if the partner is older than 18 years old
- Incest refers to sexual intercourse among family members, or those legally barred from marriage (American College of Obstetricians and Gynecologists [ACOG], 1997)

PREVALENCE

- According to a nationally representative survey from 2007:
- 10.6% of women reported experiencing forced sex at some time in their lives
- In the first rape experience of female victims, perpetrators were reported to be intimate partners (30.4%), family members (23.7%), and acquaintances (20%) (Basile et al, 2007)
- A study in 2000 found that 20% to 25% of college women experienced attempted or completed rape in college (Fisher et al, 2000)
- <25% of survivors report assault to the police (Elch et al, 2007)

MEDICAL CARE

- Treatment of the survivor should address legal, medical, and psychosocial ramifications of the assault
- Care should be coordinated with staff among all three areas
- The majority of women present to the emergency room for care following a sexual assault
- Documentation of the patient's history should include a gentle and nonjudgmental approach, and documentation in her exact words (Table 45-4)

EXAMINATION

- Physical injuries are noted in approximately half of reported assaults
- Nongenital injuries are more common than genital ones (Elch et al, 2007)
- If a patient is receiving an examination for the first time following an assault, evidence should be collected with a rape kit
- This includes collecting clothing; fingernail scrapings; head and pubic hair combings; plucked hair from the patient; swabs of oropharynx, vagina, and rectum; and blood samples

TABLE 45-4   Tips on Taking a History From Women Who Have Been Sexually Assaulted

Use the patient's exact words

Use the phrases "alleged sexual assault" or "sexual assault by history"; avoid using "rape" because it is a legal, not medical, term

Document the ages of and identifying information about the patient and the assailant; the date, time, and location of the assault; the specific circumstances of the assault, including details of sexual contact and any exposure to bodily fluids; and what the patient has done since the assault (e.g., bathing, douching, changing clothes)

Note use of restraints (e.g., weapons, drugs, alcohol)

Record the patient's gynecologic history (including most recent consensual sexual encounter)

From Petter LM, Whitehill DL: Management of female sexual assault, *Am Fam Physician* 58(4):920-926, 1998.

INFECTIOUS DISEASE TESTING, PREVENTION, AND TREATMENT

- The decision to obtain genital or other specimens should be made on an individual basis
- When specimens are obtained, they should be taken from any area of penetration, including vaginal, anal, and oral
- Trichomoniasis, bacterial vaginosis, *Neisseria gonorrhoeae*, and *Chlamydia trachomatis* are the most frequently diagnosed sexually transmitted infections (STIs) among women who have been sexually assaulted (Centers for Disease Control and Prevention et al, 2006)
- As a result of their high prevalence among sexually active women, identification following an assault does not necessarily show acquisition during the assault
- Identification of *Neisseria gonorrhoeae* and *Chlamydia trachomatis* is of particular importance because of the risk of ascending infection
- Hepatitis B infection can be prevented by postexposure vaccination

INITIAL EXAMINATION

- *Neisseria gonorrhoeae* and *Chlamydia trachomatis* testing from any site of attempted or completed penetration with nucleic acid amplification tests (NAATs); NAATs offer increased sensitivity in detecting *Chlamydia trachomatis*
- Wet mount and culture of vaginal swab specimen for *Trichomonas vaginalis* infection
- Wet mount examination of vaginal swab specimen for bacterial vaginosis (BV) and candidiasis if vaginal discharge, malodor, or itching is evident
- Serum sample for immediate evaluation for human immunodeficiency virus (HIV), hepatitis B, and syphilis
- Hepatitis C testing is not routinely recommended

FOLLOW-UP EXAMINATIONS

- If prophylaxis was administered, repeat examination for STIs should only be performed if the patient reports symptoms
- If no prophylaxis was given, examination for STIs should be repeated within 1 to 2 weeks of the assault because concentrations of organisms sufficient for detection may not have been present at the time of initial evaluation
- Serologic tests for syphilis and HIV should be repeated at 6 weeks, 3 months, and 6 months after the assault if initial tests were negative and infection in the assailant could not be ruled out

TABLE 45-5   Empiric Antimicrobial Regimen for Chlamydia, Gonorrhea, Trichomonas, and BV

Ceftriaxone 250 mg IM in a single dose

OR

Cefixime 400 mg orally in a single dose

PLUS

Metronidazole 2 g orally in a single dose

PLUS

Azithromycin 1 g orally in a single dose OR Doxycycline 100 mg orally twice a day for 7 days

From Centers for Disease Control and Prevention, Workowski KA, Berman SM: Sexually transmitted diseases treatment guidelines, 2010, *MMWR Recomm Rep* 59(RR-12):91, 2010.

STI PROPHYLAXIS

- Follow-up of survivors of sexual assault can be difficult, so the CDC recommends prophylactic treatment at the time of the initial examination (Centers for Disease Control and Prevention et al, 2006)
- The CDC recommends the following regimen:
  - Postexposure hepatitis B vaccination, without hepatitis B immune globulin, administered at time of initial examination if not previously vaccinated, with follow-up doses 1 to 2 and 4 to 6 months after the first dose
  - Empiric antimicrobial regimen for chlamydia, gonorrhea, trichomonas, and BV (Table 45-5):
- HIV seroconversion has occurred in persons whose only known risk factor was sexual assault or sexual abuse; however, the CDC states, "the frequency of this occurrence is probably low" (Centers for Disease Control and Prevention et al, 2006)
- HIV seroconversion rates for consensual vaginal intercourse are 0.1% to 0.2% and receptive rectal intercourse 0.5% to 3%

UPDATE #4

The U.S. Department of Health and Human Services recommends that an individual seeking care within 72 hours after nonoccupational exposure to blood, genital secretions, or other potentially infective body fluids of an individual known to have HIV receive a 28-day course of highly active antiretroviral therapy (HAART). This should be initiated as soon as possible after exposure (Smith et al, 2005).

TABLE 45-6   **Recommendations for Postexposure Assessment of Adolescent and Adult Survivors within 72 hours of Sexual Assault**

Assess risk for HIV infection in the assailant.

Evaluate characteristics of the assault event that might increase risk for HIV transmission.

Consult with a specialist in HIV treatment, if postexposure prophylaxis (PEP) is being considered.

If the survivor appears to be at risk for HIV transmission from the assault, discuss antiretroviral prophylaxis, including toxicity and lack of proven benefit.

If the survivor chooses to start antiretroviral PEP (*58*), provide enough medication to last until the next return visit; reevaluate the survivor 3 to 7 days after the initial assessment, and assess tolerance of medications.

If PEP is started, perform complete blood count (CBC) and serum chemistry at baseline (initiation of PEP should not be delayed, pending results).

Perform an HIV antibody test at original assessment; repeat at 6 weeks, 3 months, and 6 months.

From Centers for Disease Control and Prevention, Workowski KA, Berman SM: Sexually transmitted diseases treatment guidelines, *MMWR Recomm Rep* 59(RR-12):92-93, 2010.

- The risk for oral transmission is significantly lower
- Individuals seeking care within 72 hours of an exposure to an individual of unknown HIV status need to be evaluated on a case-by-case basis (Table 45-6)
- Factors to be assessed in the case of an assailant with unknown status include the following:
  - The likelihood of the assailant having HIV (known sexual risk factors or intravenous drug use)
  - Local epidemiology of HIV/acquired immunodeficiency syndrome (AIDS)
  - Exposure characteristics of the assault:
    - Whether vaginal or anal penetration occurred
    - If ejaculation occurred on mucous membranes
    - Whether multiple assailants were involved
  - Mucosal lesions present on assailant or survivor
- A clinician may consider prescribing nonoccupational postexposure prophylaxis (nPEP) for an individual seeking care more than 72 hours after exposure if there is a serious risk for transmission and the decreased potential benefit of treatment outweighs the potential risks for adverse effects of the antiretroviral medications

PREGNANCY

- Rape has been shown to contribute significantly to the rate of unintended pregnancies each year in the United States
- The national rape-related pregnancy rate was 5% per rape among women aged 12 to 45 years in one study over a 3-year period, equivalent to 32,000 pregnancies as a result of rape each year (Holmes et al, 1996)
- This study found that 50% of women who became pregnant opted for termination, and nearly 50% of victims received no medical attention close to the assault
- All women of reproductive age should receive a pregnancy test at the time of initial evaluation
- Upon a negative initial test, women should be offered emergency contraception (Table 45-7)

MENTAL HEALTH CONSEQUENCES

- Acute emotional reaction
  - Women may experience a wide range of emotional and physical responses during and following sexual assault

- Two studies showed that 37% and 52% of women experienced a "freeze" reaction, or tonic immobility (TI), during a sexual assault (Galliano et al, 1993; Heidt et al, 2005)
  - TI during childhood sexual abuse has been demonstrated as predictive of adult PTSD and depressive symptoms (Heidt et al, 2005)
  - TI following adult sexual or physical abuse also has been associated with increased risk of PTSD compared to women who fought back against their attacker (Rizvi et al, 2008)
  - Peritraumatic emotional responses can range from dissociation and complete loss of emotional control to an apparently well-controlled reaction; women can have acute generalized pain, headache, eating and sleep disturbances, as well as depression, anxiety and mood swings
  - About 50% of women recover from the acute reaction within 12 weeks, but many women progress to long-term symptoms of PTSD and depression (Rothbaum et al, 1991)
  - Peritraumatic dissociation has been shown by multiple longitudinal studies to be a significant risk factor for PTSD and depressive symptoms (Ozer et al, 2003)
- Posttraumatic stress disorder (PTSD)
  - Rape trauma syndrome is a subset of PTSD, first described in the 1970s, consisting of the acute phase ("disorganization"), lasting hours to days, and a delayed ("reorganization") phase that may not begin until months, or even years, following the assault (Burgess et al, 1974; Keogh, 2007)
  - PTSD symptoms include reexperiencing of the life-threatening event, typically by nightmares or flashbacks, as well as hyperarousal (increased startle response, irritability, sleep disturbance, hypervigilance) and emotional detachment (numbness and avoidance of reminders of the assault)
  - A large study showed that 31% of female rape victims developed PTSD, compared to 5% of women who were not victims of crime (Kilpatrick et al, 1992)
- Substance abuse and dependence
  - Survivors of sexual assault have been shown consistently to be at significantly increased risk of alcohol abuse (Ullman et al, 2005)

TABLE 45-7   Oral Contraceptives That Can Be Used for Emergency Contraception in the United States[a]

Brand	Company	First Dose[b]	Second Dose[b] (12 hours later)	Ulipristal Acetate per Dose (mg)	Ethinyl Estradiol per Dose (µg)	Levonorgestrel per Dose (mg)[c]
Ulipristal acetate pills						
ella	Watson	1 white pill	None[b]	30	-	-
Progestin-only pills						
Levonorgestrel Tablets	Perrigo	2 white pills	None[b]	-	-	1.5
Next Choice	Watson	2 peach pills	None[b]	-	-	1.5
Plan B One-Step	Teva	1 whilte pill	None	-	-	1.5
Combined progestin and estrogen pills						
Aviane	Teva	5 orange pills	5 orange pills	-	100	0.50
Cryselle	Teva	4 white pills	4 white pills	-	120	0.60
Enpresse	Teva	4 orange pills	4 orange pills	-	120	0.50
Jolessa	Teva	4 pink pills	4 pink pills	-	120	0.60
Lessina	Teva	5 pink pills	5 pink pills	-	100	0.50
Levora	Watson	4 white pills	4 white pills	-	120	0.60
Lo/Ovral	Akrimax	4 white pills	4 white pills	-	120	0.60
LoSeasonique	Teva	5 orange pills	5 orange pills	-	100	0.50
Low-Ogestrel	Watson	4 white pills	4 white pills	-	120	0.60
Lutera	Watson	5 white pills	5 white pills	-	100	0.50
Lybrel	Wyeth	6 yellow pills	6 yellow pills	-	120	0.54
Nordette	Teva	4 light-orange pills	4 light-orange pills	-	120	0.60
Ogestrel	Watson	2 white pills	2 white pills	-	100	0.50
Portia	Teva	4 pink pills	4 pink pills	-	120	0.60
Quasense	Watson	4 white pills	4 white pills	-	120	0.60
Seasonale	Teva	4 pink pills	4 pink pills	-	120	0.60
Seasonique	Teva	4 light-blue-green pills	4 light-blue-green pills	-	120	0.60
Sronyx	Watson	5 white pills	5 while pills	-	100	0.50
Trivora	Watson	4 pink pills	4 pink pills	-	120	0.50

[a]*ella, Plan B One-Step, Next Choice* and *Levonorgestrel Tablets* are the only dedicated product specifically marketed for emergency contraception. Aviane, Cryselle, Enpresse, Jolessa, Lessina, Levora, Lo/Ovral, LoSeasonique, Low-Ogestrel, Lutera, Lybrel, Nordette, Ogestrel, Portia, Quasense, Seasonale, Seasonique, Sronyx and Trivora have been declared safe and effective for use as ECPs by the United States Food and Drug Administration. Outside the United States, about 100 emergency contraceptive products are specifically packaged, labeled, and marketed. Levonorgestrel-only ECPs are available either over-the-counter or from a pharmacist without having to see a clinician in 60 countries. In the U.S., *Plan B One-Step* and *Next Choice* are available over-the-counter to women and men aged 17 and older. You can buy these pills by prescription if you are younger. *ella* is available by prescription only.
[b]The labels for *Next Choice* and *Levonorgestrel Tablets* say to take one pill within 72 hours after unprotected intercourse, and another pill 12 hours later. However, recent research has found that both pills can be taken at the same time. Research has also shown that that all of the brands listed here are effective when used within 120 hours after unprotected sex.
[c]The progestin in Cryselle, Lo/Ovral, Low-Ogestrel and Ogestrel is norgestrel, which contains two isomers, only one of which (levonorgestrel) is bioactive; the amount of norgestrel in each tablet is twice the amount of levonorgestrel.
Adapted from 2011 Office of Population Research and Association of Reproductive Health Professionals.

- Risk factors for alcohol abuse among survivors of sexual assault include a history of additional trauma, drinking to cope with distress, and an expectation of tension reduction with alcohol use (Ullman et al, 2005)
- Increased use of alcohol following an assault has been linked to increased posttraumatic sexual activity, which may pose a higher risk of STIs and unplanned pregnancy (Deliramich et al, 2008)
- Eating disorders
  - There are several studies demonstrating an increased risk of eating disorders among adolescent and adult survivors of sexual assault (American College of Obstetricians and Gynecologists, 2005)
- One study of adult survivors of rape without a history of childhood sexual abuse found that 67.5% of women engaged in binge eating and 47.5% of women in purging at 4 to 9 months following the assault (Faravelli et al, 2004)

SOMATIC SEQUELAE

- Women with a history of sexual assault have increased rates of chronic pelvic pain, fibromyalgia, and functional gastrointestinal disorders (Paras et al, 2009)

TABLE 45-8   Physician's Role in Evaluation of Sexual Assault Victims

Medical Issues

Ensure informed consent is obtained from patient

Assess and treat physical injuries or triage and refer

Obtain pertinent past gynecologic history

Perform physical examination, including pelvic examination (with appropriate chaperone or support person present)

Obtain appropriate specimens for sexually transmitted disease testing

Obtain baseline serologic tests for hepatitis B, human immunodeficiency virus, and syphilis

Provide appropriate infectious diseases prophylaxis as indicated

Provide or arrange for provision of emergency contraception as indicated

Provide counseling regarding findings, recommendations, and prognosis

Arrange follow-up medical care and referrals for psychosocial needs

*Legal Issues**

Provide accurate recording of events

Document injuries

Collect samples (pubic hair, fingernail scrapings, vaginal secretion and discharge samples, saliva, blood-stained clothing or other personal articles) as indicated by local protocol or regulation

Identify the presence or absence of sperm in the vaginal fluids, and make appropriate slides

Report to authorities as required

Ensure security of chain of evidence

*Many jurisdictions have prepackaged "rape kits" for the initial forensic examination that provide specific containers and instructions for the collection of physical evidence and for written and pictorial documentation of the victim's subjective and objective findings. Hospital emergency rooms or the police themselves may supply the kits when called to respond or when bringing a patient to the hospital. Most often the emergency physician or specially trained nurse response team will perform the examination, but all physicians should be familiar with the forensic examination procedure. If called to perform this examination and the physician has no or limited experience, it may be judicious to call for assistance because any break in the technique in collecting evidence, or break in the chain of custody of evidence, including improper handling of samples or mislabeling, will virtually eliminate any effort to prosecute in the future.
From American College of Obstetricians and Gynecologists: *Special issues in women's health*, Washington, DC, 2005, American College of Obstetricians and Gynecologists.

PHYSICIAN'S ROLE AND RESPONSIBILITIES
(Table 45-8)

SPECIAL CONCERNS

- Adolescents
  - The age at which an adolescent may consent to intercourse varies between states, from 14 years to 18 years; an adolescent younger than 14 years is defined as being incapable of consent
  - Young women (age 16 to 24 years) are four times as likely to be sexually assaulted as women of any other age (Danielson et al, 2004)

TABLE 45-9   Drugs Used to Facilitate Sexual Assault

Most Commonly Used

Alcohol*

Marijuana (Cannabis)*

Associated with Increased Incidence of Sexual Assault

Flunitrazepam (Rohypnol)*

γ-Hydroxybutyrate (GHB)*

γ-Butyrolactone (GBL)*

1, 4, butanediol (BD)

Ketamine*

Reported in Various Series

Alprazolam

Chloral hydrate

Clonazepam

Diazepam

Meprobamate

Midazolam

Phencyclidine*

Temazepam

Triazolam

Zolpidem

*For more information, go to www.clubdrugs.org.
Adapted from Schwartz RH, Milteer R, LeBeau MA: Drug-facilitated sexual assault ("date rape"), *South Med J* 93(6):558-561, 2000.

- Date rape or dating violence estimates are as high as 30% in this population (Wolitzky-Taylor et al, 2008)
- The risk of pregnancy is increased among adolescents because they are more likely to be repeatedly assaulted because of an incestuous relationship and low use of ongoing drug contraception
- In a California cohort study, a high proportion of infants born to adolescent mothers had fathers who were adult males: 24.3% of infants born to mothers aged 11 to 12 years, and 26.8% of infants born to mothers aged 13 to 14 years (Taylor et al, 1999)
- Sexual assault in adolescents has been linked to criminal behavior, intravenous drug use, prostitution, early initiation of consensual intercourse, unplanned pregnancy, lack of initiation and continuing use of contraception, and involvement in physically assaultive relationships (Boyer et al, 1992; Danielson et al, 2004; Elders et al, 1998; Herrera et al, 2003; Stock et al, 1997)

SUBSTANCE USE AND SEXUAL ASSAULT

- Use of alcohol and other intoxicants increases the risk for sexual assault among adolescents and college students (Howard et al, 2008)
- Alcohol and marijuana appear most consistently in screens for drug use associated with sexual assault (Scott-Ham et al, 2005)
- One study of rape treatment centers across the United States found alcohol detected in 63% of screens and marijuana in 30% (Slaughter, 2000)
- Drug-facilitated sexual assault (DFSA) involves incapacitation or loss of consciousness by the victim because of the effects of alcohol or drugs (Table 45-9)

TABLE 45-10 Screening Questions for Sexual Assault History

Because sexual violence is an enormous problem for women in this country and can affect a woman's health and well-being, I now ask all my patients about exposure to violence and about sexual assault.

1. Do you have someone special in your life? Someone you're going out with?
2. Are you now—or have you been—sexually active?
3. Think about your earliest sexual experience. Did you want this experience?
4. Has a friend, a date, or an acquaintance ever pressured or forced you into sexual activities when you did not want them? Touched you in a way that made you uncomfortable? Anyone at home? Anyone at school? Any other adult?
5. Although women are never responsible for rape, there are things they can do that may reduce their risk of sexual assault. Do you know how to reduce your risk of sexual assault?

From American Congress of Obstetrics and Gynecologists: *Screening tools—sexual assault* (website). www.acog.org/departments/dept_notice.cfm?recno=17&;bulletin=1477. Accessed May 10, 2010.

UPDATE #5

Prevalence data on DFSA related to covert administration of drugs are lacking, but the overall proportion of all sexual assaults is low. Studies have found 2% to 3% of all sexual assaults during the time studied involved covert use of medication (Hurley et al, 2006; Scott-Ham et al, 2005; Slaughter, 2000).

OTHER POPULATIONS

- Women in the military are also at elevated risk of sexual assault, termed military sexual trauma (MST), with 22% screening positive for a history of MST in a 2002 national Veterans Administration (VA) study (Suris et al, 2008)
- Incarcerated women are at risk of sexual abuse by male custodial staff,\ and have increased rates of lifetime sexual assault as well, with rates ranging from 30% to 68% (Raj et al, 2008)
- Women in areas of civil war or social disruption are also at high risk of sexual assault, as rape has been used as an act of war in many areas
- Women who have immigrated to the United States as asylum seekers have higher rates of lifetime sexual assault than the general population
- Elderly women, particularly those in long-term care facilities, can also be victims of sexual assault
- The differential diagnosis of unexplained vaginal or rectal bleeding, vaginal discharge, and vaginal foreign bodies should include sexual abuse
- Women with disabilities have been demonstrated as having a fourfold higher incidence of sexual assault than those without disabilities (Martin et al, 2006)

SCREENING

- ACOG recommends that physicians screen all patients at every visit for sexual assault (Table 45-10)

SUGGESTED READINGS

Childhood Sexual Abuse

American College of Obstetricians and Gynecologists: ACOG educational bulletin: adult manifestation of childhood sexual abuse, no. 259, July 2000: clinical management guidelines for obstetrician-gynecologists, *Int J Gynaecol Obstet* 74(3):311–320, 2001.

Ball JS, Links PS: Borderline personality disorder and childhood trauma: evidence for a causal relationship, *Curr Psychiatry Rep* 11(1):63–68, 2009.

Cougle JR, Timpano KR, Sachs-Ericsson N, et al: Examining the unique relationships between anxiety disorders and childhood physical and sexual abuse in the National Comorbidity Survey-Replication, *Psychiatry Res* 177(1-2):150–155, 2010.

Elders MJ, Albert AE: Adolescent pregnancy and sexual abuse, *JAMA* 280(7):648–649, 1998.

Grant LJ: Effects of childhood sexual abuse: issues for obstetric caregivers, *Birth* 19(4):220–221, 1991.

Grimstad H, Schei B: Pregnancy and delivery for women with a history of child abuse, *Child Abuse Negl* 23(1):81–90, 1999.

Heidt JM, Marx BP, Forsyth JP: Tonic immobility and childhood sexual abuse: a preliminary report evaluating the sequela of rape-induced paralysis, *Behav Res Ther* 43(9):1157–1171, 2005.

Leeners B, Richter-Appelt H, Imthurn B, Rath W: Influence of childhood sexual abuse on pregnancy, delivery, and the early postpartum period in adult women, *J Psychosom Res* 61(12):139–151, 2006.

Lev-Wiesel R, Daphna-Tekoah S, Hallak M: Childhood sexual abuse as a predictor of birth-related posttraumatic stress and postpartum posttraumatic stress, *Child Abuse Negl* 33(12):877–887, 2009.

Mayson B, Teichman J: The relationship between sexual abuse and interstitial cystitis/painful bladder syndrome, *Curr Urol Rep* 10(6):441–447, 2009.

McNew JA, Abell N: Posttraumatic stress symptomatology: similarities and differences between Vietnam veterans and adult survivors of childhood abuse, *Soc Work* 40(1):115–126, 1995.

Molnar B, Buka S, Kessler R: Child sexual abuse and subsequent psychopathology: results from the national comorbidity survey, *Am J Public Health* 91(5):753–760, 2001.

Noll JG, Trickett PK, Putnam FW: A prospective investigation of the impact of childhood sexual abuse on the development of sexuality, *J Consult Clin Psychol* 71(3):575–586, 2003.

Paras M, Murad MH, Chen L, et al: Sexual abuse and lifetime diagnosis of somatic disorders: a systematic review and meta-analysis, *JAMA* 302(5):550–561, 2009.

Randolph M, Reddy D: Sexual abuse and sexual functioning in a chronic pelvic pain sample, *J Child Sex Abus* 15(3):61–78, 2006.

Ross C: Childhood sexual abuse and psychosomatic symptoms of irritable bowel syndrome, *J Child Sex Abus* 14(1):27–38, 2005.

Sanci L, Coffey C, Olsson C, et al: Childhood sexual abuse and eating disorders in females: findings from the Victorian adolescent health cohort study, *Arch Pediatr Adolesc Med* 162(3):261–267, 2008.

U.S. Department of Health and Human Services, Administration for Children and Families; Administration on Children, Youth and Families; Children's Bureau and Office on Child Abuse and Neglect; *Child Abuse Prevention and Treatment Act* (website). www.acf.hhs.gov/programs/cb/laws_policies/cblaws/capta03/capta_manual.pdf2003. Accessed July 24, 2011.

Widom CS, DuMont K, Czaja SJ: A prospective investigation of major depressive disorder and comorbidity in abused and neglected children grown up, *Arch Gen Psychiatry* 64(1):49–56, 2007.

Sexual Assault

American College of Obstetricians and Gynecologists: Sexual assault, *ACOG Educ Bull* (242):1–7, 1997.

American College of Obstetricians and Gynecologists: *Special issues in women's health*, Washington, DC, 2005, American College of Obstetricians and Gynecologists.

Basile KC, Chen J, Black MC, Saltzman LE: Prevalence and characteristics of sexual violence victimization among U.S. adults, 2001-2003, *Violence Vict* 22(4):437–448, 2007.

Centers for Disease Control and Prevention, Workowski KA, Berman SM: Sexually transmitted diseases treatment guidelines, 2010, *MMWR Recomm Rep* 59(RR-12):1–110, 2010.

Danielson CK, Holmes MM: Adolescent sexual assault: an update of the literature, *Curr Opin Obstet Gynecol* 16(5):383–388, 2004.

Deliramich AN, Gray MJ: Changes in women's sexual behavior following sexual assault, *Behav Modif* 32(5):611–621, 2008.

Elch J, Mason F: Rape and sexual assault, *BMJ* 334(7604):1154–1158, 2007.

Faravelli C, Giugni A, Salvatori S, Ricca V: Psychopathology after rape, *Am J Psychiatry* 161(8):1483–1485, 2004.

Rizvi S, Kaysen D, Gutner C, et al: Beyond fear; the role of peritraumatic responses in posttraumatic stress and depressive symptoms among female crime victims, *J Interpers Violence* 23(6):853–868, 2008.

Slaughter L: Involvement of drugs in sexual assault, *J Reprod Med* 45(5):425–430, 2000.

Smith DK, Grohskopf LA, Black RJ, et al: Antiretroviral postexposure prophylaxis after sexual, injection-drug use, or other nonoccupational exposure to HIV in the United States: recommendations from the U.S. Department of Health and Human Services, *MMWR Recomm Rep* 54(RR-2):1–20, 2005.

Ullman S, Filipas H, Townsend S, Starzynski L: Trauma exposure, posttraumatic stress disorder and problem drinking in sexual assault survivors, *J Stud Alcohol* 66(5):610–619, 2005.

References

Please go to expertconsult.com to view references.

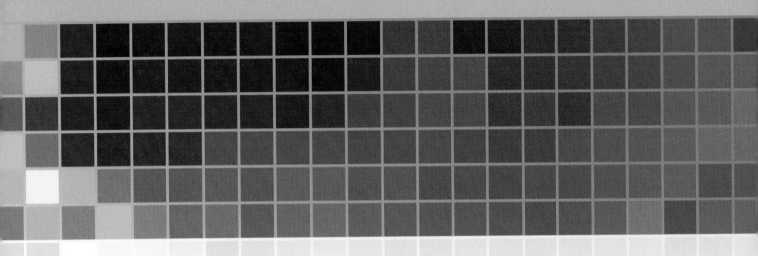

Gynecologic Health: The Postmenopausal Woman

Chapter 46

Care of Elder Women

CHRISTOPHER TARNAY

KEY UPDATES

1. Estrogen continues to be most effective option for treatment for hot flushes.
2. Gabapentin, clonidine, and selective serotonin reuptake inhibitors (SSRIs) are optional treatments for vasomotor instability in women who cannot take estrogen.
3. Local estrogen therapy is both safe and effective in alleviating symptoms of urogenital atrophy.
4. Clobetasol propionate is the treatment of choice for lichen sclerosus, but it has limited value in inducing remission in affected women over 70 years.
5. Short-course antibiotics (3 to 6 days) are sufficient for treating uncomplicated urinary tract infections (UTIs) in elderly women and improve compliance.
6. Combining an anticholinergic and behavioral therapy may treat urge incontinence more effectively than either modality alone.
7. Sacral nerve stimulation is promising therapy for the treatment of fecal incontinence
8. Organizations differ on their recommendations for the appropriate interval for mammography. Screening should be based on guidelines and individual risk.
9. Perioperative beta-blockade should be selectively given to patients with cardiac risk factors.

Introduction

- Advances in health care are contributing to women living longer, with up to a third of a woman's life occupying time after the menopause transition
- Current life expectancy of women in the United States is 80.4 years
- By 2030, more than one fifth of women in the United States will be ≥65 years
- Obstetrician-gynecologists serve in part as primary health providers to women
- Prevalence of many diseases increases as women age
- Preventive health interventions and disease screening are the foundation of care in elder women
- Quality health care in the postmenopausal woman requires a solid understanding of the age- and gender-specific issues postmenopausal women encounter
- Care of women older than 65 years of age brings a host of challenges, requiring skill sets that will equip the provider to handle the physical, emotional, and psychosocial needs of our aging population

Menopause

- Menopause is when menses ceases permanently and fundamentally because of age-related programmed loss of ovarian follicles

- Average age of menopause is 51.4 years
- Five percent of women between ages 40 to 45 years and 5% of women after age 55 will normally undergo menopause
- As opposed to age of menarche, the average age of menopause has not changed as a consequence of nutritional status or general health over the generations

Menopause Physiology

- The perimenopause, or "time around" the menopause, is notable for alterations in normal menstrual cycle bleeding and is due to unreliable fluctuating levels in estradiol and follicle-stimulating hormone (FSH)
- Hormonally associated with a marked decrease in estradiol levels and concomitant increase in FSH levels
- The postmenopausal ovary continues to secrete androgens, mostly in form of androstenedione, secondary to the stimulation of luteinizing hormone (LH)
- Androstenedione is converted to estrone in the peripheral adipose tissue and becomes the predominant circulating androgen
- The physiologic changes caused by the depletion of ovarian follicular function are directly related to much of the gender-specific disease states in women seen after the menopause

Diagnosis

- Clinically defined by absence of menstruation for 12 months after the final normal menstrual cycle
- Use of calendar to obtain menstrual history is the recommended method
- In women >45 years, no other biochemical testing is advised in absence of other symptoms

Hot Flashes

CLINICAL PROFILE

- Known to be a symptom of vasomotor instability
- It is most common symptom of menopause and occurs in at least 70% of women
  - Persists for an average of 2 to 5 years
  - Twenty percent of women continue to flush into their 70s
- Described as a sudden sensation of heat in the face, neck, and chest
- Etiology unknown, but fundamentally a disturbance of peripheral circulation
- Often accompanied by irritation, feelings of anxiety or panic, and sleep disruption
- Causes significant disruption in quality of life and is a primary reason for seeking medical attention

UPDATE #1

Hot flush symptoms are causally related to decreasing estradiol concentrations, mainly in the serum and subsequently also in the hypothalamic temperature regulating center. The lack of estrogens alters neurotransmitter activity, especially in the serotonergic and noradrenergic pathways. Because sex steroids act as potent neuromodulators, the substitution of ovarian sex steroids by hormone replacement therapy appears to be the most effective treatment option for hot flushes (Rossmanith et al, 2009).

MANAGEMENT

- Estrogen replacement therapy considered gold standard
- Oral or transdermal route
- Effective in reducing hot flushes by 75% to 95%
- No differences in conjugated equine estrogens versus 17β-estradiol
- Selective serotonin reuptake inhibitors (SSRIs)
- Randomized controlled trials (RCTs) with paroxetine and venlafaxine demonstrate reduction in symptoms with short-term use (50% to 60%)
- Other nonhormone treatments
  - Gabapentin
  - Clonidine
  - Phytoestrogens
  - Acupuncture
  - Exercise

UPDATE #2

In a meta-analysis referencing 43 trials on nonhormonal therapies for hot flushes, the SSRIs clonidine and gabapentin trials provide evidence for efficacy; however, effects are less than that for estrogen. Adverse effects and cost may restrict use for many women. These therapies may be most useful for highly symptomatic women who cannot take estrogen, but they are not optimal choices for most women (Nelson et al, 2006).

Vulvar Atrophy

CLINICAL PROFILE

- Vaginal atrophy may affect up to 75% of women
- Estrogen and progesterone receptors are present in the vagina, urethra and trigone, and pelvic floor musculature
- Estrogen deficiency contributes to decreased blood flow, a reduction in elasticity, and distensibility of the vagina
- Classic symptoms of vaginal dryness, discomfort, and dyspareunia
- Despite high prevalence, it is underdiagnosed and undertreated

DIAGNOSIS

- Examination notable for pale, thin, dry vaginal epithelium
- Loss of labia minora architecture
- Alkaline pH
- Microscopy notable for small, more spherical epithelial cells consisting of intermediate or parabasal cells lacking maturation

TREATMENT

- Local estrogen therapy (cream, ring, vaginal tablet)
- Vaginal moisturizers
- Vaginal lubricants

UPDATE #3

A prospective study of vaginal estrogen supplementation in a total of 126 women compared routes of administration: ring (EString) versus tablet (Vagifem). The study evaluated atrophy symptoms and impact on endometrial thickness. There was no statistical difference between the groups in the alleviation of symptoms and signs of urogenital estrogen deficiency. After 48 weeks of treatment, there was no statistically significant difference in endometrial thickness between the two groups (Weisberg et al, 2005).

Vulvar Disease

CLINICAL PROFILE

- Vulvar disease can affect any age group; however, some conditions are more frequent in the postmenopausal woman
- Both benign skin and premalignant conditions are more common in women over 65
- Elderly patient perineal hygiene is often compromised because of the relative immobility, urinary incontinence, body habitus, and changes in general hygiene practices
- Bowel and bladder control issues often compound the problem

Lichen Sclerosus

- Benign inflammatory dermatosis of vulvar and perianal skin
- Biphasic prevalence: prepubertal girls and postmenopausal women

- Unknown cause, likely autoimmune component
- Pruritus, soreness, burning, and pain are common symptoms
- Malignant progression to squamous cell carcinoma has been a concern in some cohort studies

DIFFERENTIAL DIAGNOSIS

- Lichen planus (LP), vulvar intraepithelial neoplasia (VIN), psoriasis, and vitiligo

DIAGNOSIS

- Clinical exam
- Biopsy is confirmatory

MANAGEMENT

- High-potency corticosteroid ointment; clobetasol propionate
- Initial dosing nightly for 4 weeks, then alternate nights for 4 weeks, then twice weekly for third month
- For symptom recurrence, return to most recent effective dosing regimen

UPDATE #4

The effectiveness and safety of long-term clobetasol use in vulvar lichen sclerosus was evaluated prospectively in 83 women. The estimated incidence of remission at 3 years was 72% in women younger than 50 years, 23% in women between 50 and 70 years of age, and 0% in women older than 70 years. Half of the relapse occurred after 16 months. There were eight observed vulvar squamous cell carcinomas (9.6%) occurring in previously untreated or irregularly treated vulvar lichen sclerosus (VLS) lesions. The authors concluded that treatment with a potent steroid cream can improve but does not cure VLS in women older than 70 years, probably because of a long disease evolution (Renaud-Vilmer et al, 2004).

Vulvar Dermatitis

CLINICAL PROFILE

- Exceedingly common in postmenopausal women, as estrogen is deficient
- Self medication and poly-use of over-the-counter preparations exacerbates the problem
- Contact dermatitis is most common type and likely caused by allergens and irritants
- Pruritus, burning, and pain
- Thickening, whitening, with associated rim of erythema and inflammation over vulva, often tracking to groin
- Suprainfection with tinea is often present

MANAGEMENT

- Remove common irritants (soaps, deodorants, feminine hygiene sprays/perfumes, unindicated antifungal creams/preparations, laundry additives such as fabric softeners)
- Gentle sitz bath cleansing
- Skin barriers with emollients
- Low to medium potency steroid ointments for 7 to 10 days

Other Vulvar Conditions

- Lichen planus
- Psoriasis
- VIN
- Paget's disease

Urinary Tract Infection (UTIs)

CLINICAL PROFILE

- UTIs account for more than 1 million emergency visits a year
- Most common bacterial infection in menopausal women
- *E. coli* is most common pathogen, with Klebsiella, Proteus, and Enterobacter more likely seen in elderly women
- Inherent risks of vaginal atrophy, altered vaginal flora, poor perineal care, voiding dysfunction, and urinary stasis all constitute risk factors leading to increased vulnerability in menopausal women
- Dysuria, frequency, urgency, and flank pain are common symptoms
- In elderly patients, low suspicion for pyelonephritis and urosepsis and, if proven, hospitalization for intravenous antibiotics

DIAGNOSIS

- Clean catch urinalysis and bacterial culture
- Sterile catheterization if specimen quality poor

MANAGEMENT

- Three-day course with nitrofurantoin or trimethoprim-sulfamethoxazole
- In patients over 65 years, fluoroquinolones are suggested
- Patients in long-term care facilities or recent hospitalization should have therapy covering Proteus and Klebsiella
- Candida should be considered in women not responsive to initial antibiotic therapy
- Women with indwelling catheters often have colonized bacteria and should be treated only if symptomatic with catheter change and antibiotics for 14 days

UPDATE #5

In a recent Cochrane review of antibiotic duration for treating uncomplicated, symptomatic lower urinary tract infections in elderly women, 15 studies (1644 elderly women) were included. In the studies that compared short-course (3 to 6 days) with long-course (7 to 14 days) treatment, short-course treatment could be sufficient for treating uncomplicated UTIs in elderly women. Shorter therapy improves compliance and reduces adverse symptoms generally associated with longer-course therapy (Lutters et al, 2008).

Urinary Incontinence (UI)

CLINICAL PROFILE

- Based on large population studies, 25% to 75% of women have urinary incontinence depending on definition
- As women age, UI becomes more prevalent with rates of moderate to severe symptoms of at least 24% in women 60 or older

- In aging women, urinary symptoms, particularly urgency, frequency, and bladder-emptying difficulty, are also extremely common and contribute to often tremendous reduction in quality of life (reduced physical activity, loss of productivity, social isolation, mood disorders, loss of intimacy, expense)
- Majority of women suffer from either stress urinary incontinence or urge-related urinary incontinence or both (mixed urinary incontinence)
- Overactive bladder (OAB) is a term that encompasses urgency and frequency with or without associated incontinence
- Predisposing risk factors of UI are multiple and varied and include vaginal delivery, postmenopausal status, obesity, pelvic surgery, chronic lung disease, smoking, diuretic use, and stress

DIAGNOSIS

- History of urinary symptoms
- Quantify severity with bladder diary and quality-of-life survey instruments
- Evaluate for presence of other pelvic floor disorders (pelvic organ prolapse, fecal incontinence)
- Cough stress test (provoking cough with semifull bladder and evaluating for leakage)
- Urine specimen for evaluation of cystitis, consider catheterization to exclude retention (>100 mL post void residual)
- Screen for potential transient or secondary causes (diet, medication, infection, atrophy, stool impaction, cognitive impairment, and mobility restriction)
- Role of cystoscopy or urodynamics; no evidence to demonstrate improved outcomes in noncomplicated patients

MANAGEMENT

- Lifestyle and behavioral changes (dietary changes, caffeine avoidance, weight reduction, fluid management)
- Pelvic floor muscle exercises are proven first-line intervention for both stress and urge-related symptoms
- Anticholinergic medications are used for urge incontinence and related symptoms and demonstrate effective improvement in reduction of urge and urge incontinence episodes
- Long-acting formulations (oxybutynin and tolterodine) of each have helped to reduce severity of side effects more associated with the immediate release forms
- Newer more bladder-specific anticholinergic medications (darifenacin, solifenacin, trospium, fesoterodine) in general show similar clinical efficacy
- Because older patients tend to be taking a number of medications, consideration should be given to additive effects

improvement. Enhanced benefit was seen in women who then had combination therapy of both with an overall reduction in incontinence. Mean improvement from baseline: BF 57.5%, BF + OX 88.5%; OX 72.7%, and OX +B F 84.3% (Burgio et al, 2000).

- Surgery with midurethral slings is the current gold standard for stress urinary incontinence, allowing short recovery with acceptably low risks
  - Safety well demonstrated in elderly cohort

Fecal Incontinence

CLINICAL PROFILE

- Generally defined as involuntary loss of flatus or stool
- Common problem in elderly with prevalence and severity increasing with age
- Prevalence is 14.4% in women over 60 years, 21.6% in women over 80 years
- In nursing homes, overall prevalence is about 45%
- Significant burden to individuals because of shame, embarrassment, and social isolation
- Risk factors include increasing age, high body mass index, limited physical activity, neurologic disease, diabetes, and inflammatory bowel disease
- Obstetrical history of episiotomy or anal sphincter injury is also associated

DIAGNOSIS

- History and physical examination
- Differentiate between structural (anal sphincter) and functional (neurologic, cognitive impairment, pharmacologic side effects) causes
- Anal sphincter defects confirmed by exam, endoanal ultrasound, or magnetic resonance imaging (MRI)
- Ancillary tests: defecography, anal manometry, and pudendal nerve terminal motor latency testing

TREATMENT

- Dietary modification: bulking with fiber
- Pharmacotherapy
  - Loperamide
  - Lomotil
- Consolidate stooling with scheduled daily enemas
- Pelvic floor therapy
  - Biofeedback
  - Electrical stimulation
- Sacral nerve stimulation

- Surgery for anal sphincter defects documented on imaging (ultrasound or MRI)
  - Anal sphincteroplasty
    - Treatment of choice: overlapping repair
    - Surgical cure rates are 50% to 80%
    - Pudendal nerve neuropathy, however, is associated with a higher failure rate
  - Postanal repair
  - Artificial anal sphincter

Cancer Screening

BREAST CANCER

Clinical Profile

- Approximately 207,000 U.S. women are diagnosed with breast cancer per year
- Approximately 40,800 U.S. women die from breast cancer per year
- Risk factors include age, family history, history of radiation exposure, carcinoma in situ, atypical hyperplasia, and history of multiple breast biopsies

Evaluation

- Screening mammography identifies breast cancers too small to palpate on physical examination and can also find ductal carcinoma in situ (DCIS), a noninvasive condition
- Sensitivity of mammography is 79%
- American Cancer Society recommends yearly mammograms starting at age 40 and continuing for as long as a woman is in good health
- Women with comorbid conditions that limit their life expectancy are unlikely to benefit from screening
- Age to discontinue screening mammography is uncertain

- Older women have higher probability of developing and dying of breast cancer but also have a greater chance of dying of other causes
- Clinical breast exam (CBE) every year in women ≥40

UPDATE #8

There is much controversy surrounding screening policy. There is no consensus among North American societies regarding the age to *initiate* screening or an optimal screening interval. The American Medical Association (AMA), the American College of Radiology (ACR), the American Cancer Society (ACS), and the American College of Obstetricians and Gynecologists (ACOG) all support screening with mammography beginning at age 40. The Canadian Task Force on Preventive Health Care (CTFPHC), the American Academy of Family Physicians (AAFP), and the American College of Preventive Medicine (ACPM) recommend beginning mammography for average-risk women at age 50.

Organizations differ on their recommendations for the *appropriate interval* for mammography. The AMA, ACR, and ACS recommend annual mammography. The CTFPHC, AAFP, and ACPM recommend mammography every 1 to 2 years. The ACOG recommends mammography every 1 to 2 years for women ages 40 to 49 and annually for women ages 50 and older (Calonge et al, 2009).

COLORECTAL CANCER

- Colorectal cancer is the third most common cancer, and the second leading cause of cancer deaths, in the United States; each year, nearly 150,000 people are newly diagnosed with colorectal cancer and 50,000 die (Table 46-1)
- Risk factors include inflammatory bowel disease, personal or family history of colorectal cancer or colorectal polyps, genetic syndrome such as familial adenomatous polyposis or hereditary nonpolyposis colorectal cancer (Lynch syndrome)

TABLE 46-1 Colorectal Cancer Screening Recommendations from the U.S. Preventive Services Task Force and the American Cancer Society–U.S. Multisociety Task Force

Screening Test	Description	U.S. Preventive Services Task Force (USPSTF)	American Cancer Society–U.S. Multi-Society Task Force (ACS-USMSTF)
Fecal occult blood test (FOBT) and fecal immunochemical test (FIT)	Examination of the stool for traces of blood not visible to the naked eye	Recommends high-sensitivity FOBT and FIT annually for ages 50-75	Recommends high-sensitivity FOBT and FIT annually for ages ≥50
Sigmoidoscopy	Internal examination of the lower part of the large intestine	Recommends every 5 years with high-sensitivity FOBT every 3 years for ages 50-75	Age ≥50, every 5 years
Double-contrast barium enema	X-ray examination of the colon	—	Age ≥50, every 5 years
Colonoscopy	Internal examination of the entire large intestine	Recommends every 10 years for ages 50-75	Age ≥50, every 10 years
Computed tomography colonography	Examination of the colon and rectum using pictures obtained using a computed tomography scanner	—	Age ≥50, every 5 years

From Holden, DJ, Harris, R, Porterfield, DS, et al: *Enhancing the use and quality of colorectal cancer screening: evidence report/technology assessment no.190.* (Prepared by the RTI International–University of North Carolina Evidence-based Practice Center under contract no. 290-2007-10056-I.) AHRQ publication no. 10-E-002, Rockville, MD, February 2010, Agency for Healthcare Research and Quality.

SKIN CANCER

Clinical Profile

- Skin cancer is the most common form of cancer in the United States
- Prevalence increases with age (most skin cancer appears after age 50)
- In 2006, 53,919 people were diagnosed with melanomas of the skin
  - 8441 deaths
- Most common types of skin cancer
  - Squamous cell carcinoma
  - Basal cell carcinoma
  - Melanoma

Risk Factors

- Ultraviolet (UV) radiation from the sun, sunlamps, tanning beds, or tanning booths; scars or burns on the skin; chronic skin inflammation or skin ulcers, personal history of skin cancer, family history of skin cancer, radiation therapy
- Conditions that make the skin sensitive to the sun, such as xeroderma pigmentosum, albinism, and basal cell nevus syndrome

Evaluation

- An annual full skin examination is recommended
- Involves a 2- to 3-minute visual inspection of the patient's entire body including the scalp, hands, and feet

- Characteristics of skin cancer lesions: asymmetry, mixed color, irregular borders, >6 mm size, rapid change in color or size, contains blood vessels

Management

- May involve surgery, chemotherapy, or radiation depending on extent

CORONARY HEART DISEASE (CHD)

Clinical Profile

- CHD causes heart attack and angina and is the single leading cause of death in America, with 425,425 deaths in the United States in 2006 (about one of every six deaths)
- More women than men die every year of CHD
- Incidence: 1,255,000 new and recurrent coronary attacks per year (34% are fatal)
- More than 330,000 women age 65 years or older died of heart disease in 2002
- Most CHD in women is preventable (Figure 46-1)
- Reduction in the death rate resulting from chronic diseases by just 2% over 1 decade would prevent 36 million deaths

Evaluation

- Medical family history
- Screen for symptoms of CHD
- Physical examination (blood pressure, body mass index [BMI], waist size)

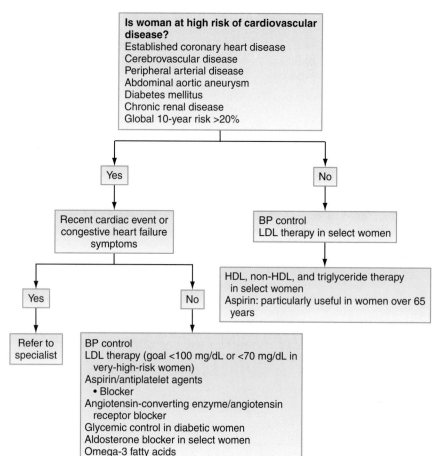

Figure 46-1. Algorithm for CVD preventive care in women. (Adapted from Mosca L, Banka CL, Benjamin EJ, et al: Evidence based guidelines for prevention of cardiovascular disease in women: update 2007, *Circulation* 115:1481-1501, 2007.)

- Laboratory tests: fasting lipoproteins (cholesterol, low-density lipoprotein [LDL], high-density lipoprotein [HDL]) and glucose

Management

- Implement lifestyle recommendations
  - Smoking cessation
  - Heart-healthy eating[*]
  - Regular physical activity: 30 minutes of moderate-intensity physical activity (e.g., brisk walking) on most, and preferably all, days of the week
  - Weight management: BMI between 18.5 and 24.9 kg/m^2 and a waist circumference <35 inches

FALLS

Clinical Profile

- Thirty-five percent to 40% of people over age 65 years old fall each year
- Approximately 16,000 seniors die each year as result of a fall
- About 1.85 million emergency visits occur annually for falls
- Twenty-five percent of women die within 1 year of sustaining hip fracture

Risk Factors

- Older age (especially ≥75 years)
- White race
- Housebound status
- Living alone
- Use of cane or walker
- Previous falls
- Acute illness
- Chronic conditions, especially neuromuscular disorders
- Medications, especially the use of four or more prescription drugs
- Cognitive impairment
- Reduced vision
- Difficulty rising from a chair
- Foot problems
- Neurologic changes

Evaluation

- Annual examination
  - Screen for history of falls
  - Review medication
  - Limb length discrepancy, foot problems
  - Vision and hearing tests
  - Neurologic exam
    - Focus on gait and balance: observe transition from sitting to standing

---

[*]Women should consume a diet rich in fruits and vegetables; choose whole-grain, high-fiber foods; consume fish, especially oily fish, at least twice a week; limit intake of saturated fat to <10% of energy, and if possible to <7%, cholesterol to <300 mg/d, alcohol intake to no more than 1 drink per day, and sodium intake to <2.3 g/d (approximately 1 tsp salt). Consumption of trans-fatty acids should be as low as possible.

Management

- Reduce risk of falls
- Home visit or review to remove tripping hazards (remove throw rugs, use nonskid mats in bathtub/showers, add handrails in bathroom and stairs, keep rooms well lit)
- Modify medications: particularly benzodiazepines and other sedating medications
- Provide balance training
- Involve the family
- Provide follow-up

Perioperative Care of the Elder Woman

- Many age-specific issues have been raised regarding the surgical management of gynecologic conditions in the elderly
- Physiologic changes that occur with age result in a global reduction in most organ functions and reserves
- "Older persons tolerate operations well, but complications poorly" (Chiang et al, 2007, page 813)
- Comprehensive perioperative assessment is critical to avoid complications
- Ensuring effective individualized communication is the key to creating optimal patient-physician interaction
- Minimum assessment should include the following:
  - Cardiovascular
  - Improved outcomes associated with perioperative beta-blockade in patients at high or intermediate risk
  - Preoperative use of statins in patients with known coronary artery disease (CAD)
  - Aspirin use potentially useful in high-risk patients
  - Respiratory
  - Identification of risk factors such as smoking, body habitus, chronic lung disease
  - Thromboembolic/pulmonary embolus prophylaxis with low-molecular-weight heparin
  - Renal
  - Function reduced related to decreases in renal and glomerular blood flow
  - Dosage adjustment often required for many medications
  - Close management of intravenous fluids because of the reduced ability to maintain sodium and hydration equilibrium

UPDATE #9

The use of perioperative beta-blockade (POBB) to reduce morbidity and death had been previously widely advocated. This general recommendation has been tempered based on recent large clinical trials in patients undergoing noncardiac surgery that demonstrated more potential risk for stroke and slightly higher mortality in the beta-blockade patients; now a more cautious and selective approach is recommended (American College of Cardiology Foundation et al, 2009). Based on the 2009 American College of Cardiology Foundation/American Heart Association guidelines, only patients currently on beta-blockers or those with risk factors such as coexisting coronary disease or ischemia will benefit from POBB (American College of Cardiology Foundation et al, 2009).

Cognitive State

- Early assessment in course of care vital
- Postoperative cognitive dysfunction is common in elderly patients and is a risk factor for postoperative delirium, falls, and mortality
- Screening can be completed with simple office testing: three-word recall, clock drawing test, or a combination of both (Mini-Cog)
- If cognitive impairment confirmed, identification of family member or person with medical power of attorney is needed
- Impairment may be subtle but may still interfere with ability to understand counseling and adhere to potentially important preoperative instructions
- General principles for preoperative preparation for postoperative setting
  - Involvement of family or patient advocate for all discussions
  - Recognizing medical literacy in elderly is generally low, repetition and using language that is simple but not patronizing
  - Use of printed materials to allow for future reference and review
  - Close communication with primary provider to partner consolidate treatment plan

SUGGESTED READINGS

Menopause Physiology/Hot Flashes

Andrikoula M, Prelevic G: Menopausal hot flushes revisited, *Climacteric* 12(1):3–15, 2009.

Bachmann GA, Schaefers M, Uddin A, Utian WH: Lowest effective transdermal 17 beta-estradiol dose for relief of hot flushes in postmenopausal women: a randomized controlled trial, *Obstet Gynecol* 110(4):771–779, 2007.

Chiuve SE, Martin LA, Campos H, Sacks FM: Effect of the combination of methyltestosterone and esterified estrogens compared with esterified estrogens alone on apolipoprotein CIII and other apolipoproteins in very low density, low density, and high density lipoproteins in surgically postmenopausal women, *J Clin Endocrinol Metab* 89(5):2207–2213, 2004.

Farquhar C, Marjoribanks J, Lethaby A, et al: Long term hormone therapy for perimenopausal and postmenopausal women, *Cochrane Database Syst Rev* (2):CD004143, 2009.

Grady D: Clinical practice: management of menopausal symptoms, *N Engl J Med* 55(22):2338–2347, 2006.

Nelson HD, Vesco KK, Haney E, Fu R: Nonhormonal therapies for menopausal hot flashes: systematic review and meta-analysis, *JAMA* 295(17):2057–2071, 2006.

Rossmanith WG, Ruebberdt W: What causes hot flushes? The neuroendocrine origin of vasomotor symptoms in the menopause, *Gynecol Endocrinol* 25(5):303–314, 2009.

Weisberg E, Ayton R, Darling G, et al: Endometrial and vaginal effects of low-dose estradiol delivered by vaginal ring or vaginal tablet, *Climacteric* 8(1):83–92, 2005.

Vulvar Disease

Olsson A, Selva-Nayagam P, Oehler MK: Postmenopausal vulval disease, *Meno Int* 12(4):169–172, 2008.

Renaud-Vilmer C, Cavelier-Balloy B, Porcher R, et al: Vulvar lichen sclerosus: effect of long-term topical application of a potent steroid on the course of the disease, *Arch Dermatol* 140(6):709–712, 2004.

Bladder/Anorectum

Bradley CS, Zimmerman MB, Qi Y, Nygaard IE: Natural history of pelvic organ prolapse in postmenopausal women, *Obstet Gynecol* 109(4):848–854, 2007.

Bugio KL, Locher JL, Goode PS: Combined behavioral and drug therapy for urge incontinence in older women, *J Am Geriatr Soc* 48(4):370–374, 2000.

Chan MK, Tjandra JJ: Sacral nerve stimulation for fecal incontinence: external anal sphincter defect vs intact anal sphincter, *Dis Colon Rectum* 51(7):1051–1055, 2008.

Goode PS, Burgio KL, Locher JL, et al: Effect of behavioral training with or without pelvic floor electrical stimulation on stress incontinence in women: a randomized controlled trial, *JAMA* 290(3):345–352, 2003.

Lutters M, Vogt-Ferrier NB: Antibiotic duration for treating uncomplicated, symptomatic lower urinary tract infections in elderly women, *Cochrane Database Syst Rev* (3):CD002111, 2008.

Norton C, Whitehead WE, Bliss DZ, et al: Management of fecal incontinence in adults, *Neurourol Urodyn* 29(1):199–206, 2010.

Norton CC, Cody JD, Hosker G: Biofeedback and/or sphincter exercises for the treatment of faecal incontinence in adults, *Cochrane Database Syst Rev* 3:CD002111, 2006.

Nygaard I, Barber MD, Burgio KL: Pelvic Floor Disorders Network: Prevalence of symptomatic pelvic floor disorders in US women, *JAMA* 300(11):1311–1316, 2008.

Pastore LM, Knightlinger RS, Hullfish K: Vaginal symptoms and urinary incontinence in elderly women, *Geriatr* 62(7):12–18, 2007.

Stav K, Dywery PL, Rosamilia A, et al: Midurethral sling procedures for stress urinary incontinence in women over 80 years, *Neurourol Urodyn* 29(7):1262–1268, 2010.

Cancer

Calonge N, Petitti DB, DeWitt TG: Screening for breast cancer: U.S. Preventive Services Task Force recommendation statement, *Ann Intern Med* 151(10):716–726, 2009.

Hay-Smith J. Mørkved S, Fairbrother KA, Herbison GP: Pelvic floor muscle training for prevention and treatment of urinary and faecal incontinence in antenatal and postnatal women, *Cochrane Database Syst Rev*. 2008 Oct 8;(4):CD007471. Review. PMID: 18843750.

Smith RA, Cokkinides V, Harmon JE: Cancer screening in the United States, 2007: a review of current guidelines, practices, and prospects, *CA Cancer J Clin* 57(2):90–104, 2007.

Cardiovascular Disease

Mosca L, Banka CL, Benjamin EJ, et al: Evidence based guidelines for cardiovascular disease prevention in women: 2007 update, *Circulation* 115(11):1481–1501, 2007.

Falls

Wenger NS, Roth CP, Shekelle PG, et al: A practice-based intervention to improve primary care for falls, urinary incontinence, and dementia, *J Am Geriatr Soc* 57(3):547–555, 2009.

Wolff T, Tai E, Miller T: Screening for skin cancer: an update of the evidence for the U.S. Preventive Services Task Force, *Ann Intern Med* 150(3):194–198, 2009.

Surgery in Postmenopausal Women

American College of Cardiology Foundation/American Heart Association Task Force on Practice Guidelines, Fleishmann, et al: 2009 ACCF/AHA focused update on perioperative beta blockade, *J Am Coll Cardiol* 54(22):2102–2128, 2009.

Chiang S, Gerten KA, Miller KL: Optimizing outcomes of surgery in advanced age: perioperative factors to consider, *Clin Obstet Gynecol* 50(3):813–825, 2007.

Devereaux PJ, Yang H, POISE Study Group, et al: POISE Study Group Effects of extended-release metoprolol succinate in patients undergoing noncardia surgery (POISE trial): a randomized trial, *Lancet* 371(9627):1839–1847, 2008.

Taylor S, Kirton OC, Staff I, Kozol RA: Postoperative day one: a high risk period for respiratory events, *Am J Surg* 190(5):752–756, 2005.

Chapter 47

Hormone Therapy

KATHLEEN BRENNAN • GAUTAM CHAUDHURI • LAUREN NATHAN

KEY UPDATES

1. Hormone therapy (HT) is associated with significantly greater increases in atheroprotective plasma high-density lipoprotein (HDL) in nondiabetic women compared to diabetic women.

2. Adding methyltestosterone to esterified estrogens in surgically postmenopausal patients may decrease triglycerides by reducing levels of apolipoprotein CIII.

3. The current recommendation from both American and European menopausal societies is to use the lowest possible dose of HT for the shortest amount of time such that symptoms are controlled yet the possible associated risks are minimized.

4. The effect of HT on nitric oxide production in vascular endothelial cells is an important component of the potential cardiovascular protection of HT and may be affected by disease states and the estrogen component of the HT.

5. A recent investigation of breast cancer risk with menopausal HT in a multicenter prospective cohort in Europe found an increased risk of breast cancer among current users of estrogen alone and a higher risk among current users of combined HT, with the highest risk found among those using a continuous combined regimen of HT.

6. In contrast to breast cancer risk, endometrial cancer risk is reduced with continuous compared to sequential HT regimens.

7. A recent study found that postmenopausal women not on estrogen with hypoactive sexual desire disorder had a higher frequency of satisfying sexual episodes with a 300-microgram testosterone patch compared to a placebo patch.

History

- Estrogen therapy (ET) was first given for treatment of menopausal vasomotor symptoms in the 1960s
- Use declined in mid-1970s when a link was made between unopposed estrogen and endometrial cancer
- Use increased in 1980s when the addition of progesterone to ET was determined to confer endometrial protection and ET was noted to be beneficial in preventing osteoporosis
- Observational studies then found users of hormone therapy (HT) to have a reduced risk of heart disease
- In 2002, HT use declined dramatically after the Women's Health Initiative trial of estrogen plus progestin (EPT) versus placebo was stopped early because of increased risk of breast cancer and cardiovascular events noted in treated patients
- The ET arm was stopped in 2004 as the risk of stroke was similar to the EPT arm and no difference in coronary heart disease was noted

Health Issues in Menopausal Women

- Vasomotor symptoms
- Urogenital atrophy
- Cardiovascular disease
- Osteoporosis
- Cancer
- Cognition and mood

Types of Hormone Therapy during Menopause

- Estrogen-only therapy
  - Should be used only in the absence of a uterus
- Estrogen progestin therapy
  - For use in women with a uterus
  - Progestins counteract the estrogenic hyperplastic effect on the endometrium
  - For women with premature ovarian insufficiency (POI), estrogen progestin therapy should be continued until age 51, the average age of menopause

- The combination HT may be in the form of combination hormonal contraceptives including oral contraceptives, the birth control patch, or vaginal ring
  - Spontaneous ovulation may occur in POI
    - Combination hormonal contraception may not prevent spontaneous ovulation and thus may not prevent pregnancy caused by excessively high follicle-stimulating hormone (FSH) levels in these women
- Local therapy
  - Vaginal ET
    - Does not result in clinically significant systemic absorption

Routes of Administration

- For vasomotor symptoms
  - Can be administered orally and nonorally
  - Different routes of administration will have differing metabolic effects
  - Oral HT produces a hepatic first-pass effect not seen with nonoral HT
    - Benefits of first-pass effects with oral HT
      - Reduction in low-density lipoprotein (LDL) cholesterol, lipoprotein(a), and insulin resistance
      - Larger increases in HDL cholesterol

UPDATE #1

A recent study investigated the effect of HT on lipoprotein profile and coronary disease progression in postmenopausal women with and without diabetes (Lamon-Fava et al, 2010). HT significantly increased the atheroprotective levels of HDL in nondiabetic women compared to diabetic women, and the coronary heart disease progressed significantly more in the diabetic women, indicating that an interaction between HT and diabetes seems to blunt the atheroprotective effect of HT-induced increases in HDL in diabetic women (Lamon-Fava et al, 2010).

- Unwanted effects of first pass effects with oral HT
  - Elevation in triglycerides
  - Activation of coagulation factors

UPDATE #2

In a randomized, double-blind trial, surgically menopausal women who were given 2.5 mg of oral methyltestosterone in addition to 1.25 mg of esterified estrogens were found to have lower triglycerides compared to women on estrogen only. The concentrations of apolipoprotein CIII, a known predictor of cardiovascular disease, were also found to be lower in the testosterone plus estrogen group. The decrease in triglycerides may be mediated through the reduced apolipoprotein CIII levels (Chiuve et al, 2004).

- Cardiovascular effects of oral and transdermal HT appear to be fairly similar
- Oral HT may be preferred in women with evidence of insulin resistance
- Transdermal HT
  - Preferred in women with coagulation disturbances

Current Indications for HT Approved by the Food and Drug Administration

- Treatment of vasomotor symptoms
- Prevention of postmenopausal osteoporosis
- Treatment of moderate to severe symptoms of vulvar and vaginal atrophy

HT for Vasomotor Symptoms

- Lowest possible dose for the shortest duration to control vasomotor symptoms

UPDATE #3

The current recommendation from both American and European menopausal societies is to use the lowest possible dose of HT for the shortest amount of time such that symptoms are controlled but the possible associated risks are minimized (Gompel et al, 2007; North American Menopause Society, 2010; Shifren et al, 2010). A recent randomized, double-blind, placebo-controlled study compared low-dose (0.023 mg/day 17β-estradiol and 0.0075 mg/day levonorgestrel), microdose (0.014 mg/day 17β-estradiol), and placebo for 12 weeks and found the frequency and severity of hot flashes decreased significantly in the microdose compared to placebo (Bachmann et al, 2007). Although a greater effect was seen in the low-dose group compared to microdose and placebo groups, 41% of microdose users had a 75% reduction in the frequency of hot flashes from baseline, and 35% had a 90% reduction in hot flashes from baseline (Bachmann et al, 2007). Given the proportion of women who responded to the microdose, this study supports the concept of starting HT at a microdose and titrating to the lowest effective dose. Another study compared oral ultra-low-dose continuous combined HT with 0.5-mg 17β-estradiol and 2.5-mg dydrogesterone to 1 mg 17β-estradiol and 5-mg dydrogesterone and placebo (Stevenson et al, 2010). The ultra-low-dose group had greater reductions in moderate to severe hot flashes than placebo, comparable to the effect of the higher-dose HT (Stevenson et al, 2010). Therefore, this study also lends support to the concept of lowest effective dose for HT. Furthermore, the concept seems to hold true for the treatment of menopausal symptoms other than hot flashes. A randomized controlled trial compared 10 and 25-mcg vaginal tablets of estradiol to placebo (Bachmann et al, 2008). Both doses of tablets improved vaginal symptoms of dryness, soreness, and irritation, dyspareunia, and discharge, as well as improved urogenital atrophy and increased the maturation index of the vaginal and urethral epithelium (Bachmann et al, 2008). Although the higher dose had a greater effect than the lower dose, both doses effectively treated atrophic vaginitis, again lending support to the concept of the lowest effective dose for HT. Similarly, another group studied the efficacy of 10-microgram vaginal tablets of estradiol compared to placebo in the treatment of vaginal atrophy and found that the ultra-low-dose estradiol improved vaginal cytology and pH and symptoms (Simon et al, 2008).

- Combined HT should be used in women with a uterus and estrogen-only HT in women without a uterus
  - Possible exceptions for combined HT in women without a uterus
    - History of endometrial cancer and no recurrence for 5 years
    - Endometrioid ovarian carcinoma
    - Malignancy arising from endometriosis

Effects of HT on Coronary Heart Disease (CHD)

- Most observational studies indicate HT reduces risk of CHD
- Randomized clinical trials (RCTs) do not support this
- Differences in results of observational studies and RCTs may in part be related to the timing of initiation of HT in relation to age and proximity to menopause

Observational Studies

- Most initiated HT around the age of menopause
- Up to 50% reduced risk of CHD in HT users
  - Protective effect of estrogen on coronary artery occlusion
  - Improved survival in women on HT at time of myocardial infarction (MI)
  - Less coronary artery calcium detected in women on HT compared to nonusers on electron beam tomography
    - Greater effect with longer duration of use
- Possible decreased risk of peripheral artery disease in HT users
- The findings of the observational studies have been questioned, arguing that HT may be a marker of a healthier lifestyle, and thus the studies were confounded by variables such as better diet demonstrating a "healthy user" effect
  - This theory has been disproved by epidemiologic studies indicating women using HT had the same health risk factors as women not using HT

Clinical Trials

- Women's Health Initiative (WHI)
  - RCT that enrolled about 27,000 postmenopausal women across the United States between the ages of 50 and 79, with the average age of 63 years
  - Combined HT arm
    - Approximately 16,000 postmenopausal women enrolled
    - Goal of study was to determine if combined HT prevented heart disease
    - Also looked at CHD, breast cancer, stroke, colorectal cancer, and hip fracture
  - Estrogen-only arm
    - Enrolled approximately 11,000 women without a uterus to study estrogen-only HT compared to placebo
- Findings
  - Estrogen-only arm
    - Reduction in CHD risk when therapy was initiated in younger and more recently postmenopausal women
    - Statistically significant reduction in the composite end points of myocardial infarction, coronary artery revascularization, and coronary arterial disease in women aged 50 to 59 who were randomized to ET
    - Younger women (<60 years) after an average of 7 years of treatment had lower levels of coronary artery calcium than those randomized to placebo
  - Combined data from both ET and EPT trials of WHI show that women who initiate HT within 10 years of menopause tend to have a lower risk of CHD
    - Healthy endothelium likely needed for beneficial steroid effects to occur

- HT is associated with an increase in CHD risk among women who are more distant from menopause at the time of HT initiation
  - In a subgroup analysis, only women 20 or more years from menopause had increased CHD risk
    - Excluding this older group, HT and placebo had the same prevalence of CHD.
- Estrogen-only HT appeared to be associated with a lower risk of CHD than combined HT
  - Many other studies have not found progestins to be detrimental in regard to cardiovascular risk

UPDATE #4

27-Hydroxycholesterol is a cholesterol metabolite that is elevated in individuals with hypercholesterolemia and is found in atherosclerotic plaques. In a mouse model, 27-hydroxycholesterol inhibited the estrogen-mediated production of nitric oxide from the vasculature, thereby decreasing the usual vasodilatory effect of estrogen (Umetani et al, 2007). 27-hydroxycholesterol, through its effects on the estrogen receptor, may be one mechanism by which the cardioprotective effect of estrogen is lost in patients with known cardiovascular disease. Interestingly, a recent study found that in human aortic endothelial cells, equine estrogens impair nitric oxide production, whereas natural 17β-estradiol enhances nitric oxide production, thereby providing a possible explanation to the differences found between various HT regimens and their effect on cardiovascular disease (Novensa et al, 2010).

HT and Stroke

- In both an observational (Nurses' Health Study) and an RCT (WHI), an increased incidence of ischemic stroke was found in HT users
  - No effect on risk of hemorrhagic stroke found in either study
- The Heart and Estrogen-Progestin Replacement Study (HERS) found no difference in stroke risk in women with preexisting coronary disease randomized to combined HT compared to placebo
- HT does not reduce the risk of recurrent stroke among women with established cardiovascular disease (CVD), particularly in women initiating HT after age 60

Venous Thromboembolism (VTE)

- Increased risk of VTE with oral HT
  - Most studies indicate a twofold increased risk
    - Supported by the combined HT arm of the WHI and to a lesser extent the estrogen-only arm (relative risk [RR] 1.47)
- Lower in women who initiate HT prior to age 60 compared to women who initiate HT at an older age
- Increased risk in women with a history of a prior VTE and women with thrombophilias
- Risk is reduced with statin and aspirin therapy
- Overall risk is low
  - Risk increased by approximately two cases per 10,000 women per year of HT use
    - Transdermal estrogen does not seem to have the same risk of VTE as oral therapy because of the lack of the first-pass effect through the liver

Breast Cancer

- Most common cancer in women
- Observational studies are conflicting regarding risk of breast cancer with HT use
  - Overall, there seems to be a slight increase in breast cancer risk with combined HT compared to estrogen-only HT
  - A meta-analysis published in 1997 found the following
    - RR 1.14 of breast cancer in ever users of HT
    - Increased risk with increased duration of use
    - No increased risk for past users
- WHI and breast cancer
  - Relative risk of invasive breast cancer in the combined HT arm was 1.24 in the updated WHI report
  - Women in the estrogen-only arm showed no increased in risk of breast cancer after an average of 7.1 years of use
  - No increase in in situ breast cancer was found
  - No differences in the histologic types of breast cancer in HT users compared to nonusers
    - Case-control studies have indicated an increased risk of invasive lobular tumors
- Family history of breast cancer is not a contraindication to HT
- Women who get breast cancer while using HT have a reduced risk of breast cancer death

UPDATE #5

An analysis of breast cancer risk among menopausal HT users in the European Prospective Investigation into Cancer and Nutrition (EPIC) cohort found that compared with menopausal HT never users, women on HT had an increased risk of breast cancer (Bakken et al, 2011). Specifically, current users of estrogen-only HT had a relative risk (RR) of 1.42 (95% confidence interval [CI] 1.23 to 1.64) compared to never users (Bakken et al, 2010). An even higher risk was noted in current users of combined HT with a RR of 1.77 (95% CI 1.4 to 2.24) compared to nonusers and a statistically significantly increased risk compared to estrogen-only users (Bakken et al, 2011). The greatest risk was seen in users of continuous combined HT regimens with a 43% increased risk of breast cancer compared to sequential regimens (Bakken et al, 2011). No significant differences were found in breast cancer risk based on the various progesterone components or the estrogen components in the sequential regimens (Bakken et al, 2011). The Women's Health Initiative (WHI) trial and observational studies have found an increased risk of breast cancer in combined HT users after approximately 5 years of use, but not in short-term or past users (Rossouw et al, 2002; Shifren et al, 2010). Interestingly, the WHI found no increased risk of breast cancer in estrogen-only users, and observational studies have found a reduced risk in users of estrogen-only compared to combined HT users, but still an associated risk compared to nonusers (Rossouw et al, 2002; Shifren et al, 2010).

- In contrast to CHD, women starting HT shortly after menopause seem to have an increased risk of breast cancer compared to those who initiated HT 5 or more years after menopause
- HT should not be prescribed to women with a history of breast cancer

Endometrial Cancer

- Most common gynecologic malignancy in American women
- Increased incidence of endometrial cancer with estrogen-only HT in women with a uterus
  - Fivefold increased risk of endometrial cancer after 5 years of 0.625 mg/day of conjugated estrogens or equivalent, and 10-fold increased risk after 10 years of use
  - Adding at least 13 days of progestin negates this effect
- HT is generally contraindicated in women with a history of endometrial cancer
  - However, data indicate that HT can be considered for very symptomatic women with early-stage endometrial cancer

UPDATE #6

A recent study found that postmenopausal Finnish women who used continuous combined HT for 3 or more years had a 76% reduced risk of endometrioid adenocarcinoma of the endometrium compared to the general population, whereas women using sequential estradiol-progestin therapy for at least 5 years had an increased risk of endometrial cancer: 69% increased risk if the progestin was added monthly and a 276% increased risk if the progestin was added every 3 months (Jaakkola et al, 2009).

Ovarian Cancer

- Fifth leading cause of cancer death in American women
- Studies are conflicting regarding the risk of ovarian cancer with HT use
  - A large prospective cohort study observed a small increased risk of ovarian cancer with HT
  - The WHI showed a nonsignificant trend toward an increased risk of ovarian cancer with combined HT; small numbers limited the statistical power
- HT does not seem to affect survival negatively in women with a history of ovarian cancer

Colorectal Cancer

- Third leading cause of cancer death in women
- Prevented by the removal of premalignant adenomas
- WHI and colorectal cancer
  - Estrogen-only therapy had no effect on colorectal cancer risk
  - Women randomized to the combined HT had a reduced risk of colorectal cancer
- Putative mechanisms for effect of HT on colorectal cancer
  - Antiproliferative activity resulting from estrogen receptor beta (ER-β) activation
  - Decrease in bile acids

Cognitive Function

- Episode memory is not substantially impacted by natural menopause
- Small observational studies have found a decreased risk of Alzheimer's disease with HT use
- The WHI Memory Study (WHIMS)

- Found an increased risk for dementia from any cause in women 65 years and older with HT use
- HT use did not prevent mild cognitive impairment but rather increased the risk of cognitive decline

Depression and Mood

- Depression affects twice the number of women as men
- Menopause does not cause depression, but clinical and subclinical depression is more common in estrogen-deficient states
- Estrogen seems to improve mood
  - May be due to beneficial effects on sleep caused by decreased vasomotor symptoms
- HT should not be used to treat psychiatric illnesses
  - Antidepressants, psychotherapy, and counseling are effective treatment modalities

Urogenital Atrophy

- Caused by estrogen deficiency
- Results in urinary symptoms such as dysuria, urinary urgency, and frequency
- Symptoms of vaginal atrophy include vaginal dryness, pruritus, bleeding, and dyspareunia
  - In premenopausal women, exfoliated vaginal squamous epithelial cells die and release glycogen, which is hydrolyzed to glucose and subsequently broken down by lactobacillus into lactic acid
  - In postmenopausal women, this exfoliation does not occur, resulting in a rise in vaginal pH and a loss of lactobacilli, with a subsequent overgrowth of other bacteria including group B streptococcus, staphylococci, and diphtheroids, which can cause symptomatic vaginal inflammation
- Treatment by local application of estrogen does lead to some systemic absorption , but generally not clinically significant
- Lower doses of vaginal estrogen have been shown to be effective in reducing symptoms of vaginal atrophy
- Whether breast cancer survivors with vulvovaginal atrophy can be safely treated with vaginal estrogens remains controversial

Testosterone Therapy and Sexual Function

- Numerous studies indicate that testosterone administered intramuscularly, orally, or transdermally to menopausal women can lead to significant improvements in libido, sexual desire and arousal, increase in frequency of sexual fantasies, and sexual pleasure compared to placebo
- Long-term safety has not been established

UPDATE #7

A recent study randomized postmenopausal women not on estrogen with hypoactive sexual desire disorder to receive either a 300-microgram or 150-microgram testosterone patch or a placebo patch. It found that the higher dose patch improved the frequency of satisfying sexual episodes compared to placebo

and that both doses were associated with increased desire (Davis et al, 2008). The higher dose was associated with more unwanted hair growth compared to placebo (Davis et al, 2008). The effect of testosterone on other health outcomes, including breast cancer risk, is still unknown.

DHEA Therapy and Menopause

- There is little convincing evidence to support the use of oral dehydroepiandrosterone (DHEA) therapy in healthy aging postmenopausal women to improve conditions synonymous with normal aging
- Vaginal DHEA may improve vaginal atrophy with concomitant improvements in sexual function in estrogen-deficient menopausal women

Bioidentical Hormones

- Generally refers to chemicals derived from plants that are modified to be structurally identical to "natural" endogenous hormones made by the ovary, specifically estradiol and progesterone
- Many bioidentical products are government approved, including oral and transdermal estradiol and oral micronized progesterone.
- No benefit and possible increased risk of custom compounded HT as purity, bioavailability, and safety are untested

Nonhormonal Therapies for Vasomotor Symptoms

- Selective serotonin reuptake inhibitors (SSRIs)
  - Overall, results are mixed with respect to efficacy in reducing the frequency and severity of vasomotor symptoms
  - Fluoxetine and paroxetine can be used as possible alternatives for hot flashes
  - SSRIs may affect the metabolism of tamoxifen to its active form through CYP2D6 of the cytochrome P450 system
    - This effect varies by the potency of the drug
    - Must use caution when using SSRIs, particularly paroxetine, in women receiving tamoxifen
- Serotonin-norepinephrine reuptake inhibitors (SNRIs)
  - Venlafaxine
    - Both 37.5-mg and 75-mg doses reduce frequency and severity of vasomotor symptoms
    - Can be used in breast cancer survivors with tamoxifen-induced vasomotor symptoms
  - Desvenlafaxine succinate
    - Active metabolite of venlafaxine
    - Best results seen with 100-mg dose
      - Sixty-four percent to 75% reduction in the number of hot flashes from baseline
    - Side effects include nausea, dizziness, and headaches
- Anticonvulsants
  - Gabapentin
    - Associated with a 50% median reduction in hot flash frequency

- Side effects include somnolence, disorientation, and headache
- Effective dose: 900 to 2700 mg/day
- Alpha$_2$ adrenergic receptor agonists
  - Modest efficacy with clonidine
  - Dose: 0.5 mg to 1.5 mg
  - Side effects include dry mouth and dizziness

Black Cohosh

- Some studies show it may be effective, but results are inconsistent
- May act as a selective estrogen receptor modifier
  - May exert an agonistic effect on serotonin receptors

SUGGESTED READINGS

Hormone Therapy and Cholesterol

Chiuve SE, Martine L, Campos H, et al: Effect of the combination of methyltestosterone and esterified estrogens compared with esterified estrogens alone on apolipoprotein CIII and other apolipoproteins in very low density, low density, and high density lipoproteins in surgically postmenopausal women, *J Clin Endocrinol Metab* 89(5):2207–2213, 2004.

Hormone Therapy and Diabetes

Lamon-Fava S, Herrington DM, Horvath KV, et al: Effect of hormone replacement therapy on plasma lipoprotein levels and coronary atherosclerosis progression in postmenopausal women according to type 2 diabetes mellitus status, *Metabolism* 59(12):1794–1800, 2010.

Hormone Replacement Therapy

Gompel A, Barlow D, Rozenberg S, et al: The EMAS 2006/2007 update on clinical recommendations on postmenopausal hormone therapy, *Maturitas* 56(2):227–229, 2007.

North American Menopause Society: Estrogen and progestogen use in postmenopausal women: 2010 position statement of the North American Menopause Society, *Menopause* 17(2):242–255, 2010.

Rossouw JE, Anderson GL, Prentice RL, et al: Risks and benefits of estrogen plus progestin in healthy postmenopausal women: principal results from the Women's Health Initiative randomized controlled trial, *JAMA* 297(3):1465–1477, 2002.

Shifren JL, Schiff I: Role of hormone therapy in the management of menopause, *Obstet Gynecol* 115(4):839–855, 2010.

Lowest Effective Dose Hormone Therapy

Bachman G, Lobo RA, Gut R, et al: Efficacy of low-dose estradiol vaginal tablets in the treatment of atrophic vaginitis, *Obstet Gynecol* 111(1):67–76, 2008.

Bachman GA, Schaefers M, Uddin A, et al: Lowest effective transdermal 17β-estradiol dose for relief of hot flushes in postmenopausal women, *Obstet Gynecol* 110(4):771–779, 2007.

Simon J, Nactigall L, Gut R, et al: Effective treatment of vaginal atrophy with an ultra-low-dose estradiol vaginal tablet, *Obstet Gynecol* 112(5):1053–1060, 2008.

Stevenson JC, Durand G, Kahler E, et al: Oral ultra-low dose continuous combined hormone replacement therapy with 0.5 mg 17β-oestradiol and 2.5 mg dydrogesterone for the treatment of vasomotor symptoms: results from a double-blind, controlled study, *Maturitas* 67(3):227–232, 2010.

Hormone Therapy and Cardiovascular Disease

American College of Obstetricians and Gynecologists Committee on Gynecologic Practice: ACOG committee opinion no. 420, November 2008: hormone therapy and heart disease, *Obstet Gynecol* 112(5):1189–1192, 2008.

Novensa L, Selent J, Pastor M, et al: Equine estrogens impair nitric oxide production and endothelial nitric oxide synthase transcription in human endothelial cells compared with the natural 17β-estradiol, *Hypertension* 56(3):405–411, 2010.

Toh S, Hernandez-Dias S, Logan R, et al: Coronary heart disease in postmenopausal recipients of estrogen plus progestin therapy: does the increased risk ever disappear? *Ann Intern Med* 152(4):211–217, 2010.

Umetani M, Domoto H, Gormley AK, et al: 27-Hydroxycholesterol is an endogenous SERM that inhibits the cardiovascular effects of estrogen, *Nat Med* 13(10):1185–1192, 2007.

Hormone Therapy and Breast Cancer Risk

Bakken K, Fournier A, Lund E, et al: Menopausal hormone therapy and breast cancer risk: impact of different treatments. The European Prospective Investigation into Cancer and Nutrition, *Int J Cancer* 128(1):144–156, 2011.

Hormone Therapy and Endometrial Cancer

Jaakola S, Lyytinen H, Pukkala E, et al: Endometrial cancer in postmenopausal women using estradiol-progestin therapy, *Obstet Gynecol* 114(6):1197–1204, 2009.

Testosterone Therapy

Davis SR, Moreau M, Kroll R, et al: Testosterone for low libido in postmenopausal women not taking estrogen, *N Engl J Med* 359(19):2005–2017, 2008.

Chapter 48

Osteoporosis and Falls

KATHLEEN BRENNAN • GAUTAM CHAUDHURI • LAUREN NATHAN

KEY UPDATES

1 As the population ages, the economic burden of osteoporosis- or osteopenia-related fractures will continue to increase, underscoring the importance of complying with screening guidelines.

2 Despite patients with type 2 diabetes mellitus having bone mineral densities similar to or greater than controls, their bones are more fragile for a given density and thus these patients are at greater risk for fracture.

3 The World Health Organization's FRAX algorithm uses clinical risk factors, bone mineral density, and country-specific fracture and mortality data to quantify a patient's 10-year risk of a hip or major osteoporotic fracture facilitating risk stratification for treatment (www.shef.ac.uk/FRAX/tool.jsp?locationValue=9).

4 Concern over a possible link between atypical fractures of the femur and long-term bisphosphonate use has not been supported by a study of a population-based registry nor a reanalysis of three randomized controlled trials of bisphosphonates, but additional research is needed to address this concern.

5 Bazedoxifene is a third-generation selective estrogen receptor modulator (SERM) currently under investigation for the prevention and treatment of postmenopausal osteoporosis that has demonstrated better selectivity of actions on estrogen receptors than the currently approved SERM, raloxifene.

6 Lasofoxifene, another SERM being investigated for treatment of osteoporosis, has been shown to decrease risk of both nonvertebral and vertebral fractures in contrast to raloxifene, which does not reduce risk of nonvertebral fractures.

7 In postmenopausal women, lower-dose hormone therapy (HT) seems to be as effective as standard dose HT in moderating bone turnover.

8 The North American Menopause Society 2010 Position Statement indicates extended use of HT for women with decreased bone mass is appropriate when other therapies are not tolerated or when the benefits of extended HT outweigh the risks.

9 Denosumab (Prolia), approved by the Food and Drug Administration (FDA) for the treatment of osteoporosis on June 1, 2010, is a humanized antibody to the osteoclastogenic receptor activator of nuclear factor-κβ ligand (RANKL); it was found to reduce the risk of vertebral, nonvertebral, and hip fractures in women with postmenopausal osteoporosis.

10 New treatment targets are being evaluated for the treatment and prevention of osteoporosis including glucagon-like peptide 2 (GLP-2), cathepsin K inhibitors, antibodies against sclerostin and Wnt pathway antagonists, as well as modulators of parathyroid hormone production.

Osteoporosis

- Skeletal disorder characterized by the following:
  - Low bone mass
  - Microarchitectural deterioration of bone tissue
  - Increased bone fragility
  - Increased fracture risk
- Defined by World Health Organization (WHO) based on bone mineral density measured by dual energy x-ray absorptiometry (DEXA) scan of the femoral neck (the reference standard), the total hip, or lumbar spine (Table 48-1)
- For postmenopausal women, diagnosis is based on a comparison to young women, ages 20 to 29 years (T score)
- For premenopausal women, low bone mineral density is diagnosed when the bone density is less than two standard deviations below the mean for a reference population matched for gender, age, and ethnicity (Z score <−2.0) without other risk factors for fracture

TABLE 48-1 **World Health Organization Definitions for Bone Mineral Density Measurements**

Diagnosis	Bone Mineral Density
Normal bone mass	Bone mineral density within one standard deviation below the mean for the young adult female reference (T score ≥–1)
Osteopenia	Bone mineral density between 2.5 and 1 standard deviations below the mean for the young adult female reference (–2.5 ≤ T score < –1)
Osteoporosis	Bone mineral density more than 2.5 standard deviations below the mean for the young adult female reference (T score < –2.5)
Severe osteoporosis	Bone mineral density more than 2.5 standard deviations below the mean for the young adult female reference (T score < –2.5) with the presence of one or more fragility fractures

From WHO Scientific Group on the Assessment of Osteoporosis at Primary Health Care Level, Summary Meeting Report; Brussels, Belgium, May 5-7, 2004.

- Fragility fractures are those fractures that occur with a fall from standing height or less or with no trauma

EPIDEMIOLOGY

- Affects more than 10 million individuals ≥50 years old in the United States alone
- Approximately 8 million women and 2 million men
- 33.6 million Americans have osteopenia
- At the time of menopause, a period of rapid bone loss ensues for 5 to 7 years
  - Vertebral bone density may decrease by 15% to 30% during this period
- Risk of osteoporosis increases with age: 19% of women 65 to 74 years of age affected, compared to >50% of women 85 years of age or older
- One of every two Caucasian women and one of every five Caucasian men will have an osteoporosis-related fracture in her or his lifetime
- In the United States, osteoporotic fractures result in the following:
  - 500,000 hospitalizations
  - 800,000 emergency room visits
  - 2.6 million physician visits
  - 180,000 nursing home placements
- Hip fractures are associated with a significant risk of morbidity and mortality
  - Twenty percent of patients with hip fracture will die within 1 year
  - Thirty percent of patients with hip fracture will have permanent disability

PATHOGENESIS

- Peak bone mass is achieved by age 18 to 25
  - Genetics account for 60% to 70% of differences in peak bone mass
  - Calcium intake, vitamin D levels, and physical activity may have small effect on peak bone mass but likely have greater effect on bone fragility later in life
- Bone loss and formation are mediated by osteoclast and osteoblast activity, respectively
  - Maintained at an equilibrium in young, healthy women
  - Increased estrogen in puberty may cause calcium reserve accumulation to prepare the body for pregnancy and lactation; this reserve is subsequently depleted with the loss of estrogen at menopause

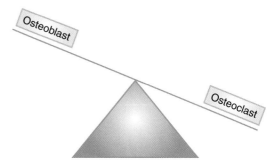

Figure 48-1. Osteoclast activity prevails in postmenopausal women.

- The mechanisms by which estrogen regulates bone remodeling are poorly understood
  - Interacts with the estrogen receptor in osteoclasts, but terminally affects osteoclastogenesis, osteoclast function, and osteoclast life span
  - Decreases the depth of erosion caused by the osteoclasts
  - May affect factors and cells in the bone marrow, especially T cells
- Osteoclast activity prevails in menopausal women (Figure 48-1)
  - Trabecular bone loss and increased cortical porosity
  - Shift to bone resorption may be secondary to rapid decrease in estrogen levels
    - No difference in any hormone levels between patients with osteoporosis and matched controls
  - Also relative decrease in bone formation
- Low bone mass may occur from low peak bone mass, excessive bone resorption, or decreased bone formation during bone remodeling
  - All three may contribute in varying degrees to the pathogenesis of osteoporosis depending on the individual patient

SCREENING

- Dual energy x-ray absorptiometry (DEXA) is the technical standard for measuring bone mineral density
  - Measures bone density at common sites of osteoporotic fracture
  - Relatively inexpensive
  - High precision and accuracy
  - Minimal radiation exposure
- Peripheral site DEXA measurements may not be as precise as central measurements with DEXA

- Can be used in lower-risk populations or when DEXA is not available
  - Less expensive
  - More portable
  - Low radiation exposure
  - Relatively precise
- Should not be used to diagnose osteoporosis or to monitor response to therapy
- Quantitative ultrasonography is increasingly being used to screen for osteoporosis
  - Assesses bone elasticity and structure peripherally (heel, tibia, patella)
    - Low cost
    - No ionizing radiation exposure
  - Should not be used to diagnose osteoporosis or to monitor response to therapy
    - Studies suggest that calcaneal ultrasound is able to predict risk of hip fracture
    - More comparative studies with central DEXA are needed
- Biochemical markers of bone turnover cannot diagnose osteoporosis or osteopenia
  - Markers of bone formation
    - Serum specific alkaline phosphatase
    - Serum osteocalcin
    - Serum procollagen 1 extension peptides
  - Markers of bone resorption
    - Urinary N-telopeptide
    - Serum C-telopeptide
    - Type 1 collagen cross-links
    - Urinary deoxypyridinoline
    - Urinary hydroxyproline
  - Cannot predict fracture risk
  - Cannot determine or predict bone density
  - Serum and urine markers can identify patients with high bone turnover
    - Could be used to monitor response to therapy
      - Can see changes in biochemical markers earlier than with bone density (weeks rather than years)
      - The value of using these markers in routine clinical practice has not been validated
    - Preferable to use serum rather than urine markers
      - Less assay variation
      - Lower likelihood for diurnal variation
- Screening guidelines
  - American College of Obstetricians and Gynecologists (ACOG)
    - Screen all women ≥65 years of age with bone mineral density testing
    - Consider screening postmenopausal women under the age of 65 with one or more risk factors for osteoporosis (see the Risk Factors for Osteoporotic Fracture in Postmenopausal Women section) with bone mineral density testing
    - Perform bone mineral density testing on all postmenopausal women with fractures to verify diagnosis and determine severity of osteoporosis
    - May screen premenopausal women that have certain diseases or medical conditions or take medications that place them at increased risk for osteoporosis (see the Risk Factors section)

- Repeat screening every 2 years in the absence of new risk factors
- Can initiate treatment without a bone mineral density test in older women with osteoporotic vertebral fracture
- U.S. Preventive Services Task Force (USPSTF)
  - Screen all women ≥65 years of age with DEXA
  - Screen women 60 to 64 years of age with increased fracture risk
  - USPSTF states that there is insufficient evidence to recommend for or against screening women under the age of 60
- National Osteoporosis Foundation
  - Screen all women ≥65 years of age
  - Screen all men ≥70 years of age
  - Screen all adults with a fracture
- North American Menopause Society
  - Screen all women ≥65 years of age
  - Screen all women with medical causes of bone loss
  - Screen younger postmenopausal women with one or more risk factors
- American Association of Clinical Endocrinologists
  - Screen all women ≥65 years of age
  - Screen all women ≥40 years of age who have a fracture unrelated to major trauma
  - Screen all peri- and postmenopausal women who have risk factors for fractures or bone loss

UPDATE #1

As our population ages, the economic burden of osteoporosis- or osteopenia-related fractures will continue to increase, underscoring the importance of complying with screening guidelines. A recent retrospective study of 809 women ≥65 years of age seen by practitioners of varying levels in different practice settings found that overall only 42.9% had evidence of bone mineral density testing (Davisson et al, 2009). In comparison to patients seen in family medicine, general internal medicine, and at the Veterans Administration, a higher proportion of patients seen in a gynecology clinic were screened (72%) (Davisson et al, 2009). Increasing age, number of medications, number of visits, and number of ICD-9 billing codes was inversely related to the proportion of women screened (Davisson et al, 2009). These findings indicate that we must be mindful of incorporating osteoporosis screening into our routine evaluation of any patient.

- Laboratory workup for secondary causes of osteoporosis
  - Serum chemistry, including calcium and phosphate
  - Twenty-four-hour urine calcium and creatinine
  - Parathyroid hormone levels
  - Thyroid-stimulating hormone
  - 25-Hydroxyvitamin D levels
  - Serum protein electrophoresis
    - Rule out multiple myeloma

RISK FACTORS

- Many lifestyle factors, diseases, genetic factors, and medications increase the risk of osteoporosis and fractures
  - Diet
    - Low calcium
    - High caffeine
    - High vitamin A
    - Low vitamin D
      - Also affected by sunlight exposure
    - High sodium

- Lifestyle factors
  - Lack of sunlight exposure
  - Immobilization
  - Low body mass index (BMI)
  - Smoking (active or passive)
  - Alcohol (three or more drinks per day)
  - Lack of physical activity
- Genetic factors
  - Cystic fibrosis
  - Ehlers-Danlos
  - Gaucher disease
  - Glycogen storage diseases
  - Hemochromatosis
  - Homocystinuria
  - Hypophosphatasia
  - Idiopathic hypercalciuria
  - Klinefelter's syndrome
  - Marfan syndrome
  - Menkes steely hair syndrome
  - Osteogenesis imperfect
  - Parental history of hip fracture
  - Porphyria
  - Riley-Day syndrome
  - Turner's syndrome
- Hypogonadal states (deficient sex steroids)
  - Androgen insensitivity
  - Anorexia nervosa and bulimia
  - Athletic amenorrhea
  - Hyperprolactinemia
  - Panhypopituitarism
  - Premature ovarian failure
- Endocrine disorders
  - Adrenal insufficiency
  - Cushing's syndrome
  - Diabetes mellitus
  - Hyperparathyroidism
  - Thyrotoxicosis

UPDATE #2

Lower bone mineral density has been noted in patients with type 1 diabetes. However, despite patients with type 2 diabetes mellitus having bone mineral densities similar to or greater than controls, their bones are more fragile for a given density and thus these patients are at greater risk for fracture (Isidro et al, 2010). Many factors may contribute to this apparent increase in fragility, including impact of insulin on bone metabolism, obesity, altered collagen formation, abnormal calcium absorption and excretion, dysregulation of vitamin D synthesis, inflammation, vascular and renal disease, and variations in growth factors (Isidro et al, 2010).

- Gastrointestinal disorders
  - Celiac disease
  - Gastric bypass
  - Inflammatory bowel disease
  - Malabsorption
  - Pancreatic disease
  - Primary biliary cirrhosis
- Hematologic disorders
  - Hemophilia
  - Leukemia
  - Lymphoma
  - Multiple myeloma

- Sickle cell disease
- Systemic mastocytosis
- Thalassemia
- Rheumatologic disorders
  - Ankylosing spondylitis
  - Lupus
  - Rheumatoid arthritis
- Other diseases or conditions
  - Alcoholism
  - Amyloidosis
  - Chronic metabolic acidosis
  - Congestive heart failure
  - Depression
  - Emphysema
  - End-stage renal disease
  - Epilepsy
  - Idiopathic scoliosis
  - Multiple sclerosis
  - Muscular dystrophy
  - Parenteral nutrition
  - Posttransplant bone disease
  - Prior fracture as an adult
  - Sarcoidosis
- Medications
  - Anticonvulsants
  - Antacids (aluminum)
  - Aromatase inhibitors
  - Barbiturates
  - Cancer chemotherapeutic drugs
    - Cyclosporine A
    - Tacrolimus
  - Depo-medroxyprogesterone
  - Glucocorticoids
    - Greater than or equal to 5 mg/day of prednisone or equivalent for more than 3 months
  - Heparin
- Risk factors for osteoporotic fracture in *postmenopausal* women specifically
  - History of prior fracture
  - Family history of osteoporosis
  - Caucasian race
  - Dementia
  - Poor nutrition
  - Smoking
  - Low weight and body mass index
  - Estrogen deficiency
    - Bilateral oophorectomy
    - Menopause before the age of 45
    - Premenopausal amenorrhea >1 year
  - Low calcium intake
  - Alcoholism
  - Impaired eyesight
  - History of falls
  - Inadequate physical activity

Falls

- The majority of osteoporosis-related fractures are the result of falls
  - Approximately 30% of people 60 years of age or older fall at least once a year, with an even higher incidence in those over the age of 80

- Must evaluate risk factors for falling
  - Strongest predictors of falls
    - Personal history of falling
    - Muscle weakness
    - Gait defects
    - Poor balance
    - Visual impairment
  - Other risk factors for falls
    - Environmental risk factors
      - No assistive devices in bathrooms
      - Loose rugs
      - Low-level lighting
      - Obstacles
      - Poor weather conditions (ice, rain, snow)
    - Medical conditions
      - Anxiety, agitation, depression
      - Arrhythmias
      - Dehydration
      - Diminished cognitive skills
      - Fear of falling
      - Female gender
      - Kyphosis
      - Malnutrition
      - Orthostatic hypotension
      - Reduced proprioception
      - Sedation from medications
      - Urge urinary incontinence

PREVENTION AND TREATMENT

- The surgeon general recommends a stepwise approach to addressing and treating bone disease
  1. Lifestyle changes
     - Nutrition
     - Physical activity
     - Fall prevention
  2. Identify and treat secondary causes of osteoporosis if present
     - Drugs
     - Diseases
  3. Begin pharmacotherapy if needed
     - Antiresorptives
     - Anabolics
- Must first maximize peak bone mass
  - Peak bone mass likely occurs in third decade of life
    - Varies based on hormonal and genetic influences
      - 60% to 70% of variability is genetic
        - Caucasian and Asian ethnicity associated with low bone mineral density (BMD)
      - 30% to 40% of variability is due to environmental factors
        - Diet
        - Vitamin D health
        - Exercise
        - Diseases
          - Inflammatory bowel disease
          - Celiac disease
          - Cystic fibrosis
        - Medications
          - Glucocorticoids
          - Anticonvulsants
        - Body weight

- Physical activity
- Cigarette smoking
- Nonpharmacologic treatment
  - Nutrition
    - Healthy diet, especially adequate intake of calcium and vitamin D from infancy through adolescence, is important to attain peak bone mass
  - Calcium
    - Recommended daily intake of calcium may change based on recent data linking calcium supplementation (without co-administration of vitamin D) to an increased risk of myocardial infarction
      - This recent meta-analysis found an approximate 30% increased risk of myocardial infarction with calcium supplementation ≥500 mg/day
    - Current recommendations are as follows:
      - U.S. surgeon general
        - Premenopausal women (18 to 50 years): 1000 mg
        - Postmenopausal women (>51 years): 1200 mg
      - Institute of Medicine
        - Age 31 to 50 years: 1000 mg
        - Age 51 years and older: 1200 mg
      - National Institutes of Health
        - Premenopausal women 25 to 50 years of age: 1000 mg
        - Postmenopausal women <65 years old on estrogen therapy: 1000 mg
        - Postmenopausal women not using estrogen therapy: 1500 mg
        - All women over 65 years of age: 1500 mg
  - Vitamin D
    - Improves absorption of calcium through the intestine
    - Important for bone mineralization, muscle function, and balance
    - Low vitamin D → poor calcium absorption → low calcium levels → increased parathyroid hormone → bone loss
    - Recommended daily intake of vitamin D (dietary and supplemental)
      - U.S. surgeon general
        - Premenopausal women (18 to 50 years): 400 IU
        - Postmenopausal women (51 to 70 years): 400 IU
        - Elderly (>70): 600 IU
        - May need more if inadequate exposure to sunlight
    - Can measure concentration of 25-hydroxy vitamin D (25 OHD) to assess adequacy of supplementation in high-risk individuals
      - Great variability in assays
    - Supplementation recommended for most men and women
    - Obesity is associated with lower vitamin D levels
      - Vitamin D seems to bind to fat cells, lowering circulating vitamin D levels
  - Physical activity
    - High impact exercise confers a benefit on bone accumulation during growth

- Extreme exercise can be harmful if associated with poor diet, low body fat, and amenorrhea
  - Weight-bearing exercise (including walking) slightly improves BMD in pre- and postmenopausal women
    - Improves muscle strength, decreasing risk of falls and thus fractures
  - Other factors
    - Minimize or eliminate tobacco use
    - Moderation of alcohol intake
    - Minimize (as able) use of drugs such as glucocorticoids and anticonvulsants
- Qualifications for pharmacologic treatment
  - National Osteoporosis Foundation (2010)
    - Postmenopausal women with BMD T scores ≤−2.5 by DEXA of the femoral neck or spine after appropriate evaluation to exclude secondary causes
    - Postmenopausal women with T scores between −1.0 and −2.5 at the femoral neck or spine and a 10-year probability of a hip fracture ≥3% or a 10-year probability of a major osteoporosis-related fracture ≥20% based on the WHO FRAX algorithm (Update #3)
    - Postmenopausal women with vertebral or hip fracture
  - American Association of Clinical Endocrinologists (2003)
    - Women with low-trauma fracture and low BMD
    - Women with BMD T scores ≤−2.5
    - Women with BMD T scores ≤−1.5 with risk factors
    - Women in whom nonpharmacologic measures are unsuccessful

UPDATE #3

The World Health Organization's FRAX algorithm uses clinical risk factors, bone mineral density, and country-specific fracture and mortality data to quantify a patient's 10-year risk of a hip or major osteoporotic fracture, which facilitates risk stratification for medically appropriate and cost-effective treatment. For the U.S. model, the risk factors used are age, sex, weight, height, previous fracture in adult life occurring spontaneously or by a trauma that would not ordinarily result in fracture, history of parental hip fracture, smoking status, use of glucocorticoids currently or for more than 3 months at a dose equivalent to 5 mg prednisolone daily, history of rheumatoid arthritis, history of secondary causes of bone loss (insulin-dependent diabetes, osteogenesis imperfecta in adults, untreated hyperthyroidism, hypogonadism or menopause before the age of 45, chronic malnutrition, gastrointestinal malabsorption, or chronic liver disease), use of alcohol (more than three beers per day or the equivalent), and BMD of the femoral neck. A BMD test is not required. Although individualization is required, treatment should be considered if a patient has a BMD T score between −1.0 and −2.5 at the femoral neck or spine and a 10-year probability of hip fracture ≥3% or a 10-year probability of a major osteoporosis-related fracture ≥20%. The algorithm can be found at www.shef.ac.uk/FRAX/tool.jsp?locationValue=9.

- Goals of treatment of osteoporosis
  - Prevent fracture
  - Stabilize or increase bone mass
  - Relieve symptoms of fracture or skeletal deformity
  - Maximize physical function
- FDA-approved pharmacologic agents for prevention or treatment of osteoporosis
  - Antiresorptive agents that target bone

- Bisphosphonates
  - Alendronate (Fosamax)
  - Risedronate (Actonel)
  - Ibandronate (Boniva)
  - Zoledronic acid (Reclast)
    - Have been shown in multiple studies to prevent bone loss, increase bone mineral density, and reduce fracture risk
    - Stable analogues of pyrophosphate that inhibit bone resorption by binding hydroxyapatite and reducing osteoclast numbers and activity and increasing apoptosis
    - Have a prolonged duration of action on the skeleton, such that there is residual benefit on BMD after discontinuing the medication
    - Bone formed during bisphosphonate treatment is histologically normal
    - Oral bisphosphonates must be taken with a glass of plain water on an empty stomach after an overnight fast, and the patient must remain upright until fast is broken 30 minutes after taking medication
      - Poor oral absorption (<1% of oral dose); absorption further impaired if medication not taken as directed
      - Esophageal irritation may occur if patient does not remain upright for at least 30 minutes after ingestion of the medication
    - Intravenous zoledronic acid may be associated with acute phase reaction with flulike symptoms
    - Osteonecrosis of the jaw has been described in patients on chronic bisphosphonate therapy
      - Estimated risk with oral bisphosphonates: 1/10,000 to 1/100,000
      - Associated with pain, swelling, exposed bone, local infection, fracture of the jaw
      - Risk factors: cancer, anti-cancer treatments, prolonged exposure, dental issues (extractions, implants, poorly fitting dentures, preexisting disease), smoking, intravenous bisphosphonates, preexisting vitamin D deficiency
    - No consensus on appropriate length of treatment
      - Can consider drug holiday after 5 years of treatment: restart treatment when there is persistent bone loss on DEXA, when bone turnover markers increase, or after 3 to 5 years

UPDATE #4

Recent case series have reported a possible link between long-term bisphosphonate use and "atypical" fractures of the femur including subtrochanteric and diaphyseal fractures of the femoral shaft, creating great concern in the media and thus the public regarding the safety of long-term use of bisphosphonates. A recent register-based national cohort study found that hip, subtrochanteric, and diaphyseal femur fractures were more common in patients taking alendronate than nonusers. However, this increased incidence was attributed to the fact that "high-risk" patients take alendronate and thus were at a higher risk of fracture, rather than the risk being attributable to the alendronate itself (Abrahamsen et al, 2009). This same group looked at cumulative alendronate dose and risk of atypical fracture in this same cohort and found that although alendronate-treated patients had a higher risk of these atypical fractures, the cumulative dose did not alter the risk (Abrahamsen et al, 2010). Again the group suggests that the atypical fractures could be due to osteoporosis rather than the bisphosphonate (Abrahamsen et al, 2010). Another group reviewed the results of three randomized trials on bisphosphonates including the Fracture Intervention Trial (FIT), the FIT Long-Term Extension (FLEX) trial, and the Health Outcomes and Reduced Incidence with Zoledronic Acid Once Yearly (HORIZON) Pivotal Fracture Trial (PFT), reviewing fracture records and radiographs when available, and found no significant increase in these atypical fractures with bisphosphonate use, even with treatment up to 10 years (Black et al, 2010).

- Approved for treatment and prevention of osteoporosis
  - Dose may vary based on indication
- Selective estrogen receptor modulators (SERMs)
  - Raloxifene (Evista)
    - Is bound with high affinity by the estrogen receptor and acts as an estrogen agonist or antagonist depending on the target tissue
      - Acts as estrogen agonist on bone
    - Inhibits bone resorption and reduces the risk of vertebral fracture, with the advantage of reducing breast cancer risk
      - Bisphosphonates increase BMD more than raloxifene and decrease incidence of hip fractures; raloxifene has only been shown to reduce vertebral fracture, not nonvertebral fractures
      - Raloxifene should be used in patients who cannot tolerate bisphosphonates or who are at increased risk for invasive breast cancer
      - SERMs do not have a prolonged duration of action in the skeleton, and thus BMD decreases significantly after discontinuation of therapy; if the patient is tolerating and benefiting from the therapy, long-term use is recommended (clinical trials have extended up to 8 years without adverse effects noted)
    - Approved for prevention and treatment of osteoporosis in *postmenopausal* women
    - Raloxifene is *not effective* for the prevention or treatment of osteoporosis in *premenopausal* women
      - Both raloxifene and tamoxifen have opposite effects on bone in pre- and postmenopausal women: BMD actually decreases in premenopausal women taking these medications

UPDATE #5

Bazedoxifene is a third-generation SERM currently under investigation for the prevention and treatment of postmenopausal osteoporosis (Pinkerton et al, 2007, 2009). Bazedoxifene has been shown to not stimulate endometrial proliferation in an animal model, but it maintains BMD in ovariectomized rats and inhibits the proliferation of a human breast adenocarcinoma cell line, demonstrating improved selectivity of actions on estrogen receptors (Komm et al, 2005; Ronkin et al, 2005). Bazedoxifene prevents bone loss and reduces bone turnover, as seen with raloxifene, and has been shown to

significantly decrease the risk of new vertebral and nonvertebral fractures in a subgroup of postmenopausal women with elevated fracture risk (Silverman et al, 2008). In postmenopausal women at risk for osteoporosis, bazedoxifene did not affect endometrial thickness, did not induce endometrial hyperplasia or malignancy, and did not cause any additional histologic findings like endometrial polyps in comparison to placebo or raloxifene (Pinkerton et al, 2009). Furthermore, bazedoxifene had no effect on ovarian volume, ovarian cyst formation, or the incidence of ovarian cancer (Pinkerton et al, 2009). Breast cancer and breast pain were rarely reported (in less than 4% and 1% of patients, respectively) and did not differ from the placebo or raloxifene group (Pinkerton et al, 2009).

UPDATE #6

Lasofoxifene was found to reduce the risks of nonvertebral and vertebral fractures, estrogen receptor-positive breast cancer, coronary heart disease, and stroke in a recent randomized trial of postmenopausal women with osteoporosis 59 to 80 years of age at a dose of 0.5 mg (Cummings et al, 2010). An increase in thromboembolic events was noted for both the 0.25-mg and 0.5-mg doses in comparison to placebo. Lasofoxifene was not associated with an increased risk of endometrial cancer.

- Hormone therapy
  - Estrogen
    - Conjugated estrogens (Premarin)
    - Estropipate (Ogen)
    - 17β-Estradiol (Alora, Climara, Estrace, Menostar, Vivelle, Vivelle Dot, Estraderm)
  - Estrogen and progesterone
    - Conjugated estrogens and medroxyprogesterone acetate (Premphase, Prempro)
    - Ethinyl estradiol and norethindrone acetate (femhrt)
    - 17β-Estradiol and norethindrone acetate (Activella)
    - 17β-Estradiol and norgestimate (Prefest)
    - 17β-Estradiol and levonorgestrel (Climara Pro)
      - Approved for prevention but not treatment of osteoporosis: data on fractures required by the FDA to be approved for treatment of osteoporosis were never submitted
      - Increases bone mineral density and reduces bone loss and risk of fractures, with the advantage of menopausal symptom relief
      - The Women's Health Initiative found a significant reduction of osteoporosis-related fractures in women on hormone therapy, as well as a reduction of colorectal cancer, but found increased odds of developing breast cancer, deep venous thrombosis, stroke, and cardiovascular disease; hip fractures were reduced by 33% in women on HT after an average follow-up of 5.6 years

UPDATE #7

The findings of the Women's Health Initiative in regard to the effects of hormone use have prompted a paradigm shift to reduce the dosages used for hormone therapy (HT) and to limit the length of HT (American College of Obstetricians and

Gynecologists, ACOG Practice Bulletin No. 50, 2004; Shifren et al, 2010). Therefore, studies have been conducted comparing the effectiveness of lower-dose HT to regular-dose HT. Low and standard doses of transdermal estradiol were found to be equally effective in controlling bone turnover in postmenopausal women (Garcia-Perez et al, 2006).

- The addition of progesterone to estrogen is necessary in treating women with uteri in situ, but it has been associated with an increased risk of adverse events
- Current recommendation is to use hormone therapy in the lowest possible dose for the shortest amount of time for relief of menopausal symptoms, which may not provide adequate bone protection
- May also be used in women who are unable to tolerate other therapeutic options
- The increase in BMD and reduction in fractures does not persist after HT is discontinued; need to consider alternative treatment in women who discontinue HT

UPDATE #8

The North American Menopause Society 2010 Position Statement indicates that the extended use of HT for women with decreased bone mass with or without menopausal symptoms is appropriate for preventing further loss of bone mass or reducing risk of fracture when other therapies are not tolerated or when the benefits of extended HT outweigh the risks (North American Menopause Society, 2010). The ideal time to initiate therapy and the most beneficial length of treatment have not been fully elucidated, but the beneficial effects of HT are quickly lost after discontinuation of treatment (North American Menopause Society, 2010).

- Calcitonin
  - Calcitonin-salmon (Fortical, Miacalcin)
    - Peptide produced by thyroid C cells
    - Inhibits osteoclast activity
  - Approved for the treatment of osteoporosis in women who have been postmenopausal for more than 5 years
    - Although FDA-approved for treatment of osteoporosis, data on fracture risk are not stated on prescribing information
      - One study showed reduced vertebral fracture risk with nasal calcitonin but no effect on hip or nonvertebral fractures
  - Generally administered as a nasal spray
    - Miacalcin also comes as a subcutaneous injection
- Denosumab (Prolia)
  - Antibody to the receptor activator of nuclear factor-κβ ligand (RANKL) that blocks binding to RANK
  - Inhibits the recruitment and activity of osteoclasts
  - Found to reduce the risk of vertebral, nonvertebral, and hip fractures in women with osteoporosis
  - FDA-approved for the treatment of osteoporosis in postmenopausal women
  - Dosage: 60 mg, injected subcutaneously twice a year

UPDATE #9

Denosumab (Prolia) was approved by the FDA for the treatment of osteoporosis in postmenopausal women on June 1, 2010. Denosumab is an antibody to the receptor activator of nuclear factor-κβ ligand (RANKL) that blocks binding to RANK and inhibits osteoclastogenesis. It was found to reduce the risk of vertebral, nonvertebral, and hip fractures in women with osteoporosis (Cummings et al, 2009). The dose is 60 mg injected subcutaneously twice yearly. In a randomized, placebo-controlled trial of the drug, flatulence and eczema were reported more commonly in the treatment group compared to the placebo group (2.2% versus 1.4%, $p < 0.001$ and 3% versus 1.7%, $p < 0.008$, respectively) (Cummings et al, 2009). More patients in the treatment group reported serious events of cellulitis (0.3%) compared to placebo (<0.1%, $p = 0.002$) (Cummings et al, 2009). There were no significant differences in the treatment and placebo groups in the number of adverse events, incidence of cancer, or cardiovascular events (Cummings et al, 2009). There were no cases of osteonecrosis of the jaw in either group (Cummings et al, 2009), although there is a potential for this with denosumab treatment as it causes suppression of bone turnover. Besides treatment for primary osteoporosis, the maker of the drug is currently seeking approval from the FDA to use the drug in cancer patients to help prevent bone complications. A recent study found that denosumab delayed skeletal-related events (including fractures, bone surgery, need for radiation, and spinal cord compression) in patients with castration-resistant prostate cancer better than zoledronic acid (Fizazi et al, 2011), a bisphosphonate that is approved for use in patients with multiple myeloma as well as those with bone metastases from breast, lung, or prostate cancer.

- Anabolic agents that target bone
  - Parathyroid hormone (PTH)
    - Teriparatide (Forteo)
      - PTH 1-34
        - Recombinant PTH fragment that maintains all of the biologic activity of the full 84-amino acid polypeptide
        - Injected subcutaneously daily at a dose of 20 mcg/day
    - PTH 1-84 (PreOs)
      - Approved in Europe but not the United States
    - PTH 1-31
      - Currently undergoing trials
    - PTH and calcitriol (1,25-dihydroxyvitamin D) are the two major hormones controlling calcium and phosphate homeostasis
      - Considered an anabolic agent for osteoporosis therapy
        - Stimulates bone formation and bone remodeling
      - Typically, PTH is released when serum calcium levels decrease, such that chronic and sustained elevation of PTH stimulates renal tubular calcium resorption and bone resorption
      - However, in the first 12 months of intermittent treatment with recombinant PTH, bone formation, rather than resorption, is stimulated
      - The increase in bone density largely occurs within the first several months of treatment, peaks at 6 to 9 months, and levels off after 18 months, but the reduction in fracture risk is seen only after at least 6 months of treatment
        - Bone resorption begins after 6 months of treatment and peaks at 12 months of treatment,

but because of the increased bone formation in the first 3 months, a positive balance persists; eventually, with long-term treatment, bone resorption will catch up to the formation of new bone such that the bone will be at equilibrium, and no further increase in BMD will occur
- Although the mechanism of action has not been fully delineated, PTH stimulates osteoblastogenesis and recruitment of bone-forming cells to the bone-remodeling unit through multiple target genes including IGF-1, amphiregulin, 1-alpha hydroxylase, Runx2, TGF-β, RANKL, and M-CSF; sclerostin, which inhibits the Wnt signaling pathway, is suppressed by treatment with PTH
  - Recruitment of osteoclasts occurs only after the activation of preosteoblasts
  - PTH may cause a reduction in apoptosis of osteoblasts
- PTH is approved for the treatment of osteoporosis but not prevention of osteoporosis
  - PTH treatment should be limited to patients with severe osteoporosis for a maximum of 2 years: potential for carcinogenicity (osteosarcoma was seen in rats given high doses of PTH throughout their lifetime; higher rate of osteosarcoma seen in patients with hyperparathyroidism); can consider treatment with a bisphosphonate after discontinuation of PTH to maintain BMD (studies have also shown treatment with estrogen and raloxifene after PTH maintains the gain in BMD)
- Combination therapy
  - Osteoporosis therapy is based largely on antiresorptive agents
    - Effectiveness is limited in that the mechanism of action targets only bone resorption
    - Combining antiresorptive therapy with anabolic agents may overcome this limit by incorporating new bone formation into the equation
    - This may lead to a greater reduction in fracture risk than either class of agents alone
      - None of the studies to date have been adequately powered to establish a decreased fracture risk with combination therapy in comparison to monotherapy despite the increased BMD observed with several combination therapy regimens
  - PTH and bisphosphonates
    - Multiple studies have shown that the sequential regimen of PTH treatment followed by bisphosphonate treatment is a viable option for osteoporosis therapy
    - Concomitant treatment has been shown to be no better than bisphosphonate therapy alone, suggesting that the bisphosphonate ameliorates the anabolic effect of the PTH
  - PTH and SERMs
    - SERMs may actually enhance the anabolic effects of PTH when given concomitantly, but further studies are needed to validate this finding
  - PTH and HT
    - This combination has been shown to increase vertebral BMD, spine, and hip bone mass, decrease vertebral fracture risk, and increase overall skeletal density
    - HT did not prevent the anabolic actions of PTH

- Bisphosphonates and SERMs
  - Although both are antiresorptive, their mechanisms of action differ
  - A comparative study found that the combination therapy of alendronate and raloxifene increased the femoral neck BMD significantly more than either therapy alone
    - The lumbar spine BMD and bone turnover were similarly significantly improved in the alendronate and combination groups in comparison to the raloxifene group
  - A study of the sequential use of alendronate and raloxifene indicated that raloxifene is less potent than alendronate, as the raloxifene group had higher levels of bone turnover markers than the alendronate group, but less than the placebo group
- Bisphosphonates and HT
  - Studies suggest that this combination may increase BMD more than either agent alone without the risk of suppressing bone remodeling
    - Should be considered in women with menopausal symptoms and continued bone loss despite HT
    - Given the paradigm shift of lowest dose HT for the shortest amount of time, the bisphosphonate/HT combination will likely be important, as the low-dose, short-term HT alone may not be sufficient treatment for osteoporosis
    - Increased BMD seen in this combination has not been clearly linked to a decrease in fracture risk
- SERMs and HT
  - Bazedoxifene and lasofoxifene, two third-generation SERMs, are currently being studied for the treatment of osteoporosis
    - Bone protection is similar to the FDA-approved SERM raloxifene
    - May prevent the HT-induced endometrial growth without affecting the efficacy of the HT on menopausal symptoms
      - May obviate the need for the addition of progesterone to estrogen therapy in women with uteri in situ, thus eliminating the associated increased incidence of adverse effects
      - The combination could potentially protect bones, the endometrium, and the breast, while improving the lipid profile and providing relief to menopausal symptoms
    - In clinical trials, patients treated with bazedoxifene and lasofoxifene had higher rates of venous thrombosis than those treated with placebo
- Tibolone
  - Not FDA approved
    - Approved in 45 countries for the prevention of osteoporosis and in 90 countries for treatment of menopausal symptoms
  - Has progestogenic, estrogenic, and androgenic properties
    - Preserves BMD
    - Reduces hot flashes
    - May increase libido and vaginal lubrication
    - Decreases HDL and triglycerides
  - Has been shown in older women (60 to 85 years) to decrease the risk of vertebral and nonvertebral fractures, reduce the risk of breast cancer and possibly colon cancer, but increase the risk of stroke (Cummings et al, 2008)

UPDATE #10

Research is ongoing for new treatment targets for osteoporosis. Glucagon-like peptide-2 (GLP-2) is released by the intestine in response to food intake and reduces bone resorption. Current investigations are finding that GLP-2 may reduce bone resorption without having an effect on bone formation (Deal, 2009). Cathepsin K is a protease expressed by osteoclasts that can degrade bone matrix in an acid environment. Balicatib and odanacatib are two cathepsin K inhibitors that have been shown to increase bone mass by inhibiting bone resorption and having less inhibition of bone formation than bisphosphonates (Deal, 2009). Wnt proteins help regulate bone formation through an accumulation of β-catenin. Antibodies to naturally occurring antagonists of Wnt signaling, sclerostin and Dickkopf-1, are being investigated as anabolic agents in the treatment of patients with low bone mass (Deal, 2009; Roux, 2010). Calcilytic agents modulate parathyroid hormone release through manipulation of the calcium-sensing receptor; studies in rats have been promising with increases in both cortical and trabecular bone, but a human study was discontinued after poor response of spine BMD after 6 months; thus further trials are ongoing (Deal, 2009; Roux, 2010).

Follow-up and Monitoring

- Repeat DEXA in untreated women after 3 to 5 years
- For women receiving therapy
  - Must use central bone densitometry
  - Repeating DEXA prior to 2 years of complete therapy may lead to incorrect assumptions regarding treatment efficacy
    - After 1 year, BMD may actually appear to decrease on DEXA
      - Likely because of the imprecision of DEXA
    - Must evaluate compliance with therapy, dosing instructions, calcium and vitamin D intake, and possible secondary causes of bone loss if BMD decreases by more than 4% to 5%

SUGGESTED READINGS

General Osteoporosis

American College of Obstetricians and Gynecologists: Women's Health Care Physicians: ACOG practice bulletin: clinical management guidelines for obstetricians-gynecologists no. 50, January 2004, *Obstet Gynecol* 103(1):203–216, 2004.

Kanis JA, McCloskey EV, Johansson H, et al: A reference standard for the description of osteoporosis, *Bone* 42(3):467–475, 2008.

National Osteoporosis Foundation: *Clinician's guide to prevention and treatment of osteoporosis*, Washington, DC, 2010, National Osteoporosis Foundation.

Sweet MG, Sweet JM, Jeremiah MP, et al: Diagnosis and treatment of osteoporosis, *Am Fam Physician* 79(3):193–200; 201–202, 2009.

World Health Organization: *WHO Scientific Group on the Assessment of Osteoporosis at Primary Health Care Level. Summary meeting report*, Brussels, Belgium, 2004, World Health Organization.

Risk Factors and Screening

Davisson L, Warden M, Manivannan S, et al: Osteoporosis screening: factors associated with bone mineral density testing of older women, *J Womens Health* 18(7):989–994, 2009.

Isidro ML, Ruano B: Bone disease in diabetes, *Curr Diabetes Rev* 6(3):144–155, 2010.

Kanis JA: Diagnosis of osteoporosis and assessment of fracture risk, *Lancet* 359(9321):1929–1936, 2002.

Siris ES, Baim S, Nattiv A: Primary care use of FRAX: absolute fracture risk assessment in postmenopausal women and older men, *Postgrad Med* 122(1):82–90, 2010.

Prevention and Treatment

Bolland MJ, Avenell A, Baron JA, et al: Effect of calcium supplements on risk of myocardial infarction and cardiovascular events: meta-analysis, *BMJ* 341:c3691, 2010.

Gass M, Dawson-Hughes B: Preventing osteoporosis-related fractures: an overview, *Am J Med* 119(4 Suppl 1):3S–11S, 2006.

Bisphosphonates

Abrahamsen B, Eiken P, Eastell R: Cumulative alendronate dose and the long-term absolute risk of subtrochanteric and diaphyseal femur fractures: a register-based national cohort analysis, *J Clin Endocrinol Metab* 95(12):5258–5265, 2010.

Abrahamsen B, Eiken P, Eastell R: Subtrochanteric and diaphyseal femur fractures in patients treated with alendronate: a register-based national cohort study, *J Bone Miner Res* 24(6):1095–1102, 2009.

Black DM, Kelly MP, Genant HK: Bisphosphonates and fractures of the subtrochanteric or diaphyseal femur, *N Eng J Med* 362(19):1761–1771, 2010.

Selective Estrogen Receptor Modulators

Cummings SR, Ensrud K, Delmas PD, et al: Lasofoxifene in postmenopausal women with osteoporosis, *N Engl J Med* 362(8):686–696, 2010.

Komm BS, Kharode YP, Bodine PV, et al: Bazedoxifene acetate: a selective estrogen receptor modulator with improved selectivity, *Endocrinology* 146(9):3999–4008, 2005.

Pinkerton JV, Archer DF, Utian WH, et al: Bazedoxifene effects on the reproductive tract in postmenopausal women at risk for osteoporosis, *Menopause* 16(6):1102–1108, 2009.

Ronkin S, Northington R, Baracat E, et al: Endometrial effects of bazedoxifene acetate, a novel selective estrogen receptor modulator, in postmenopausal women, *Obstet Gynecol* 105(6):1397–1404, 2005.

Silverman SL, Christiansen C, Genant HK, et al: Efficacy of bazedoxifene in reducing new vertebral fracture risk in postmenopausal women with osteoporosis: results from a 3-year, randomized, placebo and active-controlled clinical trial, *J Bone Miner Res* 23(12):1923–1934, 2008.

Hormone Therapy

Garcia-Perez MA, Moreno-Mercer J, Tarin JJ, et al: Similar efficacy of low and standard doses of transdermal estradiol in controlling bone turnover in postmenopausal women, *Gynecol Endocrinol* 22(4):179–184, 2006.

Lindsay R, Gallagher JC, Kleerekoper M, et al: Effect of lower doses of conjugated equine estrogens with and without medroxyprogesterone acetate on bone in early postmenopausal women, *JAMA* 287(20):2668–2676, 2002.

North American Menopause Society: Estrogen and progestogen use in postmenopausal women: 2010 position statement of the North American Menopause Society, *Menopause* 17(2):242–255, 2010.

Shifren JL, Schiff I: Role of hormone therapy in the management of menopause, *Obstet Gynecol* 115(4):839–855, 2010.

Parathyroid Hormone

Ruiz C, Abril N, Tarin JJ, et al: The new frontier of bone formation: a breakthrough in postmenopausal osteoporosis? *Climacteric* 12(4):286–300, 2009.

Combination Therapy

Pinkerton JV, Dalkin AC: Combination therapy for treatment of osteoporosis: a review, *Am J Obstet Gynecol* 197(6):559–565, 2007.

Other Therapies

Cummings SR, Ettinger B, Delmas PD, et al: The effects of tibolone in older postmenopausal women, *N Engl J Med* 359(7):697–708, 2008.

Cummings SR, San Martin J, McClung MR: Denosumab for prevention of fractures in postmenopausal women with osteoporosis, *N Engl J Med* 361(8):756–765, 2009.

Deal C: Future therapeutic targets in osteoporosis, *Curr Opin Rheumatol* 21(4):380–385, 2009.

Fizazi K, Carducci MA, Smith R, et al: A randomized phase III trial of denosumab versus zoledronic acid in patients with one metastases from castration-resistant prostate cancer, *Lancet Mar* 5; 377(9768):813–833, 2011.

Roux S: New treatment targets in osteoporosis, *Joint Bone Spine* 77(3):222–228, 2010.

Chapter 49

End-of-Life and Hospice Care

JOHN L. DALRYMPLE

KEY UPDATES

1 Ongoing, effective communication is required for successful end-of-life (EOL) care planning.

2 Systematic review of palliative care at the EOL strongly supports the use of treating many symptoms—including cancer pain, dyspnea, and depression—with proven therapies.

3 Recurrent ovarian cancer often results in intestinal blockage from carcinomatosis, for which surgical palliation may be beneficial in select cases.

4 Many barriers exist in the completion of Advanced Directive (AD), but having a clear understanding of the patient's wishes and who the surrogate decision maker is will facilitate EOL care.

5 Enrollment or transfer to hospice care is variable among terminal conditions and diagnosis but appears to be increasing.

6 The four guiding prima facie principles (autonomy, nonmaleficence, beneficence, justice) form the necessary framework for physicians to make sound ethical decisions.

7 Most cancer centers have palliative care programs.

8 Ob-gyn physicians are able to engage in effective communications focusing on future health care goals, completion of ADs, and EOL care planning.

9 Providing emotional support and clear communication to families experiencing fetal loss is essential, including the use of bereavement services and perinatal hospice.

End-of-Life (EOL) Care

GOALS AT EOL

- Adequate relief of symptoms including psychological anguish and emotional distress
- Maintain dignity and quality of life (QOL)
- Provide resources and support for patient and family, including advanced care planning and psychosocial needs of the family
- Respect patient's and family's wishes and desires
- Avoid medical futility
- Maintain autonomy and well-being of physicians and health care providers

DIAGNOSIS OF A TERMINAL CONDITION

- Understanding disease course, available treatment options, and when additional interventions are of no further benefit to patient is essential
- Avoiding harm from further treatment/interventions when clear benefit is unlikely to be achieved

- Extension of life is no longer possible with available means of therapy
- QOL (as deemed by the patient) is no longer attainable or achievable

TRANSITIONING TO PALLIATIVE CARE: WHAT TO DISCUSS WITH THE PATIENT

- Ongoing honest and open communication by treating physician or primary care physician (PCP) regarding patient's health care and disease course is essential
- Recollection of diagnosis, treatment successes and failures, and progression of symptoms may be helpful in putting terminal nature of disease into better context
- Appreciation of patient's and family's understanding of terminal condition with appropriate, sensitive full disclosure—especially when patient asks explicitly; respect of those patients who desire "not to know" should be balanced with physician's and family's need to provide appropriate care and make decisions that honor and respect the patient's preferences and wishes

- Knowledge of patient's goals of therapy and preferences about care, with specific focus on physical symptoms and psychosocial concerns of patient and family
- Appreciation of patient/family resources with sensitivity to unique cultural, religious, and socioeconomic considerations

Palliative Care: Symptom Management

PAIN

- Ongoing knowledge of level and location of pain is critical
- Narcotic versus non-narcotic medications available
  - Opioid analgesics: highly effective, but with considerable side effect profile including sedation, drowsiness, nausea, bowel dysfunction; options include morphine, oxycodone, hydromorphone, fentanyl, methadone
  - Nonopioid analgesics: often not as effective for pain at EOL; options include nonsteroidal anti-inflammatory drugs (NSAIDs), acetaminophen
  - Other agents: neurologic agents (gabapentin, carbamazepine)
- Mode of delivery of pain medication
  - Oral: short versus long-acting dosing (every 8 to 12 hours); requires ability to swallow pills/tablets with adequate absorption
  - Sublingual, buccal: liquid formulation; provides immediate effect
  - Transrectal: may be difficult with local sores/lesions or if having elimination problems
  - Transdermal: provides continuous steady-state level of effective analgesia; may be difficult to titrate if pain requirements are in flux, especially at EOL
  - Nerve blocks/epidural catheters: invasive; may be effective in alleviating focal pain
  - Intravenous (IV): patient-controlled analgesia (PCA) and subcutaneous injections can be feasible even in home settings; provide immediate effect

RESPIRATORY

- Dyspnea common from fluid overload, pleural effusions, or metastasis
- Fluid/volume status can be difficult to manage at the EOL; avoidance of IV fluids is essential with cautious use of diuretics to prevent symptomatic hypovolemia
- Pleural effusions may be managed with thoracentesis, pleurodesis, or placement of intermittent draining catheters depending on the rate of fluid accumulation and effect on symptom control; although fairly invasive, thoughtful consideration of the expected benefit and goals of palliation must be taken into account
- Medical management to alleviate the sensation of "air hunger" may be achieved with the use of morphine or other opioids; secretion buildup can be managed with atropine, and inhalers may aid in the management of airway bronchospasms; oxygen (nasal cannula) may also provide relief of symptoms related to dyspnea and hypoxia

PSYCHOLOGICAL SYMPTOMS

- Anxiety and depression common among patients with terminal conditions
- Active medical management with appropriate anxiolytic and antidepressive therapies indicated
- Supportive care by family, friends, counselors, spiritual/religious leaders

GASTROINTESTINAL (GI)

- Symptoms: nausea, vomiting, bowel dysfunction, constipation, diarrhea, incontinence
- Causes: many gynecologic malignancies result in obstruction of the GI tract during the course of the disease process, including gastric outlet, small bowel, and large bowel obstruction; often heralds final manifestation of disease process; poor prognosis
- Surgery: may alleviate terminal bowel obstruction and provide palliation of symptoms in select patients; multiple points of obstruction or "tumor ileus" often prevents consideration of surgery; options include colostomy, ileostomy, internal bypass
- Gastrostomy tube (g-tube) placement: effective at alleviating intractable nausea and vomiting from malignant, terminal bowel obstruction; insertion accomplished by interventional radiology, gastrointestinal medicine specialist, or via open surgical techniques; options include g-tube, percutaneous endoscopic gastrostomy (PEG) tube
- Nasogastric (NG) tube: provides gastric decompression as a temporary measure until more suitable method (i.e. g-tube, PEG) can be applied; long-term use may cause symptoms and complications including local pain, sinus infection, nasal septal erosion, gastritis, and general discomfort
- Antiemetic therapy: active medical management of nausea and vomiting is paramount; requires a balance of symptom relief with common sedating side effects; routes of administration: oral, sublingual, rectal, IV

- Constipation: commonly encountered at EOL from side-effect of narcotics; routine bowel regimens include stool softeners and laxatives essential; routes of administration: oral, rectal suppositories, enemas

UPDATE #3

Recurrent ovarian cancer often results in intestinal blockage from carcinomatosis and encasement of the bowel and mesentery by tumor implants. The goal of surgical palliation is preservation of QOL by restoring the patient's ability to eat, drink, and resume bowel function (tolerate a regular or low-residue diet for at least 60 days postoperatively). Factors affecting the likelihood of success include overall functional and nutritional status, other medical conditions, ability to receive additional treatment, risk of repeat obstruction, and location, number, and site of obstruction. When surgical correction is possible, successful palliation of symptoms is reported to be high (71%) with associated significantly longer median survival (11.6 versus 3.9 months) (Pothuri et al, 2003; Sun et al, 2007).

OTHER TREATMENTS

- Antibiotics: acceptable and reasonable for treatable infections; recognition that some terminal conditions may ultimately result in infections/sepsis as the natural (terminal) course of the disease process
- Blood transfusions: often not utilized; focus should be on alleviation of signs and symptoms of anemia; serologic testing and monitoring of hematologic parameters not a component of EOL care
- Intravenous (IV) fluids: controversial; often not recommended as patients unable to effectively manage additional fluid volume (e.g., pulmonary edema)
- Nutritional support: includes tube feeds and total parenteral nutrition (TPN); typically, not a component of EOL care; not shown to effectively extend life or enhance QOL except for short-term achievement of specific time-sensitive goals (e.g., use of TPN)
- Chemotherapy: universally not accepted as part of EOL care
- Radiation therapy: may provide effective palliation of symptoms when used in this context (versus as a means of active treatment for the purpose of extension of life); utilized in management of bone metastasis, pelvic tumors, brain metastasis
- Surgery: as noted earlier under management of gastrointestinal symptoms; limited use at EOL for effective palliation of symptoms such as related to bowel obstruction

Do Not Resuscitate (DNR)

A. Discussion of DNR orders should be ongoing and early on when incurable or terminal condition diagnosed
B. Patient's wishes often evolve once terminal phase realized
C. Some patients may request specific components of resuscitation in particular circumstances including the following:
  - Intubation
  - Cardio Pulmonary Resuscitation (CPR)/Advanced Cardiac Life Support (ACLS)

- Pressure support
- Intensive care unit (ICU) management
D. Outpatient discussion with documentation in the patient's medical record ideal
E. Family awareness to patient's code status will help avoid undesirable interventions when patient is unable to speak for herself

Advanced Directive

Formal mechanism by which patients express their values regarding future health status. Includes three components:

PROXY DIRECTIVES

- Durable power of attorney for health care (also known as a medical power of attorney)
- Designates surrogate to make medical decisions on behalf of patient who is no longer competent to express her choices
- Should be individual who knows, appreciates, and respects the patient's desires, wishes, and values either as written, verbally expressed, or by extrapolation (if not explicitly written or stated) based on what is known about the patient and felt to be in her best interest
- Default legal hierarchy of decision makers includes (in descending order):
  - Court-appointed guardian
  - Spouse
  - Adult children
  - Parents
  - Adult siblings
  - Relatives

INSTRUCTIONAL DIRECTIVES

- Living will
- Focuses on types of life-sustaining treatment a person would or would not accept in various clinical circumstances, including specific listing of patient's preferences regarding care at the EOL
- May address specific interventions the patient will and will not accept
  - Various aspects of DNR including intubation, CPR/ACLS, pressure support, ICU transfer and management (see section on DNR)
  - Stipulation for certain clinical scenarios (e.g., short-term intervention [intubation] if recovery from acute episode [pneumonia/Congestive Heart Failure (CHF)] highly likely)

TIMING AND LOGISTICS OF COMPLETION

- May be completed any time, especially when terminal condition not present
- If terminal diagnosis made, ideal to complete well in advance of final stages of life when patient and family can have an open and clear discussion as to patient's preferences
- Social workers and hospital personnel may provide assistance to complete
- Forms available from hospitals, clinics, and online

UPDATE #4

Many barriers exist in the completion of ADs including procrastination and time constraints, misunderstanding of terminology and process, cultural and ethnic divergence, and physician anxiety about patient's unease surrounding issues related to EOL, death, and dying. Having a clear understanding of the patient's wishes and who the surrogate decision maker is will facilitate EOL care when decisions need to be made. This is especially notable among same-sex relationships in states where gay marriage and domestic partnerships may not be legally recognized. Explicit documentation in these cases is essential to avoid unnecessary hassle, confusion, and distress (American College of Obstetricians and Gynecologists, ACOG Committee Opinion No. 403, 2008; Finnerty et al, 2002).

Hospice Care

CRITERIA

- Life expectancy of 6 months or less as deemed by treating physician
- Receiving no "active" treatment for condition with focus on palliation
- DNR order (not necessarily a requirement, but usually placed)

INPATIENT CARE SERVICES

- Can be delivered in hospital setting, palliative care unit, skilled nursing facility, or nursing home (with appropriate supervision by hospice health care providers)
- Required for higher level of acuity/care or with rapid physical deterioration (active dying process) when transition to home hospice not possible
- Inadequate relief of symptoms requiring IV administration of medication
- Unavailability of family/friends or inadequate resources to provide home care

HOME CARE

- Patient preference to die at home should be determined early on in the terminal care process
- Availability and good understanding of expectations of care by family/friends essential for patient to receive home hospice care
- Adequate resources with oversight of care from hospice health care providers

UPDATE #5

Enrollment or transfer to hospice care is variable among terminal conditions and diagnosis but appears to be increasing. In one study, 54% of ovarian cancer patients received some form of hospice support either in their home or at a hospice center, with a significant increase observed during the study period (41% between 2000 and 2002, to 70% between 2003 and 2006). Among inpatient deaths on a gynecologic oncology service, the number of patients awaiting transfer to hospice was much lower during the time frame studied one decade earlier (31%). Hospice care utilization by Medicare cancer decedents was reported to be just over 50%, compared to only 10% for other causes of death (1993 to 1998) (Dalrymple et al, 2002; Hogan et al, 2001; von Gruenigen et al, 2008).

Physician-Assisted Suicide/Euthanasia

EUTHANASIA

- Act or practice of ending the life of an individual suffering from a terminal illness or an incurable condition

PHYSICIAN-ASSISTED SUICIDE (PAS)

- Provision or supply of medication (prescription) by a physician to a patient for the known purpose or intention of ending the patient's life
- Oregon only U.S. state where legal (Death with Dignity Act, 1997; upheld by Supreme Court in 2006); legal in The Netherlands, Belgium, Australia
- Request by patients regarding PAS may indicate presence of such conditions as depression, anxiety, or inadequately treated pain

DOUBLE EFFECT

- Principle referring to the hastening of death as an expected consequence of the alleviation of pain and other symptoms with medication (e.g., sedating effects of narcotics causing respiratory depression)

Ethical Considerations

AUTONOMY

- Patient self-determination of what health care she decides for herself based on what is considered to be reasonable and sound

BENEFICENCE

- Defining feature of physician's ethical responsibility
- Health care and decisions provided to patients for their benefit, regardless of the nature of that benefit
- Includes treatment or prevention of illness, preservation of life, alleviation of pain and suffering, and avoidance of medical futility

NONMALEFICENCE

- Avoidance of harm in the context of providing beneficial health care
- Encompasses both the philosophy of intentional hastening of death (euthanasia and PAS) and the unintentional consequences of some therapies

JUSTICE

- Delivery of and access to health care should be available to all without regard to financial, social, religious, cultural, or other constraints

UPDATE #6

The four guiding prima facie principles (autonomy, nonmaleficence, beneficence, justice) form the necessary framework for physicians to make sound ethical decisions. This can be applied in all contexts, including EOL care planning. Because they are all equally significant and no one principle is more important, health care providers should take efforts to avoid or diminish the effect of any violation of these principles (Finnerty et al, 2000; Cain et al, 2005).

Role of Palliative Care Teams, Primary Care Providers (PCPs), and Other Health Care Providers

A. Consultation and transition of care to palliative care teams can provide comprehensive EOL care both in the inpatient and outpatient setting

B. PCP may be knowledgeable about an individual patient's disease course and wishes regarding EOL care planning and should be involved when appropriate

C. Specialists including oncologists, internists and associated specialties, and intensivists, as well as social workers, clergy/pastoral services, and psychologists can assist in providing a multidisciplinary approach in addressing patient and family needs and concerns

D. Consultation with ethics committees or teams may assist in addressing conflicts that might arise between the patient, family members, and various members of the health care team

UPDATE #7

Most cancer centers have palliative care programs (88%), with higher rates reported among National Cancer Institute (NCI)-designated cancer centers compared to non-NCI centers (98% versus 78%). Altogether, these cancer centers were likely to have at least one palliative care physician (84%) and inpatient palliative care consultation teams (74%). The rates of outpatient palliative care clinics (41%), dedicated palliative care beds (23%), or institution-operated hospice programs (37%) were not as high (Hui et al, 2010).

Role of the Ob-Gyn

A. Long-term relationships with women throughout their lifetime affords the ob-gyn an ideal opportunity to encourage women to formulate AD and goals for EOL care

B. Often involved in making the diagnosis of life-threatening conditions such as gynecologic malignancies and providing ongoing care alongside other health care providers, including oncologists

C. Patients may identify their ob-gyn as their "primary care provider," often seeking advice, counsel, and involvement at the EOL

UPDATE #8

Ob-gyn physicians are able to engage in effective and proactive communications focusing on future health care goals, development and completion of ADs, and even EOL care planning. Although this may be accomplished when a life-threatening illness develops, a more ideal opportunity for this to occur is at any time throughout the course of care such as during routine well-woman exams and during the course of pregnancy. The development of AD and care planning is a fluid process that will change as the patient's health status, life goals, and circumstances change (American College of Obstetricians and Gynecologists, ACOG Committee Opinion No. 403, 2008).

D. Maternal and fetal death
- Maternal death
  - Tragic and typically sudden and unexpected event

UPDATE #9

Providing emotional support and clear communication to families experiencing fetal loss is essential. This may include the use of bereavement services, pastoral/clergy services, mental health professionals (in the management of grief and depression), and other support groups. Allowing the family to build memories of their loved one is important in the grieving process and may include ultrasound visualization (during prenatal care), holding the infant, and having hand/footprints and pictures made. Avoidance of prolonged hospitalizations and recovery on postpartum wards, as well as the development and use of perinatal hospice programs, may be of significant benefit (American College of Obstetricians and Gynecologists, ACOG Practice Bulletin No. 102, 2009; Hoeldtke et al, 2001; Silver, 2007). For obstetricians caring for patients with a stillbirth, 75% have reported the large emotional toll this has taken on them personally, and 8% even considered giving up obstetric practice as a result. Seeking support from colleagues, family, and friends is a strategy physicians commonly use to help cope with this difficult situation (Gold et al, 2008).

- Likely to affect any ob-gyn during her or his professional career
- Role of ob-gyn is essential in providing medical expertise and care, guidance, and support to patient, family, and other health care providers
- Fetal/neonatal/infant death
  - The ob-gyn is often central to establishing a diagnosis of pregnancy loss, including miscarriage, missed abortion, fatal condition in utero, intrauterine fetal demise, or terminal condition of newborn (stillbirth)
  - Role in providing effective communication, support, sensitivity, and expertise of medical management is essential with utilization of a multidisciplinary team
  - Perinatal hospice programs may be beneficial
  - Effect on obstetrician can be emotionally taxing

SUGGESTED READINGS

End-of-Life Care

Cain JM, Heintz PM, Swarte NB: End of life care. In Hoskins WJ, Perez CA, Young RC, et al: *Principles and practice of gynecologic oncology*, ed 4, Philadelphia, 2005, Lippincott Williams & Wilkins, pp 1343–1359.

Sun CC, Ramirez PT, Bodurka DC: Quality of life for patients with epithelial ovarian cancer, *Nat Clin Pract Oncol* 4(1):18–29, 2007.

Palliative Care: Symptom Management

Lorenz KA, Lynn J, Dy SM, et al: Evidence for improving palliative care at the end of life: a systematic review, *Ann Intern Med* 148(2):147–159, 2008.

Norton TR, Manne SL, Ruben S, et al: Prevalence and predictors of psychological distress among women with ovarian cancer, *J Clin Oncol* 22(5):919–926, 2004.

Pothuri B, Vaidya A, Aghajanian C, et al: Palliative surgery for bowel obstruction in recurrent ovarian cancer: an updated series, *Gynecol Oncol* 89(2):306–313, 2003.

Sun CC, Ramirez PT, Bodurka DC: Quality of life for patients with epithelial ovarian cancer, *Nat Clin Pract Oncol* 4(1):18–29, 2007.

Advanced Directives

American College of Obstetricians and Gynecologists: ACOG committee opinion no. 403, April 2008: end-of-life decision making, *Obstet Gynecol* 111(4):1021–1027, 2008.

Finnerty JF, Fuerst CW, Karns LB, Pinkeron JV: End-of-life discussions for the primary care obstetrician/gynecologist, *Am J Obstet Gynecol* 187(2):296–301, 2002.

Hospice Care

Dalrymple JL, Levenback C, Wolf JK, et al: Trends among gynecologic oncology inpatient deaths: is end-of-life care improving? *Gynecol Oncol* 85(2):356–361, 2002.

Hogan C, Lunney J, Gabel J, Lynn J: Medicare beneficiaries' cost of care in the last year of life, *Health Aff* 20(4):188–195, 2001.

von Gruenigen V, Daly B, Gibbons H, et al: Indicators of survival duration in ovarian cancer and implications for aggressiveness of care, *Cancer* 112(10):2221–2227, 2008.

Physician-Assisted Suicide/Euthanasia

van der Maas PJ, van der Wal G, Haverkate I, et al: Euthanasia, physician-assisted suicide, and other medical practices involving the end of life in the Netherlands, 1990-1995, *N Engl J Med* 335(22):1699–1705, 1996.

Ethical Considerations

Cain JM, Heintz PM, Swarte NB: End of life care. In Hoskins WJ, Perez CA, Young RC, et al: *Principles and practice of gynecologic oncology*, ed 4, Philadelphia, 2005, Lippincott Williams & Wilkins, pp 1343–1359.

Finnerty JJ, Pinkerton JV, Moreno J, Ferguson JE: Ethical theory and principles: do they have any relevance to problems arising in everyday practice? *Am J Obstet Gynecol* 183(2):301–308, 2000.

Role of Palliative Care Teams, PCPs, and Other Health Care Providers

Hui D, Elsayem A, De La Cruz M, et al: Availability and integration of palliative care at US cancer centers, *JAMA* 303(11):1054–1061, 2010.

Role of the Ob-Gyn

American College of Obstetricians and Gynecologists: ACOG committee opinion no. 403, April 2008: end-of-life decision making, *Obstet Gynecol* 111(4):1021–1027, 2008.

American College of Obstetricians and Gynecologists: ACOG practice bulletin no. 102: management of stillbirth, *Obstet Gynecol* 113(3):748–761, 2009.

Gold KJ, Kuznia AL, Hayward RA: How physicians cope with stillbirth or neonatal death: a national survey of obstetricians, *Obstet Gynecol* 112(1):29–34, 2008.

Hoeldtke NJ, Calhoun BC: Perinatal hospice, *Am J Obstet Gynecol* 185(3):525–529, 2001.

Silver RM: Fetal death, *Obstet Gynecol* 109(1):153–167, 2007.

Chapter 50

Women's Endocrine Disorders (Diabetes and Metabolic Syndrome)

PETER YUAN • RUCHI MATHUR • CAROLYN J. ALEXANDER

KEY UPDATES

Diabetes

1 Diagnosis of diabetes now includes the use of hemoglobin A1C (A1C) with a cutoff point of ≥6.5%.

2 Primary A1C goal for most women with diabetes is <7%.

3 Rosiglitazone is no longer recommended for treatment of diabetes because of concerns about increased cardiovascular risk, whereas pioglitazone does not appear to have the same risk.

4 Patients with diabetes should be treated to a systolic blood pressure <130 and a diastolic <80. There is no cardiovascular benefit targeting a systolic blood pressure <120.

5 In patients with diabetes and without overt cardiovascular disease (CVD), the primary goal is a low-density lipoprotein (LDL) cholesterol level of <100 mg/dL. In individuals with overt CVD, a lower LDL cholesterol goal of <70 mg/dL is an option.

6 Aspirin therapy should be considered for those diabetic women at increased cardiovascular risk (>60 years of age with at least one additional risk factor) without contraindication.

7 Oral hormone therapy may have a protective effect on the development of diabetes mellitus and a neutral or beneficial effect on glycemic control in the setting of established diabetes mellitus.

Metabolic Syndrome

8 The National Cholesterol Education Program (NCEP/ATP III) and International Diabetes Federation definitions are the most widely used criteria for defining metabolic syndrome.

9 Though the estimates of the prevalence of metabolic syndrome are dependent on the criteria used, the overall estimated prevalence of metabolic syndrome in the literature ranges from 20% to 40% in women and increases with age.

10 The literature supports the fact that prevalence estimates may be improved by the intervention of clinicians.

11 Overnutrition leading to abdominal obesity and insulin resistance (IR) may play a role in the pathophysiology of metabolic syndrome.

12 Clinical implications of diagnosing the syndrome include risk of a prothrombotic state, a proinflammatory state, nonalcoholic fatty liver disease, diabetes, and cardiovascular disease.

13 Hyperinsulinemia is a likely common pathogenetic factor for both polycystic ovary syndrome (PCOS) and the metabolic syndrome.

14 Treatment options include weight management, increasing physical activity, and treating cardiovascular risk factors, including the goal of keeping blood pressure below 130/80 mmHg.

15 In women with impaired glucose tolerance, metformin may be beneficial in preventing diabetes.

16 Currently only orlistat has been approved by the Food and Drug Administration (FDA) for long-term use for weight loss. Sibutramine has been recently withdrawn from the U.S. market.

443

Diabetes Mellitus

INTRODUCTION

- Approximately 8.1 million women have diabetes in the United States; prevalence is two to four times higher among black, Hispanic, American Indian, and Asian Pacific Islander women than among white women
- Diabetes is classified as type 1 and type 2; type 1 diabetes results from ß-cell destruction and leads to absolute insulin deficiency, whereas type 2 diabetes results from a progressive insulin secretory defect on the background of insulin resistance
- Lower levels of estrogen, progesterone, and human growth hormone after menopause may contribute to lower metabolism and obesity, leading to type 2 diabetes
- Postmenopausal women with diabetes also have higher rates of premature death, functional disability, and coexisting illnesses such as hypertension, coronary heart disease (CHD), and stroke

DIAGNOSIS

- Testing for diabetes should begin at age 45 years in patients without other risk factors; if results are normal, testing should be repeated at least at 3-year intervals, with consideration of more frequent testing depending on initial results and risk status
- The American Diabetes Association (ADA) recommends earlier testing for all adults that are overweight and have additional risk factors such as physical inactivity, family history of diabetes, women who delivered a baby weighing >9 pounds or were diagnosed with gestational diabetes (GDM), hypertension, dyslipidemia with low high-density lipoprotein (HDL) or elevated triglycerides, women with polycystic ovarian syndrome, history of cardiovascular disease (CVD), or other clinical conditions associated with insulin resistance

UPDATE #1

The diagnosis of diabetes traditionally has been based on plasma glucose criteria, either a fasting value or with an oral glucose tolerance test. Hemoglobin A1C (A1C) is a measure of glycated hemoglobin used to identify the average plasma glucose concentration over prolonged periods of time. The ADA has now included the use of A1C ≥6.5% for diagnosis of diabetes as shown in Table 50-1 (American Diabetes Association, 2010).

TABLE 50-1   Criteria for the Diagnosis of Diabetes

1. A1C ≥6.5%
OR
2. Fasting plasma glucose ≥126 mg/dL (fasting defined as no caloric intake for at least 8 hours)
OR
3. Two-hour plasma glucose ≥200 during a 75 g OGTT
OR
4. In a patient with classic symptoms of hyperglycemia or hyperglycemia crisis, a random plasma glucose ≥200 mg/dL

From Standards of medical care in diabetes-2010, *Diabetes Care*, 33(Suppl 1), Table 2, 2010.

Diabetes Care

GLYCEMIC CONTROL

- Glycemic control is primarily assessed by patient self-monitoring of blood glucose (SMGB) and A1C
- SMBG is recommended three or more times daily to reach A1C targets safely without hypoglycemia (plasma glucose <70 mg/dL)

UPDATE #2

The glycemic goal in general is an A1C of <7%. Lowering A1C to below or around 7% has been shown to reduce microvascular and neuropathic complications. The DCCT, a prospective randomized controlled trial (RCT) of intensive versus standard glycemic control in type 1 diabetics, showed that improved glycemic control is associated with significantly decreased rates of microvascular and neuropathic complications (Diabetes Control and Complications Trial Research Group, 1993). The UK Prospective Diabetes Study (UKPDS) trial in patients with type 2 diabetes demonstrated significant reductions in microvascular and neuropathic complications with intensive therapy (UK Prospective Diabetes Study (UKPDS) Group, 1998).

- Table 50-2 demonstrates the average glucose per A1C level
- The ADVANCE study randomized type 2 diabetics to intensive glycemic control with a sulfonylurea and additional medications as needed to achieve a target A1C of ≤6.5% or to standard therapy achieving a median A1C of 7%; intensive therapy significantly reduced microvascular events and major adverse cardiovascular events
- The ACCORD study randomized 10,251 diabetic patients with CVD or significant CVD risk to an intensive control arm (target A1C <6.0%) or standard glycemic control (A1C target 7% to 7.9%); though the study was halted midway, participants with no previous CVD event and those who had a baseline A1C <8% had a statistically significant reduction in the primary CVD outcome
- It is recommended that patients with a short duration of diabetes, long life expectancy, and no significant cardiovascular disease can be considered for an even lower goal of A1C than the general goal of <7%, if this can be achieved without significant hypoglycemia
- Alternatively less stringent A1C goals than the general goal of <7% may be appropriate for patients with a history of severe hypoglycemia, limited life expectancy,

TABLE 50-2   Correlation of A1C with Average Glucose

A1C (%)	Mean Plasma Glucose (mg/dL)	Mean Plasma Glucose (mmol/l)
6	126	7.0
7	154	8.6
8	183	10.2
9	212	11.8
10	240	13.4
11	269	14.9
12	298	16.5

From Standards of medical care in diabetes-2010, *Diabetes Care*, 33(Suppl 1), Table 9, 2010.

advanced microvascular or macrovascular complications and extensive comorbid conditions, and those with long-standing diabetes in whom the general goal is difficult to achieve

THERAPY FOR TYPE 1 DIABETES

- In the DCCT study, therapy was carried out with short- and intermediate-acting human insulin; despite better microvascular outcomes, intensive insulin therapy was associated with a high rate of severe hypoglycemia (62 episodes per 100 patient-years of therapy)
- Since the time of the DCCT, a number of rapid-acting analogues have been developed, as shown in Table 50-3; they are associated with less hypoglycemia with equal A1C lower in type 1 diabetes
- Recommended therapy for type 1 diabetes therefore consists of the use of either multiple-dose insulin injections or continuous subcutaneous insulin infusion (CSII) or insulin pump therapy

THERAPY FOR TYPE 2 DIABETES

- The ADA consensus guidelines for the treatment of type 2 diabetes recommend intervening at the time of diagnosis with metformin in combination with lifestyle changes; if A1C goals are not achieved, basal insulin or a sulfonylurea can be added
- The initiation of intensive insulin therapy can ultimately be used to achieve glycemic control; less well validated therapies but still included in the ADA algorithm include the addition of pioglitazone, or a GLP-1 agonist such as exenatide
- Modest weight loss has been shown to reduce insulin resistance in overweight and obese insulin-resistant individuals
- Regular exercise has also been shown to improve blood glucose control, reduce cardiovascular risk factors, contribute to weight loss, and improve well-being
- Structured exercise interventions of at least 8-week durations have been shown to lower A1C by an average of 0.66% in type 2 diabetes patients, even with no significant change in body mass index (BMI)

- Biguanides' (metformin) major effect is to decrease hepatic glucose output and lower fasting glycemia; it is not usually accompanied by hypoglycemia and may be associated with moderate weight loss; its use is contraindicated in patients with renal dysfunction with a creatinine clearance of <30 mL/min because it can cause lactic acidosis; the UKPDS demonstrated a beneficial effect of metformin on CVD outcomes
- Sulfonylureas (glipizide, glimepiride) lower glycemia by enhancing insulin secretion; the major adverse effect is hypoglycemia, which is more severe and frequent in the elderly; sulfonylurea therapy does not appear to increase CVD mortality based on the UK prospective diabetes study (UKPDS) and ADVANCE studies (1998, 2008)
- Meglitinides (nateglinide, repaglinide) act by stimulating insulin secretion but bind to a different site within the sulfonylurea receptor; they have a shorter circulating half-life than sulfonylureas and must be administered more frequently, but hypoglycemia may be less frequent than with some sulfonylureas
- Insulin was initially developed to treat the insulin-deficient type 1 diabetic patient but is also effective in treating patients with type 2 diabetes; initial therapy is aimed at increasing basal insulin supply usually with long-acting insulin such as insulin glargine or insulin detemir; patients may also require prandial therapy with rapid-acting insulin such as insulin aspart or insulin lispro
- Insulin therapy has beneficial effects on triglycerides and HDL cholesterol levels but is associated with weight gain; insulin therapy is associated with hypoglycemia, but the risk of hypoglycemia has been reduced with the newer insulin analogues
- α-Glucosidase inhibitors (acarbose) reduce the rate of digestion of polysaccharides in the proximal small intestine, primarily lowering postprandial glucose levels, without causing hypoglycemia; its main side effect is gastrointestinal discomfort, and it should not be used in patients with liver disease
- Thiazolidinediones (TZDs: pioglitazone, rosiglitazone) are peroxisome proliferator-activated γ receptor modulators; they increase the sensitivity of muscle, fat, and liver to endogenous and exogenous insulin; the most common adverse effects are

TABLE 50-3 Insulin Comparison Chart

	Onset of Action	Peak Effect	Duration of Action
Rapid Acting			
Aspart (Novolog)	12-18 min	1-3 hours	3-5 hours
Glulisine (Apridra)	12-30 min	1.6-2.8 hours	3-4 hours
Lispro (Humalog)	15-30 min	0.5-2.5 hours	≤5 hours
Short Acting			
Regular	0.5 hour	2.5-5 hours	4-12 hours
Intermediate Acting			
NPH	1-2 hours	4-12 hours	14-24 hours
Long Acting			
Glargine (Lantus)	4-6 hours	Peakless	Generally 24 hours or longer
Detemir (Levemir)	3-4 hours	Relatively flat 3-9 hours	Dose-dependent 6-23 hours

Data from manufacturers' package inserts.

TABLE 50-4   Noninsulin Therapies for Type 2 Diabetes

Intervention	Efficacy (% Decrease in A1C)	Comments
Biguanide (metformin)	1.0-2.0	Weight neutral; GI side effects; contraindicated in renal insufficiency because of lactic acidosis; potential benefit on cardiovascular outcomes
Sulfonylurea (glipizide, glimepiride)	1.0-2.0	Rapid glucose lowering effect; weight gain, hypoglycemia; does not appear to have detrimental cardiovascular effects in large RCTs
TZD (pioglitazone)	0.5-1.4	Improves lipid profile; fluid retention, weight gain, and increased risk of bone fractures; contraindicated in CHF; pioglitazone appears to have beneficial cardiovascular outcomes
Meglitinides (nateglinide, repaglinide)	0.5-1.5	Less risk of hypoglycemia compared to sulfonylureas; weight gain
DPP-4 inhibitors (sitagliptin, saxagliptin)	0.5-0.8	Weight neutral; low risk of hypoglycemia and can be used in renal impairment
α-Glucosidase inhibitors (acarbose)	0.5-0.8	Weight neutral; frequent GI side effects; does not cause hypoglycemia as monotherapy
GLP-1 agonist (exenatide, liraglutide)	0.5 -1.0	Associated with weight loss; frequent GI side effects and increased risk for pancreatitis; requires twice daily or daily injections
Amylin Agonist (pramlintide)	0.5-1.0	Associated with weight loss; frequent GI side effects; requires three injections daily

Adapted from Medical management of hyperglycemia in type 2 diabetes: a consensus algorithm for the initiation and adjustment of therapy, *Diabetes Care* 32(1), Table 1, 2009.

weight gain and fluid retention, with peripheral edema and increased risk for congestive heart failure
- Table 50-4 reviews noninsulin therapies for type 2 diabetics

UPDATE #3

The Rosiglitazone evaluated for cardiovascular outcomes in oral agent combination therapy for type 2 diabetes (RECORD) trial found that addition of rosiglitazone increased the risk of heart failure in patients with type 2 diabetes on metformin and sulfonylurea. Recently several meta-analyses have suggested a 30% to 40% relative increase in risk for myocardial infarctions with rosiglitazone (Home et al, 2009). Given the potential for increased cardiovascular risk associated with rosiglitazone, a consensus statement from the American Diabetes Association and the European Association for the Study of Diabetes advised against the use of rosiglitazone (Nathan et al, 2009). The increased cardiovascular risk suggested with rosiglitazone does not appear to be a class effect to all TZDs. The Prospective Pioglitazone Clinical Trial in macrovascular events (PROactive) found a significant 16% reduction in death, myocardial infarction, and stroke with pioglitazone use compared with placebo (Dormandy et al, 2005).

- Glucagon-like peptide-1 agonists (exenatide, liraglutide) are long lasting agonists of naturally occurring peptides produced by the small intestine and potentiate glucose-stimulated insulin secretion; they are not associated with hypoglycemia and can cause a modest weight decrease; main side effects include nausea and vomiting, and they have been associated with an increased risk of pancreatitis
- Dipeptidyl peptidase 4 (DPP-4) inhibitors (sitagliptin, saxagliptin) are inhibitors of enzymes in the body that are responsible for degrading GLP-1 and glucose-dependent insulinotropic peptide (GIP); these medications increase the effects of the body's endogenous GLP-1 and GIPs; DPP-4 inhibitors do not cause hypoglycemia when used as monotherapy and appear to be well tolerated

- Amylin agonist (pramlintide) mimic the ß-cell hormone amylin; it is administered subcutaneously before meals and slows gastric emptying, inhibits glucagon production in a glucose-dependent fashion, and predominately decreases postprandial glucose excursions; currently pramlintide is approved for use in the United States only as adjunctive therapy with regular insulin or rapid-acting insulin analogues

Prevention and Management of Cardiovascular Disease in Women with Diabetes

CLINICAL PROFILE

- CVD is a major cause of morbidity and mortality for individuals with diabetes; the common conditions coexisting with type 2 diabetes, hypertension, and dyslipidemia are clear risk factors for CVD, and diabetes itself confers independent risk
- A meta-analysis of prospective cohort studies found that the relative risk for fatal coronary heart disease associated with diabetes is 50% higher in women than it is in men
- This greater excess risk factor for coronary heart disease may be explained by more adverse cardiovascular risk profiles among women with diabetes combined with possible disparities in treatment that favor men

HYPERTENSION

- Hypertension is a common comorbidity of diabetes that affects the majority of patients with increased prevalence as women age
- In type 1 diabetes, hypertension is often the result of underlying nephropathy, whereas in type 2 diabetes it usually coexists with other cardiometabolic risk factors

UPDATE #4

Patients with diabetes should be treated to a systolic blood pressure <130 mmHg and a diastolic blood pressure <80 mmHg. The UKPDS trial showed a 32% reduction in deaths related to diabetes, a 44% reduction in stroke, and a 37% reduction in microvascular end points in type 2 diabetes with tight blood pressure control (<150/85 mmHg) (UK Prospective Diabetes Study Group, 1998). There does not appear to be additional benefit to targeting a systolic blood pressure of less than 120 mmHg in patients with diabetes. The ACCORD blood pressure study evaluated 4733 patients with type 2 diabetes, randomly assigning them to intensive therapy targeting a systolic pressure of less than 120 mmHg or standard therapy targeting a systolic pressure of less than 140 mmHg; it showed no difference (ACCORD Study Group et al, 2010).

- Pharmacologic therapy should include either an angiotensin-converting enzyme (ACE) inhibitor or an angiotensin II receptor blocker

DYSLIPIDEMIA

- Women with type 2 diabetes have an increased prevalence of lipid abnormalities, contributing to their high risk of CVD
- Multiple clinical trials have demonstrated significant effects of pharmacologic therapy (stains) on CVD outcomes in subjects with CHD and for primary DVD prevention
- Analyses of diabetic subgroups of larger trials and trials specifically in subjects with diabetes showed a significant primary and secondary prevention of CVD events with and without CHD deaths in diabetic populations on statin therapy

UPDATE #5

- The primary goal is a low-density lipoprotein (LDL) of <100 mg/dL in individuals without overt CVD and in individuals with overt CVD; a lower LDL cholesterol goal of <70 mg/dL, using a high-dose statin, is an option, as recent clinical trials in high-risk patients, such as those with acute coronary syndromes or previous cardiovascular events, have demonstrated that more aggressive therapy with high doses of statins to achieve an LDL cholesterol of <70 mg/dL led to a significant reduction in further events (Grundy et al, 2004)
- Low levels of HDL cholesterol, often associated with elevated triglyceride levels, are the most prevalent pattern of dyslipidemia in women with type 2 diabetes
- In a large trial specific to diabetic patients, fenofibrate failed to reduce overall cardiovascular outcomes
- Lipid-lowering goals for women with type 1 diabetes should be similar to those with type 2 diabetes

ANTIPLATELET AGENTS

UPDATE #6

Consider aspirin therapy as a primary prevention strategy in diabetic women with increased cardiovascular risk (women >60 with one other cardiovascular risk) and as a secondary prevention strategy in women with diabetes and a history of CVD. Aspirin has been shown to be effective in reducing cardiovascular morbidity and mortality in high-risk patients with previous myocardial infarction (MI) or stroke (secondary prevention). A recent meta-analysis of six large trials of aspirin for primary prevention found a 12% reduction of serious vascular events, mainly the result of a reduction of nonfatal myocardial infarction and reduced stroke in women (Antithrombotic Trialists' [ATT] Collaboration, 2009).

SMOKING CESSATION

- Advise all patients not to smoke, as patients with diabetes that smoke have a heightened risk of CVD and premature death

Menopause in Women with Diabetes

INTRODUCTION

- Women commonly experience vasomotor symptoms, vaginal dryness, urinary incontinence, and sleep disturbances around the time of menopause
- These symptoms may be difficult to distinguish from hypoglycemia, and women should be educated about the need to increase the frequency of blood glucose monitoring at the beginning of the menopausal transition to help distinguish between the two
- Women with diabetes may also undergo menopause several years earlier than women without diabetes

DIABETES RISK IN POSTMENOPAUSAL WOMEN

- Diabetes risk increases with advancing age, but whether menopausal status influences diabetes risk independent of age is unclear
- One longitudinal study of 949 women investigated the natural history of the menopausal transition; in this study, 13.7% of the study group developed this syndrome by the time the women reached menopause independent of age of menopause, ethnicity, and BMI
- Menopause is also associated with changes in body composition, which lead to impairments in insulin sensitivity and glucose metabolism; postmenopausal women have increased fat mass, increased abdominal fat, and decreased lean body mass in comparison to premenopausal women independent of age leading to increased insulin resistance
- A secondary analysis of postmenopausal women in the Postmenopausal Estrogen/Progestin Intervention study found an independent association between increased BMI and waist-to-hip ratio with increased fasting and postchallenge levels of glucose and insulin

POSTMENOPAUSAL HORMONE THERAPY AND GLYCEMIC CONTROL

- Postmenopausal women with diabetes who elect to use hormone therapy to improve their vasomotor symptoms should not anticipate any deterioration in their current level of glycemic control
- Epidemiologic studies have shown that use of hormone therapy is associated with improved glycemic control; the Northern California Kaiser Permanente Diabetes registry reported that hormone therapy was associated with a reduction in HbA1C level of about 0.5%, independent of age, ethnicity, obesity, education, exercise, disease duration, treatment type, and monitoring practices
- Randomized clinical trials suggest that postmenopausal women who use hormone therapy may also have a decreased risk of developing diabetes
- The Heart and Estrogen/Progestin Replacement Study evaluated 2763 postmenopausal women with coronary

heart disease treated with 0.625 mg of conjugated estrogen plus 2.5 mg of medroxyprogesterone acetate daily versus placebo; it found that in women with coronary disease, hormone therapy was associated with a 35% reduction in the incidence of newly diagnosed diabetes when compared with women on placebo (6.2% in hormone-therapy group versus 9.5% in placebo group)

- The Women's Health Initiative Hormone Trial studied 15,641 postmenopausal women and found the cumulative incidence of type 2 diabetes was 3.5% among women randomly assigned combined conjugated equine estrogen and medroxyprogesterone acetate treatment compared to 4.2% among women on placebo; this was thought to be mediated by a decrease in insulin resistance unrelated to body size based on changes in fasting glucose and insulin, indicating a significant fall in insulin resistance in the treatment women at the first year of follow-up

UPDATE #7

Oral hormone therapy appears to have multiple beneficial effects on glycemic control in postmenopausal women with diabetes. In a randomized, blinded cross-over trial of 25 postmenopausal women with type 2 diabetes treated with conjugated equine estrogen at 0.625 mg/day, subjects were found to have lower levels of fasting glucose, HgA1C, and postprandial glucose when compared with placebo (Friday et al, 2001). Given the risks associated with the use of conventional postmenopausal hormone therapy regimes, they are not recommended for primary prevention or treatment of diabetes mellitus.

Metabolic Syndrome

DEFINITIONS

- The metabolic syndrome is defined as a clustering of components that reflects overnutrition, sedentary lifestyles, and resultant excess adiposity and includes a clustering of abdominal obesity, insulin resistance, dyslipidemia, and elevated blood pressure (Cornier et al, 2008)
- Because the metabolic syndrome is a cluster of different conditions and not a single disease, multiple concurrent definitions have resulted; there are five current definitions of metabolic syndrome:
  1. National Cholesterol Education Program's Adult Treatment Panel III (NCEP/ATP III) (Table 50-5)

  2. International Diabetes Federation (IDF) (see Table 50-5)
  3. Group for the Study of Insulin Resistance (EGIR)
  4. World Health Organization (WHO)
  4. American Association of Clinical Endocrinologists (AACE)
- In 1998, the first official definition of metabolic syndrome was published by WHO, including the presence of IR. The EGIR definition did not include microalbuminuria and the AACE definition excluded patients with type 2 diabetes

UPDATE #8

The National Cholesterol Education Program (NCEP/ATP III) and the International Diabetes Federation definitions for the metabolic syndrome are the most widely accepted. The NCEP/ATPIII definition differed from both the WHO and EGIR definition in that the presence of insulin resistance was not a necessary criterion. Its primary purpose was to identify individuals at high risk for CVD that extended beyond the traditional cardiac risk factors. The IDF definition emphasized central obesity as a necessary condition to make the diagnosis of the metabolic syndrome (MetS) (Meigs, 2006). See Table 50-5. Guidelines define the metabolic syndrome in *women* as the presence of any *three* of the following:
1. Abdominal waist circumference 35 inches in women
2. Serum hypertriglyceridemia ≥150 mg/dL or drug treatment for elevated triglycerides (treatment with one or more of fibrates or niacin)
3. Serum high-density lipoprotein (HDL) cholesterol 50 mg/dL or drug treatment for low HDL
4. Blood pressure ≥130/85 mmHg or drug treatment for elevated blood pressure
5. Fasting glucose ≥100 mg/dL (5.6 mmol/L) or drug treatment for elevated blood glucose

- Overnutrition, sedentary lifestyle, and abdominal adiposity are concerning signs of metabolic syndrome; identifying a woman with metabolic syndrome provides the opportunity to emphasize lifestyle changes that may decrease her risk of cardiovascular disease in the future

EPIDEMIOLOGY

- Metabolic syndrome is increasing in prevalence, paralleling an increasing epidemic of obesity

TABLE 50-5   The Definitions of Metabolic Syndrome for Women

Definitions	NCEP/ATP III 2005	International Diabetes Federation (IDF) 2005
Required number of abnormalities	≥3 of:	Waist circumference (WC) >88 cm* and ≥2 of:
Glucose	≥100 mg/dL or drug treatment for elevated blood glucose	≥100 mg/dL or diagnosed diabetes
HDL	<50 mg/dL or drug treatment for low HDL-C	Same
Triglycerides	≥150 mg/dL or drug treatment for elevated triglycerides	Same
Obesity	WC ≥88 cm*	
Hypertension	≥130/85 mmHg or drug treatment for hypertension	Same

*For South Asian, Chinese, and Japanese patients, ≥80 cm.
Modified from Meigs J: Metabolic syndrome and the risk for type 2 diabetes, *Expert Rev Endocrin Metab* 1:57, Table 1, 2006.

- At routine visits, clinicians should assess individuals for metabolic risk; the assessment should include a measurement of blood pressure, waist circumference, fasting lipid profile, and fasting glucose

Pathophysiology

- The infusion of FFAs into the portal vein activates the sympathetic nervous system and elevates blood pressure in the animal model
- In addition, adipose tissue is a source of proinflammatory cytokines that may play a role in liver and skeletal muscle insulin action

Risk of Cardiovascular Disease

- The majority of studies have noted that women with metabolic syndrome have a high risk of developing cardiovascular disease and dyslipidemia

- There is an ongoing debate as to whether the clustering of risk factors in metabolic syndrome is greater or simply the risk of obesity; according to three meta-analyses, the metabolic syndrome increases the risk for incident cardiovascular disease with relative risks ranging from 1.53 to 2.18 and all-cause mortality relative risks 1.27 to 1.60
- Elevated triglyceride and low HDL cholesterol levels are strong predictors of vascular events
- Ingelsson et al. evaluated the prevalence and prognostic impact of subclinical cardiovascular disease in individuals with the metabolic syndrome and diabetes; the key point of this study noted that underlying subclinical CVD—as measured by ECG, echocardiography, carotid ultrasound, and ankle-brachial blood pressure—in patients with metabolic syndrome may cause the increased risk of CVD. In the Framingham Offspring study, subclinical CVD was also predictive of overt CVD in subjects without metabolic syndrome (hazard ratio [HR] 1.93, 95% confidence interval [CI] 1.15 to 3.24)

Risk of Diabetes Mellitus

- The NCEP/ATP III and IDF definitions include elevated fasting plasma glucose as an essential, but not required, criterion for defining the presence of metabolic syndrome
- The Insulin Resistance Atherosclerosis Study found that IDF and NCEP/ATP III MetS definitions predicted incidence of diabetes as well as the WHO definition, despite the first two not requiring the use of an oral glucose tolerance test or a measure of insulin resistance
- The rise in prevalence of type 2 diabetes is worrisome, and the presence of metabolic syndrome and insulin resistance has an additive effect with a potentially six- to sevenfold increased risk (Meigs, 2006)
- The presence of metabolic syndrome in women with gestational diabetes substantially increases the risk of developing diabetes (Verma A, Boney C, Tucker R et al, 2002)

Other Conditions Possibly Associated with Metabolic Syndrome

- It is controversial whether or not to measure levels of adipokines or c-reactive protein levels

Hyperinsulinemia is likely a common pathogenetic factor for the development of both polycystic ovary syndrome (PCOS) and the metabolic syndrome (Ehrmann et al, 2006). The metabolic abnormalities of PCOS overlap with the criteria of the metabolic syndrome, a clustering of both dyslipidemia and other factors that identify patients at increased risk for coronary heart disease and type 2 diabetes mellitus. These factors include central obesity, hypertension, and elevated fasting glucose levels. A multicenter trial by Ehrmann et al. (2006), undertaken to predict the prevalence of metabolic syndrome in women with PCOS, reported the waist circumference exceeded 88 cm in 80%, HDL cholesterol was less than 50 mg/dL in 66%, triglycerides were 150 mg/dL or greater in 32%, blood pressure was 130/85 mmHg or greater in 21%, and fasting glucose concentrations were 110 mg/dL or greater in 5%. Family history of diabetes in women with PCOS may be a risk factor for the development of metabolic syndrome.

Treatment Modalities (Table 50-6)

- Lifestyle modification and weight loss are essential in the treatment plan for patients with the metabolic syndrome; modest weight loss can decrease fasting blood glucose, insulin, and hemoglobin A1C

Treatment targets include abdominal obesity, insulin resistance, dyslipidemia, hypertension, prothrombotic, and proinflammatory states. Options include weight management, increasing physical activity, and pharmacotherapy treating cardiovascular risk factors. Goals include keeping blood pressure below 130/80 mmHg, lowering LDL cholesterol, raising HDL cholesterol, and considering low-dose aspirin in high-risk patients (Cornier et al, 2008).

DIET

- A decrease in caloric intake is an avenue by which to promote a chronic negative energy balance resulting in weight loss

- Low glycemic index foods have been shown to improve components of the metabolic syndrome including hyperlipidemia and hyperglycemia
- The 2005 USDA Dietary Guidelines promote a reduction in saturated fat intake (<7% of caloric intake) and an increase in the unsaturated fatty acids, specifically linoleic (5% to 10% of caloric intake) and α-linolenic (0.7% to 1.6% of caloric intake)
- The Dietary Approaches to Stop Hypertension (DASH) diet showed that lower sodium intake reduced blood pressure in patients with high-normal blood pressure and mild hypertension; guidelines therefore recommend that daily sodium intake should be restricted to no more than 65 to 100 mmol
- Niacin has favorable effects on essentially all of the abnormalities of the metabolic dyslipidemia; combination therapy of niacin and a statin produces greater effects on lipid levels than does either agent given alone
- Supplementation with marine omega-3 polyunsaturated fatty acids (PUFAs) may be indicated in metabolic syndrome patients presenting with combined dyslipidemia

EXERCISE

- Exercise improves glucose homeostasis by enhancing glucose transport and insulin action in working skeletal muscle; higher cardiorespiratory fitness and increased physical activity have been shown to be inversely related to cardiovascular disease (CVD) mortality and to the incidence of impaired glucose tolerance (IGT) and type 2 diabetes (T2D)
- Exercise training has beneficial effects on lipids and lipoproteins and may have additional impact when combined with dietary modification and weight loss

MEDICATIONS

In women with impaired glucose tolerance, metformin may be beneficial in preventing diabetes. Metformin is a biguanide agent that has a primary mechanism of action of reducing

---

TABLE 50-6   Treatment for the Metabolic Syndrome Risk Factors

Therapeutic Target	Goals and Recommendations
Abdominal obesity	5%-10% weight loss or weight maintenance Lifestyle modification with diet and increased physical activity Pharmacologic weight loss therapy Bariatric surgery
IR/Hyperglycemia	Prevention or delay of progression to type 2 diabetes Lifestyle modification and weight loss as described above Pharmacotherapy Treatment of diabetes (appropriate glycemic control)
Metabolic dyslipidemia Primary target: LDL-C Secondary target: non-HDL-C Tertiary target: HDL-C	LDL-C lowering If TG ≥200 mg/dL, lower non-HDL-C to <30 mg/dL plus the LDL-C goal If HDL-C <50 mg/dL, consider therapy for HDL-C raising
Elevated BP	Goal BP is <140/90 mmHg (<130/80 mmHg if diabetes or CKD present)
Prothrombotic state	Consider low-dose aspirin for high-risk patients
Proinflammatory state	No specific goals; treat all of the above risk factors

Modified from Cornier M, Dabelea D, Hernandez T, et al: The metabolic syndrome, *Endocr Rev* 29(7):777-822; 2008.

hepatic glucose production and that has been shown to reduce the progression of diabetes from impaired glucose tolerance by approximately 31% in the DPP, of which 53% had the metabolic syndrome (Knowler et al, 2002). The incidence of the metabolic syndrome was also reduced by 17% in the metformin-treated group of the DPP, which was driven primarily by improvements in waist circumference (WC) and fasting glucose (Orchard et al, 2005).

- The length of time of treatment with metformin has yet to be determined
- Although thiazolidinediones may reduce waist-to-hip ratio and improve blood pressure, triglycerides, high-density lipoprotein-cholesterol complex (HDL-C), and liver-related transaminases, the use of glitazones in general has been controversial with some studies reporting an increased incidence of cardiovascular disease

UPDATE #16

Currently only orlistat is FDA approved for long-term use for weight loss. Torgerson et al. performed a 4-year randomized controlled study of orlistat and showed a significant reduction in the progression to diabetes in high-risk individuals (Torgerson et al, 2004). Sibutramine is a centrally acting serotonin-norepinephrine reuptake inhibitor structurally related to amphetamines that was approved by the FDA in 1997. The maker of the weight-loss drug sibutramine has recently agreed to withdraw it from the U.S. market, following evidence of increased cardiovascular risk among patients taking the drug. The European post-marketing Sibutramine Cardiovascular Outcomes (SCOUT) trial revealed nonfatal myocardial infarction or stroke, resuscitated cardiac arrest, or cardiovascular death rates of 11.4% among patients taking sibutramine versus 10% in the placebo group

SUGGESTED READINGS

Diabetes Suggested Readings

Diabetes Care

ACCORD Study Group, Cushman WC, Evans GW, et al: Effects of intensive blood-pressure control in type 2 diabetes mellitus, *N Engl J Med* 362(17):1575–1585, 2010.

ACCORD Study Group, et al: Effects of combination lipid therapy in type 2 diabetes mellitus, *N Engl J Med* 362(17):1563–1574, 2010.

Action to Control Cardiovascular Risk in Diabetes Study Group, Gerstein HC, Miller ME, et al: Effects of intensive glucose lowering in type 2 diabetes, *N Engl J Med* 358(24):2545–2559, 2008.

American Diabetes Association: Standards of medical care in diabetes—2010, *Diabetes Care* 33(Suppl 1):S11–S61, 2010.

Menopause in Women with Diabetes

Kanaya AM, Herrington D, Bittinghoff E, et al: Glycemic effects of postmenopausal hormone therapy: the Heart and Estrogen/Progestin Replacement Study: a randomized, double-blind, placebo-controlled trial, *Ann Intern Med* 138(1):1–9, 2003.

Margolis KL, Bonds DE, Rodabough RJ, et al: Effect of oestrogen plus progestin on the incidence of diabetes in postmenopausal women: results for the Women's Health Initiative hormone trial, *Diabetologia* 47(7):1175–1187, 2004.

Metabolic Syndrome

Cornier M, Dabelea D, Hernandez T, et al: The metabolic syndrome, *Endocr Rev* 29(7):777–822, 2008.

Ehrmann DA, Liljenquist DR, Kasza K, et al: Prevalence and predictors of the metabolic syndrome in women with polycystic ovary syndrome, *J Clin Endocrinol Metab* 91(1):48–53, 2006.

Orchard TJ, Temprosa M, Goldberg R, et al: The effect of metformin and intensive lifestyle intervention on the metabolic syndrome: the Diabetes Prevention Program randomized trial, *Ann Intern Med* 142:611–619, 2005.

Verma A, Boney C, Tucker R, et al: Insulin resistance syndrome in women with prior history of gestational diabetes mellitus, *JCEM* 87(7):3227, 2002.

References

Please go to expertconsult.com to view references.

Chapter 51

Women's Autoimmunity

DANIEL KAHN

KEY UPDATES

1 T regulatory cells are powerful subset of CD4+ T cells with the capability to suppress other T-cell activation and function through bystander effect.

2 Viral infections may serve as the antigenic bridge to the breakdown of tolerance leading to autoimmunity.

3 Female sex hormones predispose to T_H1-or T_H2-like responses, depending on the hormonal state of the woman.

4 Numerous treatments have been developed based on our growing understanding of the normal immune regulation.

Understanding autoimmune diseases and their therapies requires a basic understanding of normal immune function and the regulation of immune responses. This chapter briefly recounts basic immunology.

Immune System

IMMUNE RESPONSE

- Innate: preexisting receptor-mediated strategies to recognize and begin clearance of pathogens
  - Toll-like receptors (TLRs) bind (recognize) fundamental bacterial and viral products, resulting in an inflammatory response
- Adaptive: immune response matures into a highly efficient and specific response to limit "collateral damage"

ORGANS

- Lymph nodes: clusters of lymphoid cells bathed in interstitial fluid to provide surveillance of tissues
- Spleen: clusters of lymphoid cells to provide immune surveillance of blood
- Bone marrow: primary site of origin of lymphoid cells in order to resupply the body
- Thymus: primary site of T-lymphocyte maturation (education)

LYMPHOCYTES

- T cells
  - Bone marrow derived, these cells migrate initially to the thymus; in the thymus, these cells undergo both a positive selection process for functional T-cell receptor (TCR) expression and negative selection (elimination) for self-reactive TCR expression (central tolerance)
  - Two major classes of T cells emerge: CD8+ and CD4+
    - CD8+ T cells (cytotoxic/effector/killer) engage and eliminate host cells that express proteins that are not recognized as normal or self (e.g., viral or tumor

proteins); for example, a normal respiratory mucosal cell infected with adenovirus will express viral proteins against which the CD8+ T cell recognizes and activates; activation of a CD8+ T cell results in target destruction of the virally infected cell
  - CD4+ T cells (helper T cells) are activated by exogenous foreign or abnormal proteins that are consumed by antigen presenting cells (APC) and presented to the CD4+ T cell; CD4+ T cells are able to "decide" if proteins are self or nonself; when activated, CD4+ T cells secrete paracrine and autocrine hormones to enhance the function of lymphocytes; these "cytokines" act at the local level (though they often can be detected in circulation) to change the function of all lymphoid cell types; initially, CD4+ T cells were found to be required ("help") for CD8+ T cell ("Killer T cells") function through the secretion of interleukin – 2 (IL-2)
- B cells
  - Bone marrow derived; these cells circulate the body and populate lymph nodes and spleen
  - Activated B cells mature to plasma cells and secrete large amounts of immunoglobulin
    - Immunoglobulins consist of a *constant* domain and two *variable* domains
    - Variable domains bind (recognize) target antigens
    - Constant domains facilitate uptake by antigen-presenting cells (macrophages, dendritic cells, B cells)
  - Recognize diverse range of substances (e.g., proteins, carbohydrates, lipids) via surface-bound immunoglobulin, the B cell receptor (BCR)
- Natural killer cells
  - Semi-restricted TCR
  - Killer function autonomous of CD4+ T cell help
  - Activates against cells lacking endogenous protein expression (MHC I)
- Macrophage
  - In circulation as monocytes

- Populate organ tissues to provide immune surveillance and tissue repair (clearance of dead cells/debris)
- Resident organ macrophages
  - Brain: Microglia
  - Liver: Kupffer cells
  - Lung: type II alveolar pneumocytes
- Dendritic cells
  - Populate lymphoid tissues (e.g., lymph nodes)
  - Phagocytic behavior similar to tissue macrophages, but with enhanced capacity
  - Secrete cytokines to influence the CD4+ T cell response (prejudices the T helper response)

IMMUNE RESPONSE

- Antigen presentation
  - Every cell expresses major histocompatibility complex (MHC) class I; endogenous cellular derived peptides are expressed on the surface with MHC I; CD8+ T cells recognize peptide + MHC I
  - Exogenous proteins (cellular debris, invasive organisms such as bacteria) are consumed and broken down by macrophages/dendritic cells/B cells; these peptides are loaded (noncovalently) to MHC class II in the endosome; these complexes are subsequently trafficked to the cell surface for potential interaction with CD4+ T cells
- Cellular
  - When CD8+ T cells recognize a peptide MHC class I complex, these killer T cells up-regulate the high-affinity IL-2 receptor on their cell surfaces; when the CD4+ T cell also recognizes a peptide MHC class II complex in the same local, these cells begin to secrete large amounts of IL-2; in this manner, the CD4+ T cells provide *help* to the CD8+ *killer* T cell; The CD8+ killer T cell then induces the cell expressing antigenic peptide – MHC class I complex to undergo apoptosis
  - In addition to providing cytokine support (IL-2) to the killer T cell, the CD4+ helper T cell releases other cytokines (e.g., IFN-γ and IL-17) that activate macrophages and neutrophils to increase their phagocytic activity in order to deal with cellular debris from the action of the CD8+ *killer* T cells
- Humoral
  - When a B cell encounters an antigen to which it recognizes (via the surface-bound immunoglobulin), it will initially endocytose the antigen and attempt to "load" (noncovalently complex) onto MHC class II in the endosome
  - Subsequent display of peptide antigen – MHC class II complex has the potential to activate CD4+ T cells
  - In this environment, the CD4+ T cell will activate and release cytokine support to the B cell (primarily through the action of IL-4)
  - CD4+ T cell support of B cells enhances B cell immunoglobulin class switching and affinity maturation; additionally, B cells mature under cytokine stimulation to highly productive immunoglobulin plasma cell

Immune Regulation

SELF VERSUS NONSELF

- Immune responses limit pathogenic invasion by targeted killing; causing destruction is a necessary part of a successful immune response; the immune system has evolved to readily distinguish between harmful or benign targets through learning what is "self" (benign) and what is "nonself" (harmful)
- T cells are selected in the thymus during development for TCR that bind with sufficient avidity to either MCH class I (CD8+ T cells) or MCH class II (CD4+ T cells)
- B cells are selected (by growth advantage) for high-affinity variable chain expression in the lymph node

TOLERANCE

- Central
  - T cells
    - T cells with TCRs that recognize antigen in the thymus (that presumably displays a complete panel of self-antigens) results in activation; in this developmental context, activation through the TCR causes the cell to undergo apoptosis; thus, potentially autoreactive T cell clones are deleted (*central tolerance*)
  - B cells
    - As B cells mature in the bone marrow, immature B cells that recognize (activate through the surface-bound immunoglobin) cause the cell to undergo apoptosis (*central tolerance*)
- Peripheral
  - Despite the power of *central tolerance* to eliminate the majority of autoreactive T and B cells, it is clear that potentially autoreactive T and B cells can be identified in otherwise healthy individuals

MECHANISMS

- Cytokine deviation
  - CD4+ T cells, when stimulated, can express a pattern of cytokines to drive an immune response in a specific direction; this pattern of cytokine production is known as *immune deviation*
  - There are four distinct cytokine-producing phenotypes currently appreciated into which a naïve T cell may mature (Figure 51-1)
  - T_H1 versus T_H2
    - The initial description of immune deviation was observed for CD4+ T cells in guiding what would become either a *cellular* immune response (T_H1) or a *humoral/B cell–dominated* immune response (T_H2)
    - T_H1-like immune responses are characterized by the production of IL-1β, IL-2, IL-12, and IFN-γ; these cytokines support the action of CD8+ "killer" T cells as well as the phagocytic activities of macrophages/monocytes
    - T_H2-like immune responses are characterized by the production of IL-4, IL-5, and IL-13; these cytokines support the action of B cells in terms of the ability to produce high-affinity immunoglobulins
  - Cross-regulation

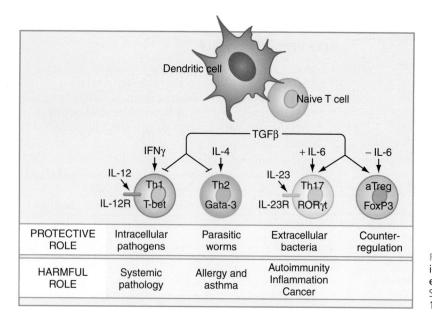

Figure 51-1. Naive CD4+ T cells may differentiate into four subtypes based on patterns of gene expression and functional capabilities. (From Reiner SL: Development in motion: helper T cells at work, *Cell* 129(1):33-36, 2007.)

- T_H1-like cytokines are known to inhibit the proliferation and function of T_H2-deviated T cells; the converse is also true, in that T_H2-like T cells are inhibitory of T_H1-like T cells
- Anergy
  - T cells require two stimuli to occur simultaneously
    - TCR–MHC interaction
    - CD28 (on the T cell) – B7 (on the antigen presenting cell)
  - CD28 – B7 interaction is known as co-stimulation
  - If co-stimulation fails to occur, then the T cell becomes refractory to further stimulation, a condition known as *anergy*
- Surface molecules
  - Fas – Fas L
    - T cells (both CD4+ and CD8+) express on the surface the molecule Fas upon activation; under certain circumstances, Fas – Ligand (Fas L) is expressed both on APC and activated T cells
    - When a T cell encounters (binds) Fas L to its Fas receptor, the consequence is apoptosis of the T cell
    - Certain immune-privileged sites (e.g., eye) express constitutively Fas L such that any activated T cell (bearing Fas) will trigger apoptosis of the invading T cell, thus limiting potentially damaging inflammatory responses in critical tissues
  - CD40 – CD40 ligand (CD40L)
    - CD40 is expressed on APC (macrophages and B cells)
    - CD40L is expressed on activated T cells
    - When CD40 is engaged by CD40L, the effect is co-stimulatory to the APC
    - APC with CD40 engagement further augments the function of the APC (increased cytokine receptor expression, increased phagocytosis, and increased antibody production)
  - CTLA – 4 (Cytotoxic T Lymphocyte–Associated protein – 4)
    - Certain activated T cells express CTLA – 4
    - CTLA – 4 binds to B7 with higher affinity than CD28, thereby depriving the T cell of the required co-stimulation leading to the state of anergy

UPDATE #1

T Regulatory Cells

1. Characterized by the constitutive expression of CD25 in the naïve state and by the expression of the transcription factor *FoxP3* (Sakaguchi et al, 2010)
2. These specialized CD4+ T cells are able to suppress, through bystander effect, other activated CD4+ and CD8+ T cells (Littman et al, 2010)
3. Tregs play an important role in the maintenance of immune homeostasis
4. Inadequate production (either through gene deletion or drug effect) results in widespread autoimmunity (Littman et al, 2010)
5. Tregs develop from naïve T cells under the local influence of TGF – β (see Figure 51-1) (Reiner, 2007)
6. In the presence of ongoing inflammation (high local concentrations of IL-6) in addition to TGF – β, these CD4+ T cells mature into a phenotype characterized by high production of IL-17; these T cells are known as T_H17; many autoimmune diseases are characterized by the presence, in abundance, of these highly inflammatory cells (Littman et al, 2010)

Reproductive Immunity

MUCOSAL IMMUNITY

- Cell types
  - The genital tract mucosa must balance the need to provide protection from invasive organisms while being permissive for the survival of a unique microbial environment
- Uterus/endometrium
  - The uterus and endometrium contain T cells (CD4+ and CD8+), macrophages, and natural killer (NK) cells
  - The endometrium also contains lymphoaggregates in premenopausal women; these unique structures, analogous to Peyer's patches in the gastrointestinal (GI) tract, contain a focus of B cells, surrounded by CD8+ (CD4-) T cells, contained within a halo of macrophages; lymphoaggregates are absent in postmenopausal women

- Fallopian tubes
  - Fallopian tubes lack lymphoaggregates; however, distributed throughout the mucosal lining are CD8+ and CD4+ T cells as well as macrophages
- Cervix and vagina
  - Similar to the fallopian tubes, the vagina and cervix lack lymphoaggregates but do contain a distribution of T cells and macrophages
- Cytolytic activity during menstrual cycle
  - Premenopause
    - Endometrium
      - The cytolytic functionality of CD3+ cells (T cells) is influenced by the timing of the menstrual cycle; during the proliferative phase, there is relatively normal activity, but during the secretory phase, there is pan suppression of the cytolytic ability of T cells; the phenomenon may exist to permit implantation
    - Cervix and vagina
      - The cytolytic activity of T cells in the vagina and cervix is unaffected by the stage of the menstrual cycle
  - Postmenopause
    - Endometrium
      - The cytolytic activity of T cells in the endometrium is greatly increased after menopause
- Susceptibility to HIV
  - The immune cellular composition of the vagina and cervix contains large numbers of the most susceptible cells to infection with human immunodeficiency virus (HIV): memory CD4+ T cells; the lower GI tract also has large numbers of these cells; because of these similarities, women are at increased risk of infection when they have intercourse with infected male partners

PREGNANCY

- Immune tolerance
  - The embryo/fetus by definition is composed of 50% paternal genetic material; as such, the fetus contains 50% of the tissue antigen from the father; if treated as a solid organ transplant, the maternal immune system would be expected to reject the fetus because of these antigenic differences; however, the fetus survives; the rationale behind this apparent immune tolerance during pregnancy has eluded explanation for more than 50 years; we do understand that the embryo has different susceptibility to maternal immune attack than does the fetus; for these apparent reasons, current theory holds that immune-mediated recurrent pregnancy loss is mechanistically distinct from intrauterine growth restriction (IUGR)/preeclampsia
    - Recurrent fetal loss
      - Early in pregnancy, subtle changes lower the immune profile of the endometrium and concepti; the endometrium, through the action of progesterone, is less inflammatory (inherent decrease in T cell cytolytic capacity); the embryo restricts the display of phosphatidylserine on the extracellular surfaces to reduce the immune profile to circulating antiphospholipid antibodies; lastly, the embryo increases the consumption of tryptophan through the action of indolamine 2,3-dioxygenase; the deprivation of T cells of tryptophan renders the T cells anergic (hypofunctional)
      - In cases of women with antiphospholipid syndrome, the high levels of circulating antibodies can lead to immune attack on a nascent implanted embryo; though the embryo gains protection from this form of attack through internalization of phosphatidylserine, it isn't clear in cases of recurrent miscarriage if the fault is with the failure of the embryo to properly internalize antigenic phospholipids or if there are sufficient numbers of high-affinity maternal antibodies to cause pregnancy failure
  - Pregnancy
    - After the embryo survives implantation, the maternal immune system must deal with the growing antigen mass; though this is the least well understood area, we do have some insight; overabundances of natural killer cells (part of the innate immune system) in the endometrium play an unclear role; interruption of the accumulation of these uterine NK cells causes adverse pregnancy outcome under experimental conditions; MHC class I expression is down-regulated on invasive placenta cells, thereby lowering the immunogenic profile of the placenta; lastly, we now understand that T regulatory cells develop in response to specific fetal antigen; through the action of Treg, potent immune regulation is achieved; however, it is yet to be elucidated exactly how pregnancy leads to changes in fundamental Treg function to achieve tolerance (Kahn et al, 2010)

Autoimmunity

DEFINITIONS

- Autoimmunity: normal host tissue becomes a target of the immune system
- Fundamental to the potential for autoimmunity is the fact that the immune system develops millions upon millions of possible TCRs and BCRs to cover potential pathogens; as described previously, deletion of those T and B cells that recognize host antigens is crucial for reducing the potential for autoimmunity *(central tolerance)*
- Because autoreactive T and B cell clones exist in otherwise healthy individuals, multiple mechanisms must exist to limit/suppress the action of these autoreactive cells *(peripheral tolerance)*
- Tissue specificity usually exists because of the inherently highly specific nature of the immune cells (T or B); however, as the disease progresses and inflammation causes ongoing tissue destruction, more T or B cell clones may become involved (as more potential antigens are exposed)

BREAKDOWN OF TOLERANCE

- Molecular mimicry

UPDATE #2

Viral infections may serve as the antigenic bridge to the breakdown of tolerance leading to autoimmunity. The proposed mechanism involves an antecedent viral infection that results in a display of viral peptides on MHC class I. These viral peptides that could cause an autoimmune disease are structurally analogous to host peptides. The resulting inflammatory action against the virally infected cells results in the expansion of T and B cell clones that also recognize normal tissue antigens resulting in an inappropriate ongoing inflammatory response (Munz et al, 2009).

- TLR activation resulting in release of normal tissue antigens, not encountered during B and T cell development
  - Pathogen infection causes APC activation through TLR activation
  - Resulting bystander tissue destruction releases normal tissue antigens
  - The now-released tissue antigens that were previously "hidden" from the host immune system activate B or T cell clones not deleted during central tolerance; thus, autoimmunity is the result of overcoming immunologic ignorance
- Genetic susceptibility
  - Certain Major Histocompatibility Complex (MHC) alleles (e.g., HLA-B27) confer increased risk in humans to autoimmunity; the mechanism is unclear but may be related to increased susceptibility to molecular mimicry
  - Treg development interference with polymorphisms in *FoxP3*; immunodysregulation polyendocrinopathy enteropathy X-linked (IPEX) syndrome results in deficiency of *FoxP3*
  - Polymorphisms in cytokines/receptors

Gender and Autoimmunity

UPDATE #3

Female sex hormones predispose to T_H1- or T_H2-like responses depending on the hormonal state of the woman. Women tend to generate a more robust T_H1 response compared with men. In part, this tendency explains the predominance of T_H1-like autoimmune disease in women (e.g., multiple sclerosis [MS], rheumatoid arthritis [RA]) (Gleicher et al, 2007; Whitacre et al, 1999). However, with the onset of the postovulatory phase of the menstrual cycle or pregnancy, where progesterone dominates, T_H2 responses are favored (Zandman-Goddard et al, 2007). In this high progesterone setting, T_H2-like autoimmune diseases dominate (e.g., systemic lupus erythematosus [SLE]).

- Gender differences in immune responses
  - Females produce a more robust antibody response to vaccination
  - Women produce a greater IgM titer (no difference in IgG)
  - Females have an increased CD4/CD8 ratio
  - Females have a greater absolute number of CD4 T cells
  - Women have increased inflammatory cytokine production in response to stimuli
  - Tendency to T_H1-like responses (Table 51-1)

FEMALE SEX HORMONES AS IMMUNOMODULATORS

- Estrogen
  - Immunostimulatory at low doses
  - Inappropriate enhancement of B cell survival (including autoreactive B cells)
  - At high doses, estrogen can ameliorate autoimmune disease in experimental animals
    - Treatment with oral contraceptives, particularly with a high estrogen/progesterone content, reduces the severity of experimental allergic encephalomyelitis (EAE) in mice
  - Early evidence suggests that estrogen may modulate immune cell homing

TABLE 51-1 Gender Prevalence Ratios for Selected Autoimmune Diseases

Autoimmune Disease Ratio	Female/Male
Hashimoto's thyroiditis/hypothyroidism	50:1
SLE	9:1
Sjögren's syndrome	9:1-20:1
Antiphospholipid antibodies	9:1
Primary biliary cirrhosis	9:1
Mixed connective tissue disease	8:1
Chronic active hepatitis	8:1
Grave disease/hyperthyroidism	7:1
Rheumatoid arthritis	3:1-4:1
Scleroderma	3:1-4:1
Myasthenia gravis	2:1-3:1
Multiple sclerosis	2:1
Autoimmune thrombocytopenic purpura	2:1
Type 1 diabetes mellitus	1:1-2:1
Ulcerative colitis	1:1
Autoimmune myocarditis	1:1.2

Adapted from Gleicher N, Barad DH: Gender as risk factor for autoimmune diseases, *J Autoimmun* 28(1):1-6, 2007.

- Prolactin
  - Increase in IFN-g production
  - Stimulated by estrogen
  - Prolactin receptors are found on B cells, monocytes, and the majority of T cells
  - The severity of many autoimmune diseases has been found to have been improved with concomitant treatment with bromocriptine
- Progesterone
  - Inhibits T cell proliferation
- Androgen
  - Treatment of female non-obese diabetic (NOD) mice (spontaneous autoimmune diabetes) with testosterone reduces the incidence of disease
  - Castration of male NOD mice increases disease incidence
  - Dehydroepiandrosterone (DHEA)
    - Decreases with aging and correlates with age-related immune senescence
    - Treatment with DHEA reverses immune senescence
    - Treatment of patients with MS or SLE, with DHEA, results in measurable benefits in small-scale trials

SYSTEMIC LUPUS ERYTHEMATOSUS (SLE)

- Preponderance of SLE in young women
- Male-to-female ratio 9:1
- Flares during pregnancy, remission after menopause
- Estrogen
  - Treatment of mice with experimental lupus with selective estrogen receptor modulators (SERMs) results in amelioration of disease
  - Males with SLE have estrogen/androgen imbalance
  - Estrogen replacement in postmenopausal women with SLE increased number of mild flares
  - Combined oral contraceptives do not worsen disease in women with inactive or stable active SLE; possible increased risk of thrombosis in women with positive

antiphospholipid antibodies and a history of oral contraceptive use (no increase in disease activity with use of progestogen-only contraceptives)
- Prolactin
  - Twenty percent to 30% of SLE patients have mild to moderate hyperprolactinemia
  - Treatment of mice with experimental lupus with bromocriptine reduces disease
- Increased symptoms in the postovulatory phase

MULTIPLE SCLEROSIS
- More common in women but more severe in men
  - Reduced survival in men
  - Shorter time to requiring assisted walking device
- MS-associated high risk HLA – D2 allele is more common in women
  - Earlier onset of disease is associated with a better prognosis
  - 3.2:1 (female/male) in patients presenting with MS <20 years old
- Premenopausal females have higher concentrations of prolactin, luteinizing hormone (LH), follicle-stimulating hormone (FSH), and testosterone but have lower levels of estrogen

RHEUMATOID ARTHRITIS
- Reduced levels of androgens and progesterone
- At the joint synovia, immune cells show a differential pattern of estrogen receptor (increased ER-α) expression during pathogenesis
- Observational evidence suggests that breast-feeding increases RA flares (potentially via the pro-inflammatory effects of prolactin)
- Increased symptoms in the postovulatory phase

Treatment of Autoimmunity

UPDATE #4
Several strategies for dealing with autoimmune disease have been developed to interfere with normal T cell activation and function (Steward-Tharp et al, 2010). Many of these therapies are based on our knowledge of normal immune regulatory mechanisms (Feldmann et al 2005; Riley et al, 2009).

DIRECT REDUCTION IN T CELLS
- Monoclonal antibodies to human T cells have been used to directly reduce T cells
  - OKT3 targets human CD3 treatment and results in a dramatic decline in the number of circulating T cells; as anticipated, the major side effect is the risk of opportunistic infection; an unanticipated major side effect results from the stimulatory effect of CD3 engagement by OKT3; when large numbers of T cells are activated all at once, large amounts of T cell–derived cytokines are released, resulting in a syndrome, cytokine storm; thus, this agent is reserved for life-threatening complications of autoimmune disease
  - Several other monoclonal antibodies to CD3 are under development to limit this stimulatory side effect (Teplizumab, Otelixizumab, Visilizumab)

- Direct deletion of CD4+ T cells has not been effective clinically; the reasons are unclear

INTERFERENCE WITH TCR SIGNALING
- Cyclosporin A and tacrolimus are used to prevent solid organ transplant rejection
- These drugs interfere with the downstream signaling of TCR signaling and thus only target activated T cells
- Tacrolimus and cyclosporin A are both effective in the treatment of a variety of autoimmune diseases, but their use is limited by the toxic side effects

INTERFERENCE WITH CO-STIMULATION
- Activation of T cells without CD28 – B7 co-stimulation leads to a refractory T cell state, anergy; some activated T cells express the surface molecule CTLA – 4 that has a higher affinity for B7 than CD28, thereby depriving activated T cells of co-stimulation resulting in T cell anergy
- Abatacept is a fusion protein of CTLA – 4 and human IgG1 constant domain; this drug works by depriving activated T cells of necessary co-stimulation by consuming B7; Abatacept is effective in a variety of autoimmune conditions
- Interference with CD40 Ligand - CD40
  - CD40 – CD40L interactions lead to increased macrophage/B cell functionality
  - A monoclonal antibody was developed against CD40L and was attempted to be used therapeutically; however, the trial was stopped early because of unacceptable thrombotic events

DIRECT TARGETING OF B CELLS
- Rituximab, a monoclonal antibody against CD20 that removes intermediate stage B cells, has remarkable efficacy in rheumatoid arthritis and several other autoimmune diseases

TARGETED CYTOKINE BLOCKADE
- Anti-TNF-α
  - Several agents have been developed to neutralize TNF-α
  - These agents (Adalimumab, Etanercept, and Infliximab) have remarkable efficacy in the treatment of autoimmune disease
- Interference with IL-2
  - Blockade of the high affinity IL-2 receptor (CD25) with monoclonal antibodies (Daclizumab or Basiliximab) has shown promise in the treatment of a variety of autoimmune diseases including RA and MS
- Interference with IL-6
  - Tocilizumab blocks the IL-6 receptor alpha subunit
  - Blockade of IL-6 has the theoretic advantage of both reducing inflammation and reducing the formation of T_H17 cells
  - Early results show this drug to be effective in the treatment of RA

REINTRODUCTION OF TOLERANCE: T REGULATORY CELL TRANSPLANTATION
- Although it might be attractive to induce an expansion of native Tregs to bring immune homeostasis back into balance, the mechanism by which such a expansion might be accomplished is not clear

- The alternative is to introduce *en masse* Tregs isolated either from healthy donors or cord blood
  - Transfer of Tregs in experimental models of diabetes (NOD mice) prevents the onset of disease
  - Barriers to this approach include tissue matching, the ability to purify the population sufficiently, and serious potential consequences of manipulation of the immune system

SUGGESTED READINGS

T Regulatory Cells

Goodnow CC, Sprent J, Fazekas de St Groth B, Vinuesa CG: Cellular and genetic mechanisms of self tolerance and autoimmunity, *Nature* 435(7042): 590–597, 2005.

Kahn DA, Baltimore D: Pregnancy induces a fetal antigen-specific maternal T regulatory cell response that contributes to tolerance, *Proc Nat Acad Sci USA* 107(20):9299–9304, 2010.

Littman DR, Rudensky AY: Th17 and regulatory T cells in mediating and restraining inflammation, *Cell* 140(3):845–858, 2010.

Martin F, Chan AC: Pathogenic roles of B cells in human autoimmunity: insights from the clinic, *Immunity* 20(5):517–527, 2004.

Reiner SL: Development in motion: helper T cells at work, *Cell* 129(1):33–36, 2007.

Sakaguchi S, Miyara M, Costantino CM, Hafler DA: FoxP3+ regulatory T cells in the human immune system, *Nat Rev Immunol* 10(7):490–500, 2010.

Molecular Mimicry

Kamradt T, Mitchison NA: Tolerance and autoimmunity, *N Engl J Med* 344(9):655–664, 2001.

Munz C, Lunemann JD, Getts MT, Miller SD: Antiviral immune responses: triggers of or triggered by autoimmunity? *Nat Rev Immunol* 9(4):246–258, 2009.

Gender and Autoimmunity

Gleicher N, Barad DH: Gender as risk factor for autoimmune diseases, *J Autoimmun* 28(1):1–6, 2007.

Whitacre CC, Reingold SC, O'Looney PA: A gender gap in autoimmunity, *Science* 283(5406):1277–1278, 1999.

Zandman-Goddard G, Peeva E, Shoenfeld Y: Gender and autoimmunity, *Autoimmun Rev* 6(6):366–372, 2007.

Treatment of Autoimmunity

Feldmann M, Steinman L: Design of effective immunotherapy for human autoimmunity, *Nature* 435(7042):612–619, 2005.

Riley JL, June CH, Blazar BR: Human T regulatory cell therapy: take a billion or so and call me in the morning, *Immunity* 30(5):656–665, 2009.

Steward-Tharp SM, Song YJ, Siegel RM, O'Shea JJ: New insights into T cell biology and T cell-directed therapy for autoimmunity, inflammation, and immunosuppression, *Ann N Y Acad Sci* 1183:123–148, 2010.

Index

Page numbers followed by "*b*" indicate boxes; "*f*" figures; "*t*" tables